A Survey of Human Diseases

A Survey
of Human Diseases

David T. Purtilo, M.D.
DEPARTMENT OF PATHOLOGY
SCHOOL OF MEDICINE, UNIVERSITY OF MASSACHUSETTS

Addison-Wesley Publishing Company
MEDICAL/NURSING DIVISION, MENLO PARK, CALIFORNIA
READING, MASSACHUSETTS · LONDON · AMSTERDAM
DON MILLS, ONTARIO · SYDNEY

To Ruth—wife, teacher,
author, and health professional extraordinaire.

About the cover: Lymphocyte from healthy person displayed in a
scanning electron micrograph. $\times$ 9300 *(left)*. By contrast, the
lymphocyte on the right is from a boy with immunodeficiency. The
scanning electron micrograph ($\times$ 7300) reveals that the surface
of the lymphocyte is abnormally smooth and convoluted (courtesy
Dr. Gary Schneider, University of Massachusetts Medical Center).
Compare the normal lymphocyte *(left)* with the abnormal lymphocyte
(right). The patient succumbed to infectious mononucleosis because
his defective lymphocytes could not defend against the virus that
causes infectious mononucleosis. These photos are representative
of the "show and tell" approach used to explain the pathophysiology
of diseases in this book.

Sponsoring Editor: James Keating
Production Editor: Pat Sorensen
Cover Design: Laurence J. Hyman
Book Design: Paul Quin
Artist: Amy Singer

Library of Congress Catalog Card No. 77-81550

ISBN 0-201-05782-4

DEFGHIJ-HA-798

Addison-Wesley Publishing Company
Medical/Nursing Division
2725 Sand Hill Road
Menlo Park, California 94025

Foreword

In its organization *A Study of Human Diseases* parallels the educational experience of the students for whom it is intended. It moves from an overview of evaluation of patients using the patient's history, a physical examination, and laboratory assessment—through etiology, pathophysiology, pathology, diagnosis, prognosis, and treatment. These steps are the same progressions used by health care practitioners in working with patients/clients.

Educational programs to prepare allied health and nursing students for professional practice are made up of incremental units arranged sequentially. With some variations in timing or order of sequence most of the programs include the following elements. The foundation consists of liberal arts and biologic and social science courses. Courses in anatomy, physiology, and neurology help the student understand the normal function of the human body. While exploring the theoretical bases for the practice of their individual health discipline (the so-called professional theory courses), students study pathology and pathophysiology to help them understand cause and effect relationships of disease and disability. Frequently this course gives them their first exposure to diagnoses, prognoses, and possible treatment regimens. The final phase of the curriculum involves the student in professional technique courses and practical experience in health care settings.

The important link between their general education and their professional education is a basic understanding of the pathogenesis of disease and disability. As they move into professional courses, learning experiences are provided that stress a logical and sequential approach to analysis of the effects of a patient's disease or disability as well as appropriate intervention strategies to be used by their particular discipline to alleviate the effects. Practice opportunities are planned to help them improve their observational skills, develop their ability to synthesize data and other pieces of related information, and increase their knowledge of disease/disability states and their consequences. The end result is to prepare competent health practitioners capable of exercising judgment and effectively transmitting their knowledge and skills into exemplary patient care.

Generally, pathology is taught to allied health and nursing students by clinicians. Nursing and medical students have been around for a long time and their educational needs and programs are well understood. The allied health students and practitioners are fairly new and young in the scheme of health care. To facilitate their learning in this important facet of their total formal education preparation pathologists must understand the function of allied health personnel, their place on the health care team, their contribution to the well-being of patients. Their reason for studying pathology is inextricably conjoined with their reason for being part of the health care delivery system —to provide services to patients/clients.

David Purtilo's book is an important milestone in the education of allied health and nursing students. The focus of the content is on the patient with whom his audience will be involved first as students and then as practitioners of their particular discipline. The book meets another of today's societal needs. There has been consumer involvement in both the development and testing of the product. And there is no doubt the book will be an important part of the armamentarium of its readers as they move through their daily responsibilities as health care providers.

Dr. Purtilo's textbook will be of invaluable help to two other audiences for whom it can help to facilitate learning. The first is allied health workers and nurses already in practice who need a ready reference to improve their patient care skills. The second, practitioners who have been inactive in their particular disciplines and who now wish to return to an active working status. *A Survey of Human Diseases* can significantly aid their reentry preparation efforts.

Students and faculty will benefit most immediately from Dr. Purtilo's book and will be grateful for his contribution to their educational experience. Long-range benefits will be experienced by the patient/clients who will be served by the allied health and nursing students and practitioners for whom his teaching and writing efforts are intended.

Helen K. Hickey, Associate Dean
Sargent College of Allied Health Professions
Boston University
   and
President-Elect, American Society of
   Allied Health Professions

Preface

A Survey of Human Diseases is the fruit of my 15 years of experience in teaching anatomy, microbiology, biology, pathophysiology, and clinical pathology to allied health, medical, and nursing students.

Written especially to meet the needs of today's nursing and allied health student, this heavily illustrated textbook provides a complete look at diseases—in the patient, under the microscope. It focuses on the major diseases and disorders which the student will actually encounter in practice, not the once-in-a-lifetime diseases. Scientific terms and disease mechanisms are introduced by use of familiar terms so that students do not have to be biochemists or physiologists to understand the book's well-explained, up-to-date content. Of particular interest, the book

● **Stresses the patient** as well as the disease.

● **Illustrates diseases** by use of numerous line drawings, photographs, and photomicrographs; then shows the effects on the individual, on organs and cells.

● **Facilitates learning** through chapter overviews and stated learning objectives at chapter beginnings, and summaries and annotated references at chapter endings.

During these years of teaching, I became increasingly frustrated by the lack of a good introductory textbook that surveyed diseases and the pathophysiologic bases of diseases. The available textbooks were designed for medical students or were too superficial for undergraduate students. I have found that students of allied health and nursing are highly motivated and are capable of understanding the pathophysiologic mechanisms of disease. Students have often been denied the opportunity to understand the diseases their patients have. Hence, in 1973, I prepared lecture outlines for physical and occupational therapy and nursing students. The outlines have evolved into the present book. The concepts and information presented in this book have been tested during a four-year period.

Focus

This book focuses on the major degenerative, neoplastic, metabolic, immunologic, and infectious diseases encountered. Rare exotic diseases are seldom mentioned (you can read about them in specialty textbooks and journals), and discussions of advanced biochemistry and basic sciences have been simplified.

Organization

I have organized the book into four sections that build on one another. Chapter 1 explains how diseases are classified, diagnosed, and treated and describes their natural course and prognosis. Chapters 2 and 3 describe and illustrate normal cells, tissues, and organs. You should know what normal tissues look like and how they behave. Many diseases occur from birth, and thus, Chapter 3 describes normal embryologic development and how birth defects ensue from faulty development.

Chapters 4 to 10 discuss cellular pathology or the basic pathologic processes of cellular injury, inflammation, repair, immunity, infectious diseases, neoplasia, genetics, and malnutrition. These basic pathophysiologic processes underlie diseases that occur in various organ systems. These, and subsequent chapters, also describe what attempts can be made to interrupt the natural course of disease.

Chapters 11 to 21 survey human diseases that commonly occur in hospitalized patients. Occasionally, unusual disorders are discussed to illustrate fundamental processes. These final chapters reinforce the concepts presented previously in the text.

Each chapter has been organized to facilitate learning. A chapter outline and extensive learning objectives have been provided at the beginning of each chapter. They serve to guide your study and provide an overview of the contents of each chapter. The learning objectives focus your attention on important items which in turn should enable you to see detailed and broad concepts. I have taken nothing for granted. Some of you will find introductory portions of the book simple, but the information will reinforce your knowledge and expand it.

An annotated bibliography is provided at the end of each chapter. I have selected three types of references: standard textbooks, which range from simple introductory works to complex subspecialty medical textbooks, are provided. Second, review articles have been selected for the clarity of their presentation and the quality of their illustrations. Finally, I have listed a few references of my own work which are germane to the text.

Medical vocabulary

Familiar words are used when possible, and when medical terms with which you may not be familiar are used, a synonym, example, or short description is given in parenthesis following the medical term. Excellent medical dictionaries are available; I have not written a glossary of terms, and extensive definitions are avoided. The medical terminology employed should help you effectively communicate with other health professionals and the patient.

Medicine is a show and tell art form; hence, I have employed two types of graphic media. Both line drawings and photographs have been used to clarify the narrative and reinforce the concepts presented. Line drawings have been used either to illustrate pathophysiologic mechanisms or, by the use of composite drawings, to show the common diseases that occur in a selected organ. These composite drawings summarize the major disease of a particular organ. Illustrations of high quality have been reproduced with permission from various textbooks and journals. I have been privileged to practice medicine in Africa, South America, and the United States and have photographed many of the patients shown herein. Also, this text contains many photographs of diseased organs to illustrate lesions in them. X-ray films, which are used for diagnosing disease in patients, and photomicrographs of diseased tissues are shown also. In summary, the illustrations in this text provide you with an opportunity to view a disease in a concrete fashion along with a narrative description.

This textbook is not a comprehensive survey of human diseases, but rather it introduces you to the pathophysiologic mechanisms of disease and describes the common diseases you will encounter in hospitalized patients. At the risk of oversimplification, I have emphasized clarity. The many biologic exceptions to the rule are not emphasized. You will learn the exceptions as you help patients. This textbook should enrich your professional experience following completion of training and should provide you with a foundation for continuing your education.

Acknowledgments

I thank Adelaide L. McGarett, Professor Emeritus of Physical Therapy of Sargent College of Allied Health Professions of Boston University who encouraged me to write this book. To my wife, Ruth, who gave valuable guidelines for the book; to Ms. Cathy Perry, Chairman of the Physical Therapy Department at Sargent College of Boston University; to the many students who used the outlines which evolved into this textbook; and to the numerous students and instructors who enhanced this book by their critical suggestions, many thanks.

I thank my colleagues for critiquing selected chapters: Drs. A. C. Templeton, Chapters 1, 8, 10 and 15; Michael Repice, Chapter 1; Gary Schneider, Chapter 2; Robert Singer, Chapter 3; Isabelle Joris, Chapters 4 and 5; James Yang, Chapters 6 and 17; Isao Katayama, Chapters 11 and 18; Arthur Like, Chapter 12; Jag Bhawan, Chapters 13, 14, and 19; Umberto DeGirolami, Chapters 20 and 21, and Ms. Karen Karni, Chapters 2 and 11, and Dr. Louise Paquin.

My secretaries who typed the manuscript are gratefully acknowledged: Mrs. Carol Nawn, Mrs. Deborah Parmenter, Ms. Jane Manzi, and Mrs. Linda Verdini.

Mrs. Amy Singer created the line drawings that illustrate the pathophysiologic mechanisms of diseases and Mr. Peter Healey developed the photographs. I thank them for their high-quality work. And a special thanks to Frank Virzi for the many hours he spent proofreading and indexing this text.

Working with Mr. James Keating and Ms. Patricia Sorensen, of the Addison-Wesley Publishing Company, has been an enriching, creative, and rewarding effort. The artistic and organizational format of this book is the result of our combined efforts.

David T. Purtilo

Table of Contents

Chapter 8
Neoplasia (oncology)   156

Chapter 9
Inherited disorders   174

Chapter 14
Pulmonary medicine   285

OBJECTIVES
INTRODUCTION

SUMMARY
BIBLIOGRAPHY

Chapter 15
Gastrointestinal disorders   308

OBJECTIVES
INTRODUCTION

SUMMARY
BIBLIOGRAPHY

A Survey of Human Diseases

CHAPTER 1

Causes, Diagnosis, Prevention, and Treatment of Disease

Chapter Outline

Objectives

After reading this chapter you should be able to

Define the terms health and disease.

List the factors determining the severity of a disease.

Compare the definitions of the terms symptoms and signs and also disease and syndrome.

Describe the medical model.

Discuss the relationship and contribution of inheritance and environment to disease.

List factors important in our life styles that determine the diseases we are prone to develop.

List the ten leading causes of death in order of frequency.

Define the terms etiology and pathology.

Compare the periods of life—prenatal, neonatal, and infancy—with respect to time.

Define the terms mutation and metabolic disease.

List several examples of degenerative diseases.

Define the terms mutation and metabolic disease.

List several examples of degenerative diseases.

Define the terms neoplasm, prognosis, autoimmunity, hypersensitivity, iatrogenic, and idiopathic.

List the three major groups of information that provide the data base for achieving a diagnosis.

Compare the relative importance of the clinical history, physical examination, and laboratory findings in achieving a diagnosis.

List the major components of a clinical history.

Know why a family history is important.

List the systems of the body.

Describe the senses used during a physical examination.

List the vital signs.

Define the terms auscultation and percussion.

Describe the importance of a rectal examination.

List the laboratory studies required for all hospitalized patients.

Describe the value of laboratory screening for disease.

List the usual laboratory tests ordered for various disorders including infections, arteriosclerosis, liver disease, renal failure, blood disorders, gastrointestinal disorders, and cancer.

Describe methods of preventive medicine.

Define internal medicine, surgery, pediatrics, and physical medicine specialties.

List several types of therapy used for treating diseases.

List an etiologic classification of disease.

Introduction

"Health" is a state of soundness or vigor of the body and mind. Being in good health means that a person may indulge in physical and mental activities without undue distress and that he or she is free from diseases that threaten well-being. The World Health Organization defines health as complete physical, mental, and social well-being. For most people, however, health implies perhaps even more the ability to do what they regard as worthwhile and conduct their lives as they want.

We are normal when our genetic constitution provides us with protoplasm (living molecules) that harmonize with the environment. When genes and molecules are normal, there is well-being, activity, longevity, and the capability to reproduce a like being. Conversely, when genes and molecules are abnormal, disease* may ensue.

Critical issues in the evaluation of the severity of disease include: How many individuals suffer from a disease? Is the disease of short duration (acute) or of long duration (chronic)? Does the disease need treatment? How high is the relapse (recurrence) rate? To what extent is the person's life expectancy shortened? Finally, can the disease be diagnosed and cured, and can it be prevented?

The severity of a disease depends on many factors: genetic constitution, nutrition, physical fitness, age, prior exposure and immunity, and quality of sanitation and housing, as well as other socioeconomic factors. These factors determine whether an individual will die of the disease or only suffer temporary impairment. Most diseases produce some morbidity, which is defined as an "unhealthful" state induced by disease. At the extreme, a disease can be lethal—it causes death.

To conquer and understand diseases, we must identify their causes (etiology). In this chapter, discussion focuses on the etiology of some diseases with examples provided. Other chapters will consider common diseases and pathophysiologic processes in greater depth.

The specific signs and symptoms manifested by a person with a disease include objective evidence of disease (signs) and specific recognizable abnormalities (symptoms); both suggest the diagnosis and etiology. For example, a person with acute appendicitis experiences pain in the right lower quadrant of the abdomen; tenderness is noted overlying the inflamed appendix—this is a sign of acute appendicitis.

A syndrome refers to a group of symptoms and signs occurring in a characteristic pattern. For example, the Mallory-Weiss syndrome is due to a tear of the esophagus and is associated with extensive bleeding that is usually caused by severe retching

and vomiting of a person who is drunk, but this syndrome may also be caused by vomiting associated with pregnancy or from ingestion of toxic chemicals. Hence, a syndrome usually has several causes; a disease has only one.

The Medical Model

To understand diseases, we will use what is called the medical model. The medical model seeks to cope with disease by (1) identifying causal factors, (2) diagnosing structural and molecular abnormalities, and (3) administering acceptable therapies for either arresting, palliating (temporarily relieving), or curing an individual of the disease.

The medical model employs the technique of differential diagnosis. The physician assesses all of the clinical findings and thoughtfully lists different diseases that would most likely cause the signs and symptoms. Then, selective laboratory studies and X-rays are done to confirm or rule out a diagnosis. Later, rational therapy is given to restore health.

Causes of Diseases

No single textbook can describe all of the diseases experienced by human beings. Hundreds of diseases are inherited, and more than 1400 skin diseases and 100 different types of cancer can occur. Of the thousands of diseases occurring in persons living in the United States, 95% are encompassed by only 200 different disease entities. The study of the cause and distribution of diseases is epidemiology.

The emphasis of this book concerns primarily common and lethal diseases, but nonlethal diseases, such as deafness, diseases of the skin, dental caries, and anxiety, markedly decrease the quality of life and effectiveness of millions of persons. For example, over one hundred thousand diseased teeth are extracted each day in the United States. Although these diseases are important, they will not be emphasized.

*Disease: morbus; illness; sickness; an interruption, cessation, or disorder of body functions, systems, or organs. (Definition from Stedman's Medical Dictionary, ed. 23. 1976. Baltimore: The Williams & Wilkins Company.)

Inheritance and Environment

The cause of human disease is intimately linked with two factors—genetic makeup and environment. Some persons regard disease as a means by which nature judges the desirability of an individual's genetic makeup in a given environment. "Survival of the fittest" the theme of Darwinian evolution, or the struggle between nature (genetic makeup or inheritance) and nurture (environment), is ongoing. This struggle is encompassed by the term ecogenetics.

The relative impact of genes and environment varies with each disease (Fig. 1-1); for example, retrolental fibroplasia results from exposure of a

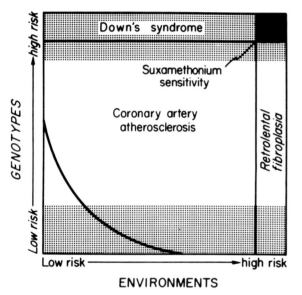

Figure 1-1   *Shown are the relative contribution of inheritance (genotypes) and environmental factors in determining four diseases. Retrolental fibroplasia requires the unusual environment of premature birth and high-oxygen concentration; this causes damage to the retina resulting in blindness. In contrast, Down's syndrome is expressed in all environments. Succinylcholine (or suxamethonium chloride, a muscle relaxant) sensitivity requires a high-risk genotype as well as exposure to an unusual environmental agent, namely suxamethonium during surgery. Coronary artery arteriosclerosis is a common disease involving many genotypes and a variety of environmental agents. (From Martin, G., and Hoehn, H. 1974. Human Pathology. Philadelphia: W. B. Saunders Company).*

premature newborn to a high-oxygen concentration and is almost entirely environmentally induced. In contrast, Down's syndrome (mongolism) results from an extra chromosome and occurs in all environments. Mongolism has a genetic basis only. A hypersensitivity disease can result when the muscle relaxant succinylcholine, or suxamethonium chloride, is being used; both inheritance and exposure to this drug during surgery are required for the disease to occur. Finally, coronary arteriosclerosis results from many predisposing genetic and environmental factors. This widely occurring disease has multifactorial causes.

Geneticists have taught us that we are unique genetically and biochemically. Agents present in our environment may be helpful to one individual but harmful to another. Unfortunate combinations and instances of hereditary factors combining with environmental factors, such as the abnormal hemoglobin of sickle cell anemia with exposure to low-oxygen concentrations, may induce unconsciousness in a black pilot flying in a nonpressurized cockpit. That pilot's erythrocytes immediately form sickle shapes when the oxygen concentration is low. This leads to headache, dizziness, and pain in the abdomen when the sickled erythrocytes plug small blood vessels in the brain and liver.

Life Style and Age-Associated Diseases

The environment and the political climate of countries determine how people live and the health problems that are likely to ensue. Persons living in the United States, for instance, *consume* too much food, alcohol, and tobacco and do not exercise enough. Arteriosclerosis; cancer; diseases of the kidney, liver, and lungs; and accidents cause most deaths in the United States. By contrast, persons living in developing nations suffer and frequently die from undernutrition and infectious diseases.

Not only a person's life style but age and ethnic group determine what diseases might develop. To underscore these concepts, consider the following vital statistics in the United States: in 1974, the infant mortality rate was about 16.5 per 1000 for white infants, but 31 per 1000 among black infants.

Incidentally, on a worldwide basis the United States ranks fifteenth in infant mortality.

In the United States, approximately 6% of the children have defective distant vision and 10% have defective near vision. By 11 years of age, 17% of American children have defective distant vision. About 700,000 children have lower front teeth that bite into their palates and another 1.5 million children have less severe malocclusion.

Among young adults, violent deaths, such as accidents, suicides, and homicides, nearly equal deaths from *all* other causes. Beyond the age of 19 years, a marked decline in physical fitness occurs in many young American adults.

Good physical conditioning provides resistance against colds, surgery, and heart attacks. Oftentimes, individuals who do not exercise also overconsume food, alcohol, and cigarettes.

In the United States, from 10% to 20% of adult men and 3% to 5% of adult women are heavy drinkers, and between 1950 and 1973, death rates from cirrhosis of the liver—associated with alcoholism—doubled. Deaths from bronchitis, emphysema, and asthma, aggravated by smoking and air pollution, tripled during the same period. During 1975, 38% of the deaths in the United States were from coronary arteriosclerosis ("hardening" of the arteries) and 19.5% of the deaths were caused by cancer. Environmental agents probably caused the cancers in 85% of the cases.

Following is a discussion of the classification and *etiology* of disease. Subsequent chapters will discuss cellular and systemic pathology of various organs. *Pathology* (the study of disease) concerns itself with finding the mechanisms, diagnosis, and causes of disease. Table 1-1 lists an etiologic classification of diseases; no single classification of disease is truly comprehensive. Only common, important diseases and their etiologic agents are described in this book.

Congenital (Inborn) Diseases

Prenatal influences are responsible for most neonatal deaths. *Prenatal* denotes the period of in utero life, whereas *neonatal* means the first two months of life. During infancy, the first 2 years of life, birth defects arising from the pregnant mother having taken drugs, such as thalidomide, or infection by viruses are the major cause of death. These agents can deform the brain or other organs (see Chapter 3, Development and Birth Defects).

Inherited Diseases

Previously, emphasis has been placed on the fact

Table 1-1
Etiologic Classification of Diseases

Type	Chapters
Congenital (inborn) diseases or birth defects	3
Inherited diseases	9
Metabolic diseases	9 and 12
Degenerative diseases	4, 13, 14, 20, and 21
Neoplastic diseases	8
Immunologic diseases	6
Infectious diseases	7
Physical agent–induced diseases	4 and 5
Nutritional deficiency diseases	10
Iatrogenic diseases	(Iatrogenic, psychogenic, and
Psychogenic diseases	idiopathic diseases are discussed in
Idiopathic diseases	virtually every chapter.)

that inheritance provides certain conditions for diseases that are induced by environmental agents. Many abortions are caused by *mutations* (permanent alterations in genes induced by chemicals, irradiation, etc.). Most mutations are lethal, but other mutations cause problems only when the person is exposed to certain environmental agents. Other mutations cause problems without any environmental contribution (Fig. 1-2). Chapter 9 discusses common inherited diseases.

Metabolic Diseases

Metabolic diseases arise from abnormalities in the chemistry of the body. Over 100 deficiencies of vital enzymes have genetic bases. Screening for metabolic disorders is an important aspect of preventive medicine for childhood diseases, such as phenylketonuria (PKU). Children having this enzyme deficiency suffer brain damage when toxic chemicals accumulate in the brain. PKU must be diagnosed and the infant placed on a special diet before reaching the age of 1 year.

Abnormalities in the biochemistry of bodily functions are discussed in Chapter 12, Endocrine and Metabolic Disorders.

Degenerative Diseases

Degenerative diseases are increasing in frequency as persons are living beyond the fifth decade (Fig. 1-3). Heart attacks and strokes combined account for over one-half of all deaths in the United States. Other degenerative diseases, including cirrhosis of the liver and emphysema of the lungs, cause chronic illness and numerous deaths. These diseases are discussed in detail in subsequent chapters.

Aging and degeneration have been linked with excessive caloric intake, radiation, winding down of biologic clocks, errors in gene function, and a loss of immunologic vigor. Most medicine practiced in the United States is centered in hospitals and clinics that diagnose and treat individuals with degenerative diseases. The average life span in the United States of 75 years in women and 68 years in men is not likely to be extended much because

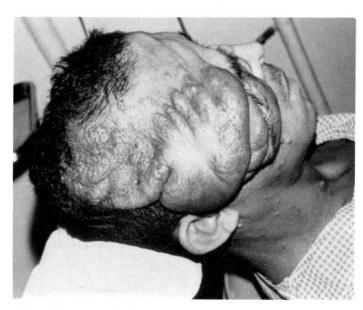

Figure 1-2 *Neurofibromatosis. This man has an inherited disorder characterized by neurofibromas on the skin. Many small neurofibromas are seen on his neck, and one large neurofibroma extends down from his eyebrow.*

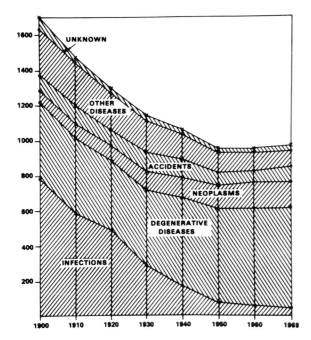

Figure 1-3   *Death rates for all causes—United States 1900–1969 by major types. Note the decrease in infectious diseases and increase in most of the chronic diseases. (From Peery, T. M. 1975. The new and old diseases.* Am. J. Clin. Pathol. *April, p. 458, J. B. Lippincott Company.)*

degenerative and neoplastic diseases are difficult to prevent and cure.

Neoplastic Diseases

Neoplastic diseases (tumors), especially the malignant variety (see Chapter 8), are a menace: One in five persons dies of cancer (Fig. 1-3). Cancers cause death when they spread from their site of origin. Generally, cancers are signaled by a lump (Fig. 1-4), an increase in the size of an ulcer, loss of weight, anemia, or pain.

Of the deaths attributable to the 100 different types of cancer, more than 60% are caused by a few common types, involving the breast, lung, colon, stomach, and uterus.

One measure of the impact of a cancer is the determination of the percent of patients who survive a given type of cancer for five years. This information enables a prediction of survival (*prognosis*) for patients with cancer. The curability of various cancers is shown in Figure 1-5.

Cancer probably arises from mutations induced by mutagenic agents such as chemicals, viruses, sunlight, irradiation, and chronic irritation. The clustering of cancer in selective geographic areas

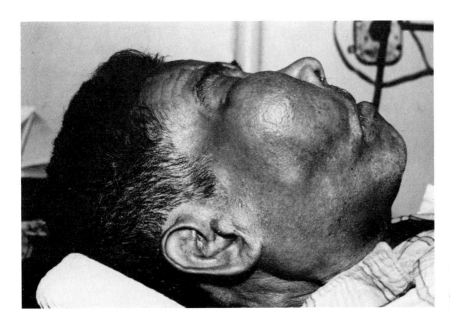

Figure 1-1   *Shown is a man with cancer arising in a bone. The swelling (tumor) prompted this man to go to the hospital.*

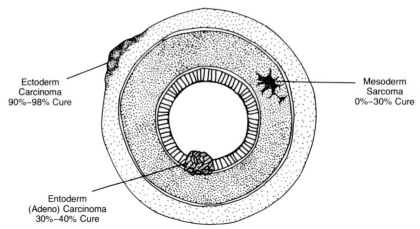

Ectoderm
Carcinoma
90%–98% Cure

Mesoderm
Sarcoma
0%–30% Cure

Entoderm
(Adeno) Carcinoma
30%–40% Cure

Figure 1-5   *Curability of cancers depends on early recognition and accessibility of the cancer to inspection, palpation, and biopsy. The highest cure rate is skin cancer (90%–98%). The skin rises from ectoderm. The curability rate drops to about 30% to 40% in cancers of the hollow organs (carcinoma and adenocarcinoma arising from entoderm). When diagnoses are delayed until symptoms of obstruction or bleeding occur (as in cancers arising in mesoderm), the curability ranges from 0% to 30%.*

implicates environmental factors as the cause of cancer. For example, Burkitt's malignant lymphoma, a rare cancer, occurs more frequently in tropical Africa where specific humidity, temperature, and altitude provide an optimal environment for this cancer.

Immunologic Diseases

Our immune system gives us a license for survival by protecting us against infectious agents that surround us and from cancers that may arise. In some instances, the immune system may attack one's own body *(autoimmunity)* or overreact *(hypersensitivity)*. See Chapter 6 on Immunology. Illustrated in Figure 1-6 is an allergic conjunctivitis, which causes only irritation. Anaphylactic immunologic reactions to allergins such as venom of a bee could be lethal in hypersensitive persons. Immunologic reactions are responsible for allergies; asthma; rheumatic heart disease; and many kidney, skin, and endocrine diseases.

Infectious Diseases

Infectious diseases were the major cause of death in the United States until the 1940s. At the turn of

the century, almost half of American children died before the age of 5 years. Even today, they cause much morbidity. For example, the common cold can cause death in a debilitated individual, in the newborn, and the elderly and misery in all.

On a worldwide basis, infectious diseases and malnutrition are the two most important health problems. Improvements in sanitation and nutri-

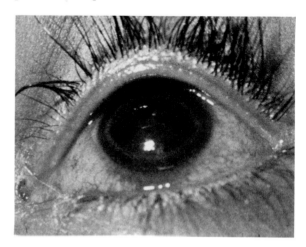

Figure 1-6   *Conjunctivitis. The redness and itching of the eye were caused by an immunologic hypersensitivity response to pollen from flowering trees.*

tion, the use of vaccination, plus the advent of antibiotics have lessened the impact of infectious diseases (Fig. 1-7).

Physical Agents

Violent injury (trauma) or death from mechanical, chemical, or physical agents are common among young people. Traffic accidents, homicide, suicide, and trauma from accidents at home, work, and war are examples. In addition, some genetically predisposed persons react adversely to certain drugs or chemicals. Such persons may injure their skin, lungs, intestinal tract, liver, and kidneys from such adverse reactions to drugs. The liver and kidneys are often damaged because these organs concentrate and excrete toxic drugs and chemicals.

Within the body, mechanical failures can occur. An intestinal loop can slip through a defect in the abdominal wall and become trapped. This is called a *hernia*. The intestine can also become twisted or telescoped within itself. Pain in the abdomen and

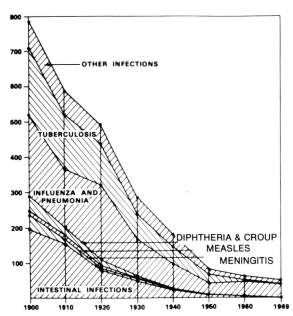

Figure 1-7 *Declining death rates for infectious diseases in the United States from 1900–1969, by major types. (From Peery, T. M. 1975. The new and old diseases.* Am. J. Clin. Pathol. *April, p. 459, J. B. Lippincott Company.)*

urinary tract infection occurs when a blood vessel or stricture blocks the flow of urine (Fig. 1-8). Similarly, gallstones commonly form in the gallbladder; they can pass into the bile ducts and mechanically obstruct them, causing abdominal pain, nausea, and vomiting.

Nutritional Deficiency Diseases

Deficiencies in nutrients are responsible for many diseases. On a worldwide basis, deficiencies of proteins, calories, and vitamins are rampant; over 300 million preschool-aged children are malnourished and vulnerable to infectious diseases. In developing countries, tuberculosis and malnutrition are the most common causes of death. Also deficiencies in vitamins or iodine may induce nutritional deficiency diseases (Fig. 1-7).

Iatrogenic Diseases

Many diseases are caused by a physician or health professional; such diseases are *iatrogenic* in origin. The first dictum of health care is "do no harm"; violation of this dictum results in iatrogenic disease. Five percent of patients entering a hospital, for instance, become infected from a procedure performed on them. The slip of a surgeon's knife or an incorrect diagnosis by a physician can cause disease.

Moreover, numerous drugs cause disease. One tragic example still cries out. Formerly, pregnant women who were threatening to abort were given the drug diethylstilbestrol, or stilbestrol. Approximately 20 to 25 years later, many young women born of these pregnancies developed cancer of the vagina.

A subcategory of drug-induced iatrogenic disease is growing in importance. Approximately 2% to 5% of hospitalized patients are ill because of a drug-induced disease. In addition, 5% to 30% of patients experience adverse reactions to drugs while being treated in the hospital. Allergy to penicillin resulting in a rash is a common example.

The misuse of radiation by those not realizing its potential danger has resulted in the development

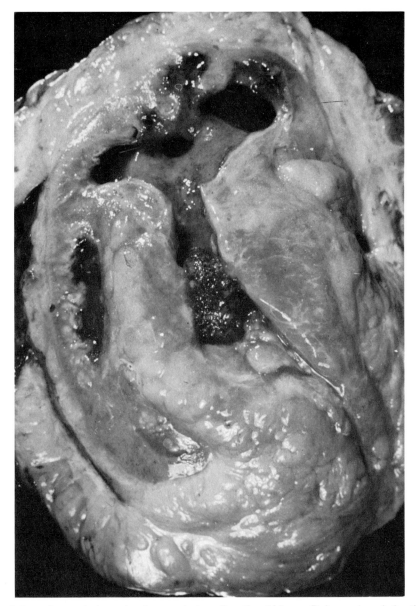

Figure 1-8   *A renal stone is shown obstructing the kidney. Pain and an infection in the urinary tract led to the diagnosis and removal of the kidney.*

of cancers of the liver, skin, thyroid gland, and blood (Fig. 1-9).

Psychogenic Diseases

Psychogenic or emotional factors contribute to many diseases. Moreover, psychogenic factors are ex-

tremely important in determining the course of the disease. Many diseases are encompassed by psychosomatic medicine, the discipline involving the physiologic impact of psychic stress on the emergence of disease. A variety of gastrointestinal disorders, such as peptic ulcer, ulcerative colitis, spastic colon, and pruritus ani (itchy anus), are either

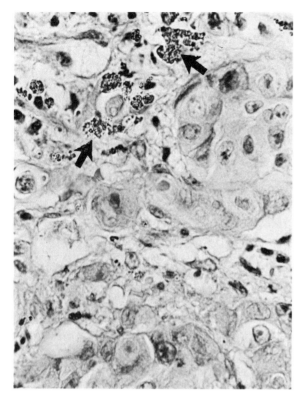

Figure 1-9   *Photomicrograph of liver showing a radioactive substance, thorotrast (arrows), which caused cancer in this liver 20 years after thorotrast was used in an X-ray study.*

caused by or associated with psychic stress. In addition, asthma and dermatitis have important psychologic components.

Idiopathic Diseases

A textbook such as this one, as well as some educators, especially physicians, may give one the idea that much is known about disease. The truth is we do not know what *causes* most diseases!

The term *idiopathic* means undetermined cause. Examples of diseases with unknown causes abound; one example is hypertension. Elevation of blood pressure, above 140/90mm Hg, is a sign of an underlying disease. Only 10% of persons with hypertension have an identifiable cause; approximately 90% have no discernible cause for hypertension; they have *idiopathic hypertension.*

Diagnosis of Disease

The physician obtains a history and physical findings. Then, that physician considers all of the possible diseases or conditions that might cause these complaints. Putting complaints, history, and physical examination together with laboratory findings, the most probable diagnosis is made. This process is termed *differential diagnosis.*

First, crude estimates are made of the probability of occurrence of a disease in a person of a given age, sex, and race with a typical history and physical findings. Uncommon diseases are usually eliminated, narrowing the differential diagnosis to a highly probable disease. For example, a 25-year-old white woman taking birth control pills complains of coughing up blood (hemoptysis) and shortness of breath. The physician might eliminate many of the known causes for the symptoms, for example, such symptoms in a man might indicate cancer of the lungs. The physician knows that women taking birth control pills have a higher incidence of thrombophlebitis (inflammation of veins in the legs) and pulmonary embolism (blood clot in the lungs). The pulmonary embolism is the most likely cause of hemoptysis in a young woman taking birth control pills. Through the process of elimination, the physician makes a presumptive diagnosis of pulmonary embolism. Then the physician uses X-ray and laboratory studies to confirm or rule out the diagnosis.

The following discussion offers a brief presentation of the clinical method used for diagnosing disease from the clinical history, physical examination, and laboratory studies.

Clinical Methods of Diagnosis

Clinical History   A carefully obtained clinical history is the *most* valuable tool health professionals have for diagnosing disease. The clinical history pinpoints the source of many medical problems and suggests a diagnosis. Diseases have predictable, even stereotyped, clinical histories.

Several years ago a study was conducted in which three groups of physicians were given either the clinical history, physical examination findings, or laboratory data. Pause and think for a moment: Which is most important for diagnosis? Physicians were asked to diagnose diseases based only on the information provided. Approximately 85% of diagnoses were correct based on clinical history alone, 15% were correct based on physical examination findings alone, and only 7% of diagnoses were achieved from laboratory findings alone.

A clinical history includes general information about the person, age, sex, race, and home; the chief complaint or complaints; history of present illness; family history; and social history. A review of the bodily systems is then taken, entered in the patient's clinical record, and further studied for clues to the diagnosis.

Chief Complaint or Complaints   The chief complaint or complaints focus on the major problem as *viewed by the patient*. Complaints are recorded by the physician in the words of the patient, for example, "bellyache."

History of Present Illness   The history of the present illness draws out associations related to the chief complaint. For example, an individual complaining of jaundice (yellow discoloration of the skin and eyes) is asked about the onset, the duration, and intensity of the symptom. The individual will be asked whether jaundice has previously occurred and whether there has been any recent travel overseas, about receiving any blood transfusions, taking of drugs, and if other family members have experienced jaundice. All of these questions are geared toward determining the etiology of the jaundice. The physician wants to know whether the jaundice is drug-induced, infectious, or inherited, for example.

The remainder of the clinical history and the physical examination, although systematic and broad in scope, is problem-oriented, that is, focused on the chief complaint.

Family History   The family history ascertains what the patient's family members died from as well as the health of survivors. In the family his-

tory, a search is made for any possible inherited disorders.

Social History   The social history of the individual concerns the occupation and habits of the person, such as cigarette and alcohol consumption, including the amount and duration. Moreover, the individual is questioned concerning drugs and previous operations, medical problems, and hospitalizations. The occupational history of the individual is investigated, especially as it relates to exposure to possible toxins.

Review of Body Systems   A verbal review of body systems is pursued to assure that no significant information is missed. An inquiry is made about each organ system; this begins with the individual's general constitution, such as changes in weight, appetite, anxiety, and amount of sleep. Concern about the skin includes information about rashes, spots, lumps, and sensitivity to sunlight. The individual is questioned about blurred or double vision and the use of glasses. The person is questioned about hearing, earaches, discharge and ringing in the ears, obstructed breathing, allergies, sore throats, or speech problems. The condition of the teeth and the presence of ulcers or sores in the mouth are investigated.

The function of the central nervous system is assessed by asking whether headaches, dizziness, double vision, weakness, numbness, tingling of extremities, blackout spells (syncope), injury to the head, prior strokes (cerebrovascular accidents), or seizures have occurred. In addition, information about previous hospitalizations for psychiatric illness or a psychiatric illness in the family is sought. Questions concerning the musculoskeletal system focus on the presence of aches and pains, stiffness, weakness, deformities, and fractures.

In populations living in Western societies the cardiovascular system is frequently damaged by arteriosclerosis (hardening of the arteries). Thus the following associated conditions are sought: presence of high blood pressure (hypertension), shortness of breath and pain in the chest with exertion, blueness of the mouth or extremities (cyanosis), swelling of ankles (edema), irregularities in the heartbeat (arrhythmias), fainting spells, flushing, and pain in the legs occurring with exercise.

Regarding the respiratory tract, shortness of breath, wheezing, hay fever, coughing, pain in the chest on breathing, and previous tuberculosis are searched for.

A review of the gastrointestinal tract includes questions about the individual's weight, appetite, diet and presence of nausea, vomiting, diarrhea, or constipation. Color of feces is important; for instance, black or tarry stools might signify gastrointestinal hemorrhage. Prior jaundice, blood transfusion (for hepatitis), pain in the abdomen (for ulcers and cancer), intolerance to fatty foods (for gallbladder disease), and excessive production of gas are noted.

Women are queried about the age of onset of their menstrual period (menarche), number of days of menstrual flow, amount of flow, and whether vaginal discharge or pain are present. In addition, number of pregnancies, live births, and abortions are recorded. Women are also asked about discharge from the breasts, masses, and ulceration or discoloration of the nipple.

Men are asked whether they have pain, lumps, or discharge from their penis, testes, or scrotum. The urinary tract is investigated by asking the individual whether he experiences a burning sensation on urination (dysuria), how often voiding occurs (frequency), whether he voids during the night (nocturia), and whether pain in the back over the kidneys is experienced.

The endocrine system is investigated by asking questions concerning the person's constitution; does the individual experience weakness, heat intolerance, weight gain or loss, frequency of urination, and desire for sugar.

Function of the immune system is probed by asking about vaccinations, frequency of infectious diseases, allergies, enlargement of lymph glands, and malignancies. Concerning the blood, a person is asked about pallor, weakness, shortness of breath, and whether any disorders of the blood have occurred.

At the conclusion of the clinical history, the patient may again be asked to restate major complaints before the physical examination begins.

Physical Examination

The physician or other health professional who examines the patient uses all senses—eyes, ears, nose, and touch—to detect any abnormalities in structure and function of a patient.

The examiner scrutinizes the patient, first noting general appearance, then body build, state of nutrition and development, and whether the patient is in acute, chronic, or no distress. Also the individual's approximate intelligence is assessed.

Vital Signs   Vital signs include blood pressure (recorded in mm of Hg on a sphygmomanometer), temperature (recorded in degrees Fahrenheit or Celsius), heart rate (recorded in beats per minute), and respiratory rate (recorded in respirations per minute). These are taken on all patients. These data call attention to disorders of the cardiovascular and respiratory systems, infections, and many other diseases.

Skin   Inspection of the individual's skin often provides clues not only to skin disorders but also to *systemic* diseases (diseases involving many organ systems). Pallor (due to anemia), rashes (from allergies), and lumps (possibly from malignancies) are searched for. The distribution of pigment and hair, the quality (moisture and texture) of skin and hair give clues to disorders of the endocrine system. For examples, loose skin is a clue to weight loss that could be caused by cancer. Discoloration of the skin or collection of fluid under the skin (edema) in the lower legs can indicate heart, liver, or renal failure.

The breasts of women are thoroughly evaluated for discharges, masses, ulcers, and retraction. The axillary lymph glands are examined for possible enlargement, which could indicate spread (metastasis) of cancer from the breast to the lymph glands.

Head   The individual is evaluated literally from head to foot. Ears, eyes, nose, and throat are systematically examined. Symmetry of muscles, moisture, texture, masses, ulcers, and weakness are looked for. Also the individual's arteries are evaluated by looking into the eyes with an ophthalmoscope. The condition of small arteries can be seen directly in the retina and the condition of the optic nerve can be seen also. Next the pulse (throbbing rush of blood through an artery with heart beat) of the neck and the size, texture, and contour of the thyroid gland and lymph glands of the neck are palpated with the examiner's fingertips.

Heart   Notation is made as to whether the chest is symmetrical and if it has a normal shape. Attention is then focused on the heart; it is inspected, palpated, ausculated, and percussed. In *percussion* the fingers are used to tap the chest, and one listens to the sound that resonates from the chest. *Palpation* is feeling with fingertips and to *auscultate* is to listen to the heart with a stethoscope. Size of the heart is noted and assessment of the quality of the sound of blood rushing through the heart helps detect heart murmurs. One searches for pulses in the neck, abdomen, arms, inguinal and popliteal regions, and the feet to determine whether arteriosclerosis is present.

Lungs   The lungs are also assessed by inspection, auscultation, palpation, and percussion; abnormal breath sounds, the presence of dullness (indicating fluid), and a wheezing sound signal underlying pulmonary diseases.

Abdomen   The abdominal cavity is evaluated with the individual lying in a dorsal position (on the back). The shape of the abdomen and the presence of scars, dilated veins, and protruding masses can be noted. On palpating the abdomen, the examiner can search for the liver and spleen. Normally, only the edges of these organs can be felt; thus enlargement can be determined by palpating the liver and spleen. Masses, tenderness, and the presence of fluid are also detected by palpation.

Rectum   A rectal examination is done with a gloved finger; hemorrhoids and neoplasms (some of which may be malignant) are searched for. For example, one-half of rectal cancers can be palpated with the finger (Fig. 1-10). In individuals over 40 years of age, a proctoscopic examination should be done. This is accomplished by using a long hollow tube with a light (proctoscope), which enables the physician to see ulcers and tumors. About 75% of all colorectal cancers can be detected by rectal examination plus proctoscopy.

Pelvic Examination   A pelvic examination is

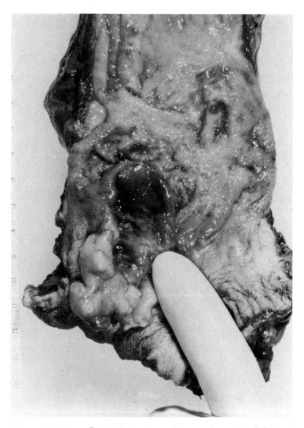

Figure 1-10   *Rectal cancer. Approximately 50% of cancers of the rectum can be palpated with a gloved finger.*

performed to find discharge of pus and ulcers, and palpation of the uterus and ovaries is done to detect masses. A pap smear should be done during a pelvic examination to diagnose any possible uterine cancer. Examination for hernia is also done by palpating for masses in the inguinal region. In men, the penis and scrotum are examined and hernias are noted in the inguinal region.

Neuropsychiatric Examination   A neurologic examination assesses the individual's orientation —name, place of examination, and date. Also, memory and reasoning capacity of a person are evaluated, and a brief psychiatric examination is performed. The function of the cranial nerves and peripheral nerves are evaluated by noting symmetry, development of muscles, and the sensations of touch, vibration, and position. Reflexes are also tested, and the strength and coordination of the individual noted.

Musculoskeletal Examination   The musculoskeletal system is evaluated by determining the muscular development, range of motion of the joints, strength, coordination, and presence of masses and deformities.

A thorough physical examination may also reveal findings of which the person is unaware. I recall a young boy who was brought to me because he had been kicked in the shins while playing hockey. Indeed, he had swelling over his shin bone (tibia); in addition, a mass below his mandible was seen. Surgical removal revealed a lymphoma (malignancy of the lymph gland). Early diagnosis and removal of the lymphoma led to the boy's cure.

Following the clinical history and physical examination, laboratory studies are usually ordered to confirm or eliminate presumptive diagnoses made from the clinical history and physical examination. Differential diagnosis permits the examiner to sort out the one correct diagnosis from numerous possibilities.

Laboratory Studies

Laboratory tests are performed to diagnose a disease, monitor the course of a disease, determine whether therapy is successful, and detect complications arising from drugs or surgical procedures. Laboratory studies, together with the clinical history and physical examination, provide the data base used for managing the patient's disease. Moreover, some diseases require a specific laboratory test for diagnosis.

Evaluation of blood and other body fluids, bacteriologic culturing of fluids and orifices for infectious agents, and X-raying of parts of the body are all performed to substantiate diagnoses suspected from the clinical history and physical examination findings.

Screening   Additional diagnostic screening can reveal unsuspected diseases. The American Hospital Association requires accredited hospitals to perform the following three routine tests: CBC, urinalysis, and chest X-ray.* The CBC, complete blood count, consists of a hematocrit, hemoglobin, white blood count, and white cell differential count of cell types. A urinalysis is used to search for urine sugar, protein, and cells. A chest X-ray is used to detect pulmonary infection, primarily tuberculosis, and lung cancer. Automation of laboratory procedures has motivated physicians to screen extensively for disease. For example, only 5 ml of blood are necessary to perform as many as 25 different laboratory determinations when one is using certain automated laboratory instruments. During 1976, 6 billion dollars were spent for laboratory tests in the United States; the cost is rising at an appalling rate. Many of the laboratory tests are not needed.

Beyond the use of the routine tests (CBC, urinalysis, and chest X-ray), specific laboratory tests are chosen to differentiate diagnoses of patients who exhibit signs and symptoms of various groups of common diseases.

Infectious Diseases   When an individual experi-

---

*Though technically the term that should be used here for chest X-ray is *roentgenogram* or *roentgenography*, I will use X-ray throughout in discussing both the end product and the process.

ences a fever and weakness, infectious disease is usually suspected. Cultures of the individual's throat, blood, urine, cerebrospinal fluid, or other body fluids are obtained selectively depending on the organ affected. In addition X-rays of the chest may be performed to rule out pneumonia, or an intravenous pyelogram may be done to identify infection in the kidney (pyelonephritis).

Arteriosclerosis When arteriosclerosis is suspected, an electrocardiogram (ECG) is performed to indicate whether the heart has sustained damage. If acute (recent) damage to the heart is suspected, certain enzymes are elevated in the patient's serum. These enzymes are released from damaged heart muscle (see Chapter 13, Cardiology). Metabolic disorders that could be responsible for the arteriosclerosis are searched for by checking the individual's blood cholesterol, triglycerides, and blood sugar concentrations.

In the event the person suffering from coronary artery disease has a blocked coronary artery, it may be necessary to evaluate for possible corrective surgery, that is, to bypass that blocked artery. Cardiac catheterization is performed, and coronary arteriograms are made. In the arteriogram, dye is injected into the coronary arteries, and X-rays demonstrate the extent of the blockage (occlusion).

Patients suffering from stroke, seizures, or stiff neck may have a lumbar puncture performed for diagnosis. Cerebrospinal fluid is removed and evaluated for the presence of tumor cells, protein, or microorganisms. In addition, the electrical activity of the brain can be determined via an electroencephalogram (EEG) and an arteriogram is often performed to search for a blocked artery, blood clots, tumor, or other lesions.

Jaundice Caused by Liver Disease Individuals with jaundice are usually evaluated by tests of liver function. The tests include quantification of enzymes released by damaged liver, bilirubin, and testing for the presence of hepatitis B virus in the patient's serum. If the individual has a mass in the liver or when certain infectious or inherited diseases are suspected, a biopsy specimen can be obtained for

microscopic examination. To obtain a biopsy, a needle is passed through the skin into the liver, a small piece of the liver is removed, and examination is made by the pathologist.

Renal Failure Renal failure is determined by testing the blood to see whether the individual has a normal concentration of electrolytes (K^+, Na^+, Cl^-, Ca^{++}) and blood urea nitrogen. Whether protein and red blood cells are passing through damaged kidneys into the urine is also noted; urine can also be cultured for bacteria. Occasionally the kidney may be biopsied. X-ray studies are used to evaluate the liver, gallbladder, and kidneys of persons exhibiting hepatic or renal failure.

Blood Disorders Individuals having disorders of the blood such as anemia (decreased hemoglobin concentration), bleeding, or recurrent infections are studied by examining blood smears and determining various blood clotting times. Occasionally, the bone marrow is examined to see if blood cells are developing normally or pathologically.

Gastrointestinal Disorders Abdominal discomfort is evaluated with CBC, urinalysis, measurement of blood serum enzyme concentration, and by special X-ray studies. For these X-ray studies, a solution of barium sulfate is used since it appears opaque on X-ray film (Fig. 1-11). The barium sulfate can be introduced into the gastrointestinal tract by swallowing or by enema; the barium coats and outlines the wall of the tract revealing a stricture, ulcer, tumor, or other defects. In a more direct examination, the physician inserts a long flexible tube (gastroscope or proctoscope) into the gastrointestinal tract; a lesion is seen directly and can be biopsied for diagnosis.

Cancer Persons suspected of having cancer are evaluated by X-rays, organ scans, serum enzymes, mammography, cytology, and biopsy. The biopsy is usually the most definitive diagnostic tool available. In special instances, physiologic tests of the function of lungs, heart, kidney, liver, and muscles are performed. Mention will be made of other laboratory tests in subsequent chapters (see Chapter 8).

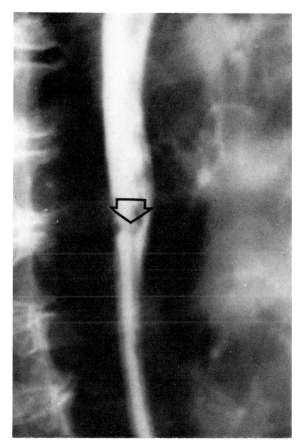

Figure 1-11 *X-ray of carcinoma of the esophagus was detected by noting narrowing of the barium sulfate stream at the site of the tumor. (The barium was swallowed.)*

A pathologist (physician specialist) is responsible for the diagnosis of disease by studying tissues and cells under the microscope, and body fluids chemically and microbiologically within the clinical laboratory.

Prevention of Disease

Prolongation of life has resulted largely from decreased mortality from infectious disease (Fig. 1-8). Improvements in nutrition, economy, housing, and sanitation of persons living in developed countries are responsible for increased longevity. For example, incidence of tuberculosis has declined drastically because of better socioeconomic conditions and because of early detection by skin testing, chest X-rays, and the introduction of antituberculosis medication. Also, vaccination (immunization) against viral infectious diseases has virtually eliminated smallpox and polio. Quarantine of infected persons and animals, as well as other public health measures, to assure clean food, air, and water prevent many diseases. Regrettably, we are bathing in a sea of industrial pollutants which poison our lungs, as well as other organs. Some experts fear an epidemic of cancer due to the carcinogenic chemicals blighting our environment.

Yearly physical examinations can lead to early diagnosis of disease and permit cures. The routine use of Papanicolaou (Pap) smears has led to a gratifying decline in the incidence of invasive cancer of the uterine cervix. Also, more women are examining their own breasts monthly for cancer; thus earlier diagnoses are achieved. Adherence to safety precautions such as the posted speed on highways and precautions in the use of chemicals and machinery likewise prevent accidental deaths. Simply lowering the speed limits to 55 mph on the highway has led to a significant decline in highway fatalities.

Prenatal diagnosis of certain genetic diseases is possible (see Chapter 3). New diagnostic laboratory techniques provide definitive information for the genetic counseling of parents. This information can aid in predicting chances of involvement or noninvolvement of offspring for a given genetic disorder, for example, mongolism. One technique, *amniocentesis*, consists of removing a small amount of fluid from the amniotic sac that surrounds the fetus and analysing the cells and chemicals in the fluid. Blood samples can also be obtained from the fetus by amniocentesis; the amniotic fluid and fetal blood are then studied for defects in enzymes, determination of sex, and measurement of substances associated with defects in the spinal cord and brain.

Diagnosis of genetic defects aims to provide a choice for the family to abort the child or to prepare for the extra responsibilities of having a defective child. Parents can also choose to avoid future pregnancies.

Treatment of Disease

Medicine is divided into two major disciplines, medicine and surgery. Numerous other subspecialties of medicine and surgery have evolved to more effectively serve humanity. Both internists and surgeons diagnose and treat patients. Also, a growing number of subspecialists who focus on a given organ or technique provide diagnoses and treatment.

Surgery

Surgeons are oriented toward coping with diseases in which they can alter anatomical structures (usually by cutting them) and thereby provide lifesaving intervention or a more healthful state. Surgeons perform a service which is the only means of therapy in certain instances of trauma, congenital birth defects, most malignancies, and in many diseases that fail to respond to medical care.

The surgeon can also perform surgery to diagnose, cure, palliate (improve temporarily), or reconstruct. Although surgeons employ the use of a scalpel blade, scissors, and sutures primarily, they also can use electrocauterization (burning of the abnormal tissue) or cryotomy (freezing abnormal tissues). Other specialized tools such as the laser beam are used by surgeons, for example, for attaching detached retinas of the eye.

Internal Medicine and Pediatrics

In contrast to the surgeon, the internist and pediatrician use drugs and a variety of techniques to improve the health of an individual. Drugs such as antibiotics can cure an individual of certain bacterial infections. Other drugs such as digitalis improve the function of the failing heart, whereas insulin replaces a defective hormone in a diabetic patient.

The physician also serves as counselor to help individuals cope with their diseases or disabilities. If needed, psychotherapy, with or without drugs, is used for psychiatric disorders.

The internist has a comprehensive understanding of most disorders of the human body. Pedia-

tricians function similarly in caring for children. A reemphasis on family practice as a desirable approach to providing primary health care has come into vogue.

Physical Medicine

Numerous physical modalities such as heat, light, cold, electricity, massage, and exercise are employed to improve the well-being of individuals suffering from disease. The physiatrist (MD specialist in physical medicine) and physical therapist, especially, use these therapeutic modalities for victims of stroke, accidents, or poliomyelitis, for example.

Radiotherapy

Radiologists are medical specialists either in diagnostic radiology or radiotherapy. Diagnostic radiology employs examination of X-rays of patients, and radiotherapists are concerned with the treatment of persons with malignant neoplasms using radiation. Radiologists work in a treatment team that employs chemicals, radiation, and surgery for the treatment of cancer.

Chemotherapy

Chemicals have been developed during the past two decades that can destroy certain malignancies. Chemotherapeutic agents kill tumors because they are highly toxic to fast growing tumors and thus control their growth; in contrast, normal tissues are not severely affected and the patient usually survives. Oncologists are medical specialists who employ chemotherapy in treating patients with cancer. During the past decade, a dramatic improvement has occurred in the survival of some young patients, especially those with acute lymphocytic leukemia who are treated with several drugs simultaneously.

Immunotherapy

One additional therapeutic modality is now being employed, immunotherapy. Herein, an attempt is made to enhance the normal immune response of persons against their own tumors. Each patient's immune system (lymphocytes, macrophages, and antibodies) is provoked to attack the tumor (see Chapter 6): Immunotherapy is also employed in restoring immunity in immunodeficient patients who fail to develop immunity against infectious diseases. This can be done, for example, by giving gammaglobulin injections to persons who lack gammaglobulin or antibodies.

Summary

This chapter provides a general summary of this book and medicine in general. An etiologic classification of diseases is described that is applicable to each organ or system. The medical model, which seeks to cope with diseases by identifying causal factors, diagnosing structural and molecular abnormalties, and providing acceptable therapies, is the theme of this book.

Students (and patients) are often confused by a seeming lack of promptness in providing treatment. The master clinician Sir William Osler cautioned, "There are three types of therapy, diagnosis, Diagnosis, DIAGNOSIS!" Symptomatic treatment is often irresponsible and can cover up diagnosis of treatable conditions. We also must admit, however, that not all diseases are diagnosable, and often definitive treatment is lacking. Rene Dubos in 1976 summed up the situation, "To cure, sometimes—to help, often—to comfort, always."

Bibliography

Beeson, P. B., and McDermott, W., Eds. 1974. *Textbook of Medicine*, ed. 13. Philadelphia: W. B. Saunders Company. Comprehensive reference used by all physicians. Not recommended for the novice.

Cairns, J. 1975. The cancer problem. *Sci. Am.* 233:64–78. Global view of the cancer problem including causes, frequency, and biologic behavior of malignancy.

Davidsohn, I., and Henry, J. B. 1975. *Clinical diagnosis by laboratory methods*, ed. 15. Philadelphia: W. B. Saunders Company. The standard reference textbook describing most of the clinical laboratory tests used for diagnosis of disease.

Delp, M. H., and Manning, R. T. 1968. *Physical diagnosis*, ed. 7. Philadelphia: W. B. Saunders Company. Describes the methods used in taking a clinical history with emphasis on how to perform a physical examination of the patient.

Douthwaite, A. H., Ed. 1967. *French's index of differential diagnosis*, ed. 9. Bristol: John Wright & Sons, Ltd. Encyclopedia of differential diagnosis of many diseases which can cause given symptoms or signs of disease.

Dubos, R. 1976. To cure, sometimes—to help, often—to comfort, always. *Dialogue* 3:4–5. Philosophic discussion of the proper orientation of modern medicine by an eminent experimental pathologist.

Health in the United States 1975. U.S. Public Health Service. Provides a statistical, epidemiologic overview of disease in the United States.

McKusick, V. A. 1975. *Mendelian inheritance in man*, ed. 4. Baltimore: The Johns Hopkins University Press. Catalog of over 1200 inherited disorders which includes an abstract of the disease and key references.

Peery, T. M. 1975. The new and old diseases: a study of morality trends in the United States, 1900–1969. *Am. J. Clin. Pathol.* 63:458–474. The source of several graphs used in this chapter. Written by a physician who lived and taught medicine during the period.

Squire, L. F. 1974. *Fundamentals of roentgenology*, ed. 2. Cambridge: Harvard University Press. A provocative and well-illustrated book suitable for the uninitiated student.

Stanbury, J. B.; Wyngaarden, J. B.; and Fredrickson, D. S., Eds. 1972. *The metabolic basis of inherited disease*, ed. 3. New York: McGraw-Hill Book Company. Sophisticated but complete source of information on metabolic diseases.

Syme, S. L., and Berkman, L. F. 1976. Social class, susceptibility and sickness. *Am. J. Epidemiol.* 104:1–8.

Wishnow, R. M. 1976. The conquest of the major infectious diseases in the United States. *Annu. Rev. Microbiol.* 30:427–450.

CHAPTER 2

Normal Cells, Tissues, and Organs

Chapter Outline

Introduction

The Cell (cytology) / Membranes / Cytoplasmic organelles /
Cytoplasmic inclusions / The nucleus / Cell division /
Diagnostic cytology

Tissues (histology) / Chemicals in tissues / Epithelium /
Connective tissue / Adipose tissue / Cartilage / Bone /
Blood-forming (hematopoietic) tissues / Lymphoid
organs / Muscular tissues / Nervous tissue

Organs (organology) / The kidneys / The liver / The
gastrointestinal tract / The pancreas / The lungs

Summary

Objectives

After reading this chapter you should be able to

Define the terms cytology, histology, and organology.

Know the fundamental characteristics of living cells.

Compare cellular organelles with inclusions.

Describe the fluid mosaic model of membranes.

Define the role of granular endoplasmic reticulum.

Understand how cells adapt to alcohol, phenobarbitol, and other drugs.

List characteristics of mitochondria, suggesting they have "invaded" the cell as
discrete living microbes.

Describe the organelle responsible for autolysis of cells.

Compare the function of the Golgi complex with the granular endoplasmic reticulum.

List supporting structures of cytoplasm.

List cytoplasmic inclusions.

Identify the "conductor" that "orchestrates" the function of cells.

Compare chromosomes of men and women.

Describe the chemical composition of the nucleolus.

Compare mitotic division with meiotic division.

Know how a Papanicolaou smear is taken and its value in diagnosis.

List cytologic features characteristic of malignant cells as seen in a Pap smear.

Name the three primary germ layers in the embryo.

List the four major groups of tissues.

Distinguish between the three types of muscle in structure and control.

Compare hyaline cartilage, elastic cartilage, and fibrocartilage.

List the percentage of water, protein, minerals, and fat in an "ideal" person.

List important anions and cations in the body.

Define the term epithelium.

Know the distribution of simple epithelium in the body.

Compare a mucosal epithelium with skin.

Recognize that the liver, pancreas, and many other organs are composed of epithelial tissues.

List the three major categories of connective tissues.

Compare collagen and reticulin fibers.

Know the name of the cell that produces fiber.

Recognize that collagen constitutes one-third of the protein in the human body and is rich in connective tissues.

List the locations and composition of the three types of cartilage.

List the chemical ingredients of bone.

Distinguish between endochondral and membranous bone.

List the hematopoietic tissues.

List the three major types of cells of the immune system.

Know the function of T-lymphocytes.

List the two major functions of the spleen.

List the two contractile proteins in all muscles.

Compare "voluntary" with involuntary muscles.

List the divisions of the nervous system.

Describe the connective tissue cells in nervous tissue.

List organ systems of the body.

Define the two parts of a nephron.

List structures in the kidney in which plasma is filtered and water reabsorbed.

Know function of Kupffer's cells in the liver.

List layers of hollow organs.

Describe the two components of the pancreas.

Introduction

A prerequisite to understanding the structural basis of disease and abnormal tissues is knowing what normal cells and tissues look like; the normal structure and function of cells and tissues will thus be described in this chapter. For example, diagnoses, especially in diagnostic cytology, are based on the microscopic appearance of cells. A Pap smear of the uterine cervix is examined under a microscope to evaluate for cervical cancer. Recognition of normal cervical cells must be made so that cancer cells can be identified.

The most primitive forms of life, protozoa, are unicellular. In one cell, this microorganism shows all of the four fundamental characteristics of living protoplasm: motility (mobility), irritability or responsiveness to stimuli, metabolism, and reproduction. Virtually all the cells in our bodies exhibit these characteristics.

The cell is the basic structural and functional unit of life. Highly developed multicellular animals possess specialized cells. Tissues having common specialized functions such as the skin, heart, brain, and liver evolved to provide diverse form and function in multicellular creatures. In order of complexity, we will study cells (cytology), tissues (histology), and organs (organology). Before considering tissue structure and function, we first need to discuss the cell.

The Cell (cytology)

Cells are variable in size, shape and function. Yet common biologic elements are obvious. The living substance of cells, protoplasm, is divided into two major compartments: the *nucleus* (nucleoplasm) and the *cytoplasm* (surrounding the nucleus). Both the nucleoplasm and cytoplasm contain highly organized subunits called organelles and inclusions. Division of labor within the cell is comparable to the different roles organs play in the body.

Organelles are living structures which occur in nearly all types of cells. These small internal organs of the cell carry out special functions. By contrast, *inclusions* are building blocks or sources of energy, including stored protein, fat, carbohydrates, pigment, secretory droplets, or debris. Inclusions are not vital to the cell, but organelles are required for normal function. *Membranes* enclose the cell and its organelles and contain the enzymes that control the biochemical (metabolic) processes of cells. Membranes are the "gatekeepers" of the cell; they determine what goes in and out.

A typical schematized cell displaying organelles and inclusions is shown in Figure 2-1. The structure and function of normal membranes, organelles, and inclusions will be considered in the fol-

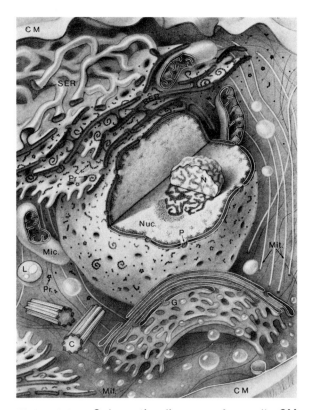

Figure 2-1   *Schematic diagram of a cell.* CM, *cytoplasmic membrane;* SER, *smooth endoplasmic reticulum;* RER, *rough, endoplasmic reticulum;* Pr, *protein;* Mic, *mitochondria;* L, *lysosomes;* C, *centrioles;* Nuc, *nucleus;* N, *nucleolus;* Mit, *microtubules; and* G, *Golgi complex. (From Hogan, M. J. 1971.* Histology of the human eye. *Philadelphia: W. B. Saunders Company.)*

lowing discussion; many diseases result from underlying defects in organelles and/or membranes.

Membranes

Most important physiologic processes are carried out on the surfaces of membranes. Thousands of enzymes vital for chemical activities (metabolism) in the cell are locked within membranes. In addition, the membranes give form and structure to the cell and surround the organelles. If membranes did not surround organelles, the enzymes in these sacs would digest the cell from within or autolysis (self-digestion) would occur. Membranes form compartments separating the organelles from their reaction products. Useful substances (O_2, glucose) enter the cell and waste products (CO_2, urea) leave the cell for export. Traffic in cells is directed by selective permeability.

A thin limiting membrane, called the *plasmalemma* (cell membrane), surrounds cells. It is too thin to be seen with a light microscope. Electron micrographs suggest that membranes are composed of a bimolecular layer of lipids sandwiched between two layers of protein (Fig. 2-2). Recent studies show that this *trilaminar model* of cell membranes is too simplistic. More sophisticated and accurate biophysical studies reveal that living membranes are composed of fluid containing a suspension of linked proteins, lipids, and carbohydrates of varying size and shape. The high lipid content makes the cell pliable and water repellent.

The *fluid mosaic model* is depicted in Figure 2-2, with the proteins depicted as vegetables and fruit floating in fluid. Certain chemical compounds, for example, proteins, are found only on the inner or outer surface of the membrane, whereas others penetrate entirely through the membrane. The position and depth of penetration of the proteins in membranes is important. Selective permeability, or the passage of electrolytes and other substances through the membranes is governed by the arrangement of the compounds. Thus the structure and biochemical organization of membranes determines the selective permeability of electrolytes, the function of enzymes, and the conduction of nervous electrical impulses in certain cells, as in nerves and muscles. Each organelle, including the nucleus, is covered by membranes.

Cytoplasmic Organelles

Organelles visible under the light microscope are the mitochondria, Golgi complex, and ergastoplasm (Fig. 2-1). The organelles are composed mostly of membranes, and contain *enzymes* that are appropriately released under the direction of the nucleus. Enzymes are proteins that induce or accelerate specific chemical reactions. The location of enzymes on the inner or outer surface of membranes regulates the direction of traffic of substances into or out of the cells.

Organelles provide the cell with the vital functions of living organisms, namely, metabolism (mitochondria and ergastoplasm), reproduction (centrisome), and growth (nucleus); other cytoplasmic components provide a matrix (support) structure and contraction (motility and irritability).

Ergastoplasm   The *ergastoplasm* ("granular" endoplasmic reticulum) consists of a complex network of delicate membranes dotted by numerous small particles called *ribosomes* that synthesize new protein in the cell. Cells producing protein for secretion or release from the cell, such as plasma cells (which produce antibodies to fight infections) or pancreatic cells (which produce enzymes that digest food), contain many ribosomes on their endoplasmic reticulum.

Agranular endoplasmic reticulum is also seen in cells. This special organelle consists of membranes that are agranular (smooth) because they lack ribosomes. Muscle cells have abundant agranular endoplasmic reticulum. Other cells with diverse function, such as liver cells, are rich in agranular and granular endoplasmic reticulum.

The ergastoplasm can undergo proliferation (growth) when stimulated by drugs. Hence, an individual may become tolerant (require greater quantities to achieve the same effect) when taking alcohol or phenobarbital because repeated exposure to these drugs causes the smooth endoplasmic re-

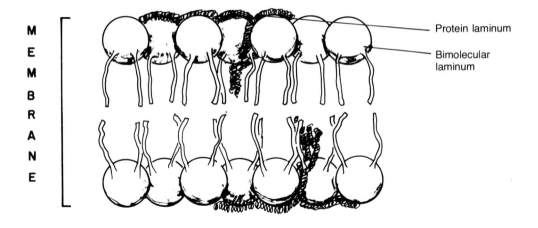

Trilaminar model of cell membrane

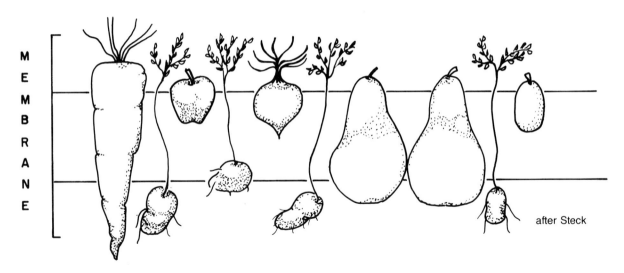

after Steck

Arrangement of proteins in cell membrane ("food model")

Figure 2-2 *Hypothetical models of cell membranes. Trilaminar model of cell membrane* (top) *and fluid mosaic model of cell membrane* (bottom). *(Adapted from Steck, T. L. 1974. J. Cell Biol. 62:12.)*

ticulum to proliferate to detoxify* these drugs. Thereby, the body adapts to changes in environment, and cell injury is prevented (see Chapter 4, Adaptation, Injury and Death of Cells). Adaptation

*The process of converting one compound, drug, or metabolite into another is called *detoxification*.

cannot occur when abuse is severe or of long duration.

Mitochondria The mitochondria generate energy that supports metabolic functions of the cell. The slender mitochondria (Fig. 2-1) have internal plates that add to their membrane area. These "powerhouses" are rich in enzymes that trap energy in high energy phosphate compounds. For example, adenosine triphosphate (ATP), a rich source of energy, is concentrated in the mitochondria. Possibly mitochondria are descendents of primitive bacteria that long ago invaded cells. Mitochondria possess characteristics of bacteria: they can move in the cytoplasm, reproduce, and even have their own deoxyribonucleic acid (DNA).

Cells with high metabolic activities (kidney tubules, for example) are rich in mitochondria. Differences in the number of mitochondria even account for the color as well as the function of cells. For example, the breast meat of a chicken is white whereas that of the thighs is red. This is due to numerous mitochondria being present in red meat —giving great strength to the red thigh muscles. In contrast, white muscle has few mitochondria.

Lysosomes   The name of these organelles is descriptive of their function. *Lyso*—to dissolve and let loose, *some*—a body. Lysosomes (minute dense bodies that are scattered throughout the cytoplasm) are shown in Figure 2-1. These membrane-bound sacs contain more than 20 different powerful hydrolytic enzymes capable of splitting polypeptide, lipid, and carbohydrate bonds. The cell is safe as long as these enzymes are contained within membranes, but with cellular injury from trauma or exposure to certain noxious agents, the lysosomes release their enzymes, which rapidly hydrolyze (digest) the cells.

Cells capable of *phagocytosis* (engulfment of solid extracellular material, such as bacteria) use lysosomes to digest bacteria. The phagocytosed vacuoles become fused with lysosomes to form phagolysosomes. The lysosome spills its enzymes onto the phagocytosed bacterium, killing and digesting it (see diagram in Chapter 7, Infectious Diseases).

Frequently, many diseases arise from abnormalities in lysosome function. The inflammation of rheumatoid arthritis, for instance, occurs when lysosomes are released from granulocytes into the joints. Moreover, many lysosomal disorders are inherited, and the resulting deficiency of certain lysosomal enzymes results in accumulation of toxic compounds. Such storage diseases are inherited.

They are discussed in Chapter 9, Inherited Disorders.

Golgi Complex   The Golgi complex, residing adjacent to the nucleus, is contiguous with the ergastoplasm in the cytoplasm and exports secretory products, such as antibodies, into the blood or mucus into the intestinal glands. This apparatus is composed of complex membranous plates that condense proteins or mucus from the ergastoplasm and package them in secretory vacuoles for export from the cell (Fig. 2-1). The Golgi complex is prominent in pancreatic cells, which produce enzymes that are packaged in the Golgi complex as secretory droplets that flow into the pancreatic duct. By this mechanism, digestive enzymes are moved from the pancreatic cell into the pancreatic duct and duodenum where they can digest foods.

In addition to packaging, the Golgi complex in secretory cells (the lining cells of the intestinal and respiratory tracts, for example) can also synthesize a portion of the secretory products, such as mucus. Secretions line the surfaces of the gastrointestinal and respiratory tracts and protect them from dust and microorganisms.

Centrioles   The centrosome is an organelle (Fig. 2-1) essential for cell division. Prior to cell division, the centrosome divides into two centrioles, which anchor contractile spindle fibers in the cytoplasm and permit daughter chromosomes to pull apart during mitotic division into two daughter cells.

Cytoplasmic Support System   Filaments of protein provide the cytoskeleton of cells and contractile protein give cells their motility. The cytoplasm of virtually all cells, especially muscle cells, contains numerous thin filaments composed of the two contractile proteins—*actin*, and a thicker protein, *myosin*. These filaments are arranged in parallel bundles that interdigitate; the chemical interaction of actin with myosin is converted into mechanical contraction.

Filaments binding cells together are termed *desmosomes*. These specialized dense plaques maintain cell-to-cell contact and tissue integrity. In certain cancers the desmosomes may be deficient. Tumor cells often lack desmosomes and this defect is thought to account for the separation of tumor cells from a primary cancer site to distant sites, spreading (metastasizing) the cancer.

In addition to contractile filaments, microtubules (submicroscopic filaments) pass through the cytoplasm of cells. Microtubules are numerous in cells of the endocrine system, which secretes hormones. For example, insulin produced in the pancreas is thought to pass through the microtubules in small membrane-bound packages into the blood. Microtubules form a cytoskeleton for supporting the cell. Moreover, they direct the flow of cytoplasm in the cell, moving nutrients to and from cells.

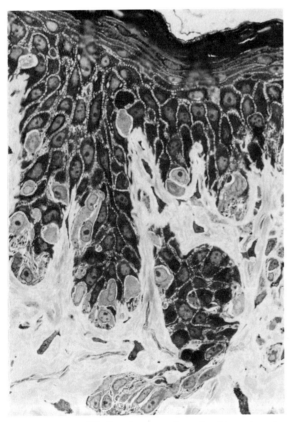

Figure 2-3 *Photomicrograph of skin showing light-staining melanocytes containing melanin pigment (black particles) and numerous keratinocytes in the epidermis. (Courtesy Dr. Jag Bhawan).*

Cytoplasmic Inclusions

The nonliving cytoplasmic inclusions include pigment granules, fat, and glycogen. Melanin pigment granules within melanocytes in skin (Fig. 2-3) are examples of cytoplasmic inclusions. Melanin pigment is responsible for tanning following exposure to sunlight and skin color in pigmented races.

Glycogen is a carbohydrate stored primarily in liver and skeletal muscle. There is glycogen, sufficient for approximately 11 hours of energy use, stored in human muscle and liver; fat and protein energy reserves are not drawn on until these stores are depleted. Many glycogen-associated diseases (glycogenoses) have abnormalities in deposition or release of glycogen from cells.

Fat is found in most cells as lipid droplets within the cytoplasm. Certain conditions (starvation or alcoholism, for example) are associated with a marked increase in deposition of fat in liver cells. Specialized fat cells called *adipose cells* normally store large quantities of fat.

The Nucleus

The nucleus orchestrates the function of the organelles in the cells as demands arise. Most metabolic and synthetic activities are controlled by the nucleus and are carried out in or by organelles in the cytoplasm.*

The nucleus is composed predominantly of deoxyribonucleic acid (DNA) (Fig. 2-1). All genetic information is stored in the thousands of genes bound together to form chromosomes. Humans have 46 chromosomes, including 22 pairs of autosomes and 2 sex chromosomes. A woman has XX and a man XY sex chromosomes. The chromosomes in the nuclei of most cells are either heterochromatin (clumped) or euchromatin (dispersed) in arrangement, as seen in Fig. 2-4.

Amazingly, each cell in the human body contains all of the genetic material that an individual possesses—each cell has the capacity to express all

*The reader is spared here from having to read about the complex biochemical processes which are responsible for the synthesis of protein. *The Molecular Biology of the Gene* by J. Watson describes the process they discovered.

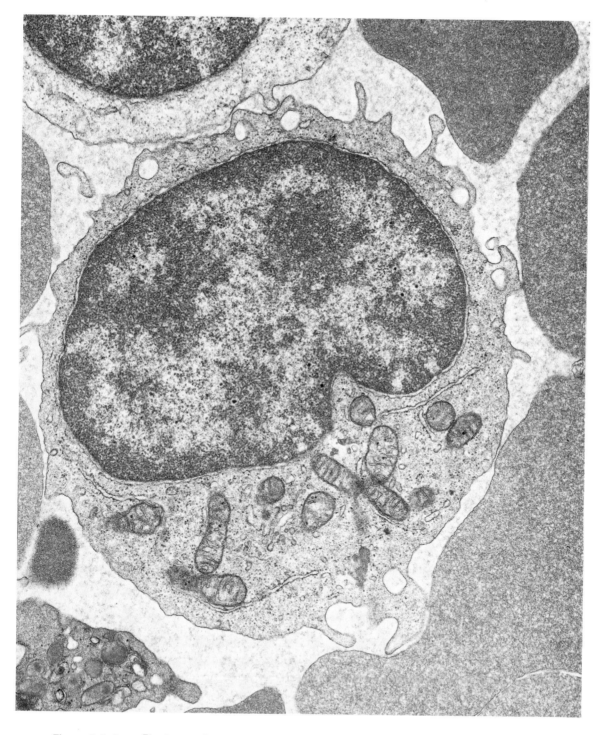

Figure 2-4, A   *Electron micrograph. Lymphocyte showing mitochondria and endo-plasmic reticulum. × 20,000. (Courtesy Dr. Jag Bhawan.)*

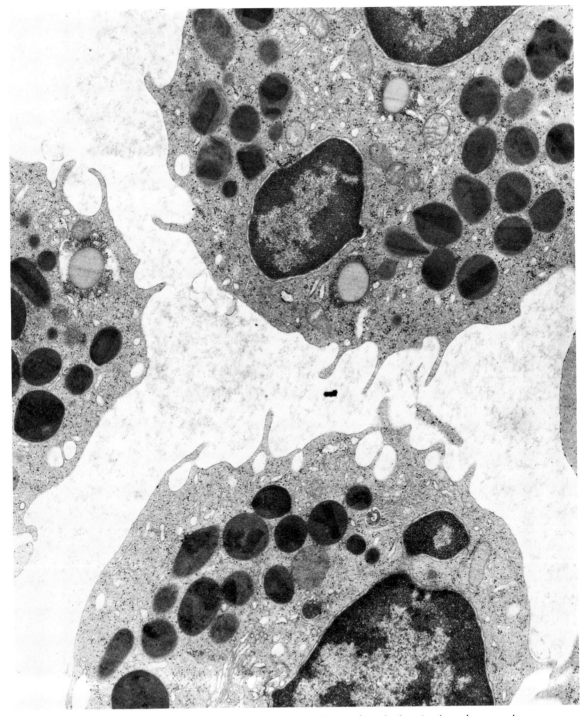

Figure 2-4, B *Electron micrograph. Eosinophil showing dark cytoplasmic granules.* × *14,400. (Courtesy Dr. Salvatore Allegra.)*

functions and activities of all cells. But during fetal development, individual cells undergo specialization, certain genes become inactive (depressed), whereas other genes continue to function. This permits specialized intestinal cells to secrete mucus while neurons (nerve cells) transmit nerve impulses. In Chapter 3, the process of specialization of cells, tissues, and organs—differentiation (developmental anatomy)—will be described.

The Nucleolus The nucleolus is a conspicuous rounded body within the nucleus. It stains intensely owing to its high content of ribonucleoprotein. A rim of heterochromatin (condensed chromatin) surrounds the edge of the nucleolus. The nucleolus assists in directing the synthesis of protein in the cytoplasm. Cells that secrete protein often have large nucleoli. Large nucleoli are also seen in malignant cells and in growing immature cells (Fig. 2-5).

Cell Division Cell division and growth is important to the developing embryo and also for growth and repair of normal tissues. Moreover, abnormal cell division and growth is characteristic of many diseases, especially malignancy. Most orga-

nisms have a limited life span; cells grown in tissue culture (Fig. 2-5) possess approximately 50 cell divisions (generations) and then die. Proponents of a major theory of aging state that we have a limited life span and that we are programmed by our genetic material to have only a limited number of divisions before aging and death ensue.

Mitosis Somatic (body) cells multiply by mitosis. During this process the chromosomes double in number and separate with precision, giving nearly two exact sets of chromosomes to daughter cells (Fig. 2-6). The actual mitotic division extends over a period of 30 to 60 minutes in most human cells, with variable intervals of time between cell division ranging from hours to years. Yet, some cells, such as neurons in the brain, are never replaced throughout life. Other cells are programmed to function for finite periods of time—in circulation, red blood cells live 120 days, and white blood cells, two to five hours. Thus, individual tissues and cells have their own built-in reproduction and life cycles.

Meiosis Meiosis is a second type of cell division. It occurs in spermatozoa and ova. This process is similar to mitosis but consists of two successive cel-

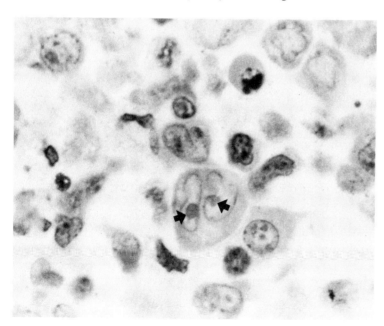

Figure 2-5 *Cultured lymphocytes showing nuclei and nucleoli* (arrows).

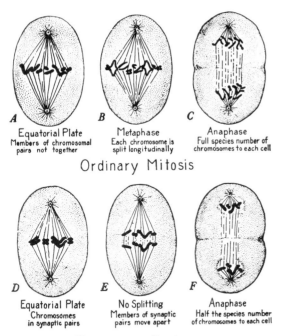

A — Equatorial Plate
Members of chromosomal pairs not together

B — Metaphase
Each chromosome is split longitudinally

C — Anaphase
Full species number of chromosomes to each cell

Ordinary Mitosis

D — Equatorial Plate
Chromosomes in synaptic pairs

E — No Splitting
Members of synaptic pairs move apart

F — Anaphase
Half the species number of chromosomes to each cell

Reduction Division

Figure 2-6   *Mitosis and meiosis. (From Bradley Patten. 1929. Early embryology of the chick. Copyright 1929 by McGraw-Hill Book Company. Used with permission of McGraw-Hill Book Company.)*

lular divisions with only a single replication of the chromosomes. Meiosis reduces the number of chromosomes in the daughter cells to one-half (haploid) the normal number (23). When the egg (23 chromosomes) is fertilized by the sperm (23 chromosomes), the 46 chromosomes (diploid) are restored. We will now briefly discuss how cytology contributes to the diagnosis of disease.

Diagnostic Cytology

Cells scraped from surfaces of the body or removed from body fluids are studied in the microscope to provide diagnostic information. Diagnostic cytology is the diagnosis of malignancy by examining cells from body surfaces or fluids. In addition, numerous inflammatory, infectious, and degenerative diseases, as well as other disorders, can be ascertained cytologically.

A woman who has itching in the vaginal area and a milky discharge can be examined by touching a spatula to the fluid in the vagina and smearing it on a slide. Following fixation of the cells to the slide with methyl alcohol, it is possible to stain and study these cells. If the woman has a yeast infection, yeast cells can be seen under the microscope and appropriate therapy given. Cells from the cervix, as well as urine, spinal fluid, other fluids, and sputum, can be examined cytologically for diagnoses (Fig. 2-7).

Routine cytologic examination employing the Papanicolaou test (Pap smear) has resulted in a marked reduction in the occurrence of advanced uterine cervical cancer. In this procedure, the cervix is gently scraped with a wooden spatula; cells are scraped off and smeared on a slide. Based on the size, shape, and other characteristics of the nucleus, a judgment is made as to whether the cervix is malignant.

Certain cytologic features are described in detail in Chapter 8, Neoplasia (Oncology). In the Pap smear, the nuclei of malignant cells show enlargement and marked distortion of their shapes; in addition, abundant heterochromatin is found. Moreover, the nucleoli may be enlarged as compared to surrounding normal cells.

Diagnostic cytology is a form of preventive medicine since some cancers can be detected early and cured. Cervical cancer appears gradually over a 10- to 20-year period. Thus, yearly Pap smears can result in early diagnosis of malignancy, which can be treated before it reaches an advanced stage.

Tissues (histology)

A *tissue* is a group of cells and their cell products that have similar appearance and function. Histology, the study of tissues, also commonly includes the study of cells and organs as well. Examples of tissues are listed in Table 2-1. In the following brief section, normal tissues are described to give an understanding of the structural basis of diseases discussed in subsequent chapters.

Tissues are best understood by tracing their development from the time of conception. The study of development of a new being is termed *embryology*. After an ovum (egg) is fertilized by a sper-

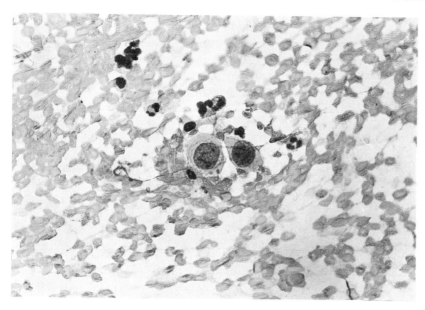

Figure 2-7 *Photomicrograph of Pap smear showing squamous cell carcinoma of lung in sputum.*

matozoan (sperm cell), it then divides into smaller cells. The daughter cells rapidly segregate into three superimposed germ layers. These layers are logically named according to their position—*ectoderm* (external); *mesoderm* (middle portion); *entoderm* (internal). A tubular embryo forms through processes of folding, budding, resorption, migration, and growth of tissues and organs (Fig. 2-8).

The three primary germ layers further differentiate forming tissues and organs. The growth of specialized tissue is called *histogenesis*. During histogenesis four major groups of tissues form: (1) epithelium, which arises from all three germ layers; (2) supporting tissues (connective) from mesoderm; (3) muscle tissues from mesoderm; and (4) nervous tissue from ectoderm (Table 2-1).

An *epithelium* is a sheetlike covering having one surface free and the other attached. Examples of epithelium include the skin; linings of the respiratory, gastrointestinal, reproductive, and genitourinary tracts; and linings of the thoracic and abdominal cavities, as well as the joints, blood vessels, and covering of the brain.

Supporting tissues connect, bind, and support the human body. They are composed chiefly of the special protein *collagen*. The connective tissues arise from mesoderm and include bones, tendons, and ligaments; and sheaths of dense connective tissue

separating muscles (fascia) also constitute supporting tissues. Lymphoid tissues are really organs, but they are loosely considered tissues. They arise from the mesoderm and are distributed throughout the body in the thymus gland, spleen, lymph nodes, tonsils, bone marrow, and the intestinal tract.

Muscle cells all contain the specialized intracellular proteins *actin* and *myosin*. Muscle cells respond to stimulation by contracting.

Nerve cells are "irritable." They conduct nerve impulses and move our bodies by stimulating skeletal muscle and causing it to contract. In addition, nerve tissue serves autonomic (subconscious) functions of digestion, respiration, and cardiovascular activity; protects; and provides pleasurable and painful sensations.

Chemicals in Tissues

Fluid is an extremely important component of the body. *Water* comprises approximately 70% of the body weight of an "ideal" young man; 14% is protein, 7% minerals, and 7% fat. Fat tissue contains less water than other tissues. Women are generally fatter than men because of their breasts and buttocks. The average water content of most persons is closer to 60% of the body weight because of obesity.

Table 2-1
Tissues Forming the Human Body

Epithelium
Simple
  Squamous
  Cuboidal
  Columnar
Pseudostratified
Stratified
Simple branched
Compound tubuloalveolar }   Glands of the body
Compound alveolar
Connective tissues
Loose
  Reticular (framework of hematopoietic organs)
  Areolar (soft tissues filling spaces between cells and tissues)
  Adipose (fat)
Hematopoietic
  Blood cells
  Bone marrow
  Lymphoid tissues
Strong
  Bone—compact and cancellous
  Joints
  Tendons
  Ligaments
  Cartilage—hyaline, fibrocartilage, and elastic
Muscular tissues
Smooth involuntary muscle
Striated involuntary muscle (myocardium)
Striated voluntary muscle (skeletal)
Nervous tissues
Tissue of central nervous system—gray matter and white matter
Tissue of peripheral nervous system—nerves, ganglion, and nerve endings

Water within cells (intracellular) makes up 33% of the body weight, or about 55% of the total body water. In contrast, the fluid between cells (extracellular fluid) and within blood vessels and lymphatics comprises 27% of the body weight and 45% of the total body water. Extracellular water is divided into plasma water, tissue water, cerebrospinal fluid, aqueous humor of the eye, and water trapped in the intestinal tract.

Some water is present in a free state, but much water is bound to components in the cell, to proteins, for example. Every living cell is bathed with fluid on at least one surface. Active cells (myocardium, or heart muscle, for example) are bathed and nourished by blood from adjacent capillaries.

The nonliving formed material between cells is termed *ground substance* or *matrix*. This material, called *connective tissues,* is composed of a mixture

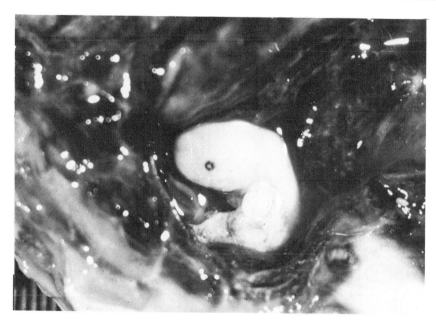

Figure 2-8   *Human embryo in tubular stage.*

of protein, carbohydrates, and calcified salts, which provides form and rigidity to bone and cartilage.

Electrolytes are minerals that contain positive or negative charges (ions). Important electrolytes include Na^+, K^+, Ca^{++}, and Mg^{++} among the positive-charged electrolytes *(cations)*. Na^+ is most abundant in blood plasma, whereas K^+ is the major electrolyte within cells. The important *anions* (negative-charged electrolytes) are HCO_3^-, Cl^-, HPO_4^-, SO_4^-, organic acid, and certain proteins. In cells, total content of cations and anions must be in balance for metabolism to be maintained. In normal homeostasis, the pH of the blood is slightly alkaline, 7.39. (A pH of 7.00 represents neutrality.)

Additional chemical elements of importance include nitrogen, hydrogen, oxygen, and carbon. These four elements form the basis of the primary foods, carbohydrate, protein, and fat. Also, sulfur, phosphorus, magnesium, zinc, cobalt, and iron are present in small quantities. Iron, zinc, and cobalt are important constituents of proteins, especially enzymes. The enzymes are important since they function as biologic catalysts; they enhance biochemical reactions in the cells.

Tissues are "the fabric of life." The following is a brief description of the structure and distribution of the four major types of tissues that fabricate our body.

Epithelium

Epithelial tissue covers external or internal surfaces of the body. Typically, one surface of epithelium is free, facing either against air or fluid, while the opposite surface almost always rests on a thin *basement membrane*, which connects the cell attaching it to connective tissue.

Epithelial cells are always packed tightly together and are held together by specialized junctions and *desmosomes*. No space occurs between the cells. Hence, epithelium forms a barrier which blocks the passage of fluid and thus helps to maintain body fluid and electrolyte concentrations in various compartments of the body.

Classification   The three main groups of epithelia are classified by the number of layers they possess: (1) *simple epithelium* is one layer thick, (2) *pseudostratified epithelium* is one layer thick but appears to be two or three layers thick because the nuclei are staggered in rows, and (3) *stratified epi-*

thelium consists of many layers of cells superimposed on each other (Table 2-1 and Fig. 2-9).

Subclassification of the epithelium is then based on cell shape: (1) *simple squamous epithelium* consists of flat cells and lines the blood vessels (endothelium) and body cavities (mesothelium), (2) *simple cuboidal epithelium* is composed of cells that have the same height and width and, (3) *simple columnar epithelial cells* are taller than they are wide. Columnar epithelium can be specialized; it can contain cilia (minute "hairs") or secrete mucus, for example. Cilia are found in the respiratory and reproductive tracts. In the lungs, particles such as dust are moved along in mucus by the ciliated epithelium.

The mouth, esophagus, and vagina are covered by moist epithelial surfaces (mucosa). *Mucosal surfaces* are moist because they are bathed by fluid from glands. By contrast, a thick horny layer of a special type of protein, keratin, makes the skin dry

and resistant to invasion by microbes and fluid (Fig. 2-10). Areas of the body that are exposed to friction thicken. For example, the palms and soles of the feet are heavily keratinized from rubbing by friction.

The skin is a complex organ covered by stratified squamous epithelium and has numerous accessory appendages, namely, hairs, sweat glands, and sebaceous glands (oil glands) (Fig. 2-10).

Glands of Secretion The epithelium can become tubular and form either a simple gland or a complex branching gland (Fig. 2-11). Glands can be specialized to secrete oil, mucus, enzymes, or other substances. Glands are often specialized for the production and release of fluids. Surprisingly, both the liver and pancreas are specialized epithelial glands. Secretion of bile is one of the many functions of the liver. The pancreas secretes the enzymes lipase, trypsin, and amylase, which help digest fat, protein, and carbohydrate, respectively.

When epithelial tissues undergo malignant transformation, the malignant epithelium is termed *carcinoma*. The word carcinoma will be used often in subsequent chapters, as carcinomas are the most common types of cancer (see Chapter 8).

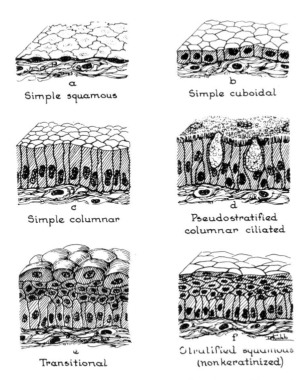

Simple squamous

Simple cuboidal

Simple columnar

Pseudostratified columnar ciliated

Transitional

Stratified squamous (nonkeratinized)

Figure 2-9 *Types of epithelia. (From Ham, A. 1975.* Histology, *ed. 7. Philadelphia: J. B. Lippincott.)*

Connective Tissues

Connective tissues include bone, cartilage, tendons, ligaments, fascia, and adipose tissue. They perform certain mechanical functions, for example, connect and anchor parts of the body, and support the body and its organs. Therefore, they are often called supporting tissues.

Connective tissues consist of cells and extracellular fibers embedded in a gellike ground substance. The number of cells, fibers, and ground substance vary greatly in different types of connective tissues. The fibers are either *collagen* or thinner units of collagen termed *reticulin*. Collagen and reticulin fibers are composed of the same fibrous protein; they differ only in thickness. Connective tissues arise from mesoderm in the embryo.

In adults, the cell capable of producing fibers is called a *fibroblast*. The fibroblasts are capable of

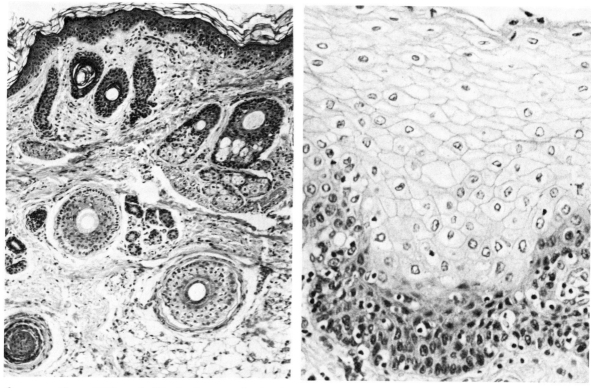

A   **B**

Figure 2-10   A, *Photomicrograph of skin —numerous hair shafts are seen as well as their attached sebaceous glands;* **B,** *Mucosa lining the esophagus.*

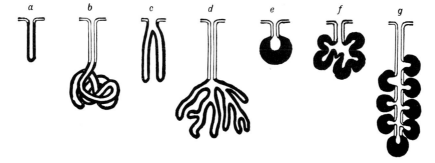

Figure 2-11   *Diagrams of simple exocrine glands.* **A,** *Simple tubular;* **B,** *simple coiled tubular;* **C** *and* **D,** *simple branched tubular;* **E,** *simple alveolar; and* **F** *and* **G,** *simple branched acinar. Secretory portions are black; ducts are double contoured. (From Fawcett, D. 1975. A textbook of histology. Philadelphia: W. B. Saunders Company.)*

producing matrix material as well. The fibroblasts synthesize bundles of collagen fibers, which are present in many connective tissues.

Fibrous connective tissue, composed chiefly of collagen, performs a variety of functions including anchoring internal organs in place, forming the elastic outer walls of blood vessels, and binding together nerves and muscles. Fibrous connective tissue also forms *tendons*, which connect muscle to bone, and *ligaments*, which connect bone to bone.

Approximately one-third of the protein in the human body is collagen; collagen, then, is the predominant fiber of connective tissue.

The following sections describe the three major types of connective tissue—cartilage, bone, and fat.

Adipose Tissue

About 7% to 10% of the total body weight of an average person is fat. Energy reserves are stored in adipose (fat) tissue sufficient to last approximately 40 days. Fat varies in color from white to brown; however, most often it is pale yellow. Individual fat cells are usually spherical but may assume other shapes. Fat cells can range up to 120μ in diameter. (The average red blood cell is 7μ in diameter.) Adipose tissue is often subdivided into small lobules by connective tissue partitions.

When adipose tissue is fixed in formalin, the fat dissolves during processing. Thus the cells only show nuclei and outlines of cells (Fig. 2-12). Special laboratory techniques, such as using osmic acid stain, reveal the fat. Delicate blood vessels and capillaries pass randomly through adipose tissue to nourish it. Miles of new capillaries and blood vessels are required to feed each pound of fat, thus placing a burden on the heart. As a consequence of prolonged fasting or chronic illness, adipose tissue loses its stored lipid and becomes a thin strand of vascular connective tissue.

Distribution   Fat is widely distributed in subcutaneous tissue, and the large continuous subcutaneous layer of fat is termed *panniculus adiposus.* Differences in age and sex of an individual dictate the distribution of body fat. The secondary sexual characteristics of women are mainly due to an accumulation of adipose tissue in the breasts, buttocks, hips, and anterior aspects of the thigh. Also, fat accumulates in the mesenteric membrane, which attaches the intestinal tract to the back, the omentum, and behind the peritoneal membrane.

Cartilage

Cartilage is a specialized form of connective tissue consisting of cells, called *chondrocytes,* and extracellular fibers embedded in a gellike cementing matrix. The intercellular matrix predominates over the cells. Unlike other connective tissues, cartilage lacks nerves and blood vessels of its own. Three types of cartilage are hyaline, elastic, and fibrocartilage. The specific types of cartilage are named according to the fibers found in their matrix.

Hyaline Cartilage   Hyaline cartilage is found at the sternal end of the ribs, tracheal rings, larynx, and at the joint surfaces of bones. Also in the embryo, hyaline cartilage forms a model on which bone forms. Hyaline cartilage is composed largely of chondrocytes and matrix and contains many collagen fibers. Shown in Fig. 2-13 is an epiphyseal plate (the growing end) of a rib. Note the transition from cartilage to bone as the cartilage matures and is replaced by bone in the lower shaft.

Elastic Cartilage   Elastic cartilage is found in the external ear, the walls of the ear canal, Eustachian tubes, and the epiglottis. It differs from hyaline cartilage by being penetrated by branching elastin fibers. The elastin fibers give elasticity to the structures formed by it; the ear is flexible, for example.

Fibrocartilage   Fibrocartilage occurs in the intervertebral discs, pubic symphysis, and areas where tendons insert into bones. Fibrocartilage differs from hyaline cartilage in its parallel arrangement of collagen fibers and in composition of its matrix.

Bone

Osseous (bone) tissue is the most highly differentiated of the supporting tissues. This rigid tissue constitutes most of the skeleton, whose rigidity results from the calcified salts contained in its matrix. Eighty-five percent of bone is calcium phosphate, 10% calcium carbonate, and 5% a mixture of various chemicals and proteins. The bone cells are called *osteocytes.* Bone growth arises from *osteoblasts,* which line or cover the bone. Internally, osteoblasts that line the bone give rise to *endosteum;* osteoblasts that cover the bone produce *periosteum.*

Bone is considered to be either *compact* or *spongy.*

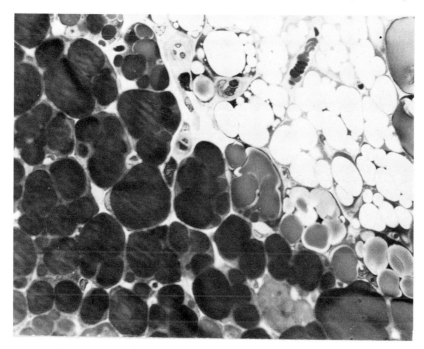

Figure 2-12   *Photomicrograph of adipose tissue. Osmic acid has stained the fat black. Clear spaces are where fat has dissolved during the processing.*

Compact bone forms the thick cortex of the shaft of long bones; spongy bone lines the hollow shafts and ends of bones. Spongy bone is also termed *cancellous bone* and contains bone marrow.

In the embryo, bone forms in two ways. Cartilagenous models are formed for most bones of the body, and this is termed *endochondral bone* formation. The models are formed prior to the activation of osteoblasts to produce bone. The second mode of bone formation is *membranous bone* formation; flat bones of the skull, jaw, and the clavicle are formed directly from osteoblast membranes.

Bones are metabolically active. Two cells are involved primarily—*osteoblasts* and *osteoclasts*. The osteoblasts produce collagen fibers, which later become calcified new bone *(osteoid)*. Osteoclasts then work in synchrony with osteoblasts—osteoclasts resorb old bone and osteoblasts remodel it. The osteoclasts are activated by a hormone (parathormone) produced in the parathyroid gland. The bone produced by the osteoblasts is layed down in concentric sheets or lamellae. So-called lamellar bone is found in the compact bone forming the

shafts of long bones (Fig. 2-14). The spongy bone cells forming the soft ends of bones have thin spicules of bone and are rich in bone marrow.

Blood-forming (hematopoietic) Tissues

Hematopoietic tissues form blood. They are not actually connective tissue, but they are discussed following connective tissues since they have a common origin in mesoderm. Hematopoietic tissue produces blood cells. These blood cells are responsible for carrying oxygen (erythrocytes or red blood cells), for providing an inflammatory response to infection (neutrophils and monocytes), and for providing an immune response to other infections (lymphoid cells). Platelets, a formed element of blood that serve in coagulating blood, are also formed in bone marrow.

Bone marrow   The bone marrow is one of the largest organs in the body. It is distributed primarily in the cancellous (spongy) bones at the ends of the long bones, sternum, vertebrae, and hips.

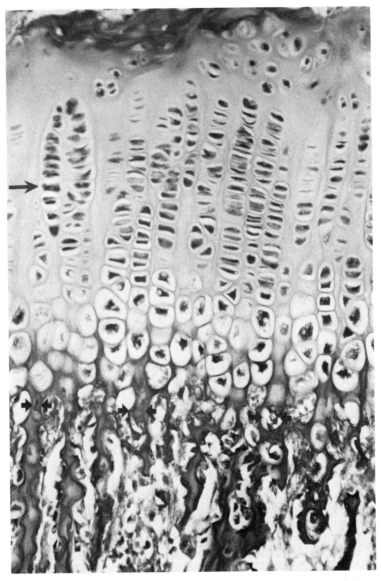

Figure 2-13 *Photomicrograph of epiphyseal plate (growing end) of bone showing hyaline cartilage* (arrow). *The matrix is gray and located between chondrocytes. A transition to bony cells* (double arrows) *is seen below.*

The formed elements of the blood (erythrocytes, leukocytes, and platelets) grow from an original stem cell. This stem cell gives rise to three major types of cells that form the blood cells—*erythroblasts* form erythrocytes, *myeloblasts* form leukocytes, and the *megakaryocytes* form platelets (Fig. 2-15). Additional aspects about the hematopoietic organs, blood, and diseases of the blood are described in Chapter 11, Hematology.

Lymphoid Organs

The thymus gland, spleen, lymph nodes, tonsils, and lymphoid nodules distributed in the gastroin-

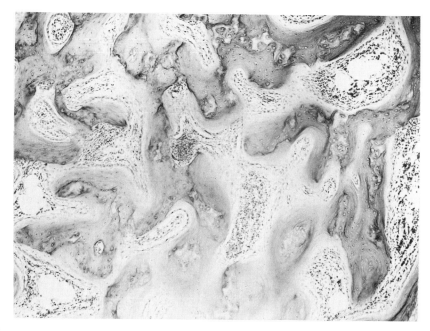

Figure 2-14   *Photomicrograph of lamellar bone, sheets (lamellae) of irregularly-shaped bone are seen. The spaces between bone are filled with fat and bone marrow cells.*

testinal tract constitute lymphoid organs or the immune system. The cells composing these organs contain lymphocytes, plasma cells, and macrophages; these cells provide an immune defense against infection and invasion by malignant cells (see Chapter 6, Immunology).

The Thymus Gland   The thymus gland is a broad, flat, bilobed lymphoid organ located just beneath the upper sternum. This gland arises from the pharyngeal pouches of the embryo, which are lined by epithelium. The adult gland is lobulated; each lobule is divided into a medulla and cortex (Fig. 2-16). The medulla or central core contains remnants of the epithelium formed from the lining of the pharyngeal pouches, the thymic corpuscles. The corpuscles are the site of production of the hormone thymosin, which maintains function of thymus-dependent lymphocytes (T-lymphocytes). T-lymphocytes defend against intracellular microorganisms and malignancies. The cortex surrounds the medulla and is populated by numerous T-lymphocytes formed there. With aging, the thymus

gland becomes atrophic (withered) and is replaced by adipose tissue; concurrent with aging and atrophy of the thymus, immunity declines.

The Spleen   The spleen has two major functions. It serves as a filter for cleaning debris from erythrocytes (including malarial parasites) and destroying damaged erythrocytes, and it is the site of production of lymphocytes and antibodies. The spleen is located in the upper left side of the abdominal cavity and is approximately the size of a fist, weighing 150 gm. This gland is composed of two parts—sinuses, which filter blood, and lymphoid tissue. Lymphoid tissue surrounds the arteries that enter from the surface of the spleen. The lymphoid tissue is termed white pulp and the surrounding tissue red pulp. The red pulp obtains its color from the presence of numerous erythrocytes that pass through the splenic filter from the sinuses (Fig. 2-17).

Lymph Nodes   Numerous tiny lymph nodes (glands) filter lymph fluid from the extremities,

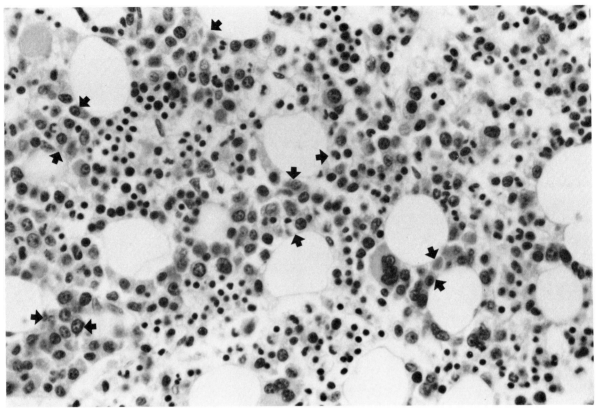

Figure 2-15   *Photomicrograph of bone marrow showing the three major cellular elements—megakaryocytes (largest cells), erythroblasts (small black nuclei in clusters), and myeloblasts (arrows), which constitute the majority of cells. Lymphocytes are scattered among these cells.*

head, and other organs of the body. The lymph nodes are the sites from which immune responses originate. Each node is divided into *cortical* and *medullary* regions (Fig. 2-18). The cortex is surrounded by a delicate connective tissue capsule. Beneath the capsule, lymphoid nodules that may contain active germinal centers are seen. The germinal centers are the sites from which new lymphocytes and *plasma cells* are formed; plasma cells synthesize antibodies for immune defense. Surrounding the follicles are other types of lymphocytes. In addition, macrophages, cells capable of engulfing foreign invaders, are scattered throughout the lymph node. Macrophages are especially concentrated in sinuses, where they "patrol" and engulf invading particles in lymph fluid.

Tonsils   Three different pairs of tonsils form a ring of lymphoid tissue at the back of the mouth in the oropharynx—the *palatine* tonsils are located at both sides of the mouth, the *lingual* tonsil is located at the base of the tongue, and the *adenoids* surround the roof of the oropharynx.

The tonsils are covered by squamous epithelium and are composed of lymphoid tissue, and germinal centers are occasionally seen. The tonsils and other lymphoid tissues reach their maximal size at approximately 10 years of age and thereafter decrease in size. The tonsils and thymus gland atrophy more than the other lymphoid organs for an unknown reason.

Other organs in the body contain lymphoid tissues in association with epithelium. Especially rich

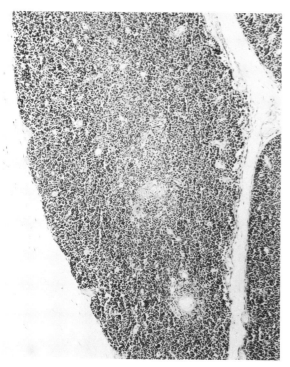

Figure 2-16 *Photomicrograph of thymus gland showing the cortex populated by numerous small lymphocytes and a central (medullary) clearer area containing epithelial corpuscles of Hassall.*

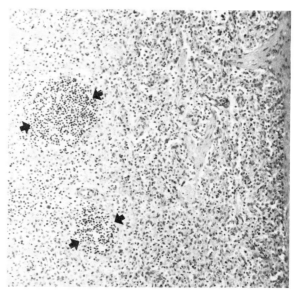

Figure 2-17 *Photomicrograph of spleen showing lymphoid tissue surrounding central arteriole (arrows). The tissue surrounding the white pulp is the red pulp, consisting of sinuses that filter particles from erythrocytes. The capsule of the spleen is seen to the right.*

in lymphoid nodules is the small intestine. The appendix, colon, and stomach also contain lymphoid nodules.

Muscular Tissues

The flesh of the body is composed of muscle. Morphologically, muscles are of three types—smooth muscle, striated skeletal muscle, and striated cardiac muscle (Fig. 2-19). The heart is composed mostly of cardiac striated muscle; in contrast, the walls of many hollow tubular organs are lined by smooth muscle. Muscular tissue contracts and moves the skeleton and internal organs to permit physiologic processes.

The unit of muscle tissue is the muscle fiber, which contains actin and myosin filaments—these slide over each other and interact chemically during contraction.

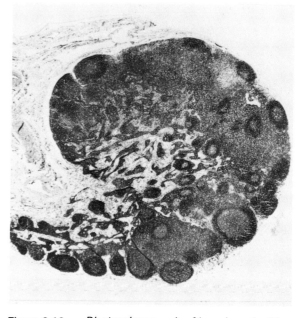

Figure 2-18 *Photomicrograph of lymph node. The lymph node shows large round germinal centers in the cortex and sinuses in the medulla.*

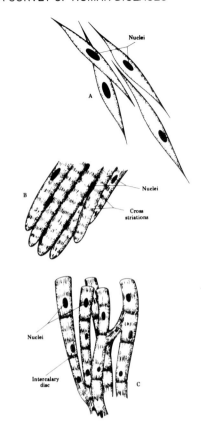

Figure 2-19 *Muscle types* **A**, *smooth;* **B**, *skeletal; and* **C**, *cardiac muscle. (From Wasserman, A. O. 1975.* Biology. *Reading, Mass.: Addison-Wesley Publishing Company, Inc.)*

Smooth Muscle   Smooth muscle has the simplest structure of the three kinds of muscle. It comprises the walls of all hollow visceral organs, except the heart, and forms the walls of ducts and blood vessels. In addition, it is found in the skin, spleen, eye, penis, and many other organs.

Smooth muscle fibers are elongated and are tapered at their ends. They contain actin and myosin filaments. Striations are not seen, and hence, smooth muscle is also called nonstriated muscle.

Smooth muscle is under *involuntary* (autonomic) control; autonomic nerve fibers can be seen ending on the surface of smooth muscle fibers. Chemicals liberated either by the nerve endings or by the endocrine glands (hormones, epinephrine, and acetylcholine, for example) will provoke smooth mus-

cle to either contract or relax. The smooth muscle in blood vessels stabilizes blood pressure by contracting appropriately after each heartbeat. Also, smooth muscle propels digesting food through the intestinal tract.

Striated Skeletal Muscle   In contrast to smooth muscle, skeletal muscle is under *voluntary* control. Motor nerve plates attach peripheral and cranial nerves to skeletal muscle and transmit nerve impulses that initiate muscle contraction. The basic unit of structure of skeletal muscle is the skeletal muscle fiber. Muscle fibers can be extremely long (up to 4 cm) and usually contain several nuclei. The striations of skeletal muscles are due to the arrangement of the actin and myosin filaments. Muscle fibers are then bound together by connective tissue to form individual muscles.

Skeletal muscle contracts more rapidly than smooth muscle, but skeletal muscle also fatigues more readily. The most active skeletal muscles are red; they are rich in mitochondria. Muscle fibers, unlike cartilage and epithelium, have their own blood supply; active cells, especially striated cardiac muscle, have an especially rich blood supply.

Striated Cardiac Muscle   Cardiac muscle is under autonomic control and forms the bulk of the heart. Cardiac muscle consists of a syncytium (network) of interconnected myocardial fibers. Nuclei of muscle cells are located centrally in the cells, and striations are present. Both types of autonomic nerves, namely, sympathetic and parasympathetic (vagus) nerves, innervate the heart. Thus, the heart contracts according to the stimulation supplied by the nerves—the sympathetic nerves speed up the heartbeat, and parasympathetic nerves slow down the heartbeat.

Nervous Tissue

Irritability and conductivity are vital processes inherent in protoplasm. Irritability is the ability to sense stimuli, thus setting up a stimulus-response that can be lifesaving. Nervous tissues also have the capacity to conduct or transmit waves of excitation, conductivity. The qualities of *irritability* and *con-*

ductivity reach their highest expression in the nervous system.

A neuron is the cell unit of the nervous system (see Chapter 21, Neurology). The neuron contains a nucleus and surrounding cytoplasm. In addition, dendrites, nerve processes that receive impulses, and axones, long processes that send impulses, are seen passing from the surface of the cell (Fig. 2-20).

Nerve cells are concentrated in the *central nervous system* (CNS), which consists of the brain and spinal cord. Collections of nerve cells outside the central nervous system are termed *ganglia.* Extending from the central nervous system are numerous *nerve tracks* and *fibers.* The nerves extending from the central nervous system constitute the *peripheral nervous system.*

Nervous tissue is supplied by numerous blood vessels and is equipped with *neuroglia and Schwann cells,* specialized connective tissue cells that are unique to nervous tissue. The Schwann cells often lay down a fatty lipoprotein spiral array of membrane (myelin) to coat the axon. This coating is called a *myelin sheath.* The myelin sheath insulates nerves, permitting impulses to travel accurately down a fiber. Special nerve stains, such as osmic acid, blacken the nerve cell and demonstrate the myelin sheath (Fig. 2-21).

The connective tissue cells of the nervous system can proliferate through the life span of an individual; thus, recovery from injury is possible (see nerve injury in Chapter 21). By contrast, neurons lose all reproductive function around the time of

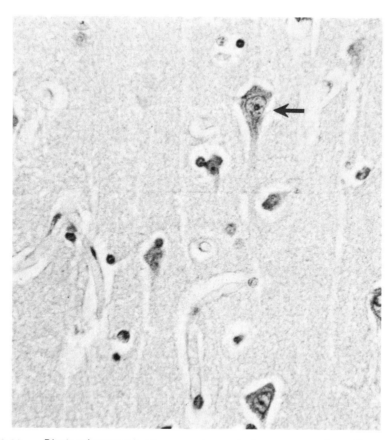

Figure 2-20 *Photomicrograph of neuron in central nervous system. The nucleus is centrally located and large. Dendrites (branchlike processes) leave the surface of the cell and an axon (long process) extends from the cell.*

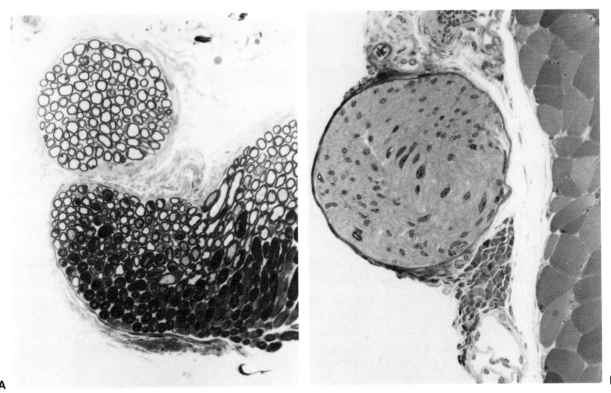

A　　　　　　　　　　　　　　　　　　　　　　　　　　　　　　**B**

Figure 2-21 **A,** *Photomicrograph of nerve fibers showing myelin sheaths. These sheaths are composed of fat, which stains black with osmic acid.* **B,** *Photomicrograph cross section of nerve and skeletal muscle* (right).

birth; as individuals age, or suffer brain damage from injury, they lose neurons, which are never replaced.

Organs (organology)

The study of organs is designated *special history* or *organology*. This science deals with the architecture and adaptations of tissues to form organs. Each organ is composed of two or more tissues that function together to perform a specific function. Within organs, one tissue usually predominates and is of functional importance; other tissues are secondary or supportive. For example, the epithelium lining the stomach and the glands that grow from it are primary components, whereas the connective tissue, muscular wall, and peritoneal covering are secondary features.

Organ systems include the digestive, genital, urinary, respiratory, and reproductive tracts; the nervous system; hematopoietic tissue; organs of special sense; and skin. In addition, the endocrine system, which releases hormones directly into the blood, is considered an organ system. A few organs —the kidney, liver, intestinal tract, pancreas, and lung—are described here because in subsequent chapters we will discuss abnormal histology (histopathology) and abnormal function (pathophysiology) of the organs as a graphic method of assisting you in understanding human disease.

The Kidneys

The urinary system consists of the kidneys and the passages that drain the kidneys—the renal pelvis, the ureter, the urinary bladder, and the urethra, its drainage duct. In adults, each kidney weighs approximately 180 gm. The functional unit of the kidney is the nephron and its excretory duct. Approximately 1.3 million nephrons are found in each kidney; the combined length of nephrons in the body totals about 80 miles.

A *nephron* consists of two major parts—the glomerulus, which acts as a filter of blood plasma (Fig. 2-22), and the renal tubules. Surrounding the glomerulus is Bowman's capsule, which collects filtered urine. Attached to the capsule is the proximal convoluted tubule, which drains into the loop of Henle; the distal convoluted tubule and the collecting ducts then connect and drain into the caliceal collecting system.

The function of the kidneys is to rid the body of nitrogenous wastes and to establish electrolyte balance. Eighty-five percent of the filtered plasma is reabsorbed in the proximal convoluted tubule; the

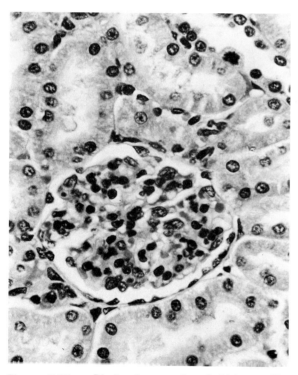

Figure 2-22 *Photomicrograph of kidney. The glomerulus, which filters blood, is seen in the center. Surrounding the glomerulus are renal tubules cut on cross section.*

remaining fluid is reabsorbed in the distal convoluted tubule, which acts under the influence of the antidiuretic hormone ADH. This hormone is produced in the pituitary gland, circulates in the blood, and causes the distal tubule to resorb water (see Chapter 12, Endocrine and Metabolic Disorders).

The kidneys are richly supplied with blood, as one-fifth of all blood pumped by the heart passes through the kidney each minute; the glomerular filtration rate is about 125 ml per minute. On the other hand, urinary output approximates 1200 ml each 24 hours owing to the great amount of reabsorption of the original glomerular filtrate.

The renal epithelium, especially the proximal convoluted tubule, can repair injuries by regeneration; however, glomeruli are unable to regenerate. Defective kidney function is not demonstrable by tests of function until almost 90% of the renal substance is lost. Thus, the kidney is remarkable in its ability to function even with extensive damage.

The Liver

The liver is an accessory gland of the intestinal tract. It is formed by epithelium arising from the entoderm lining the gut of the embryo. It is the largest gland of the body, weighing approximately 1200 gm.

The function of the liver is, in some ways, analogous to mitochondria; it is the metabolic "factory" of the body. It is strategically placed to capture nutrients from digested food draining from the intestine via the portal vein. The liver is capable of metabolizing fats, carbohydrates, and proteins and is the major site of *synthesis* of many of the plasma proteins, especially blood-clotting factors and serum albumin. The liver also serves as a storage depot for carbohydrates, such as glycogen, and vitamins A, D, E, and K. Finally, another major function of the liver is to *catabolize* (break down) old red blood cells and to convert the heme from within these red cells into bilirubin. Bilirubin, in turn, is detoxified by conjugation in the liver and is excreted in bile. Bile, then, is excreted through the common bile duct into the small intestine (see Chapter 11, Hematology).

Structure   The liver is separated into *lobular anatomical units*. The lobular units are composed of two components—parenchyma and blood sinusoids. The parenchyma is composed of closely packed glandular hepatocyte epithelium. *Hepatocytes* are arranged in plates that radiate outward from the central vein. The *sinusoids* converge radially into the central vein. These sinusoids are lined by *Kupffer's cells*, the phagocytic cells of the liver. The arrangement of the hepatic lobule is such that blood enters the lobule from the portal vein in the portal triad and drains through the sinusoids to the central veins. The *portal triads*, areas in the liver, are bile ductules, arterioles, and portal venules (Fig. 2-23). Tributaries gather from the portal venules to form the hepatic vein, which eventually returns blood to the inferior vena cava and subsequently to the heart. Blood passing through the sinusoids comes into intimate contact with Kupffer's cells and the hepatocytes. The hepatocytes actively carry on more than 500 biochemical reactions, including production of plasma proteins, fats, and bile. Kupffer's cells filter foreign particles and debris from the blood.

The liver has a marked capacity for repairing itself even after extensive tissue destruction. Up to 90% of the liver can be removed and regeneration occurs promptly, within two weeks, for example. New lobules form from old ones; hepatic cells enlarge and increase by mitotic division. Repeated and extensive cellular injury, however, may take its toll on the liver. For example, excessive alcohol abuse can result in destruction of hepatocytes and cause scarring. When scarring (fibrosis) has occurred from the activation of the fibroblasts, which produce collagen, the liver then fails to regenerate and scar tissue persists. Serious consequences arise. These consequences are elaborated in Chapter 16, Diseases of the Liver and Pancreas.

The Gastrointestinal Tract

The gastrointestinal tract is a canal beginning at the mouth and extending through the anus. This tract is typical of the *hollow organs* (gastrointestinal tract, gallbladder, ureter, urinary bladder, and reproductive ducts) of the body, since most tubular and sac-

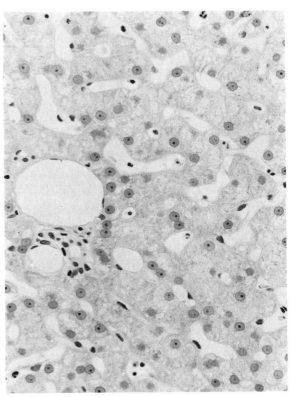

Figure 2-23   *Photomicrograph of liver showing, on cross section, a portal triad consisting of (1) a large portal venule, (2) a bile ductule composed of cuboidal-shaped cells, and (3) a smaller blood vessel, an arteriole. The hepatocytes, which are polyhedral-shaped cells and the Kupffer cells, which are small spindle-shaped endothelial cells lining the sinuses are the cells surrounding the portal triad.*

cular organs are constructed according to a common design. Four coats form the wall of the gastrointestinal tract—mucosal, submucosal, muscularis, and adventitia.

The epithelium bordering the cavity or lumen of a hollow organ can be folded (Fig. 2-24) or relatively smooth, and is named the *mucosa*. Folded epithelium is found in the small intestine and is smoother in the stomach. The epithelium is attached to a basement membrane; beneath it, loose connective tissue containing numerous lymphocytes, lymphatic vessels, blood vessels, and nerves is seen. Simple or compound glands may also be present in some areas of the intestine. A thin layer

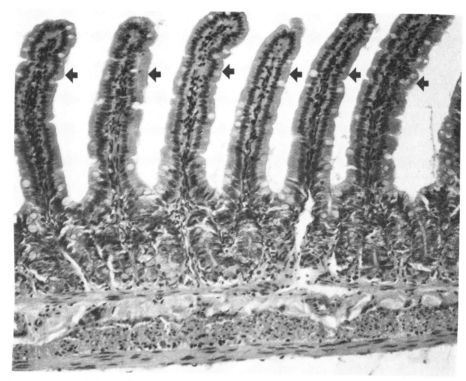

Figure 2-24   *Photomicrograph of ileum (small intestine). The mucosal surface is folded into villi* (arrows) *and composed of tall columnar epithelium. Loose connective tissue, termed lamina propria, and smooth muscle complete the organ.*

of smooth muscle, usually only two layers in thickness, surrounds an area termed the *lamina muscularis*.

The *submucosal coat* is composed of moderately dense connective tissue that is elastic and provides mobility to the mucosa. It contains and supports larger blood vessels, lymphatics, and nerves. It also contains glands, in some areas (the duodenum, for example), and autonomic ganglion cells.

The *muscular coat* is relatively thick; almost without exception it is composed entirely of smooth muscle. Commonly, two concentric tubes of smooth muscle, an inner circular layer and an outer longitudinal layer, are seen. Between the two muscle coats, vascular and nerve collections are found. The muscularis maintains the tone of the tube and propels the contents from within the tube onward.

The outermost coat (*adventitia*) of hollow tubes is commonly fibrous. In a few specialized organs, such as the lungs, this may be strengthened with cartilage (bronchial cartilage, for example). Through the adventitia, blood vessels and nerves pass to deeper levels of the wall.

The Pancreas

The pancreas has been chosen for illustration because it is both an exocrine and endocrine gland. The *exocrine* part elaborates enzymes and digestive juices, whereas the endocrine part secretes insulin and glucagon hormones directly into the blood. The cells responsible for enzyme production are glandular epithelial cells (Fig. 2-25). The *pancreatic cells* have prominent granular endoplasmic reticulum and secrete *zymogen* granules. Zymogen granules are rich in the enzymes lipase, trypsin, and amylase, which break down fats, proteins, and carbohydrates in food.

The *endocrine* part of the pancreas is diffusely scattered among the epithelial cells. The *islets of*

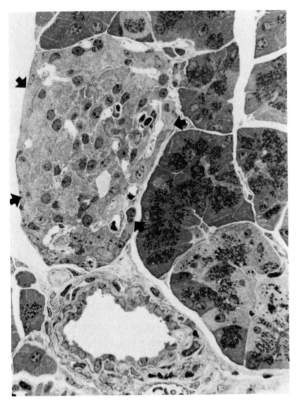

Figure 2-25 *Photomicrograph of pancreas showing an islet of Langerhans* (arrow) *composed of beta and alpha cells. Nearby, the exocrine pancreas composed of glands containing numerous black zymogen protein granules are seen.*

Langerhans are composed of two cell types, β and α cells. The β cells secrete insulin, and the α cells secrete glucagon. Insulin acts to drive blood sugar (glucose) from the blood into cells (see Chapter 12, Endocrine and Metabolic Disorders). By contrast, glucagon offsets the influence of insulin.

The exocrine and endocrine portions of the pancreas appear to function independently. The exocrine gland releases the digestive juices into ducts, which drain into the duodenum. By contrast, the endocrine cells empty insulin and glucagon hormones directly into the blood stream.

The Lungs

The lung is designed to exchange O_2 and CO_2 be-

tween blood and air. The oropharynx, trachea, bronchi, and bronchioles are lined by ciliated columnar epithelium. Small glands beneath the mucosa secrete mucus onto the mucosa, which together with the cilia in the mucosa, cleanse the airways of dust and bacteria.

Cartilage supports and maintains an open airway. Smooth muscles surround the bronchioles and constrict under the influence of nerves and hormones. Blood is pumped from the right ventricle, enters immediately into the lung, branches (a treelike arrangement) and then proceeds into the small arterioles and capillaries that line the alveolar (Fig. 2-26) air sacs. Numerous fine elastin fibers surround the air sacs giving the lungs elasticity. This discussion of normal structures should serve as a reference for pathologically altered cells in subsequent chapters.

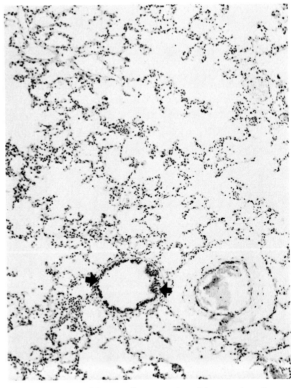

Figure 2-26 *Photomicrograph of lung showing a bronchiole* (arrows) *and numerous small alveolar air sacs.*

Summary

This book emphasizes the structural basis of disease and the clinical implications of structural as well as biochemical defects are stressed. You should, therefore, recognize the normal structure of cells, tissues and organs. Reference will be made to various cell organelles and cells that are vulnerable to damage from changes in their environment.

For example, mitochondria swell and release enzymes when the myocardium is deprived of oxygen, as occurs when a coronary artery is blocked by a blood clot. It is essential that you recognize that the myocardial cells release mitochondrial enzymes from cells damaged during a heart attack. Subsequent discussions of diseases requires that you understand basic facts about the fabric of our body. You will thereby understand why certain enzymes become elevated when a myocardial infarction ensues as described previously. Also, it will become apparent why the physician orders blood tests to detect these enzymes to confirm a suspected diagnosis of myocardial infarction in a middle aged man with severe chest pain.

Bibliography

Arey, L. B. 1970. *Human histology*, ed. 6. Philadelphia: W. B. Saunders Company. In outline form.

Bloom, W., and Fawcett, D. W. 1975. *A textbook of histology*. ed. 10, Philadelphia: W. B. Saunders Company. A standard textbook of cytology, histology and organology.

DeDuve, D. 1963. The lysosome. *Sci. Am.* 208(5):64–72. Good illustrations.

DiFiore, M. S. 1971. *Atlas of human histology*, ed. 4. Philadelphia: Lea & Febiger. Excellent colored illustrations of tissues.

Fox, C. F. 1972. The structure of cell membranes. *Sci. Am.* 226(2):31–38. Good illustrations.

Ham, A. W. 1974. *Histology*, ed. 7. Philadelphia: J. B. Lippincott Company. A thorough discussion of bones.

Koss, L. G. 1968. *Diagnostic cytology and its histopathologic bases*, ed. 2. Philadelphia: J. B. Lippincott Company. Standard textbook.

Rhodin, J. A. G. 1974. *Histology: a text and atlas*. London: Oxford University Press. Chiefly discusses ultrastructure of cells and tissues.

Swanson, C. P. 1969. *The cell*, ed. 3. Englewood Cliffs, New Jersey: Prentice Hall, Inc. Chiefly discusses ultrastructure.

Thomas, L. 1974. *Lives of a cell*. New York: The Viking Press, Inc. This book of essays provides provocative glimpses into the function and structure of cells and broad views of humankind and the world.

Warwick, R. ed. 1973. *Gray's anatomy*, ed. 35. Philadelphia: W. B. Saunders Company. Beautifully illustrated standard textbook of gross and microscopic anatomy.

Watson, J. 1975. *The molecular biology of the gene*, ed. 3. Menlo Park, California: W. A. Benjamin, Inc. This book describes the complexities of DNA and molecular bases for genetic disorders.

CHAPTER 3

Development and Birth Defects

Chapter Outline

Objectives

After reading this chapter you should be able to

Define the term congenital defect.

Describe the frequency of birth defects.

Define the terms karyotype, genotype, phenotype, and embryology.

Understand the principal stages of human prenatal development.

Describe the formation of the genitalia.

List examples of gonadal dysgenesis.

List the three primary germ layers and some adult tissues derived from them.

Know the fetal ages at which most organs are formed and when development is advanced sufficiently to permit extrauterine life.

Define the term mutant.

Define the terms monosomy, trisomy, and teratogenesis.

List three groups of etiologic agents of birth defects.

Describe when and what birth defects occur from rubella infection.

Describe the defect in development resulting from cytomegalovirus or toxoplasmosis infection.

Define the term abortion and its frequency of occurrence.

Define the term prematurity.

Know which single organ is most critical for extrauterine survival.

Describe mechanisms responsible for birth defects.

List the common birth defects in descending order of frequency.

Define and describe spina bifida.

Compare anencephaly and microcephaly.

List two reasons for developing hydrocephalus.

Compare cleft lip and cleft palate in terms of etiology.

Define the term tracheoesophageal fistula.

Define the term atresia.

List common birth defects of the urogenital system.

Describe four cardiac birth defects.

List the common skeletal abnormalities.

Describe techniques used for the antenatal detection of birth defects.

Understand how an amniocentesis is performed.

List information obtainable from an amniocentesis.

Discuss indications for doing an amniocentesis.

Describe the value of α-fetoprotein for detection of birth defects.

Introduction

The genes of two persons blend together when a sperm unites with an egg. Within the short period of eight weeks, organs form from the fertilized egg. Following differentiation into organs, rapid growth occurs and, eventually, birth ensues. The baby must be equipped to survive the transition from an intrauterine fluid-filled environment to an extrauterine gaseous environment. The gaseous environment is far more dangerous with its infectious agents, pollutants, and other hostile elements. This chapter first summarizes normal development and then considers the etiology of abnormal development and mechanisms responsible for birth defects.*

Major inborn errors of development occur in approximately 2% of all newborn infants. These are termed *congenital*, meaning the disease is present at birth. Congenital diseases can result from a variety of causes including mutation (an error in genes) or from in utero influences. Most of us have one or more minor birth defects that have trivial or no significance. For example, approximately 10% of all humans have a minor malformation in the genitourinary tract. More commonly, congenital malformations can cause disease with loss of function and well-being.

Approximately 0.6% of all individuals have some abnormality in their chromosomes that is discernible by studying their chromosome number and

---

* The National Foundation, a research organization devoted to the prevention of birth defects, defines a birth defect as an abnormality of structure, function or metabolism, whether genetically determined or a result of environmental interference during embryonic or fetal life. A congenital defect may cause disease from the time of conception through birth or later in life.

appearance, or *karyotype*. The normal karyotype consists of a total of 46 chromosomes, including two sex chromosomes and 22 autosomes (see Chapter 9, Inherited Disorders). Thousands of individual genes are bound together in double strands of DNA and form the chromosomes. The genes are so small that they cannot be seen even with electron microscopy. The genetic makeup, or *genotype*, determines the many genetic expressions, or *phenotypes*, that provide individuality, such as blue or brown eyes.

Prevention of malformations concerns all of us. Health workers who often work with persons born with malformations include physical, occupational, and speech therapists; public health nurses; maternal nurse practitioners; obstetricians; pediatricians; geneticists; and neonatalogists. (Neonatalogists specialize solely in problems of newborn infants.)

Localized malformations usually result from the inheritance of several minor gene defects together with exposure of the fetus to certain environmental factors. Thus genetic and environmental factors cause most of the common malformations including cardiac abnormalities, cleft lip and palate, and clubfoot deformities.

Within the past two decades, two etiologic agents of birth defects have been identified—the drug thalidomide, which has been identified as a cause of birth defects and the infectious disease rubella (German measles). Rubella has so often caused severe abnormalities in development that when it occurs during early pregnancy, infection justifies abortion. The consequences of rubella infection in pregnant women have moved scientists to develop a vaccine that is given to girls to prevent future rubella during pregnancy. Fortunately, a few malformations previously lethal or disabling, particularly heart malformations, are now treated surgically. In spite of these advances, infant death due to malformations remains the leading cause of death in the first 2 years of life.

Later in the chapter, consideration will be given to the diagnosis of birth defects in utero as well as some efforts being used to surgically correct and to rehabilitate persons with malformations.

Normal Development

Embryology is the study of processes and mechanisms that transform the fertilized egg into a new individual. Embryologic development is directed (programmed) by genetic mechanisms that mold and form a person in a characteristic fashion. Survival of the fertilized egg, its implantation in the endometrial lining of the uterus, and the adaptation of the mother to the fetus are possible because maternal hormones, such as estrogen and progesterone, govern the formation and fertilization of the egg, implantation of the embryo in the uterus, and suppression of the mother's immunity to the embryo. Prevention of rejection of the embryo by maternal immune responses is necessary because the embryo is foreign material to the mother.

The term *conceptus* refers to the embryo (or fetus) and membranes; in total they are called the products of conception. Figure 3-1 summarizes the significant stages of human prenatal development.*

Development of Reproductive Organs

As can be seen in Figure 3-2, genital development occurs from a sexually indifferent or neuter gonad. The neuter gonad can become either a male or female sex organ; potentially all human embryos are bisexual. At the neuter stage, two pairs of ducts, the wolffian and müllerian ducts form the internal genitalia. In males, the müllerian ducts become inhibited by estrogen in females. Concurrently, the cortex (outer portion) of the neuter gonad becomes differentiated or changed into the ovary, whereas the medulla (inner portion) of the neuter gonad becomes differentiated into the testes.

The sex of the fetus is not distinguishable by microscopic examination of the gonad until the seventh week following conception; sex becomes distinguishable externally at about twelve weeks.

Gonadal differentiation into testes or ovaries commences during the fifth week under the influ-

*A more thorough presentation is found in Moore, K. L. 1974. *Before we are born: basic embryology and birth defects*. Philadelphia: W. B. Saunders Company.

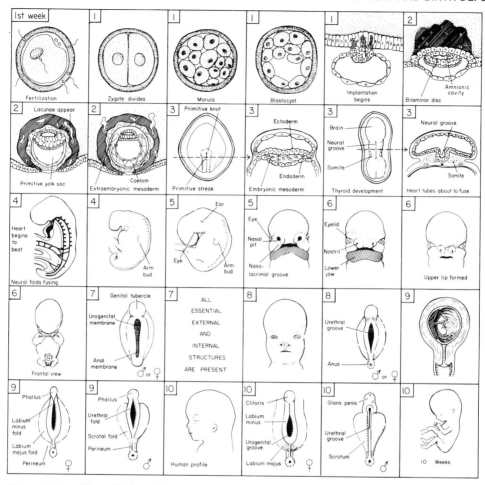

Figure 3-1   *Time table of human embryologic development. Shown are the major stages of development of the human embryo (to eight weeks) and fetus (eight weeks to birth). (The drawings are modifications of illustrations by Glen Reid in Moore, K. L. 1977. The developing human. Clinically oriented embryology, ed. 2. Philadelphia: W. B. Saunders Company.)*

ence of the sex chromosomes. A female has XX sex chromosomes and 44 autosomes. The X chromosome and estrogens (female hormones) cause the cortex (outer part) of the neuter gonad to form an ovary. A male embryo has XY sex chromosomes and 44 autosomes. Under the impact of the Y chromosome and androgens (male hormones), the medulla (inner part) differentiates into a testis while the cortex regresses. Illustrated in Figures 3-3 and 3-4 are a testis and an ovary.

Gonadal Dysgenesis

Because the fetus can potentially develop into a man or a woman, errors in development of the sex organs (gonadal dysgenesis) can occur. Disorders of sexual development are divisible into three main types—infertility without ambiguity in genital development, infertility with ambiguity in genital development, and ambiguity without infertility. (Ambiguity is the lack of sexual differentiation.)

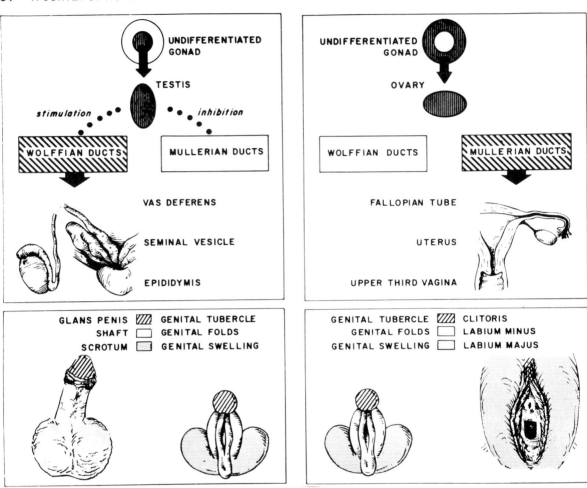

Figure 3-2 *Outline of genital development in the male and female. Note that the gonadal development occurs from a common indifferent (neuter) gonad. The internal genitalia develop from separate primitive structures present in both sexes (wolffian ducts and müllerian ducts). The external genitalia develop in a continuous transformation from common sources. (Reprinted by permission from the* New England Journal of Medicine 277, *No. 7).*

The first type, infertility without genital ambiguity, encompasses individuals with an abnormal number of X chromosomes. *Klinefelter's syndrome* is an example in which a person has 44 autosomes and XXY sex chromosomes. The extra X chromosome causes the person to have a slender build, breast enlargement (gynecomastia), and extremely small testes, which measure less than 1.5 cm in length (normal being 4 cm).

Another gonadal dysgenic disorder, *Turner's syndrome,* results from a lack of an X chromosome. The karyotype of a person with Turner's syndrome is 44 autosomes, and they are X0. Persons with Turner's syndrome have a characteristic appearance (phenotype) of short stature, lack of menses, and breast development, as well as abnormalities of the aorta and gonads. The gonads remain undifferentiated (Fig. 3-5). Persons with Klinefelter's or Turner's syndromes are usually infertile.

Mixed gonadal dysgenesis constitutes the second group of persons who have infertility and ambiguity of sex. Within this classification, an individual may have true hermaphroditism—possess gonads of both sexes. Alternatively, an undif-

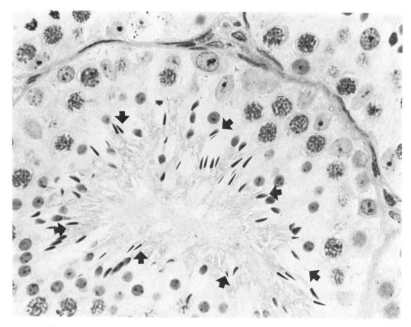

Figure 3-3   *Photomicrograph of normal testis showing a cross section of a tubule. Primitive germ cells located at the periphery progressively mature towards the center to form spermatozoa* (arrow).

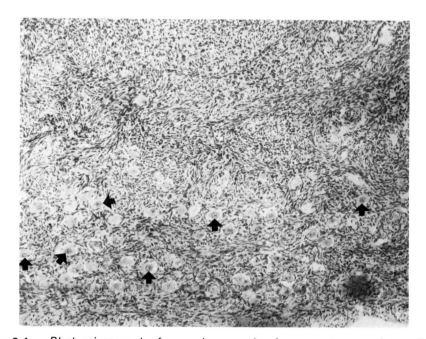

Figure 3-4   *Photomicrograph of normal ovary, showing numerous ova* (arrows) *embedded in stromal cells. Approximately 400,000 eggs are normally present at birth. Thus a woman has a great storehouse of eggs for reproduction.*

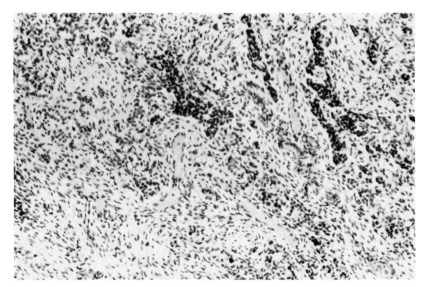

Figure 3-5 *Photomicrograph of undifferentiated fibrous ovary seen in Turner's syndrome. No eggs are seen in this XO individual.*

ferentiated ovary may develop on one side and a testis on the other side.

Included in the classification of ambiguity without infertility is the condition of dysgenic male pseudohermaphroditism. This occurs either when a person has two abnormally developed testes or when a person is a dysgenetic male pseudohermaphrodite.

Germ Cells

During spermatogenesis and oogenesis, sex cells divide and form germ cells (spermatozoa or ova, Figs. 3-3 and 3-4) each of which contain 23 chromosomes. Germ cells unite at conception (fertilization) to restore the individual to the normal 46 chromosome content (see Chapter 2).

The menstrual cycle of a woman is carefully orchestrated to prepare the endometrial lining of her uterus to receive the embryo. Actual fertilization, however, occurs while the egg is still within the uterine tube.

Fertilization

Fertilization occurs in the dilated portion of the uterine tube. Only one sperm can penetrate the egg; after fertilization occurs, the egg stiffens to prevent further penetration. Fertilization restores the chromosomal number to 46, determines the sex, and provides all the genetic information the person will ever have. The fertilized egg is then termed a zygote.

Cleavage

As the zygote passes down the uterine tube, it undergoes cleavage (cellular division) into smaller and smaller cells called *blastomeres* (Fig. 3-1). Morula (a ball) forms after about three days and enters the uterus. A cavity forms in the morula causing its conversion to a blastocyst. Next, placental trophoblastic cells appear; these provide a link with the mother by invading the uterine endometrium. The placenta provides nutrition and transfers carbon dioxide and oxygen between the mother and fetus. One week after conception the blastocyst is superficially implanted in the uterus and is then dependent on the mother for nutrition.

Formation of the Embryo

During the time placental trophoblastic tissue is developing, primitive connective tissue arises from the outside of the embryo from tissue termed mesoderm. As the mesoderm grows inward, the size of the blastocyst cavity reduces. A slitlike amniotic cavity appears between the placental trophoblast and the inner cell mass. The amniotic cavity fills with amniotic fluid, which bathes the fetus; this amniotic fluid is derived from secretion of fluid from the placenta and from urine produced by the fetus. The inner cell mass then differentiates into two layers—the embryonic ectoderm and entoderm. Mesoderm penetrates between the ectoderm and the entoderm to complete the differentiation into an embryo containing three primary germ layers. Gradually these layers differentiate into all of the tissues and organs of the body (Fig. 3-6).

After the three germ layers form, the midline of the embryo differentiates. The head portion devel-

ops first. The primitive streak, the forerunner of the brain and spinal cord, forms from ectoderm in the midline of the embryo during the third week.

Meanwhile, the mesoderm forms supporting structures—the vertebral column and the vault of the skull. These fuse across the midline of the back to protect the central nervous system. Forming laterally to the neural tube are neural crest cells, which migrate into the skin to form melanin pigment.

Muscles arise from somites (primitive blocks of mesoderm) situated laterally to the neural tube. One special block of mesoderm tissue gives rise to the heart.

Blood vessels appear initially in the yolk sac and later within all parts of the embryo. Vascular channels arise from aggregates (blood islands) of me-

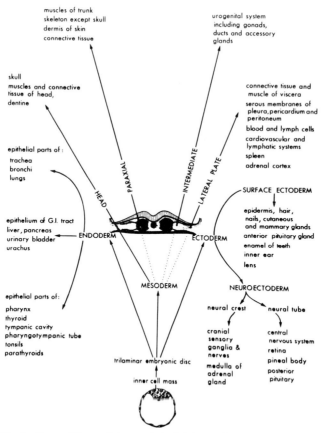

Figure 3-6   *Illustration of the origin and derivitives of the three primary germ layers. (Moore, K. L. 1977.* The developing human. Clinically oriented embryology, *ed. 2. Philadelphia: W. B. Saunders Company.)*

soderm, which become lined by endothelium. The islands unite to form a primitive cardiovascular system. At the end of the third week, the heart is composed of a pair of tubes that then fuse. The heart begins to beat during the fourth week.

During the ensuing fourth to seventh weeks, rapid embryonic development and differentiation of organs occurs. Exposure of an embryo to certain agents such as drugs, viruses, or radiation during this period of organ development may cause major birth defects.

Major organ systems are established by the end of the embryonic period. Beyond this time (eighth week) the conceptus is less vulnerable to teratogenic (deforming) agents.

The Fetal Period

Between the eighth week following conception and birth, the conceptus is called a fetus, signifying it has become a recognizable human being. The fetal period is concerned chiefly with growth and maturation of tissues and organs that have formed in the embryonic period. A few new structures appear during the fetal period.

At about the eighth week, longitudinal and transverse folding of the fetus converts the flat trilayer embryonic disk into a C-shaped cylinder. A primitive gut, gastrointestinal tract, forms from the back portion of the yolk sac, and the liver and pancreas grow out from the gut as buds. The major theme of this fetal period is rapid growth in size. Marked growth occurs between weeks 12 and 16.

The fetus is generally incapable of sustaining life outside the uterus before week 24. This is due chiefly to immaturity of the lungs. Before 24 to 26 weeks, the lungs consist of thick glands that do not transmit air (Fig. 3-7). Thus the age of *viability* (life) is regarded as being about 24 weeks. Prior to 24 weeks, the fetus is generally nonviable; it cannot sustain extrauterine life because its lungs are immature.

The fetus is far less vulnerable to the teratogenic effects of drugs, viruses, and radiation than is the embryo. Nevertheless, these agents can interfere with the growth and development of certain organs, especially the brain.

Birth Defects

Two in 100 of all live-born infants have some form of congenital defect. Stillbirth (a fetus born dead), prematurity, and immaturity are associated with higher incidences of congenital malformations. In the United States approximately 22,000 newborn deaths occur yearly due to congenital malformations.

Birth defects are usually localized to a specific anatomical area. Many localized malformations are due to a single *mutant* (altered) gene; these are considered inborn errors of embryogenesis. Other malformations can be widespread, involving two or more organ systems. Many birth defects can be cured only with surgery.

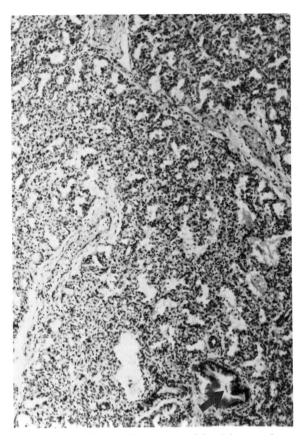

Figure 3-7 *Photomicrograph of fetal lungs at approximately 20 weeks gestation. Note the absence of large air sacs. Instead, primitive glandlike solid tissue is seen. A bronchus is shown (arrow).*

The two major groups of factors associated with congenital malformations are *genetic factors* and *environmental factors*. Genetic factors include abnormalities in chromosome number or structure and mutant genes. Environmental factors include infectious agents, chemicals, and radiation. Most common malformations are thought to result from an interaction between genetic and environmental factors.*

Chromosomal Abnormalities

Genetic abnormalities can arise from a decrease in or excessive number of chromosomes, changes in a part of a chromosome, and/or a mutation of one gene.

Approximately 0.6% of live-born infants have a noteworthy *chromosomal* abnormality, such as having an extra chromosome. About 70% of chromosomal abnormalities are subtle and are, therefore, not detectable on routine physical examination of the patient. Many genetic abnormalities cause inborn errors of metabolism, errors in the biochemical function of cells. A metabolic error, usually an enzyme deficiency, arises from a *mutant gene*. Metabolic error results in an abnormality in amino acid metabolism or accumulation of certain substances (storage disease) in various tissues (see Chapter 9, Inherited Disorders). More than 100 different enzyme deficiencies have resulted from mutant genes.

McKusick's catalog of human genetic disorders includes nearly 2100 other inherited abnormalities. Many of the 2100 genetic defects are trivial, others significantly alter an individual's well-being, and some are lethal.

Monosomy   Monosomy occurs from an absence of an entire chromosome. Embryos missing an autosome frequently die; monosomy of an autosome is extremely rare in living persons. In contrast, monosomy of sex chromosomes is more frequent. Turner's syndrome previously mentioned, occurs when only one X chromosome is present. About 97% of embryos lacking an X chromosome die, the remaining 3% survive and have Turner's syndrome.

*Most diseases arise on an ecogenetic basis, that is, from an interaction between genetic and environmental factors.

Trisomy   Trisomy is more common than monosomy. Rather than having a pair of chromosomes, the individual with trisomy has an extra chromosome. Trisomy arises from an unequal separation of daughter cells during oogenesis or spermatogenesis, giving a germ cell with 24 instead of 23 chromosomes.

Best known among the trisomies is Down's syndrome, caused by an extra autosome chromosome, number 21. Numerous birth defects in the heart and other vital organs occur and the person generally has low intelligence as well as characteristic facial features. Shown in Figure 3-8 is an infant with trisomy 13 with multiple birth defects.

Malformations From Mutant Genes   About 12% of all congenital malformations are recognized as being caused by mutations. These malformations are inherited according to mendelian laws (see Chapter 9). The possibilities of genetic counseling and the detection of certain genetic diseases prior to birth have captured the attention of both lay and medical persons. For those parents who require genetic counseling, reasonable predictions can be given of the probability of a malformation occurring in their future offspring.

Teratogenesis   Teratology is the science devoted to the diagnosis, treatment, and prevention of malformations. Cellular injury in the embryo causes developmental malformations. Teratogenesis then is the process of development of birth defects. Embryogenesis is a precisely controlled process involving cell division, growth, cell death, differentiation or specialization of cells to form specific specialized functions, and movement of cells to form organs. These phenomena occur in a chronologic order controlled by the activity of genes and the environment. Both the genes or environment may alter the normal development of the fetus, giving rise to birth defects. Mechanisms responsible for birth defects are shown in Table 3-1.

Etiology of Malformations

The three leading groups of etiologic agents responsible for birth defects are *maternal infection,*

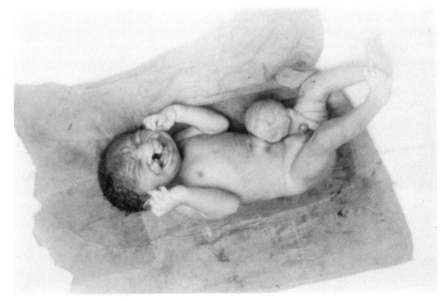

Figure 3-8   *Child with trisomy 13, showing cleft lip and palate and large umbilical hernia.*

Table 3-1
Mechanisms Responsible for Congenital Malformations

Mechanism	Examples
Too little growth	Agenesis (of kidney, brain, etc.)
Too little resorption	Double aortic arch
Failure to close	Spina bifida and cleft palate
Failure to open	Imperforate anus
Failure to unite	Double uterus
Failure to divide	Syndactyly (fusion of fingers)
Failure to divide properly	Polydactyly (extra fingers) and heart defects
Failure to differentiate properly	Achondroplastic dwarfs
Failure to locate properly	Ectopic tissue
Overgrowth of tissue or structure	Pyloric stenosis

drugs, and *physical agents*, especially irradiation. Shown in Table 3-2 are some common teratogenic agents. Inspection of the table reveals that many of the agents responsible for congenital malformations can be prevented. For example, with proper prenatal care, most infectious agents and drugs will be eliminated as sources of birth defects.

Rubella-induced Malformations   Although vaccination is available against rubella (German measles) some women remain unvaccinated. About 15% to 20% of the infants born of women with rubella infection during the first one-third of pregnancy (first trimester) have malformations. In the infected fetus, a triad usually occurs. This consists of (1) cataract (opacification of lens of the eye), (2) cardiac malformations, and (3) deafness.

The earlier in pregnancy that the infection occurs, the greater the danger there is to the embryo. Virtually *all* infants infected by rubella during the first five weeks following fertilization have malformations; development of the eye, ear, heart, and brain are most easily damaged during this period. In contrast, malformations are much less common when rubella infection occurs during the second and third trimesters of pregnancy. Less severe functional defects of the central nervous system and ears result when rubella infections occur during the last half of pregnancy.

Cytomegalovirus-induced Malformations   Cytomegalovirus (CMV) is a herpes-type virus that can also cause malformations. Cytomegalovirus infection of the fetus that occurs in the second and third trimester often results in abnormalities of the brain, such as microcephaly and, in the eyes, microphthalmia. Calcification of the brain can also occur. A diagnosis is usually made by examining the cellular sediment of a newborn's urine. Finding cytomegaloviral inclusions within renal tubule cells, which are shed into the urine, confirms the diagnosis. CMV infection is the most common teratogenic infection occurring in pregnant women. Recent studies reveal that children infected with CMV in utero have lower intelligence quotients than noninfected children.

Toxoplasmosis-induced Malformations   *Toxoplasma gondii*, a protozoan, can infect the fetus when the pregnant mother eats raw or poorly cooked meat or comes in contact with an infected animal. I recall diagnosing the disease in an unfortunate baby whose mother admitted to having eaten raw sirloin steak while pregnant. The child had toxoplasmosis and failed to form a brain; when a flashlight was directed against its head, light was transmitted through the skull, and the empty skull glowed as a pink balloon. The infant died of pneumonia five months later. Other common malformations induced by toxoplasmosis are microcephaly, microphthalmia, and hydrocephaly (water on the brain).

Other Infection-induced Malformations   Other infectious agents may induce malformations. One example, chickenpox (varicella) occurring in a

Table 3-2
Teratogenic Agents

Physical agents—radiation, hypoxia, excessive carbon dioxide, and mechanical trauma
Maternal infection—(TORCH complex) toxoplasmosis, other agents, rubella, cytomegalovirus, and herpes simplex
Hormones—sex and corticosteroids
Vitamin deficiencies—riboflavin, niacin, folic acid, and vitamin E
Chemotherapy drugs—used for treating malignancies
Antibiotics—mitomycin, dactinomycin, and puromycin (used as chemotherapy agent)
Tranquilizers—thalidomide, diazepam (Valium), and chlordiazepoxide HCl (Librium)

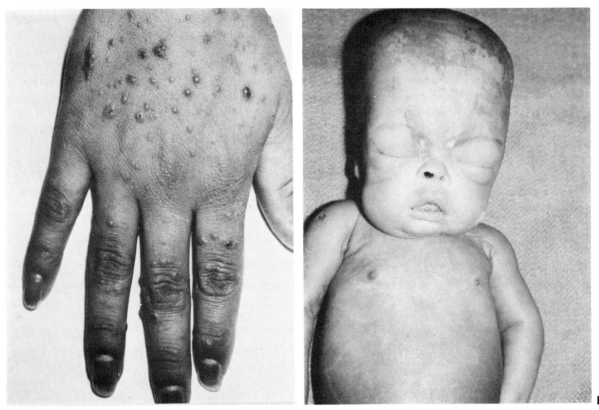

Figure 3-9 **A,** *Rash of chickenpox (varicella) occurring in a pregnant woman.* **B,** *Hydrocephalus (water on the brain) occuring in the child born of the infected mother. Hydrocephalus occurred because the flow of cerebrospinal fluid was obstructed by inflammation in the brain.*

pregnant woman, is seen in Figure 3-9. The woman died of widespread chickenpox shortly after childbirth. Her baby daughter lived for approximately two months but then developed blocked drainage of cerebrospinal fluid. The infant's head swelled with fluid, hydrocephalus ensued, and the girl died two months later from infection of the brain (encephalitis) and hydrocephalus.

Irradiation Radiation is a potent teratogen. In pregnant women who have had malignancies, X-ray treatment has caused microcephaly, mental retardation, and malformations of the child's skeleton. No definitive proof is available, however, that congenital malformations have been caused by the low doses of radiation used in diagnostic X-rays. Nonetheless, avoidance of X-rays during the first trimester is an intelligent precaution.

Genetic Factors Knowledge of a genetic basis of certain malformations enables the prediction of future malformations in additional offspring. After the birth of one malformed child, the frequency of malformations in subsequent offspring is increased about tenfold. For example, the usual frequency of cardiac malformation in the general population is 1 in 500, but a sibling of an affected child has a 1 in 50 chance of developing a similar malformation. Correspondingly, malformations of the central nervous system occur in 1 in 200 infants; the chances of this is increased to 1 in 20 for a sibling of one such affected child.

Drugs Such drugs as thalidomide, cortisone, chemotherapeutic drugs used against malignancies, alcohol, anticonvulsants, and anticoagulants have been implicated in malformations. Women who work in operating rooms and hence are exposed to anesthetics give birth to excessive numbers of malformed babies.

Closely linked to malformations are spontaneous abortions. Malformed fetuses are often spontaneously aborted. This event may be nature's way of ridding humankind of unfortunate, unfit persons.

Abortion   Abortion is defined as the expulsion of a fetus from the uterus prior to the period of viability—generally considered to be about 24 weeks. Often mutagenic or teratogenic agents are responsible for bringing on an abortion. Approximately 10% to 15% of all pregnancies end as spontaneous abortions before 20 weeks of gestation, the period of embryonic development; whereas only 1.5% of pregnancies abort after 20 weeks of gestation. Many aborted fetuses are malformed and show chromosomal abnormalities.

The incidence of chromosomal abnormalities is approximately 20% to 25% in those spontaneous abortions that occur to the fifth month of pregnancy. Chromosomal abnormalities, for instance, cause Down's and Turner's syndromes, and approximately 97% of fetuses with Turner's syndrome and 65% of fetuses with Down's syndrome are spontaneously aborted.

Abortions and malformations are more common with increasing maternal age. Well known is the occurrence of Down's syndrome in pregnant women who are beyond 35 years of age. The syndrome occurs thirtyfold more in offspring of a 40-year-old woman than in that of a 20-year-old woman. The reason for the genetic mistake is not known, although some suggest that older women may have "tired eggs" and old men, "tired spermatozoa."

Local environmental disturbances, for example, an inadequate blood supply or an incompetent cervix, may also cause a fetus to die.

Prematurity   Prematurity depends on three findings—length of gestation, birth weight, and infant body length. Newborns are expected to weigh greater than 2500 gm (5 lb 8 oz) at birth or they are considered premature; mortality rates are higher for infants weighing less than 2500 gm. Nevertheless, a few fetuses of less than 500 gm have survived

in neonatal intensive care nurseries. Generally, the longer the gestation period, the greater the chance of survival; normally 30 to 32 weeks of gestation are the lower limits to infant survival.

Prematurity is the major factor responsible for death during the initial 2 months of life. The primary cause of death is immaturity of lungs (Fig. 3-7). Prevention of premature births and better clinical care for infants born prematurely have decreased the frequency of neonatal deaths.

Legally, an abortion may be performed until week 24 of gestation. In recent years, the salvaging of premature infants—of less than 24 weeks of gestation—has raised significant religious, ethical, and medical-legal issues as to whether the definition of age of viability should not be extended downward.*

Common Malformations

Approximately 14% of fetuses who die in utero, 26% who die during delivery, and 30% of infants who die during the first 30 days of life have severe malformations. Again, the overall incidence of malformations in *all* newborns is about 2%.

Commonly malformed are the heart, neural tube, face, gastrointestinal tract, and skeleton. In most instances, only a single system is involved. Shown in Table 3-3 are the relative frequencies and sex ratios of common major congenital malformations.

Central Nervous System (neural tube)   Common congenital malformations of the brain include microcephaly; mental retardation; motor, speech and learning deficits; anencephaly; hydrocephalus; and meningomyelocele. Meningomyelocele is a midline bony birth defect permitting meninges and neural tissue to be exposed to the outside.

Most major congenital malformations of the central nervous system (CNS, which includes the brain and spinal cord) result from defective formation of the neural tube. This occurs usually at the end of the first month of gestation. Abnormalities may be

---

*A physician in Boston was convicted in 1975 of manslaughter for aborting a baby (fetus?) of approximately 24 weeks gestation. The jury ruled the conceptus was a baby (not a fetus) and that the obstetrician took the life of the baby. The conviction was reversed on appeal.

limited to the CNS, or they may involve overlying tissues, especially bone.

As with malformations of other organs, CNS defects can be caused by genetic or environmental factors. Infectious diseases are the most frequent cause of malformations of the CNS (Table 3-1). Severe abnormalities of the CNS are incompatible with life. Minor CNS malformations can cause functional disabilities in speech, control of muscles, and behavior.

Spina Bifida   Failure of fusion of the neural tube and the bones that encase the central nervous system (the skull and vertebral column, for example) can result in major neural deficits. The term spina bifida refers to a defect in the vertebral column (Fig. 3-10). Spina bifida occurs most commonly in the lower thoracic, lumbar, and sacral regions.

Spina bifida can be obvious or hidden (occult). The only evidence of an occult spinal malformation is a tuft of hair over the site. On X-ray examination, the vertebral defect is seen. Fortunately, the occult form of spina bifida seldom causes problems.

When a portion of the spinal cord and meninges protrude through the defective vertebrae, the condition is called spina bifida with *meningomyelocele*. When the brain protrudes through a bony defect in the skull, the condition is called *meningoencephalocele*.

The incidence of meningomyelocele is slightly more than 1 in 1000 live births. The extent of neurologic impairment the child has depends on the position and extent of the lesion. Usually a loss of sensation (anesthesia) and muscular deficit results from the defect.

Anencephaly   Anencephaly literally means "without a brain." Anencephaly occurs as commonly as meningomyelocele, 1 per 1000 live births. Extrauterine life is impossible for anencephalic individuals because they do not have a brain. Their heart, lungs, and other organs cannot properly function; and shortly after birth, they die. Anencephaly results from a failure of the cranial neural folds to develop, fuse, and form the front portion of the brain.

Microcephaly   Microcephaly is a relatively uncommon condition in which the cranium is small and the face has a normal size. Such infants usually have marked mental retardation (Fig. 3-11).

Hydrocephalus   Hydrocephalus is characterized by an accumulation of cerebrospinal fluid in the brain under increased pressure (Fig. 3-9). Hydrocephalus may result from an *overproduction* of cerebrospinal fluid, from *failure of resorption* of the fluid, or from *obstruction* of fluid flow. Hydrocephalus can be associated with spina bifida or it can occur alone. It is often not obvious at birth but will be when subsequent expansion of the head occurs. The cerebral cortex becomes progressively thinner, and mental retardation usually ensues. However, if a shunt that bypasses the site obstruction is inserted by a neurosurgeon, the fluid drains releasing the pressure.

Mental Retardation   Mental retardation can result from prenatal infection, birth trauma, or a variety of inherited conditions. The brain is damaged by infections, lack of oxygen in utero or during birth,

Table 3-3
Frequency and Sex Ratio of Common Major Congenital Malformations*

Malformations	Frequency per 1000 total births	Sex ratio (male to female)
Spina bifida	2.5	0.6
Anencephaly	2.0	0.3
Congenital heart defects	6.0	1.0
Pyloric stenosis	3.0	4.0
Cleft lip (and/or cleft palate)	1.0	1.8
Congenital dislocation of hip	1.0	0.1

*From Carter, C. O. 1976. *Br. Med. Bull.* 32:21.

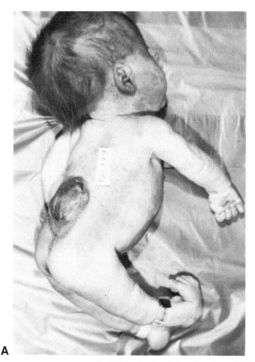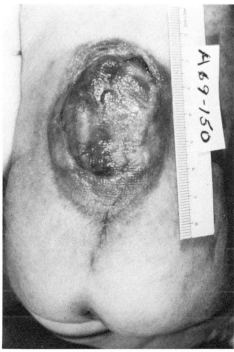

A   B

Figure 3-10   **A,** *This infant had spina bifida and clubfeet.* **B,** *Close-up view of spina bifida with meningomyelocele in the lumbar region. Note the nerve involvement affecting the lower extremities. (Courtesy Dr. A. C. Templeton).*

or injury during birth. Inherited abnormalities usually result in an accumulation of fatty compounds, such as sphingomyelin.

Women who have one child with a central nervous system defect have a 5% chance of giving birth to a second child with the same defect. In about 60% of such cases, the second child will be affected with a defect similar to the first sibling. For parents who have had two affected children, the chance of recurrence in future pregnancies is between 10% and 25%.

Cleft Lip and Palate   Cleft lip, and malformation of the upper lip with or without cleft palate, occurs in about 1 in 900 births (Fig. 3-12). The defect may be located on one or both sides of the upper lip. It may be simply a small notch in the upper lip or a complete division of the lip and maxilla. The location of these various defects depends on when during development of the face the lesion occurs. Embryologically and etiologically, cleft lip and cleft palate are distinct malformations that

originate at different times during embryogenesis and involve different developmental processes.

Cleft palate, with or without cleft lip, occurs less commonly, 1 in 25,000 births. The cleft may be unilateral or bilateral and may or may not extend through the hard and soft palates.

The embryologic basis of cleft palate is a failure of the mesodermal masses of the maxilla to fuse in the midline. With respect to the failure of fusion of the bone in the midline, cleft palate is comparable to spina bifida.

Cleft lip and cleft palate have mixed genetic and environmental etiologies. A sibling of a child with cleft palate has an increased risk of having a cleft palate but no increased risk of having a cleft lip.

Respiratory Tract   *Tracheoesophageal fistula* is an abnormal passage connecting the trachea and esophagus. It occurs in approximately 1 in 2500 births (Fig. 3-13). This condition results from incomplete division of the primitive foregut into the respiratory and digestive tracts during the fourth

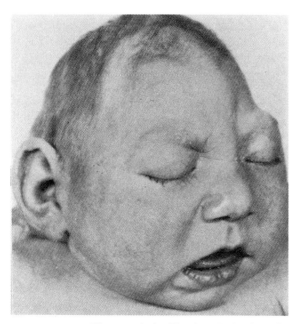

Figure 3-11   *Microcephaly. The head of this child is extremely small resulting from premature fusion of the cranial bones. (From Laurence, K. M. and Weeks, R. 1971. Abnormalities of the central nervous system. In A. P. Norman, ed. Congenital abnormalities in infancy, ed. 2. Blackwell Scientific Publications, Ltd.)*

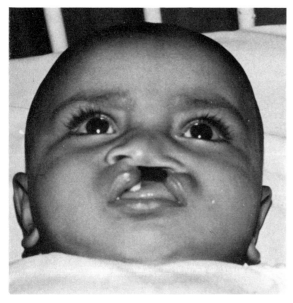

Figure 3-12   *Child with cleft lip and cleft palate. The cleft lip and palate is exceptionally wide.*

and fifth weeks of gestation. Following birth, when the infant is fed, choking and blueness (cyanosis) ensues; milk flows through the fistula into the lungs rather than into the stomach.

Digestive Tract   The term *atresia* is used to denote the failure of any portion of the gastrointestinal tract to form a channel for the passage of food. It occurs throughout the intestinal tract, especially in the esophagus, small intestine, and biliary tract. One extreme form of atresia is failure to form an anus; this is called *imperforate anus*.

Narrowing of the outlet of the stomach to the duodenum results when the muscular mass surrounding the pylorus enlarges; this produces pyloric stenosis or a narrowing of the distal (pylorus) end of the stomach (Fig. 3-14). This abnormality affects approximately 1 in 200 newborn boys and 1 in 1000 girls. Vomiting following feeding of the infant is a symptom of pyloric stenosis and palpation of the baby's abdomen reveals an olive-sized mass caused by the muscular band of the pylorus.

Additional defects of the gastrointestinal tract include faulty rotation of the gut; herniation (displacement of a portion of the intestine through the abdominal wall or diaphragm), and reduplication of a portion of the tract. Very occasionally primitive embryologic structures persist. For example, the cloaca, a common orifice for the urinary and digestive tracts, may remain.

Urogenital Tract   A congenital abnormality of the urogenital tract is very common—one of ten persons has one. Most, however, are not easily recognizable. Malformations include variations in supply of blood, abnormal position of kidneys or ureters, duplication, or failure of formation of structures. Duplications of ureters are relatively common; they cause a problem only when they obstruct the flow of urine, permitting urinary tract infections to occur.

Agenesis denotes a failure of formation; and renal agenesis on one side of the body is relatively common. Rather notorious is the discovery that, following removal of one diseased kidney, a kidney is congenitally missing on the other side.

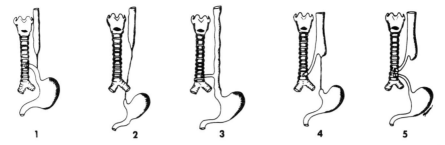

Figure 3-13   *Five types of esophageal atresia with or without tracheoesophageal fistula. (From Kissane, J. M. 1975.* Pathology of infancy and childhood, *ed. 2. St. Louis: The C. V. Mosby Co.)*

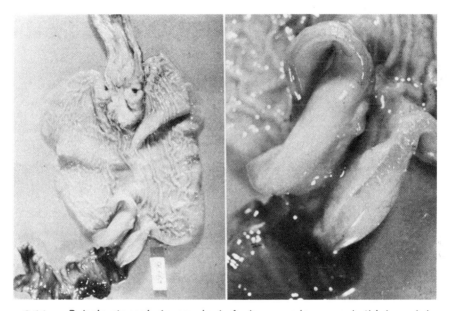

Figure 3-14   *Pyloric stenosis (narrowing). A close-up view reveals thickened, hypertrophied muscular layer. (From Kissane, J. M. 1975.* Pathology of infancy and childhood, *ed. 2. St. Louis: The C. V. Mosby Co.)*

Genitalia   Numerous malformations can occur in male and female genitalia. In the penis, a malpositioning of the opening of the urinary tract, termed *hypospadia*, is a common defect which arises when the urethra fails to fuse in the midline; the urinary stream flows from the base of the penis. In addition, the abdominal wall and urinary bladder can also fail to fuse in the midline and may protrude through the abdominal wall.

The uterus is formed from a fusion of paired müllerian ducts. If the fusion does not occur properly, duplication of the uterus can occur. The du-

plication may be complete or incomplete; nevertheless, reproduction is impaired since the uterus does not properly accommodate the fetus.

Cardiac Malformations   Cardiac and great vessel development are complex; therefore, congenital heart malformations are relatively common. Approximately 0.7% of live births and 2.7% of stillbirths show cardiac abnormalities.

The heart consists of four chambers. Blood normally flows from the right atrium → right ventricle → lungs → left atrium → left ventricle and out

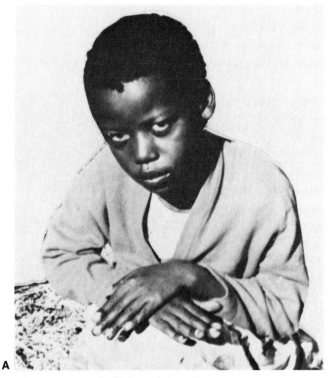
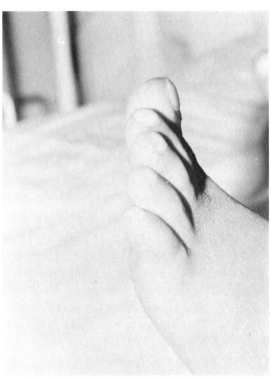

A   B

Figure 3-15   **A,** *This child had a severe cyanotic cardiac defect. Note the crouched posture and the swelling of finger tips and toes into clublike configuration;* **B,** *note clubbing of the toes.*

the aorta. The heart is formed from a pair of tubes that fuse and then divide into four chambers when septa (partitions) form.

Individuals with cardiac abnormalities may suffer from inadequate oxygenation of the blood. This is termed *cyanotic congenital heart disease.* The cardiac defects cause blood to be shunted away from the lungs. Insufficient oxygenation and blueness of the blood occurs, and the individual develops shortness of breath, which can be progressive with time and is aggravated by exercise. A newborn blue at birth is called a "blue baby."

Children with cyanotic congenital heart disease appear dusky gray because the blood lacks oxygen (Fig. 3-15); these children often assume a characteristic sitting posture at rest and show clubbing of their fingers and toes. Cardiac defects can be heard with a stethoscope. They cause murmurs as blood rushes through the defect.

Ventricular septal defects occur most commonly of all cardiac defects. They are found in about 30%

of infants with congenital heart disease. A persistent open (or patent) ductus arteriosus connecting the aorta and the pulmonary artery accounts for 10% of congenital heart defects; six other lesions account for the remaining defects of the heart (Fig. 3-16). Fortunately, during the past 40 years, cardiac surgery has developed to the point where many cardiac malformations can be surgically corrected.

Septal Cardiac Defects   Partitions can fail to form between atria or ventricles; this causes a septal defect (a hole, for example). These defects are termed atrial septal defects or ventricular septal defects (Fig. 3-16, *B* and *C*). Ordinarily, ventricular septal defects are more devastating than atrial septal defects. Blood in the left ventricle is under high pressure, thus blood passes under great pressure into the right ventricle and damages the lungs. The size of the septal defect as well as location determine whether the individual will become symptomatic.

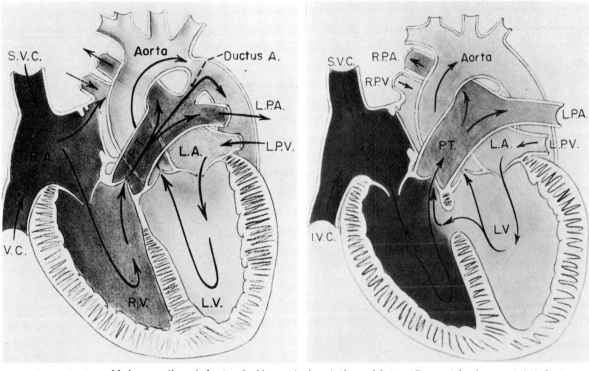

Figure 3-16   *Major cardiac defects.* **A,** *Normal circulation of fetus;* **B,** *ventricular septal defect.*

Defects of Great Arteries (Aorta and Pulmonary Arteries)   Defects in the great vessels consist chiefly of "persistence of the common truncus arteriosus." Persistence of the common trunk occurs when the septum that normally forms between the aorta and pulmonary arteries fails to form (Fig. 3-16, *C*). The result is a common aorta-pulmonary artery. The blood mixes and fails to become properly oxygenated.

Another significant defect is a complete transposition of the great arteries (Fig. 3-16, *D*). In typical cases the aorta lies in front of the pulmonary artery and arises from the right ventricle, rather than from the left ventricle. For newborn survival, a septal defect that permits an exchange of blood between the pulmonary and systemic circulations must also occur; otherwise heart failure and insufficient oxygenation of blood ensues.

Tetralogy of Fallot (Fig. 3-16, *E*) is a common cardiac abnormality consisting of the following four defects: (1) pulmonary stenosis (narrowing), (2) a ventricular septal defect, (3) an overriding aorta,

and (4) hypertrophy (thickening of the right ventricle). The tetralogy causes cyanosis (Fig. 3-15). In rare cases surgery corrects the tetralogy.

Skeletal Abnormalities   Previously mentioned were midline defects in fusion of bones, which can result in cleft palate and spina bifida. Other common skeletal abnormalities involve the hips and feet and give major problems in walking.

Clubfoot   Approximately 1% of children have a positional deformity of their feet at birth. Most of these deformities quickly correct themselves. Clubfoot is the general term used to describe abnormalities of the feet. Approximately 0.3% of individuals develop *talipes equinovarus*, wherein the foot turns inward and downward.

Dislocation of Hip   Dislocation of the hip occurs in about 1 in 1000 children. In this condition, the head of the femur is unstable and may slip from its epiphyseal plate. Instability of the hips at birth is

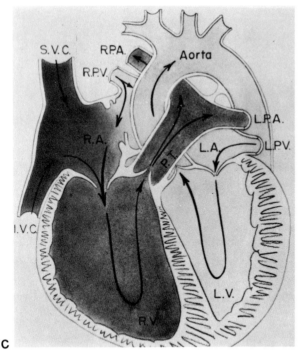

C

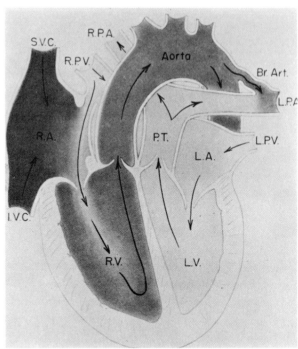

D

Figure 3-16 *C, atrial septal defect; D, transposition of the aorta and pulmonary artery.*

thought to be brought about during intrauterine molding of the bones, as are clubfoot abnormalities.

Prenatal Detection of Fetal Abnormalities

Anatomical fetal defects account for about 20% of all deaths in newborns. Prenatal diagnosis of severe defects with the consequent termination of pregnancy could reduce the suffering arising from these abnormalities in children. More importantly, prenatal diagnosis could potentially lead to the development of fetal intrauterine surgery to correct the defects before the organ is entirely developed. Moreover, diagnosis would enable the family and medical staff to anticipate the need for surgery following delivery. Finally, the information gained could be used for genetic counseling, which could eliminate the risk of future pregnancies if the individuals chose contraceptive measures.

The only means of preventing hereditary malformations is to diagnose the affected unborn fetus in utero. An antenatal diagnosis would help provide the option of a therapeutic abortion or carrying the conceptus to term. Several methods, including diagnosis from history and physical examination and the use of X-rays, fetoscopy, and amniocentesis, can be used for the diagnosis of malformations and genetic defects in the unborn fetus. The examination of cells obtained by drawing fluid (amniocentesis) from the amniotic sac surrounding the fetus can be studied to determine the sex of the baby and chromosome and biochemical abnormalities can be detected (Table 3-4).

Table 3-4
Indications for Prenatal Diagnosis by Amniocentesis

Maternal age over 40 years
A parent known to carry a chromosomal defect
Previous child with Down's syndrome (trisomy 21)
Mother with X-linked disease in family
Previous child with anencephaly or
  meningomyelocele
Assessment of fetal maturity

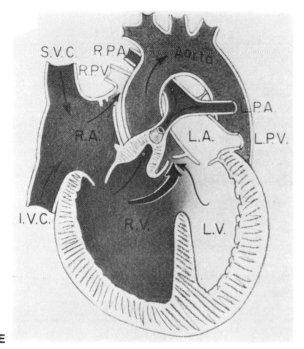

E

Figure 3-16 **E,** *tetralogy of Fallot. (From Moller, J. H., Amplatz, K., and Edwards, J. E. 1974. Congenital heart disease. Bethesda, Maryland: Universities Associated for Research and Education in Pathology, Inc.)*

History and Physical Examination The occurrence of a viral infection, especially rubella, the taking of drugs, or exposure to irradiation during pregnancy may forebode a possible malformed fetus. A history of prior malformations could also signal inherited defects. A physical examination of the pregnant woman can reveal excessive fluid in the uterus (polyhydramnios). Amniotic fluid accumulates when atresia of the esophagus or intestinal tract have occurred. A too small or too large fetus with regard to gestational age can also provide physical evidence of such conditions as hydrocephaly or microcephaly.

Diagnosis of Malformation by X-ray The fetal skeleton can be visualized on a plain X-ray film of the mother's abdomen at 15 to 16 weeks of pregnancy. The only bony abnormality that can be seen at this time is anencephaly, in which an X-ray reveals that the fetal skull is absent. Hydrocephaly

of a large magnitude can also be seen and abnormalities of the limbs, such as dwarfism, can be recognized.

Amniocentesis Of the techniques used in the early prenatal diagnosis of birth defects, amniocentesis offers the best chance for accurately achieving a diagnosis. In amniocentesis a sample of amniotic fluid is obtained by passing a long needle through the abdominal wall of the mother into the amniotic sac. A sample of 10 to 20 ml of fluid can be obtained optimally at 15 to 16 weeks. (The risk involves a 1% to 2% chance of precipitating an abortion.) Viable cells from the fetus can be grown in tissue culture to assay for chromosome number, for certain enzymes, for determination of sex, and for karyotyping. Certain compounds associated with neural tube defects can also be detected.

Amniocentesis provides important information concerning the maturity of the fetus, sex, chromosomal abnormalities, the presence of metabolic disorders (inborn errors of metabolism), and certain malformations, such as anencephaly and spina bifida.

In theory, all "known" chromosomal abnormalities can be identified prenatally, including the monosomies and trisomies. Down's syndrome (trisomy 21), which occurs in approximately 1 in 700 births is detectable via amniocentesis. Likewise, the sex of the fetus can be determined for sex-linked inherited diseases.

Presently, certain conditions indicate using amniocentesis for prenatal diagnosis (Table 3-4). Suspected malformations of the central nervous system, especially anencephaly and spina bifida, are clear indications for amniocentesis. A fetal protein produced by the fetal liver, *α-fetoprotein* (AFP), is markedly increased in the amniotic fluid when the fetus has an open neural tube defect such as anencephaly or spina bifida with meningomyelocele. Detection of AFP in the amniotic fluid provides clear evidence that these defects are present in the fetus.

Extensive ethical discussions are raging about the moral impact of prenatal diagnosis of disease which could lead to abortion. Most parents who face the risk of having malformed, diseased children are generally receptive to information that will aid them in making important decisions.

Therapy

Currently, surgery is the only means for correcting some malformations. The surgical subspecialties of plastic surgery and pediatric surgery have developed to cope with congenital malformations that require special reconstruction of small organs. In the future, surgery will probably be performed on the fetus in utero when a birth defect is suspected.

Biologic genetic engineering ultimately should correct some enzyme deficiencies by inserting new genes into defective cells. Currently, the best "treatment" of birth defects is by preventing them. Other measures include the vaccination of young women against viruses, prevention of exposure of pregnant women to drugs, and planned parenthood.

Summary

Birth defects involve all organs and range in severity from trivial to profound deformity. Fetal death is often associated with severe chromosomal and congenital defects. Birth defects often arise from mutations caused by radiation, drugs, and maternal infections. They can be inherited too and may not necessarily cause physical deformity; inborn errors of metabolism are another very common type of birth defect. Remember that most organs are formed by eight weeks, and thus, the fetus is most vulnerable to teratogens early on. Prevention remains the best mode of treatment of birth defects; surgery can be lifesaving when mechanical defects are present, and biologic engineering offers hope for correcting inborn errors of metabolism.

Bibliography

Bergsma, B., ed. 1973. *Birth defects: atlas and compendium.* The March of Dimes. Baltimore: The Williams & Wilkins Company. Numerous photographs of virtually all birth defects are shown.

Berry, C. L., ed. 1976. *Human malformation, Br. Med. Bull.* 32:1–94. The entire issue on malformations.

Federman, D. D. 1967. Disorders of sexual development. *N. Engl. J. Med.* 277:351–361. Describes the pathogenesis of defects in gonadal development.

Gustavson, K. H., and Jorulf, H. 1976. Recurrence risks in a consecutive series of congenitally malformed children dying in the perinatal period. *Clin. Genet.* 9:307–314. Describes chances of inherited birth defects.

Holmes, L. B. 1974. Inborn errors of morphogenesis. *N. Engl. J. Med.* 291:763–776. The pathogenesis of common birth defects are shown.

Kissane, J. M. 1975. *Pathology of infancy and childhood.* St. Louis: The C. V. Mosby Company. Standard textbook with chapters on malformations.

Lev, M. 1971. Congenital Heart Disease. In *Pathology,* ed. W. A. D. Anderson, pp. 706–727. St. Louis: The C. V. Mosby Company. Chapter on heart defects.

Martin, G. M., and Hoehn, H. 1974. Genetics in human disease. *Hum. Pathol.* 5:387–405. Describes inherited diseases.

Milunsky, A.; Macn, J. N.; Weiss, R.; Alpert, E.; McIsaac, D. C.; and Joshi, M. S. 1975. Prenatal detection of neural tube defects. *American J. Obstet. Gynecol.* 122:313–315. Describes amniocentesis.

Moore, K. L. 1974. *Before we are born: basic embryology and birth defects.* Philadelphia: W. B. Saunders Company. Excellent concise descriptions.

Purtilo, D. T., and Bhawan, J. 1976. Fatal varicella in a pregnant woman and hydrocephalus in a baby. *Am. J. Obstet. Gynecol.* 15:208–209. Describes fatal chickenpox in a pregnant woman and a birth defect–hydrocephalus in her baby.

Wagatsuma, T. 1976. Amniotic fluid analysis in diagnosing fetal abnormalities. *Diagnostica* 35:12–15. Describes how and why amniocentesis is used for the antenatal diagnosis of birth defects.

CHAPTER 4

Adaptation, Injury, and Death of Cells

Chapter Outline

Objectives

After reading this chapter you should be able to

Name the "father" of pathology.

Describe the two phases of cell injury.

Define the term hypertrophy and describe two mechanisms permitting this cellular
adaptation.

Define the term hyperplasia.

Describe and compare the phenomena of hypertrophy and malignancy.

Define the term atrophy and list five factors associated with atrophy.

Define the term metaplasia.

Describe the sequence of changes occurring during injury of the cell.

List etiologic agents that can injure cells.

List physical agents capable of injuring tissues.

Describe three types of burns.

Understand why third degree burns fail to heal without skin grafting.

Define and describe the cause of retrolental fibrous dysplasia.

Compare and define the terms wound, abrasion, laceration, and contusion.

Describe why persons can succumb to a sudden loss of blood or from hemorrhage into a closed space (brain or pericardial sac, for example).

Define the term acute tubular necrosis.

Identify the color of a person with carbon monoxide poisoning.

List the two factors determining the extent of injury induced by ionizing radiation.

Describe the clinical signs and symptoms of radiation sickness.

List three factors that determine the availability of oxygen in tissues.

Define the term ischemic injury.

List three common causes of death resulting from ischemic injury.

Compare the duration of time the following cells can survive in anoxia: fibroblast, myocardium, renal tubules, and neurons.

Give an example of microbial-induced injury.

Define the terms necrosis and autolysis.

List the two special types of necrosis and cite examples of each.

Define the terms decubitus ulcer and "wet" and "dry" gangrene.

Introduction

More than a century ago Rudolph Virchow (1865) made a great impact on the basic philosophy of scientific medicine by recognizing that the cell is the basic unit of life. His microscopic studies showed how cellular alterations correlate with clinical disease. He concluded that all diseases are in the last analysis reducible to groups of living units, whose functional capacity is altered in accordance with the state of their molecular composition and is thus dependent on physical and chemical changes of their contents. For his tremendous insight, Rudolph Virchow is considered the father of pathology.

The cell is a complex unit providing vital processes; these depend on precise integration of many metabolic processes. A cell's response to adverse environmental conditions depends on its ability to *adapt* itself to new conditions; when it fails to adapt, the cell undergoes a series of alterations that can end in cell death. Hence, cell injury can be *lethal* or *sublethal*. Lethal injury causes cell death; sublethal injury alters function without killing the cell.

Two phases of *cell injury* can be recognized: (1) *altered homeostasis*, in which the structural and functional changes are reversible if the injurious stimuli is removed, and (2) *necrosis*, in which cell components are broken down largely by digestion of itself (*autolysis*) by hydrolytic enzymes. The "point of no return" in this process is a point of transition from the first to the second phase of injury. Cell death is the "point of no return."

The cellular adaptations of cells responding to injurious stimuli that prevent injury and necrosis will now be discussed.

Cellular Adaptations (sublethal reactions to injury)

The capacity of cells to adapt to unusual or injurious stimuli by undergoing structural or functional changes allows survival. Such adaptations are extremely common and are part of many physiologic and disease processes. For instance, the forearm muscles of a tennis player enlarge because of exercise. The enlargement of the muscles results from new synthesis of the constituents of the muscle fibers, especially mitochondria and myofilaments. The newly adapted muscle cell thus escapes potential injury and is able to respond to the work demands.

The environment makes a tremendous impact on cells. Prolonged exposure to sunlight stimulates synthesis of melanin, and tanning of the skin ensues. Likewise, mechanical friction to the skin stimulates synthesis of a special fibrous protein, keratin, which forms a horny (cornified) protective callous (Fig. 4-1).

Hormones act on sensitive "target organs" and stimulate the synthesis of new proteins. For example, the breasts of pregnant women markedly increase in size; cells increase in size as they prepare to produce milk in response to the hormones estrogen, progesterone, and prolactin. This process is a physiologic adaptation to hormones.

Before considering cell necrosis in detail, we will discuss the mechanisms whereby cells adapt to potentially injurious stimuli: hypertrophy, metaplasia, hyperplasia, and atrophy. The following chapter describes the body's response to injury by inflammation and the healing process that attempts to restore the injured tissue.

Hypertrophy

Hypertrophy occurs without cell division and refers to the increased size of cells resulting from increased synthesis of macromolecules including protein, nucleic acids, lipid, and the various intracellular organelles that they constitute. Adaptive cell reactions can be considered to be a response of two general types: *compensatory* and *hormonal*. The most commonly encountered examples of compensatory hypertrophy are increases in the cell mass of skeletal and cardiac muscle or kidney tissue as a result of increased work demand. The heart of a person with hypertension (high blood pressure) can hypertrophy to pump blood against the raised pressure to meet the tissue requirements for blood (Fig. 4-2). The volume of the myocardial (cardiac muscle) cell is increased, and ultrastructural studies show increased numbers of myofilaments and mitochondria.

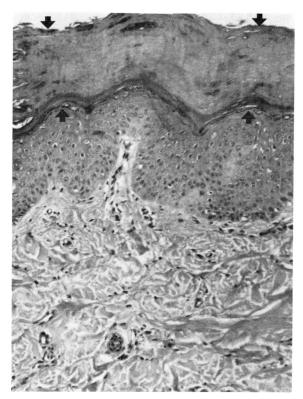

Figure 4-1 *Photomicrograph of a callous. Note the thick layer of cornified cells (between the arrows) formed in response to mechanical friction.*

Compensatory hypertrophy of kidney tissue occurs when renal disease affects one kidney or following the removal of a kidney. A compensatory increase in the mass of the remaining functional kidney ensues to compensate for the loss. During the process, the weight of the compensating kidney usually increases from a normal weight of 180 gm to a compensatory weight of about 350 gm.

The increased size of the uterus that occurs during pregnancy results from stimulation by estrogenic hormones, the size of uterine smooth muscle cells increasing about one hundred–fold from the hormone-induced hypertrophy.

Hyperplasia

Various stimuli increase the frequency of mitotic divisions in cells causing new cells to grow. The resulting greater number of cells is termed *hyper-*

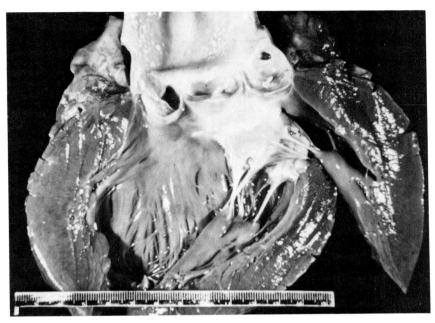

Figure 4-2 *Hypertrophy of the heart. The left ventricle is markedly thickened as a response to high blood pressure.*

plasia. The process of hyperplasia is reversible when the stimulus is removed, whereas malignant neoplasms continue to grow autonomously even when the stimulus is removed.

Hyperplasia occurs as an adaptive mechanism for restoring a tissue or organ. For example, removal of part of the liver leads to *regeneration*, or hyperplasia, of remaining liver cells to compensate for the loss. After removal of 70% of the liver, numerous mitoses of hepatocytes occurs, reaching a peak at 33 hours. By the twelfth day, the mass of liver excised is totally restored.

Hormonally-induced hyperplasia occurs especially in estrogen-dependent organs such as the uterus and breast. For example, under continued estrogen stimulation, the endometrium proliferates (grows) and thickens to become suitable for receiving the fertilized egg. In rare instances of prolonged stimulation by estrogenic hormones, a hyperplastic endometrium can undergo *malignant neoplastic transformation;* cell proliferation will no longer be under control and cell growth continues to the detriment of the patient. This concept has been substantiated by a several–fold increase in endometrial carci-noma in women who have been on long term oral contraceptive hormone therapy.

Atrophy

Atrophy refers to a decreased size of cells with consequent decrease in size of the affected organ. Atrophy occurs in any organ but is more recognizable in skeletal muscle, heart, secondary sex organs, and the brain (Fig. 4-3). In early stages, atrophy results solely from a decrease in cell size, whereas in later stages an actual loss of cells occurs, as in cerebral atrophy. Atrophy is a cellular adaptation to decreased (1) use, (2) workload, (3) blood supply, (4) nutrition, or (5) hormonal stimulation.

Atrophy is a physiologic reaction in which a group of cells, a tissue, or an organ, having served its function, returns to basal (resting) function. On proper restimulation, the tissues return to normal or even undergo hypertrophy. Atrophy in a tissue or organ can also be the consequence of a disease and be so marked that it is a pathologic reaction.

Characteristically, *disuse atrophy* occurs when the workload diminishes. The legs of an individual who does not get sufficient physical exercise become atrophic; the muscles become thin and weak. Decreased numbers of mitochondria and myofilaments are seen in atrophic muscle.

During the process of *aging* many cells naturally die *(necrobiosis)*. Lack of blood supply can lead to senile atrophy of the brain (Fig. 4-3). Concurrently, *senility* in elderly persons, characterized by loss of memory, inappropriate behavior, and/or orientation, often occurs.

Metaplasia

Another adaptive phenomenon of cells is *metaplasia,* the transformation of one cell into another. Generally, metaplasia results in the change of highly specialized cells into less specialized cells. For example, metaplasia occurs in the bronchi of cigarette smokers as an adaptation to smoke. The normal highly specialized ciliated columnar epithelium lining the bronchial airways changes into or is replaced by squamous epithelium (Fig. 4-4). The squamous epithelium is more resistant or adaptive to injury from smoke. Metaplasia is usually reversible when the inducing stimulus is removed; when a cigarette smoker quits smoking, the bronchial lining reverts back to its normal ciliated columnar epithelium.

Cellular changes in response to injury, including adaptation, injury, and death, occur along a continuum. When adaptive measures fail, cell injury develops.

Cell Injury

Common responses of cells to diverse forms of injury usually consist of the following sequence of reactions: (1) loss of cell volume control (cell swelling or shrinking, for example), (2) a decrease in the density of the cytoplasm due to swelling of organelles, (3) accumulation of lipid droplets in the cytoplasm, (4) violent movements and distortion of the plasma membranes, (5) nuclear edema, (6) pyknosis (a condensation of the cell nucleus to a clumped mass of chromatin), and (7) karyolysis (dissolution of the nucleus and its contents). These cellular reactions range from mild swelling, which is reversible, to cell death—structural dissolution of the nucleus and cell.

Many agents and factors injure cells. These include (1) physical agents, (2) chemicals, (3) hypoxia, (4) microbial agents (see Chapter 7, Infectious Diseases), (5) immunologic hypersensitivity reactions (see Chapter 6, Immunology), (6) malnutrition (see Chapter 10, Nutritional Deficiency

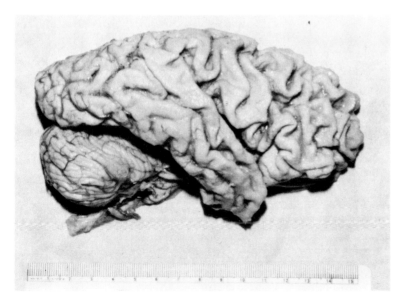

Figure 4-3 *Atrophy of the cerebral cortex. Note the increased width of the sulci (valleys) and narrowing of the gyri (hills). (Courtesy Dr. Umberto DeGirolami.)*

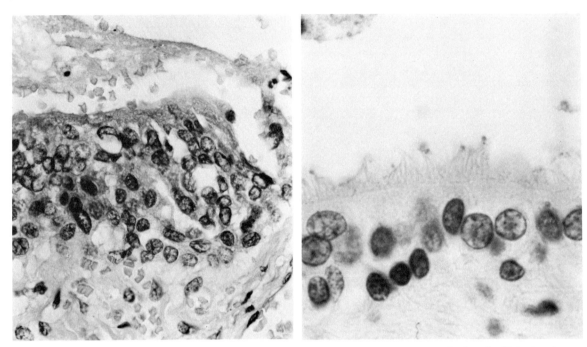

Figure 4-4   *Photomicrograph of lining of bronchus showing squamous metaplasia of ciliated columnar epithelium. Normal ciliated columnar epithelium is shown at the right for comparison.*

Diseases), (7) inherited defects (see Chapter 9, Inherited Disorders), and (8) aging.

Energy Deficit

Cell injury often occurs because more energy is needed than is available. If the energy deficit is mild or transient, functional and metabolic adjustments occur. If the deficit is severe or prolonged, the cell dies. Energy deficit occurs if the cell has insufficient glucose, or insufficient oxygen to support glucose combustion.

Intracellular glucose deficiency occurs if circulating levels of blood glucose are low (hypoglycemia); if blood is not reaching the cell (because of defective circulation); or if glucose cannot cross the membrane to enter the cell (as in diabetes mellitus). The liver and skeletal muscles have intracellular reserves of glycogen, the storage form of glucose, but these reserves are readily depleted. Some cells can transiently burn fatty acids instead of glucose, but this alternative is self-limited because toxic waste products are produced. As short-term measures fail, the cell must adjust to a lowered total energy supply.

Deficient Oxygen (hypoxia-induced injury)

Following the blockage of blood flow in a coronary artery by a blood clot, myocardial cell injury develops. The earliest event in oxygen deficiency is slowing of oxidative metabolism, and decreased production of ATP by mitochondria is noted in the hypoxic myocardial cell. The myocardial cell must remain engaged in contraction and continues to use energy and to consume ATP. The result is that the ADP:ATP ratio rises, and the extraneous phosphate group accumulates in the cytoplasm as more and more ATP is converted to ADP. In cardiac muscle, high concentrations of phosphate induce conversion to an alternate pathway of energy production (anaerobic glycolysis). As ATP levels fall, enzymes have access to less energy. Reduced energy sources cause membranes to lose their selective permeability leading to increased permeability to sodium and water. Also lactic acid accumulates in the cell. The endoplasmic reticulum and mitochondria swell and nuclear chromatin clumps. If the oxygen supply is not restored, then lysosomal enzymes spill out and cell death follows.

Injurious Physical Agents

Injury can result from excessive exposure to many physical environmental changes. Also, these agents, when employed for diagnosing and treating patients, can be injurious. Potential injurious physical agents include extremes of temperature, radiant energy, luminous ultraviolet and ionizing radiation, hydrotherapy, mechanical factors (therapeutic physical exercise, for example), diathermy, and ultrasound. If any of these physical modalities are used excessively, for too long a period or in great intensity, then cellular injury can result.

Temperature Extremes   Extremes of temperature can cause cell injury and death. Tissues sustain themselves better at cooler temperatures (a decrease of 15 C is tolerated). Beyond these limits, cell injury occurs and cell death may ensue.

Fever or Exposure to Extreme Heat   Respiratory rate, heart rate, and metabolism accelerate when temperatures are elevated. Eventually, proteins in cells coagulate, and cells die. Heat stroke, for instance, occurs when the body temperature reaches approximately 42 C. I recall running the Boston marathon on a hot day (35.5 C). Many runners fainted (heat stroke) when their body temperatures increased. They either fainted (became unconscious) or became stuporous (incoherent and confused). In some cases, minor reversible brain damage resulted from hyperthermia. Thus, efforts should be made to decrease the body temperature in victims of heat stroke with ice packs, intravenous fluids, and ventilation.

Circulation slows when the temperature of blood is reduced to 20 C. Hypothermia (cooling of the body) is beneficial during open heart surgery. When the body is cooled, the oxygen requirements of the tissues are decreased, and long periods of hypoxia are tolerated without damage to the tissue.

Cold (Frostbite)   Rapid or prolonged chilling causes injury to tissues because the blood vessels can become clotted (a thrombosis). *Ischemia* (lack of oxygen) results from the blood clots induced by frostbite, and in extreme cases, ice crystals form and burst the cells. If the ischemia persists, cell death occurs.

Burns   *Cutaneous burns* are classified as first, second, or third degree burns. A *first degree burn* is manifested by a redness (erythema) without significant alterations of the epidermis. By contrast, *second degree burns* are characterized by destruction of the epidermis with minor injury to the dermis. Second degree burns become vesiculated (blistered), and the skin regenerates because the dermis is slightly injured (Fig. 4-5). The severest burn, the *third degree burn*, causes damage to both the dermis and the epidermis. Damage to the deep dermis interferes with the epithelial regeneration.

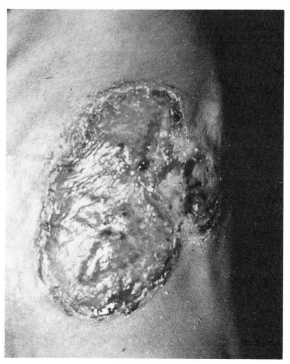

Figure 4-5   *Second degree burn on chest of a child. The epidermis has undergone necrosis, and minor injury to the dermis has occurred. It healed without skin grafting.*

Shock is a major complication of extensive cutaneous burns. It results from a loss of circulating blood volume, as blood concentrates with the oozing of blood plasma from the burn site. Another complication can arise later, cutaneous infection by *Pseudomonas* or *Staphylococcus* bacteria. Individuals at the extremes of life (infants and elderly persons) are vulnerable to cutaneous burns; infants and octogenarians who sustain third degree burns covering more than 50% of their body surfaces will invariably die.

Electrothermal Injury   Profound injury results from being struck by lightning. When the current passes through a vital organ such as the heart, it induces fibrillation (an uncoordinated contraction of the heart) and instantly kills the person. Occasionally, the victim escapes only with burns where the lightning bolt exits. *Coagulative necrosis* can be extensive in the skin and skeletal muscles. In coagulative necrosis, chemical bonds of proteins in the cells become altered permanently and die.

Contact with alternating current (AC) at 110 volts is frequently the source for individuals sustaining electrothermal injury. The harmful effects that develop depend on (1) the amount, (2) the kind, (3) the path, and (4) the duration of the current. Alternating current produces greater cellular injury than does direct current. Alternating current produces coagulative necrosis of the skin. When the current passes through the vital cardiorespiratory centers of the brain, circulation and respiration cease and death follows.

Ultrasound Injury   Deafness can result from loud sustained tones that damage the hearing apparatus, the cochlea. This is a common occupational problem for persons working in industries having loud noises and poor safety standards. Permanent loss of hearing results from prolonged exposure to loud music (100 decibel volume, for example). Music played on powerful amplifiers, such as "Rock" music, has been shown to cause permanent hearing loss.

Ultrasound is used to treat physical disabilities by inducing hyperthermia in tissues; if improperly used, ultrasound injures tissues. *Supersonic radiation (ultrasound)* can raise the temperature in the liver 25 C in just 30 seconds. Cellular injury results from disruption of the cells with subsequent edema, redness, and degeneration of cells.

Oxygen-induced Injury   The use of 100% oxygen in incubators for neonates with "respiratory distress syndrome" can bring about blindness. Oxygen at 100% was formerly used to treat infants with respiratory distress, and on occasion, this form of therapy induced fibrosis in the retina (*retrolental fibrous dysplasia*) and permanent blindness. This disease has virtually disappeared now that we finally recognize that oxygen can be toxic.

Also, patients who are placed on automated respiratory devices that deliver large volumes of oxygen can develop oxygen-induced damage to their lungs ("pump lung"). Subsequent fibrosis can follow—diffusion of gases across the alveoli becomes impaired and the patients fail to oxygenate their blood.

Mechanical Injury

Mechanical injury occurs when an individual is hit or struck by a moving object and a wound results. A *wound* is an interruption in the continuity of tissues. Wounds range in severity from an *abrasion*, a superficial scratch or tearing of epidermal cells by friction with the epidermis remaining intact, to a *laceration*, which disrupts the integrity of the organ or tissue by tearing of tissues. Laceration of the spleen or liver, for instance, often results from crushing injuries such as those occurring in automobile accidents. Extensive loss of blood (hemorrhage) from the site of the laceration can be life-threatening.

A *contusion* (bruise) is an injury in which the force of impact is transmitted through the skin to the underlying tissues, resulting in the disruption of small blood vessels with bleeding into the skin, brain, or any other organ underlying the impact. A contusion of the brain results in loss of consciousness and, usually, temporary amnesia (loss of memory).

Hemorrhage and Shock   Hemorrhage occurs when blood vessels are disrupted in tissues. Blood flows from tissues, and clotting causes the bleeding

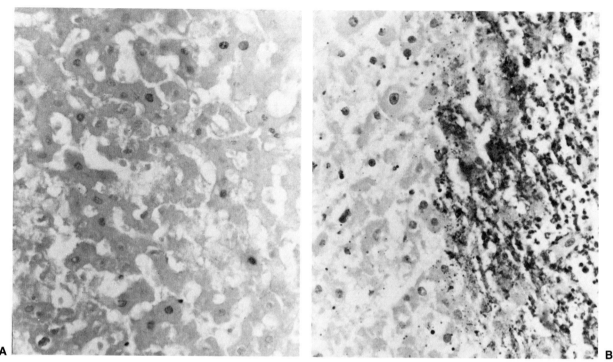

Figure 4-6   **A,** *Photomicrograph of liver with necrosis 48 hours following obstruction of the hepatic artery. It shows a slight loss of nuclear staining and swelling of cytoplasm of hepatocytes.* **B,** *Photomicrograph showing necrosis of same liver at 72 hours. Nuclear staining has decreased and cells have autolyzed; calcification of dead tissue has occurred.*

to stop (see Chapter 11, Hematology). If bleeding occurs gradually, it generally causes no significant problem. However, if an individual suddenly loses 1 liter of blood, shock and death often result if a blood transfusion or intravenous fluids are not given. If the hemorrhage occurs into a *closed space,* such as the brain (that is, subdural hematoma), as little as 300 ml of blood can compress vital cardiac and respiratory centers in the brain, and the heart and lungs will cease functioning. Similarly, a hemorrhage into the closed pericardial sac from a ruptured heart rapidly fills the sac, compressing the heart and obstructing filling and pumping of blood by the heart. The process is termed *cardiac tamponade.*

Mechanical injuries can trigger events that terminate in a collapse of blood pressure (cardiac shock), loss of consciousness, and in some instances, death. Secondary (hemorrhagic) shock results from a reduction in blood volume. Symptoms and signs of shock are a rapid weak pulse and cool,

moist, and pale extremities resulting from the decreased circulation of blood. Subsequently, injury can result from anoxia (lack of oxygen), and ischemic necrosis of tissues may follow. The kidney, brain, and liver (Fig. 4-6) are vulnerable to hypotension (drop in blood pressure) and anoxia. For example, *acute tubular necrosis* of the kidney can take place when hypotension occurs. During a surgical procedure, stimulation of the nerves in the abdomen or a loss of blood volume from hemorrhage can elicit hypotension, renal tubules can undergo necrosis, and only ghostlike outlines of the necrotic renal tubules are visible (see Chapter 17, Urology and Renal Medicine).

Chemical Injury

Accidental poisoning or suicide produces numerous deaths in the United States. Suicide from taking an overdose of drugs, especially sleeping medication such as barbiturates, from alcohol intoxication, and from carbon monoxide poisoning are common causes of chemical injury. Suicide is the leading cause of death in young people in their late teens. Also, many drugs used to treat illness have side effects—they often injure the intestinal tract or liver.

Poisoning from the ingestion of *corrosive poisons*, such as lye, causes coagulative necrosis in the esophagus, and scars and strictures can follow during the healing process. *Heavy metals*, such as lead, can cause poisoning in children who eat paint containing lead. The brains of such children become edematous (swollen), and the children may become mentally retarded. Anemia may develop as lead is deposited in bones; injury to peripheral nerves occurs, especially to motor nerves; and muscular weakness can develop. The lead level can be measured in the child's blood or urine. The child should be removed from exposure to the lead paint, and drugs that bind (chelate) the lead in the child's body should be given to eliminate the lead. Most of the problems caused by lead poisoning eventually remit after treatment.

Carbon Monoxide Injury   Carbon monoxide has a three hundred–fold greater binding affinity for hemoglobin than oxygen; an individual exposed to carbon monoxide binds carbon monoxide to hemoglobin rather than to oxygen. The exhaust coming from an automobile contains approximately 5% to 15% carbon monoxide, and gas heaters emit about 5% carbon monoxide. Hence, an automobile left in a closed, single-car garage for five minutes will rapidly produce a deadly atmosphere.

Pathologically, individuals suffering from carbon monoxide poisoning develop pink to red skin because carbon monoxide is bound to their hemoglobin. Carboxyhemoglobin is bright red, and hence, persons poisoned severely with carbon monoxide are bright red.

Radiation Injury

Ionizing radiation includes gamma rays emitted from an X-ray machine or alpha and beta particles, neutrons, deuterons, protons, and pions emitted from cobalt or linear accelerators. Radioactive rays or particles introduce electrons into molecules in cells and ionize the tissues. The degenerative and atrophic changes ensuing in a radiated tissue are comparable to necrosis induced by heat, cold, electric current, drugs, or other protoplasmic poisons.

The extent of injury from ionizing radiation depends on two factors: the *intensity* and the *duration* of radiation exposure. Redness usually appears in the skin 6 to 48 hours after exposure to radiation. Significant damage to the skin appears after 6 to 14 days. The blood vessels are especially vulnerable to radiation; they undergo swelling of their lining endothelial cells, and later fibrous connective tissue can block the lumen of blood channels.

The injurious impact of radiation is accumulative in effect. When ionizing radiation is given for therapeutic purposes (radiotherapy), small doses are focused on a malignant tumor over a period of many days to prevent cellular injury (Fig. 4-7); the focusing of the rays on the tumor shields normal tissues from exposure.

Tissues have marked differences in their sensitivity to radiation. Rapidly growing cells of the bone marrow, the intestinal mucosal cells, and the germ cells are highly sensitive; whereas cells no longer growing, such as neurons (brain cells), are much less sensitive to radiation injury.

Radiation Sickness   Radiation sickness often occurs when an abdominal or pelvic neoplasm is irradiated. Radiation sickness is characterized by vomiting, nausea, and depression coming on promptly, or within a few hours, after exposure; it seldom lasts beyond 48 hours. Diarrhea can also occur, especially when the pelvic organs have been irradiated, as the intestinal tract mucosa can become injured.

Ischemic Injury

The amount of oxygen available to tissues depends on (1) the oxygen-carrying capacity of hemoglobin in the blood, (2) the lung's capacity to exchange carbon dioxide and oxygen, and (3) the ability of the heart and the blood vessels to deliver blood to

Impact of Radiotherapy
on Normal and Cancerous Cells

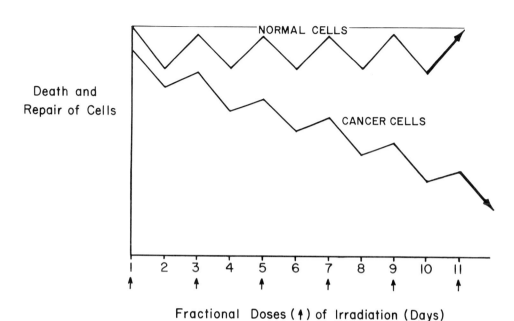

Death and
Repair of Cells

Fractional Doses (↑) of Irradiation (Days)

Figure 4-7   *Dividing the doses of irradiation given during radiotherapy into small exposures allows normal tissues surrounding a tumor to recover from injury. The tumor cells, because they can be rapidly dividing, are sensitive to the radiation and thus die. (Reprinted, by permission from the* New England Journal of Medicine *293:81, 1975).*

tissues. A defect in any of these can compromise metabolism of the tissues enough to cause cell death (Fig. 4-6).

Our bodies tolerate a gradual onset of anoxia more successfully than acute anoxia. For instance, gradual blockage of a coronary artery of the heart due to arteriosclerosis is well tolerated; whereas, when the channel is suddenly blocked by a thrombus, anoxia dramatically occurs and the lack of oxygen causes *ischemic injury*. Myocardial fibers die within minutes if the blood supplying is not restored (see Chapter 13, Cardiology).

The ability of tissues of the body to survive hypoxia is remarkably variable. As little as two minutes of hypoxia can kill some neurons of the brain. The kidney and heart undergo necrosis after about 30 minutes of anoxia.

Most deaths in the United States result from ischemic injury: (1) stroke, (2) heart attack, and (3) pulmonary infarction. The heart, lungs, and brain are vulnerable to hypoxia; when the blood vessels that supply them are blocked by arteriosclerotic plaques, thrombi, or emboli and when collateral (alternate routes of supply) blood vessels become unable to carry blood around the blocked site, tissues die.

By contrast, the robust fibroblasts of connective tissues can survive hypoxia for up to two weeks. In fact, tails from wild animals have been sent by mail from Alaska to New England and have survived to grow in tissue culture after being en route for up to two weeks.

Microbial Injury

Nearly 1000 different microbes can produce disease in human beings; they are termed *pathogens*. Cellular injury from microbes results from a variety of

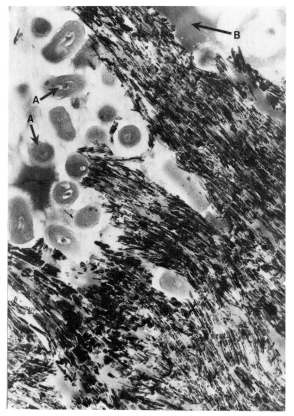

Figure 4-8 *Electron micrograph of human tooth infected with caries. A swarm of bacteria, A, are shown burrowing into the black enamel segments, B, the enamel is being dissolved by lactic acid produced by the bacteria. Enlarged × 21,000. (Courtesy Dr. Guido Majno and Harvard University Press.)*

mechanisms. Some bacteria produce enzymes that digest tissues (collagenase from streptococci digests collagen, for example). Another example of microbial injury is *dental caries*, which are caused by an infection in teeth; bacteria produce lactic acid, which then dissolves the enamel (Fig. 4-8). Microbes also injure tissues from the associated inflammatory and immune responses of the infected person. Neutrophils invade tissues harboring bacteria and spill their lysosomal enzymes into the tissues digesting them (see Chapter 5, Acute Inflammation and Repair). Similarly, macrophages and lymphocytes can injure tissues during an immune response to microbes (see Chapter 6, Immunol-

ogy). The vulnerable site of injury is the cell membrane.

Injury to Membranes

Anything that interferes with membrane function causes severe cell damage or death (necrosis). Any of the preceding agents can paralyze membrane function. Depending on which enzymes in membranes are inactivated, the membrane becomes indiscriminately permeable, or it may selectively lose the ability to regulate permeability of few critical substances.

Indiscriminate increased permeability allows sodium and calcium ions to enter and potassium and magnesium ions to exit, causing large amounts of water to enter the cell. The endoplasmic reticulum and the mitochondria swell, and membranes fragment or distort their contours. Dilution of cytoplasmic and nuclear fluid by water interferes with enzymic reactions and interrupts function. The cumulative effects of these changes lead, within a short time, to cell death.

Selective impairment of membrane function can prevent nerve cells from transmitting impulses, or muscles from contracting, without actually killing the cell. These functional defects result from interference with specific enzyme activities and is more likely to be reversible than indiscriminate loss of selective permeability of cells.

Necrosis

Necrosis is the manifestation of cell death. Agents that severely injure cells can lead to cell death. Membranes are the vulnerable point of cells, especially membranes surrounding mitochondria. Enzymes embedded in mitochondrial membranes are readily inactivated by changes in temperature, oxygen, and pH.

As cells die, their mitochondria swell and develop coarse granules, and the endoplasmic reticulum in the surrounding cytoplasm become disrupted (Fig. 4-9). The metabolic pumps that maintain the selective permeability to sodium, potassium, chloride, and bicarbonate ions in the cells

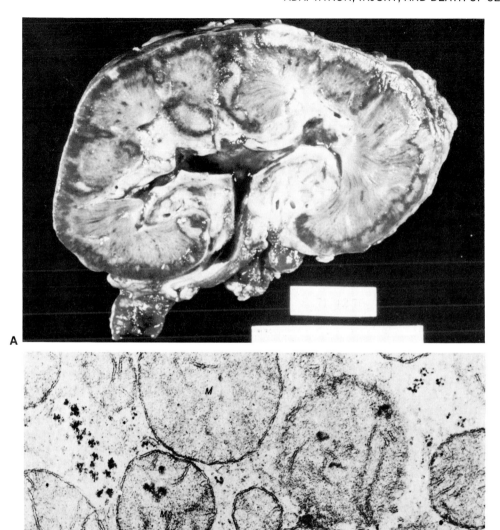

Figure 4-9   A, *Hypotension causing acute tubular necrosis of kidney.* **B,** *Proximal tubule of kidney with acute tubular necrosis after irreversible shock. The features are typical of irreversible cell damage. Note the dilated endoplasmic reticulum, ER; the mitochondria, which are swollen and contain dense dark bodies; and the general pallor of the cell sap. (From Kashgarian, M.; Hayslett, J. P.; and Spargo, B. H. 1974. Renal disease. Bethesda, Maryland: Universities Associated for Research and Education in Pathology, Inc.)*

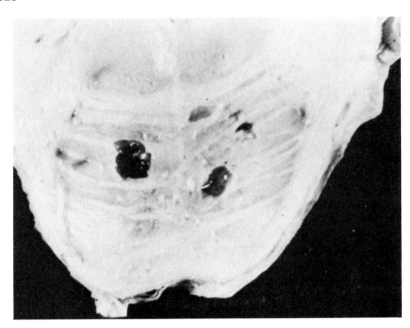

Figure 4-10   *Brain with bilateral infarction and liquefaction necrosis. Note the cystic cavities that were filled with liquid material* (arrows).

deteriorate; the membranes fragment; and fluids flow freely into the cell causing edema. The enzymes in the cells that are stored in *lysosomes* break apart and release enzymes that destroy the tissues. Lysosomal rupture usually occurs late in a generalized process that damages the cells. These "suicide bags" self-destroy the cell *(autolysis)*.

Concurrently, the nucleus may undergo one of three fates: (1) dissolution *(karyolysis)* from the action of hydrolytic enzymes, (2) break up *(karyorrhexis)*, or (3) nuclear *pyknosis*.

During the process of cell death, water enters the cells, and small clear vacuoles (hydropic degeneration) are seen. In other cells, lipid accumulates (fatty metamorphosis). This occurs especially in the liver damaged by alcohol. Other cells "mummify" or undergo hyaline degeneration. The word *hyaline* is used to describe the pink-staining glass-like appearance of portions of cells and tissues in some conditions of cell degeneration. Two special types of necrosis occur: *liquefaction necrosis* and *coagulative necrosis*.

Liquefaction Necrosis

In the central nervous system, *ischemic necrosis* is characterized by softening, which rapidly pro-

gresses to *liquefaction necrosis* (Fig. 4-10). The surrounding uninvolved tissue defines the limits of a cystic space in which fluid collects. Liquefaction necrosis probably results in the brain because it contains cells rich in digestive enzymes, has an abundant supply of lipid, and contains few connective tissue cells. Likewise, when bacteria infect necrotic tissue, acute inflammation ensues; invading neutrophils usually release lysosomal enzymes and digest the tissues. This results in liquefaction necrosis.

Coagulative Necrosis

During coagulative necrosis, proteins are denatured in the cells—the proteins link together (polymerize) and enzymes lose their function. Coagulation of protein occurs, for instance, when an egg is cooked. Realignment of protein linkages causes the albumin to change from a gelatinous transparent material to an opaque firm material. The vast majority of tissues of the body can undergo coagulative necrosis.

Gangrenous necrosis results from severe hypoxia and subsequent ischemic injury (see Chapter 13, Cardiology). This commonly occurs in the lower leg or foot from arteriosclerotic blockage of major arteries. *"Dry" gangrene* results from the coagulative necrosis of the tissues deprived of oxygen. If the gangrenous tissue becomes infected, *"wet" gangrene* develops because liquefaction of the necrotic tissue commences when neutrophils invade and inflame the site.

Decubitus Ulcer   A decubitus is an ulcer of the skin that develops over the bony prominences, such as the sacrum, hips, and heels, in debilitated patients. It results from anoxia to the skin when pressure blocks the flow of blood to the skin. If the blood supply is not restored by moving the patient, ischemic necrosis can develop. Oftentimes, a decubitus ulcer becomes secondarily infected. Attentive nursing care can usually prevent decubitus ulcers from occurring.

Summary

When cells fail to adapt to potentially injurious stimuli by undergoing hypertrophy, hyperplasia, metaplasia, or atrophy, necrosis ensues. The agents that can injure or kill cells include physical changes, chemicals, hypoxia, microbes, and a variety of other factors. Membranes of cells are the structure of cells vulnerable to injury. Only two basic types of necrosis occur, coagulative or liquefactive necrosis. But organs suffering from the death of cells have amazing capacities for restoring themselves and defending against destruction. The products of necrosis are irritating to normal tissues, so that inflammation commonly follows necrosis. The necrotic debris is removed by neutrophils and macrophages so the injury can heal.

Bibliography

Auerbach, O.; Gere, J. B.; Forman, J. B.; Petnick, T. A.; Smolin, H. J.; Muehsom, G. E.; Kassouny, D. Y.; and Stout, A. P. 1957. Changes in the bronchial epithelium in relation to smoking and cancer of the lung. *N. Engl. J. Med.* 256:97. Describes the metaplastic, hyperplastic, and neoplastic changes seen throughout the lining of airways of smokers.

Bogt, M. T., and Farber, E. 1968. On the molecular pathology of the ischemic renal cell death. Reversible and irreversible cellular and mitochondrial metabolic alterations. *Am. J. Pathol.* 53:1. Defines the ultrastructural alterations seen in dying mitochondria.

Cochrane, C. G. 1968. Immunologic tissue injury mediated by neutrophilic leukocytes. *Advanc. Immunol.* 9:97. Describes the role of neutrophils in inducing tissue injury during immunologic hypersensitivity reactions.

Hanawalt, P. C., and Haynes, R. H., eds. The chemical life: an introduction to molecular and cell biology. Readings from Scientific American 1953–1973. This is a superb collection of summary articles.

Haylick, L. 1976. The cell biology of human aging. *N. Engl. J. Med.* 295:1302–1308. A concise summary by an authority who suggests that normal cells and persons have a predetermined life span of about 100 years.

Jennings, R. B., et al. 1969. Ischemic injury of myocardium. *Ann. N. Y. Acad. Sci.* 156:61. Describes experimental studies that define the limits of time the heart can be bloodless and survive.

Jones, A. L., and Fawcett, D. W. 1966. Hypertrophy of the agranular endoplasmic reticulum in hamster liver induced by phenobarbital. *Histochemistry and Cytochemistry* 14:215. Illustrates a cellular adaptation to a drug and provides an ultrastructural basis for explaining development of tolerance to drugs.

Kohn, R. R. 1973. *Aging.* Published by the Upjohn Company. Injury can result from the processes of aging. This monograph concisely reviews theories of aging.

Majno, G., et al. 1960. Death and necrosis: chemical, physical, and morphologic changes in rat liver. *Virchows Archiv* (Cell Pathol) 333:421. A classical article describing the death process and injury of hepatocytes.

Malt, R. A. 1969. Compensatory growth of the kidney. *N. Engl. J. Med.* 280:1446. Regeneration or hyperplastic adoptive changes are described in the kidney.

Scarpelli, D. G., and Trump, B. F. 1971. *Cell injury.* Published by The Upjohn Company, Kalamazoo. The one best concise reference on cell injury.

Trump, B. F., and Arstila, A. U. 1975. Cellular reaction to injury. In *Principles of pathobiology*, eds. M. F. La Via and R. B. Hill, Jr., pp. 9–96. ed. 2. New York: Oxford University Press. Intracellular events that follow lethal and sublethal injury are considered.

Weissman, G. 1972. Lysosomal mechanisms of tissue injury in arthritis. *N. Engl. J. Med.* 286:141. Describes the destructive changes brought about by lysosomes in arthritis.

CHAPTER 5

Inflammation and Repair

Chapter Outline

Objectives

After reading this chapter you should be able to

Define the terms acute and chronic inflammation.

Know what fibroblasts form.

List the three major structures or factors involved in acute inflammation.

Know the signs of inflammation.

List the sequential events transpiring during acute inflammation.

Define the term edema.

Compare the three types of endothelium and their location in the body.

Define the terms pinocytosis, oncotic pressure, and transudate.

Compare characteristics of transudates and exudates.

Compare the mechanisms of direct and indirect histamine-type injury to endothelium.

Describe how histamine makes venules "leaky."

List and give examples of various types of exudates.

Compare acute and chronic inflammation with respect to time of occurrence.

Describe the type of leukocytes involved in acute and chronic inflammation.

List anti-inflammatory drugs.

Define the terms abscess and cellulitis.

Recognize a granulomatous inflammation.

Describe one local and one systemic effect of acute inflammation.

Define the terms chemotaxis and phagocytosis.

List the three phases of phagocytosis.

Define the process of opsonization of bacteria.

List three possible defects of neutrophil function.

Define lysosome and describe what it is capable of doing to bacteria or tissues.

Describe granulation tissue.

Describe what a myofibroblast does in the process of wound healing.

Compare healing of wounds by primary and secondary intention.

List possible complications in wound healing.

Define the term contracture and give examples.

List factors that modify wound healing.

Introduction

Infection, injury, and necrosis induce inflammation, which begins as an acute reaction, may continue as a chronic reaction, and ultimately ends in healing. Both inflammation and repair are vital processes permitting recovery from injury. Inflammation is a process central to the practice of medicine for two reasons. (1) Numerous signs and symptoms of diseases result from inflammatory or reparative processes in our bodies. (2) Attempts to treat diseases are often focused on either enhancing or diminishing inflammation or repair.

The consequences of inadequate inflammatory responses can be drastic; for example, individuals can become overwhelmed by bacterial infections. In contrast, overgrowth of reparative processes disfigures individuals; ugly scars can ensue, such as a keloid (a hypertrophic thick scar, Figure 5-1). Fortunately, inflammation and repair almost always harmonize and restore injured tissues to a nearly normal condition.

Inflammation

Definitions

Inflammation ("fire") is an ancient term coined because injured parts are flaming, red, hot, and painful. Technically, inflammation is a biochemical and cellular process provoked by injurious stimuli in vascularized tissues; subsequently, fluid and white blood cells (WBCs) accumulate at the site of injury. Inflammation is a defense mechanism that can occur in two forms: (1) *Acute inflammation* is present when the process is of two weeks or less duration, and it is generally *suppurative* (or *purulent*); that is, neutrophils are the predominant cell type producing the pus. (2) *Chronic inflammation* lasts for weeks, months, or even years and is characterized by a lymphocytic infiltration.

The *repair* process begins simultaneously following injury. Repair processes replace dead tissues with newly formed healthy cells derived either from surviving cells or from connective tissue *fibroblasts*

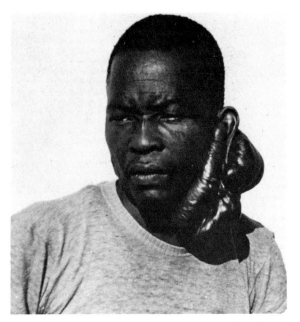

Figure 5-1 *Keloid of ear from simple piercing of the ear. Black persons are genetically predisposed to keloids. (Courtesy Dr. Clitus Olson.)*

("fiber makers"). The fibroblasts synthesize collagen fibers and scars form. Reparative mechanisms will be discussed after inflammatory processes are considered.

Acute Inflammation

Cornelius Celsus, a first century Roman, noted the four major signs of inflammation; *rubor et tumor cum calore et dolore* (redness and swelling with heat and pain). Many centuries later, the father of modern cellular pathology, Rudolph Virchow (1821–1902), added a fifth sign, *functio laesa* (disturbed function); an inflamed organ does not function properly. Whether all signs of inflammation occur depends on the site and extent of injury.

Inflammatory Cells   A dazzling array of changes in the distribution of blood plasma and cells is triggered by injury. Three major "actors" perform in this drama: (1) the *endothelium* lining venules, (2) *plasma proteins*, which passively leak through injured endothelium, and (3) white blood cells (WBCs), which actively travel to the site of injury

and engulf (phagocytose) particles (unwary bacteria, for example).

During inflammation, the following events transpire in sequence: (1) dilation of arterioles, (2) acceleration of blood flow through the arterioles, (3) slowing of the blood flow and engorgement of veins, (4) leakage of fluid (plasma) through the venule wall into surrounding tissues, (5) sticking of neutrophils to the venules, (6) emigration of neutrophils from the venules into the injured area (Fig. 5-2), and finally, (7) phagocytosis and killing of particles by neutrophils.

The foregoing cellular changes help us to understand the signs of inflammation: vasodilatation accounts for rubor (redness); increased blood flow yields calor (heat); and the exudation of fluid pro-

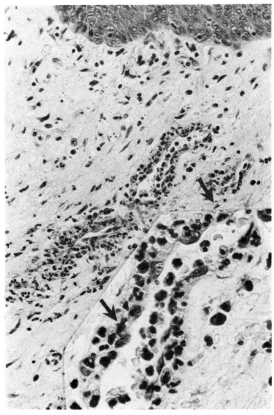

Figure 5-2 *Photomicrograph of acute inflammation. The venule in the center is being invaded by neutrophils. The tissue is separated by edema fluid (clear areas). The inset shows the neutrophils at higher magnification in the wall of the venule.*

duces the tumor (swelling). The pain and loss of function that often accompany inflammation are less well understood—pressure from fluid passing into a closed compartment may press and distort nerves and impair function. In summary, inflammation is divisible into three major events: (1) changes in vascular caliber and blood flow, (2) increased vascular permeability, and (3) infiltration of the tissues by neutrophils and other blood cells.

Edema   Edema (swelling of tissues) due to accumulation of fluid in tissues is always present to some degree in acute inflammation because fluid accumulates within hours following injury (Fig. 5-2). Edematous tissues are soft to touch; when healing has occurred and new connective tissue is produced, the injured site becomes firm.

How does fluid leave the vascular space and get into injured tissue? To answer this question, it is first necessary to examine the normal structure of endothelium (Fig. 5-2). Three types of endothelium are found in various organs: (1) *Continuous endothelium* is continuously attached around the periphery of each endothelial cell. It commonly lines the vessels of skin, muscle, brain, and lungs. (2) *Fenestrated endothelium* contains numerous holes (windows) in the cytoplasm. It is found in certain vessels that filter plasma, such as the glomerulus of kidneys and in endocrine and exocrine glands. (3) Finally, *discontinuous endothelium* has openings between cells and is found in splenic filter tissue and bone marrow.

Ordinarily, *continuous endothelium* filters the blood in most organs of our bodies. Fluid passes either directly across the endothelium itself by *pinocytosis* (microscopic sipping) or between endothelial junctions. Fluid leaks out of vessels when the opposing forces, consisting of (1) the *oncotic pressure* due to plasma proteins retaining water and (2) the force of blood pressure pushing fluid through the vessel walls, become unbalanced. *Edema* ensues when fluid flows from the vascular channels and accumulates in tissues.

A *transudate* forms when fluid passes through normal noninjured microcirculation. For instance, a transudate forms when a cuff, which obstructs the return of fluid in the lymphatics and veins, is

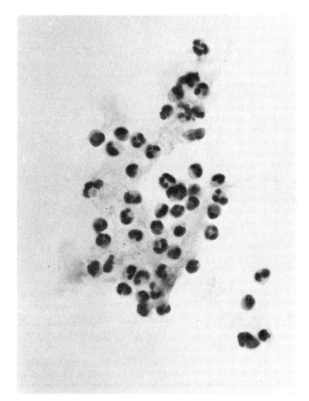

Figure 5-3   *Photomicrograph of exudate. The exudate is rich in neutrophils; protein in the exudate forms a hazy background.*

placed around a limb. This fluid contains only 0.2 to 0.5 gm of protein per 100 ml. Persons with heart failure often accumulate transudate (pleural fluid, for example) in their pleural cavities. In contrast, an *exudate* is a fluid richer in protein (4 to 5 gm of protein per 100 ml) that accumulates in various compartments in the body (chest, abdomen, or joints, for example) when vessels are inflamed. Often exudates are also rich in WBCs and cellular debris (Fig. 5-3).

Mechanism of Vascular Leakage

Either *direct injury* to the endothelium or *indirect histamine-type injury* elicits leakage of fluid from the microcirculation. It is fortunate that blood vessels leak when injury occurs; this process allows antibodies and phagocytes to flood the area and prevent infection from occurring.

Direct Vascular Injury   Leakage by *direct vascular injury* is easily understood. A burn or direct trauma (burns or razor cuts, for example) to an artery, capillary, or venule tears the wall of the blood vessel apart permitting fluid (plasma) to escape. Direct vascular injury can persist up to a day or more, or until the vessel is plugged by a thrombus or is repaired. The blood clotting system, the platelets and plasma clotting factors, forms a fibrin clot (thrombus) which blocks small leaks in the microcirculation, thus preventing hemorrhage and loss of fluid (see Chapter 11, Hematology).

A common example of direct injury is sunburn. On the evening following a day of exposure to the bright sun, the damaged microcirculation in the exposed skin leaks fluid from venules. It is critical for individuals treating patients with ultraviolet light to recognize that a "minimal erythemal dose" (the time of ultraviolet light exposure required to induce minimal redness) can, if extended, damage endothelial cells of venules and cause injury and edema.

Indirect   Histamine-type   Vascular   Leakage   *Histamine-type vascular leakage* takes place when histamine and a variety of chemical *mediators* are released from tissue mast cells during injury and cause venules to leak. Among the mediators capable of this action are histamine, serotonin, and bradykinin. Histamine vascular leakage is transient (15–30 minutes) and affects primarily the venules. Almost all of the mediators cause actin contractile filaments in the endothelial lining cells of venules to contract. Hence, they may pull away from each other (Fig. 5-4).

Histamine-type leakage is commonly seen in allergic conditions (hives, for example). Histamine is stored in all persons within tissue mast cells; but in sensitized persons, these cells are coated by antibodies (against ragweed pollen, for example). Histamine spills from the mast cells into the tissues surrounding blood vessels when antigen (ragweed pollen, for example) reacts with antibody coating mast cells. The histamine, which diffuses onto the surface of the venules, causes the actin to contract. Plasma fluid then passes from the blood vessel into the tissues, producing edema, swelling, and itching

(see Chapter 6, Immunology). To a certain extent the mechanical disruption of mast cells occurring during a direct injury to tissues also contributes to the leakage.

Types of Inflammatory Exudates

An exudate results from the passage of both fluid and neutrophils from the vascular space into an extravascular compartment (Fig. 5-3). Exudates contain varying concentrations of cells and proteins. An inflammatory lesion dominated by fluid is termed *serous;* if large amounts of fibrin and fibrinogen are present, *fibrinous;* or if blood is prominent, *hemorrhagic.* Generally most of the common acute inflammatory reactions contain large numbers of neutrophils and are termed *suppurative.*

The following are examples of clinical conditions in which these exudates occur: (1) Mild vascular injury is responsible for a *serous exudate,* and thus, cells do not pass through the endothelial spaces. (2) A *purulent exudate* arises from a large concentration of neutrophils as provoked by nearby bacteria. Certain bacteria are called pyogenic (pus-forming) organisms. For example, staphylococci can cause an extensive neutrophilic infiltrate (exudate) in the chest cavity, a condition termed *empyema.* (3) Severe injury to endothelium results in a *hemorrhagic exudate* rich in red blood cells. (4) A *fibrinous exudate* is characteristically seen on moist serous surfaces of the heart (pericardium) and lungs (pleura). A white coat of fibrin develops when blood plasma seeps onto these surfaces. Thus a firm, rigid encasement forms restricting the action of the heart or lungs. Individuals with profound uremia due to renal failure may develop fibrinous pericarditis (Fig. 5-5).

Chronic Inflammation

Acute inflammation gradually subsides and chronic inflammation and reparative processes ensue. The term *chronic inflammation* refers to a condition prolonged beyond two weeks. A persistent infection may result in a chronic condition that may last for a lifetime, but chronic inflammation can occur without a preceding acute inflammation. Regard-

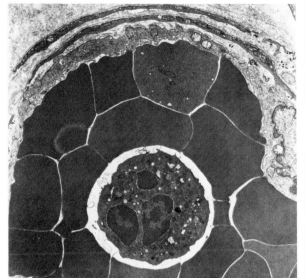

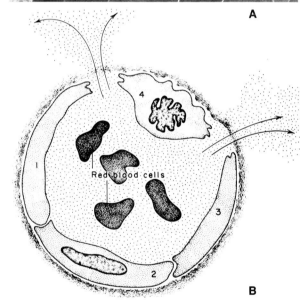

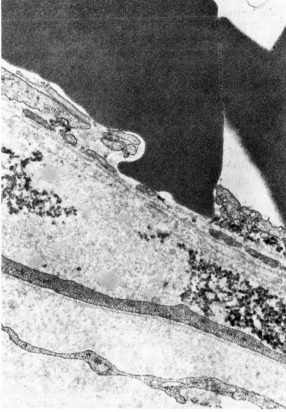

Figure 5-4   A, *Electron micrograph of cross section of normal venule. A neutrophil is surrounded by dark erythrocytes. × 10,500.* **B,** *Cross section of venule showing histamine-type vascular leakage. The endothelial cells undergo muscular contraction from histamine stimulation, and the cells pull away from each other. × 5000. (Courtesy Dr. Guido Majno and Harvard University Press.)* **C,** *Electron micrograph of wall of venule stimulated to contract by histamine. Particles of India ink are seen leaking through gaps between endothelial cells, which have pulled apart by the contraction. × 30,000. (Courtesy Dr. Isabelle Joris.)*

less of the condition leading to chronic inflammation, it results from a response to foreign bodies or sensitization of lymphocytes to foreign proteins (antigens). These antigens are processed by macrophages in regional lymph nodes. There, new sensitized lymphocytes are formed that subsequently travel to the site of the antigens and form a chronic inflammatory response. Most chronic inflammatory reactions contain mononuclear cells (lymphocytes, plasma cells, and macrophages) rather than neutrophils. This subject is discussed in detail in Chapter 6, Immunology.

Anti-inflammatory Drugs

Anti-inflammatory drugs, aspirin and aspirinlike drugs (indomethacin, phenylbutazone), and steroids such as cortisone and prednisolone decrease inflammatory responses. Aspirin and aspirinlike drugs inhibit the synthesis of certain prostaglandins, hormones active in inflammation. Likewise, steroid hormones stabilize lysosomal membranes in neutrophils and prevent them from liberating their enzymes into tissues.

Inflammation in Special Sites

Abscess   An *abscess* is a confined collection of pus (neutrophils and necrotic tissues, for example) and is surrounded by a wall of proliferating fibroblasts that produce collagen. The introduction of a bacterium, foreign object, or necrotic tissue deep within an organ or tissue provokes neutrophils to move into the site and surround these objects. In the process of healing, an abscess may resolve by rupturing through a surface and discharge its pus. Alternatively, gradual resorption of the pus and proliferation of fibroblasts may close the space, leaving a scar.

Cellulitis   Cellulitis is a special inflammatory reaction which generally results from a beta hemolytic streptococcus infection. This streptococcus infection produces proteolytic enzymes (collagenase and hyaluronidase, for example) and invades the tissue, penetrating in a linear direction. Cellulitis dissects through spaces and passes along fascial surfaces. The fascia are natural barriers against infection (see Chapter 7, Infectious Diseases).

Granulomatous Inflammation   Granulomatous inflammation is a special type of chronic inflammation composed of lymphocytes and macrophages (see Chapter 6, Immunology). It can be due to an immune response to foreign protein *(antigens)* or to foreign nonorganic bodies, such as glass. Classically, a granulomatous immune response occurs in a sensitized person (delayed-type hypersensitivity) to protein of the *Mycobacterium tuberculosis*, bacillus. Numerous lymphocytes, macrophages, and giant cells occur in this response and central caseous (cheeselike) necrosis is seen as a hallmark of this inflammatory response (see Chapter 7, Infectious Diseases).

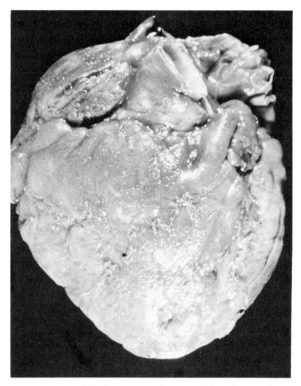

Figure 5-5   *Fibrinous exudate coating the surface of the heart from a patient with uremia.*

A second type of granulomatous inflammation enlists the same cells and eliminates foreign bodies or particles. *Foreign body granulomatous response* is similar in appearance to granulomatous inflammation, but the multinucleated giant cells respond to foreign particles rather than protein antigens of bacteria. Oftentimes, giant cells can be seen surrounding and engulfing the foreign material (Fig. 5-6).

Local and Regional Effects   The inflammatory reaction causes damage at the site of inflammation. This is a small price to pay for survival. Damage can occur, for instance, when extensive stasis of blood flow occurs and the tissues become oxygen starved and die. Likewise, infiltrating neutrophils may be destructive because they release enzymes (collagenase and elastase, for example) capable of digesting collagen and elastic fibers. For example, when the glomeruli in the kidneys are inflamed

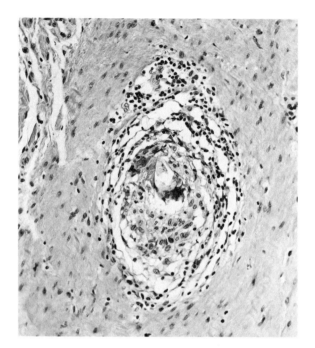

Figure 5-6 *Photomicrograph of foreign body granulomatous inflammatory response. A multinucleated giant cell has engulfed a piece of glass (center).*

(acute glomerulonephritis), the enzymes escaping from neutrophils damage the glomeruli, and protein leaks from blood into urine.

Also, when the healing process attempts to restore an organ following an exudate, a fibrinous exudate may "glue" together adjacent surfaces (fibrinous pericarditis, for example, Fig. 5-5). Moreover, adjacent surfaces of joints can become fused.

Bacteria, necrotic tissue, and neutrophils may drain into regional lymph nodes. The lymphatic channels may become inflamed and infected, and a red streak may be noted along the arm, hence *lymphangitis* occurs. Lymphadenitis develops when the lymph node draining the inflamed lymphatic vessel becomes infected. In addition, systemic signs may arise as a result of the release of *pyrogens* (fever generators) from neutrophils and leukocytosis (increased WBC) may occur.

Systemic Effects The vital signs (heart rate, respiratory rate, and temperature) generally in-

crease as a result of infection and thus provide clues to the cause of the underlying infection or inflammatory responses to an infection. Fever, an abnormally high body temperature (usually greater than 37.8 C), and leukocytosis, an abnormally high WBC count, are characteristic responses to inflammation. Likewise, an increased erythrocyte sedimentation rate (ESR) is noted. In the ESR the erythrocytes more rapidly sediment to the bottom of a tube in persons suffering from inflammatory conditions. An increase in plasma proteins can be responsible for the increased ESR in inflammation.

The normal body temperature is approximately 37 C. The temperature regulatory center is located just above the pituitary gland, in the hypothalamus. This thermostat can be offset by the release of pyrogens—blood vessels in the skin constrict and shivering chills commence. Neutrophils and macrophages release pyrogens when they phagocytose bacteria or cellular debris and are exposed to other stimuli such as antigens and antibody complexes. Fever is probably beneficial; it may enhance immune responses and increase the flow of blood; thus, more WBCs and antibodies are carried to damaged or infected tissue. Further, mobilization of noncirculating WBCs from the bone marrow, spleen, and other organs provides additional neutrophils to the inflammatory response.

Leukocytes and Inflammation

The neutrophils and macrophages are *phagocytic* cells, which fight against infectious agents. During inflammation, neutrophils stick to the walls of blood vessels and then emigrate toward the injured site in the tissues. They move slowly toward bacteria (Fig. 5-7) or damaged cells. The process directing their movement is termed *chemotaxis*. In unknown ways the neutrophils respond to tissue antigens-antibodies and fragments of serum complement (see Chapter 6, Immunology). Thus, the process of chemotaxis prompts neutrophils to invade the site of injury.

Phagocytosis (engulfment) and killing of the offending agent then occurs (see Chapter 7, Infectious Diseases). The process of passage of blood cells across the walls of veins is *diapedesis*. Neutrophils pass through interendothelial junctions within 2 to 12 minutes. In the early stages of acute inflammation, neutrophils predominate (Fig. 5-4), especially in the first six hours; and thereafter, mononuclear phagocytes appear and predominate.

Phagocytosis   The major goal of acute inflammation is disposing of dead cells and killing of invading bacteria. Cellular eating (phagocytosis) was discovered by a Russian, Élie Metchnikoff, approximately one century ago. Neutrophils and mononuclear phagocytes (monocytes) most avidly phagocytose material. In their cytoplasm, these cells contain numerous granules rich in lysosomal enzymes. Likewise, glycogen, the major source of energy for these active cells, is plentiful. Glycogen provides fuel for metabolism in the damaged oxygen-deprived tissues in which certain bacteria like to grow.

Three phases of phagocytosis are (1) *attachment* of particles to the surface of the cell and (2) *ingestion* of material in small sacs, termed *phagosomes*, by the leukocytes. The phagocyte extends pseudopods (footlike processes) that attach to the bacteria. These feet form a vacuole, termed a *phagosome*, around the particle. (3) *Destruction* of the material occurs when the phagosomes fuse with lysosomes, forming phagolysomes; enzymes then digest the particles (see Chapter 6, Immunology). Large quantities of hydrogen peroxide (H_2O_2) and acid are produced in the cell; and various enzymes, including myeloperoxidase, assist iodine, bromide, and chloride in binding tightly to the bacterial cell wall to kill them.

The bacteria are easily recognized and phagocytosed by neutrophils after an antibody (*opsonin*) reacts with the bacteria coating it. This antibody coating process (*opsonization*) enables the phagocyte to vigorously engulf the particle. Also specific antibodies against antigens on the bacteria bind serum complement and enhance phagocytosis.

Impairment of Neutrophil Function   Many clinical disorders impair neutrophil function. A decreased number of circulating neutrophils is termed *neutropenia*. This condition commonly oc-

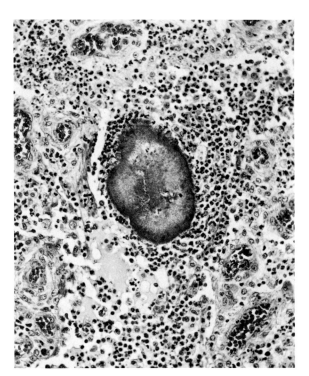

Figure 5-7   *Photomicrograph showing neutrophils surrounding a colony of bacteria. Chemotaxis directed the neutrophil to the bacteria.*

curs in leukemia or can be induced by toxic drugs. Likewise, *disorders of migration* and of *chemotaxis* occasionally occur. Metabolic diseases, such as diabetes mellitus, malnutrition, and acute alcoholism, depress the migration (locomotion) of neutrophils and killing of bacteria. Deficiencies in serum complement or opsonizing antibodies can also impair neutrophil function and phagocytosis. These disorders all make the person vulnerable to infection.

Lysosomal Disorders   Certain diseases are partly due to an excessive release of lysosomes from neutrophils. These released enzymes destroy tissues. Best known examples are *gout* and *silicosis*. In gout, sodium urate crystals (uric acid) deposit in and around joints. Neutrophils phagocytize the crystals and lysosomes fuse with the phagosomes forming phagolysosomes. The phagolysosomes rupture allowing enzymes to spill into the tissues and thereby causing damage (see Chapter 12, Endocrine and

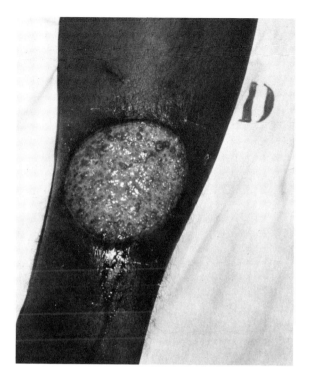

Figure 5-8   *Granulation tissue healing over an ulcer of the leg. The ulcer has a granular surface. Note the serum exuding from the wound.*

Metabolic Disorders). Silicosis occurs in some persons who grind stones or mine coal. The lungs become damaged when lysosomes are ruptured by the silica spicules that they have phagocytosed. The enzymes destroy pulmonary tissue.

Repair

Granulation Tissue

The repair of wounds occurs initially by the formation of granulation tissue. On gross inspection, granulation tissue has a granular red appearance (Fig. 5-8). Granulation tissue is red because it contains numerous capillaries, which bud from nearby surviving blood vessels. It is composed of proliferating fibroblasts, capillaries, neutrophils, fibrin, and cellular debris.

When tissue is lost, for instance, in a cut or when an epithelial surface is lost (ulcerated), new tissue

is formed and temporarily covers this defect (Fig. 5-8). Epithelial cells grow from the cut margins and slide over the surface of the granulation to fill the defect (Fig. 5-9). Granulation tissue forms proliferating fibroblasts, capillaries grow outward from blood vessel walls, and other larger vessels form. Later, the new vessels become wider and acquire thick walls. Meanwhile, the macrophages and neutrophils clean up the debris and fibrin.

The remarkable contraction of wounds occurs because the granulation tissue contains *myofibroblasts*, or newly formed fibroblasts, which are rich in actin filaments and capable of contracting (Fig. 5-10). Myofibroblasts pull the margins of the wound together enabling the wound to close. At about four or five days following the injury, newly formed collagen is deposited by the fibroblasts. By three or four weeks, approximately two-thirds of the maximal strength of the wound is achieved.

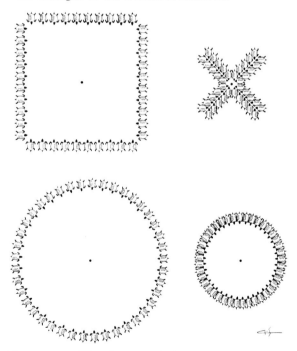

Figure 5-9   *The shape and size of a wound determine how efficiently it heals. This "turtle" model illustrates perhaps why a square wound heals more efficiently than a round wound. The squamous cells in contact monitor the speed of their growth. (Courtesy of Dr. Guido Majno and Harvard University Press.)*

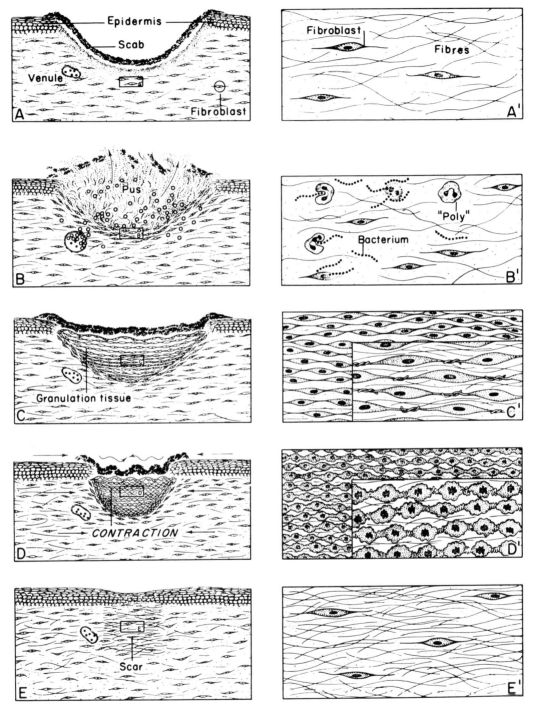

Figure 5-10   *Stages in the healing of a wound as seen through the microscope. The column at the right shows details of the figure at the left. Myofibroblasts are seen contracting in* **D.** *(Courtesy Dr. Guido Majno and Harvard University Press.)*

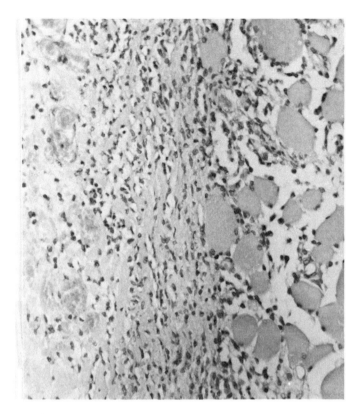

Figure 5-11 *Photomicrograph showing growing fibroblasts forming a wound. Between the cells, collagen fibers are being deposited. Skeletal muscle fibers are seen on cross section at the right.*

When at the outset the edges of the wound are approximated by artificial means, such as sutures, the process of healing is speeded and is said to have occurred by *primary or first intention*. The apposition of the wound simply reduces the size of the cavity that the granulation tissue must fill. When the healing is by *secondary intention*, the wound heals on its own from the base upward until the defect is filled in with new granulation tissue. Slowly the wound contracts and pulls the margins together. The surface becomes epithelialized as the epithelial cells move to cover the wound (Fig. 5-11). In other organs (kidney or liver, for example) if the fine supporting reticulin network is maintained, the epithelial cells can regenerate into the network. If the network is destroyed, collagen forms excessively and the liver can become fibrotic.

Complications

Many complications result when interference with wound healing occurs. The wound may become gangrenous if the blood supply is inadequate, leading to massive death of tissues. The wound may spread when it is infected; excessive formation of granulation tissue can occur (Fig. 5-12). Most of the complications of wound healing are caused by bacterial infection of the wound.

The shape of the wound determines how efficiently the wound will close; for instance, a square-shaped defect in the skin is able to close more effectively than a round lesion. Adjacent epithelial cells in a round lesion transmit pressure in an outward fashion; thus resistance to closure of the defect occurs. The maximal size of defect of skin that can regenerate without skin grafting is approximately the size of a 50¢ piece.

Inflammation and repair can be a two-edged sword: (1) it prevents invasion by bacteria and other infectious agents, and it heals damaged tissue; (2) but the inflammatory response per se can destroy tissues, as for instance, in immune complex disease of the kidney in which neutrophils infiltrate the kidney and release enzymes causing destruction

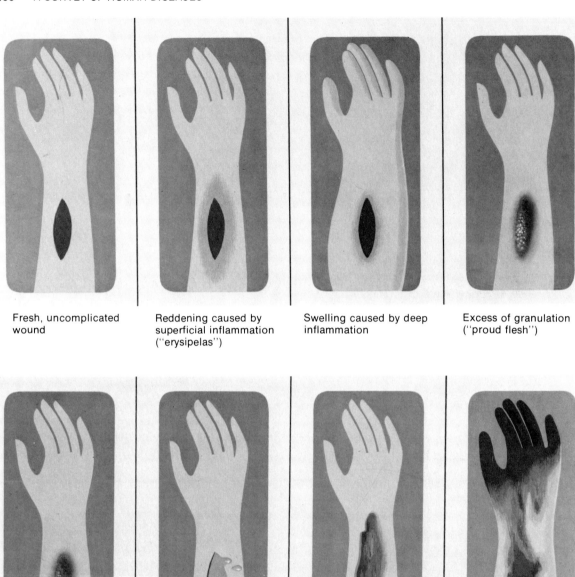

| Fresh, uncomplicated wound | Reddening caused by superficial inflammation ("erysipelas") | Swelling caused by deep inflammation | Excess of granulation ("proud flesh") |

| Excess of granulation ("pround flesh") | Suppuration | Spreading ulcer | Gangrene |

Figure 5-12   *Six major complications that can occur in a wound. The majority of these complications results from bacterial infection. (Courtesy Dr. Guido Majno and the Harvard University Press.)*

(see Chapter 6, Immunology). Likewise, a variety of chronic inflammatory conditions can cause severe permanent scars and contractures. In contractures, a shortening in the normal length of a tissue occurs.

Scarring and contractures can occur in organs such as liver. For example, in chronic liver disease (cirrhosis), granulation tissue, fibrosis, and regenerative nodules produce a shrunken liver as a result of the contracting granulation tissue (Fig. 5-13). Likewise, chronic "endstage" renal disease occurs from extensive scars; renal function becomes defective.

Inflammation and repair of the lining of the heart (endocardium) from rheumatic fever shortens and deforms the cords that restrain the heart valves (Fig. 5-14). Likewise, fibrosis of the palmar fascia (*Dupuytren's contracture*) can result in severe contractures of the palmar fascia in the hands. Contractures can result from burns over the forearm flexors at the elbow and in the hands when scars form.

Range of motion exercises are given to patients who have injuries in or over joints to maintain normal joint function. Also anti-inflammatory agents, such as cortisone, are occasionally given to impair the formation of collagen and prevent disfiguring scars.

Factors that Modify Healing

The presence of *foreign bodies* impedes healing because these foreign bodies form mechanical barriers. Immobilization of healing wounds is necessary, especially in fractured bones (see Chapter 20, Diseases of Muscles, Bones, and Joints). *Advanced age* slows the formation of collagen by fibroblasts; elderly patients tend to heal more slowly than children.

Nutritional status is important to the healing process; vitamin C, for instance, is important in the formation of collagen. Scurvy (see Chapter 10, Nutritional Diseases) is caused by a deficiency of vitamin C. Scorbutic individuals have poor healing of wounds.

An *adequate blood supply* to a wound is necessary to enable inflammation and repair to proceed normally. Likewise, an *intact immune system* with functioning neutrophils which clean up dead cells and lymphocytes and plasma cells which defend against

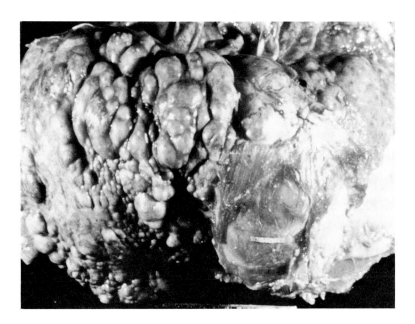

Figure 5-13 *Cirrhosis of the liver. Scars are seen in deep crevices between the regenerative modules.*

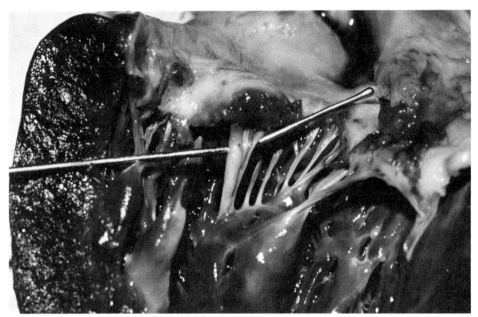

Figure 5-14 *A heart damaged by rheumatic fever. The heart valve and chordae tendineae have been deformed by scar tissue. A probe passes beneath a cord. This heart valve became incompetent (leaked) and was later infected by bacteria.*

bacteria are necessary. Finally, the *excessive* use of *antibiotics* and *corticosteroids* can impair the healing process.

It is unfortunate that many patients requiring surgery have one or more conditions that impair inflammatory responses and healing (malnutrition and poor blood supply associated with aging). Hence, these persons often develop postoperative wound infections and wound healing is slowed. For this reason preoperative care is very important to prepare the patient for optimal inflammation and repair of surgical wounds.

Summary

When tissues are injured, mast cells quickly release mediators that cause vasodilatation and vascular leakage. The mast cells, when injured, sound the alarm to the endothelial cells of blood vessels. Histamine is the major mediator released by the mast cells which causes endothelial cells to contract. The endothelial cells separate and hence, blood plasma and inflammatory cells leak out. The leukocytes phagocytize bacteria and mop up cellular debris during acute inflammation. Later lymphocytes may come in and provide chronic inflammation. Mediators (pyrogens) are also released into the circulation and cause systemic effects such as fever. If the irritant persists, the process will become chronic. Otherwise, the process settles down and repair ensues.

The formation of granulation tissue composed of proliferating fibroblasts, capillaries, neutrophils, and cellular debris is essential to repair and wound healing. Granulation tissue covers wounds and growing epithelial cells glide over the surface to cover the defect. Fibroblasts in granulation tissue contain contractile protein and cause wounds to contract. They also produce collagen which gives scars strength. Wounds can become complicated by excessive scar formation to produce keloids or contractures. Many factors can impair wound healing.

Bibliography

Fisher, E. R. 1969. Repair by regeneration. In *Pathology annual*, ed., S. C. Sommers. New York: Appleton-Century Crofts. Describes regeneration of tissues.

Florey, H. W., ed. 1970. *General pathology.* Philadelphia: W. B. Saunders Company. A standard textbook discussing cellular pathology.

Hurley, J. V. 1972. *Acute inflammation.* Baltimore: The Williams & Wilkins Company. Describes acute aspects of inflammation.

Lepow, I. H., and Ward, P. S., eds. 1972. *Inflammation.* New York: Academic Press. Monograph summarizing inflammation.

Macleod, A. G. 1973. *Aspects of acute inflammation.* Kalamazoo: Upjohn Company. A beautifully illustrated concise monograph.

Majno, G. 1975. *The healing hand.* Cambridge: Harvard University Press. The history of wound healing in the ancient world is described in detail and depicted with artistic clarity.

Panner, B. J., and Orbison, J. L. 1973. *Chronic inflammation and healing.* Kalamazoo: Upjohn Company. A concise monograph depicting various types of chronic inflammatory processes.

Purtilo, D. T., and Connor, D. H. 1975. Fatal infections in protein-calorie malnourished children with thymolymphatic atrophy. *Arch. Dis. Child.* 50:149–152. Atrophy of the thymus and immune system caused by undernutrition can render persons vulnerable to fatal infectious diseases.

Ryan, G. B., Majno, G. 1977. *Inflammation.* Kalamazoo: Upjohn Company. Current, concise, and beautifully illustrated 80-page monograph.

Zweifach, B. W.; Grant, L.; and McCluskey, R. T., eds. 1965. *The inflammatory process.* New York: Academic Press. A scholarly presentation.

Immunology

Chapter Outline

Objectives

After reading this chapter you should be able to

Identify the organs of the immune system.

Compare characteristics of B-lymphocytes and T-lymphocytes.

Describe the two key attributes of immunity.

Define the terms antigen and antibody.

Compare humoral and cellular immunity.

List the functions of T-lymphocytes.

Know what type of cell is produced in germinal centers.

Describe the chemical subunits of an immunoglobulin molecule.

List the five classes of immunoglobulins.

Compare the functions of the various classes of immunoglobulins.

Describe the origin and structure of the thymus gland.

Know the relative frequency of primary and secondary immunodeficiency.

List the six most common primary immunodeficiency syndromes of children.

Define the DiGeorge syndrome.

Describe the inheritance and method of treatment of agammaglobulinemia.

Name the most common primary immunodeficiency.

List common causes of acquired immunodeficiency.

Describe the immune response occurring during tetanus vaccination.

Distinguish between a primary and secondary (anamnestic) immune response.

Discuss the mechanisms whereby humoral immunity becomes amplified.

Define the function of serum complement.

Describe the process of opsonization.

List the four hypersensitivity responses responsible for diseases.

Define the term immediate hypersensitivity.

Describe the mechanism whereby histamine is liberated from mast cells.

List the pathologic findings seen in bronchi of asthmatic patients.

List the clinical symptoms induced by histamine released during acute anaphylaxis.

Recognize that hives result from localized anaphylaxis.

Define and give one example of cytotoxic hypersensitivity.

Describe how immune complexes injure tissues.

List four diseases caused by immune complexes.

Describe the function of serum complement and neutrophils in inducing tissue injury in immune complex diseases.

List clinical findings of serum sickness.

Name the reaction responsible for most hypersensitivity diseases of the lung.

Define the term autoimmunity.

Describe the typical clinical features of systemic lupus erythematosus.

List the laboratory tests aiding in the diagnosis of systemic lupus erythematosus.

Name the organ which, when involved by systemic lupus erythematosus, usually signals a poor prognosis.

Define rheumatoid arthritis.

Define the terms rheumatoid factor and pannus.

Compare cell-mediated immunity with humoral immunity.

Describe the events transpiring when a tubercle bacillum enters the lung of an unsensitized person.

Define the term granuloma. What does it signify?

Know the potential consequences of depressed cellular immunity.

List factors causing immunosuppression.

Define the term histocompatibility antigen.

Define first-set rejection of a transplant.

Compare hypersensitivity reactions occurring in first- and second-set rejection reactions.

Define immunologic surveillance.

List evidence for immunologic surveillance.

Define the clinical use for carcinoembryonic antigen and α-fetoprotein.

Introduction

Consider for a moment that although we live in a sea of microorganisms, we survive. The immune system defends us against invasion by microorganisms and malignancy. When our immunity is *hypoactive* (underactive), we are said to be immunodeficient. The immunodeficient person is easily invaded by microorganisms and malignancy. Paradoxically, when the immune system becomes *hyperactive* (overactive), immunologic diseases of hypersensitivity, such as allergies, occur.

Specific recognition of nonself (foreign infectious agents and malignancy) and *memory* for nonself are the two key attributes of immunity. The protection afforded us by an immune response to microorganisms permits survival. We rarely suffer twice from the same infectious disease (mumps or chickenpox, for example). Protection is provided by antibodies evoked in response to *antigens* (foreign objects or microorganisms capable of stimulating lymphoid cells to generate *antibodies*). Combination of antigen with antibody leads to the elimination of the antigen. *Memory* for the antigens persists because lymphocytes imprinted with the capacity to recognize an antigen live for many years. In this chapter, we will consider the basic function of the normal immune system and then we will discuss clinical immunology.

Anatomy of the Immune System

Immunity is provided by lymphoid cells residing in the immune system. This system is composed of central and peripheral lymphoid organs. The *central lymphoid organs* are the thymus gland and the bone marrow, and *peripheral lymphoid organs* are the tonsils, gut-associated lymphoid tissue, spleen, and lymph nodes (Fig. 6-1).

Lymphoid Cells

The lymphoid cells providing immunity include macrophages and two types of lymphocytes that arise from primitive stem cells in the embryo. They function together to eliminate antigens. *Macrophages* ("large eaters") can invade tissues and phagocytize particulate antigens. Within lymph nodes, macrophages prepare, or process, antigens so that lymphocytes can mount a specific immune response, which further eliminates the antigens. Some sensitized lymphocytes live for years retaining a memory for the antigen (Fig. 6-2).

The two types of lymphocytes providing immunity are designated T-lymphocytes and B-lymphocytes. When an antigen enters the body, two immunologic reactions can occur: (1) synthesis of *antibody* by B-lymphocytes (following cloning and maturation into plasma cells), which is released into the blood or body fluids, and (2) growth of new T-lymphocytes having receptors on their surfaces for the antigen. Often T- and B-lymphocytes respond simultaneously. Sensitized T-lymphocytes release special chemicals (lymphokines) on contact with an antigen, such as a microorganism. The lymphokines either directly kill the microorganism or amplify the immune response by recruiting macrophages and other nearby lymphocytes to amplify their response. B-lymphocytes, on stimulation by

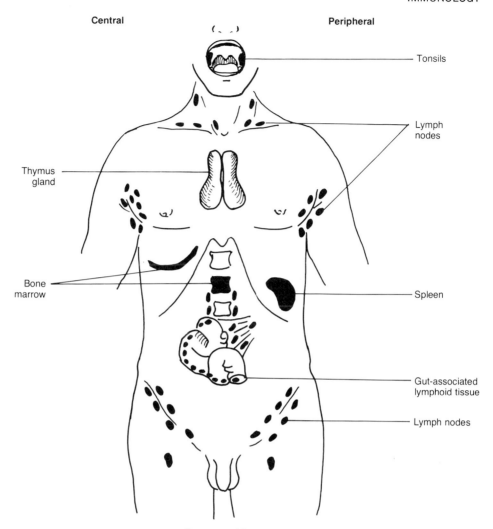

Figure 6-1   *Organs of immune system.*

an antigen, can mature to become plasma cells capable of producing antibodies. The immunity provided by antibodies is *humoral immunity*, and T-lymphocytes provide *cell-mediated immunity* (cell-bound immunity).

All lymphocytes recirculate from the blood to lymph nodes. Lymphocytes move from the tissues via lymphatic vessels, which then flow into the thoracic duct lymphatic, and are returned to the blood. Lymphocytes are either short-lived (weeks) or long-lived (years). The finding of damaged chromosomes in lymphocytes from victims of the Hiroshima and Nagasaki atomic bomb explosions dem-

onstrates that some lymphocytes survive 30 years or more. The long-lived cells have a "memory" imprinted against infectious agents that they have previously been exposed to. Memory cells make vaccination and prolonged immunity to infectious agents possible.

At this point in the chapter you are probably wondering where the designations T- and B-lymphocytes originate. The thymus gland controls a subpopulation of lymphocytes providing cell-mediated immunity (CMI), and therefore, the lymphocytes responsible for CMI are termed T-lymphocytes or thymus-derived lymphocytes. Humoral

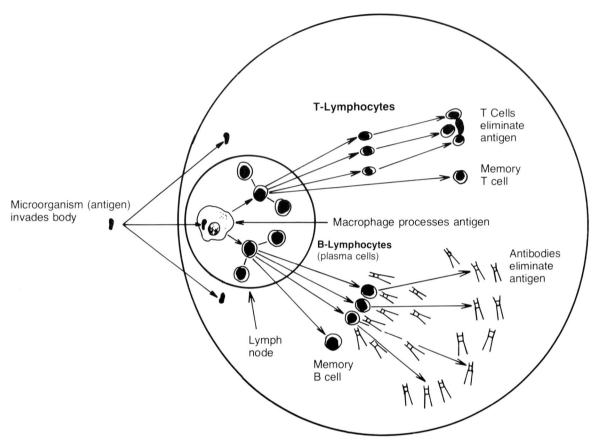

Figure 6-2   *Cooperation between macrophages, T-lymphocytes, and B-lymphocytes in mounting an immune response to antigen.*

immunity is mediated by antibodies formed by plasma cells that arise from B-lymphocytes following antigenic stimulation of these lymphocytes. The B-lymphocytes are named after the bursa, a lymphoid organ in chicks that contains lymphoid cells capable of forming antibodies. The equivalent to the bursa of chicks in human beings is probably the bone marrow (Fig. 6-3), and hence, the B-lymphocytes in mammals are bone marrow-derived.

T-Lymphocytes

T-lymphocytes are formed from primitive stem cells that have circulated through the thymus gland and are capable of (1) killing intracellular viruses, bacteria, and fungi; (2) rejecting transplanted organs; and (3) defending against cancer by providing

immunologic surveillance that eliminates cancer cells (Fig. 6-4). Following processing in the thymus gland, T cells circulate to special regions within the lymph nodes (paracortical) and spleen (periarterial), where they await challenge by antigens. Approximately two-thirds of lymphocytes circulating in the peripheral blood are T-lymphocytes, 15% are B-lymphocytes and uncommitted lymphocytes, termed *null cells* comprise the remaining lymphocytes.

B-Lymphocytes

As previously mentioned, B-lymphocytes were so named because studies in chicks revealed that B-lymphocytes arise in the chick bursa lymphoid organ. Following challenge by antigens, the sensi-

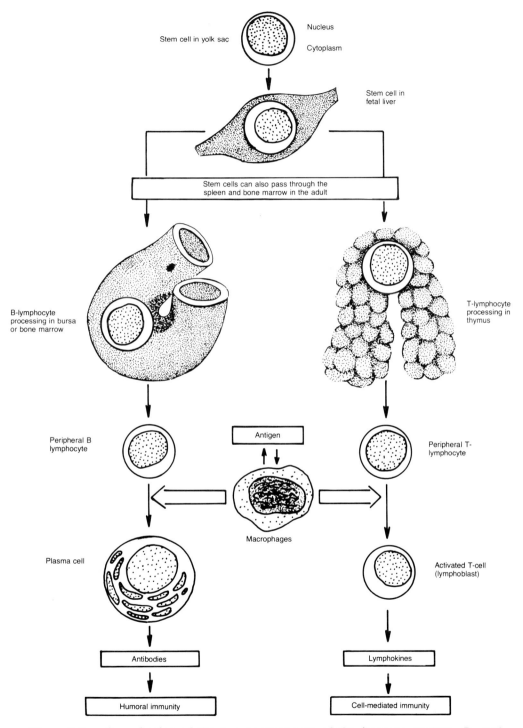

Figure 6-3   *Organization of the two components of the immune system: B- and T-lymphocytes respond to antigen processed by macrophages.*

Humoral immunity

1. Anaphylactic
2. Complex-mediated
3. Cytotoxic-type

Cellular immunity

1. Killing of intracellular microorganisms
2. Transplantation immunity
3. Immunologic surveillance

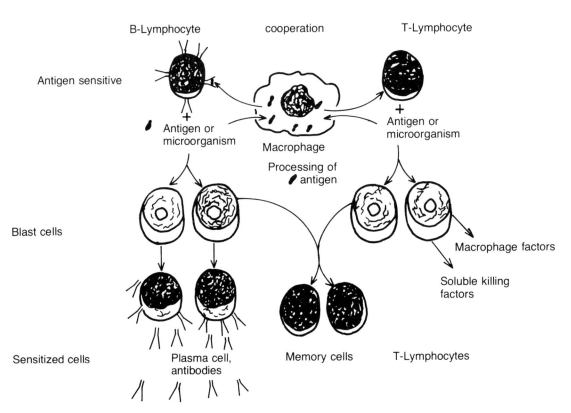

Figure 6-4   *Summary of functions and relationships between macrophages and T- and B-lymphocytes in mounting an immune response to an antigen.*

tized B-lymphocytes divide and mature into *plasma cells* that produce specific antibodies. B-lymphocytes in human beings probably arise from the bone marrow or lymphoid tissue in the gut. B-lymphocytes do not circulate through the thymus but pass directly from the bone marrow or gut to reside in special areas adjacent to T cells in the lymph nodes (in germinal centers and medulla), spleen (germinal centers and red pulp), and intestinal tract (germinal centers). In general, B-lymphocytes arise in germinal centers in lymphoid organs.

When B cells become stimulated by various antigens, they mature into plasma cells capable of

producing antibodies against an antigen (Fig. 6-4). The antibodies are proteins that are synthesized on endoplasmic reticulum membranes in the cytoplasm of plasma cells. These antibodies (immunoglobulins) circulate in the blood or coat mucous membranes. Antibody-synthesizing plasma cells are capable of producing only one immunoglobulin at a time.

The antibody molecule, or immunoglobulin, consists of four polypeptide (small units of protein) chains: two heavy chains (H-chains) and two light chains (L-chains) linked together to form an immunoglobulin molecule.

There are *five classes of immunoglobulins:* immunoglobulin G (IgG), IgA, IgM, IgD, and IgE. Specific heavy chains of each immunoglobulin molecule determines its specific class. That is, portions of the H-chains of all IgM molecules are identical.

Special functions are served by each class of immunoglobulin. *IgG* is the only immunoglobulin capable of passing the placenta to protect the fetus. Also, it is present in serum in greatest concentration and helps to defend against bacteria and other microbes. *IgM* is the largest immunoglobulin molecule and helps to destroy some viruses and other microbes. It is the first immunoglobulin to appear in the serum in a primary immune response following antigenic challenge. *IgA* is secreted not only into the blood but also onto mucosal surfaces lining the respiratory, gastrointestinal, and genitourinary tracts. It prevents invasion of these organs by microbes.

The remaining two classes of immunoglobulin are less well understood. *IgD* is present in low concentrations in serum but is commonly found on the surface of B-lymphocytes; perhaps it serves as a receptor for antigens. *IgE,* or reaginic antibody, is important in allergic diseases. It is present in serum in very low concentrations, and its normal function remains unknown.

Development

The primitive stem cells of the blood appear first in the yolk sac of the embryo (Fig. 6-3). These stem cells give rise to all blood cells, including lymphocytes. The *human thymus gland* grows from pharyngeal pouches in the embryo's neck region commencing at eight weeks of gestation. The epithelial lining of the pouches becomes *Hassall's* corpuscles in the thymus and is the source of an important hormone, *thymosin,* which somehow maintains T cell function. Lymphocytes migrate into the thymus gland and surround the corpuscles (Figs. 6-3 and 6-5). The ability of T-lymphocytes to respond to antigenic stimuli is well developed by 12 weeks gestation in the fetus. Therefore, the fetus has the immune capacity to defend itself in utero. The B-lymphocytes also function early in fetal life. However, because the fetus is in a protected environment, antibodies are not formed; instead, IgG antibodies pass through the placenta from the mother's blood to the fetus to provide passive immunity, thereby protecting the fetus against infection. Antibodies (immunoglobulins) are synthesized by the newborn immediately on exposure to antigens. During the first 3 months of life, the baby is protected by the mother's IgG antibodies, which were received in utero.

Immunodeficiency

Primary Immunodeficiency

Rarely, children are born with a *primary immunodeficiency disease* (Fig. 6-6). The primary immunodeficiencies arise usually from an inherited lack of development of one or more components of the immune system. The earliest and most devastating immune defect is bone marrow *stem-cell deficiency.* In stem-cell deficiency, extrauterine survival is impossible, and fatal infections ensue within days of birth. In another immunodeficiency, the *DiGeorge syndrome,* the thymus gland does not develop. T-lymphocytes are lacking, and the infant is highly susceptible to intracellular microorganisms (viruses, tuberculosis, and fungi, for example). Children with the DiGeorge syndrome have normal B-lymphocytes and form antibodies. These children also suffer from hypoparathyroidism because the parathyroid gland fails to develop from pharyngeal pouches in the neck of the embryo. Transplantation of a thymus gland can restore their T-lymphocyte immunity.

Likewise, a selective deficiency of B-lymphocytes can occur resulting in *agammaglobulinemia* (absence of immunoglobulins). It often has a sex-linked recessive hereditary transmission. Only 50% of boys born of mothers who carry the defective genes are affected; girls are unaffected but 50% may carry the defective gene on their X chromosome and transmit it to one-half of their male offspring (see Chapter 9, Inherited Disorders). The affected boys lack B cells and immunoglobulins (Fig. 6-7). Persons with agammaglobulinemia are

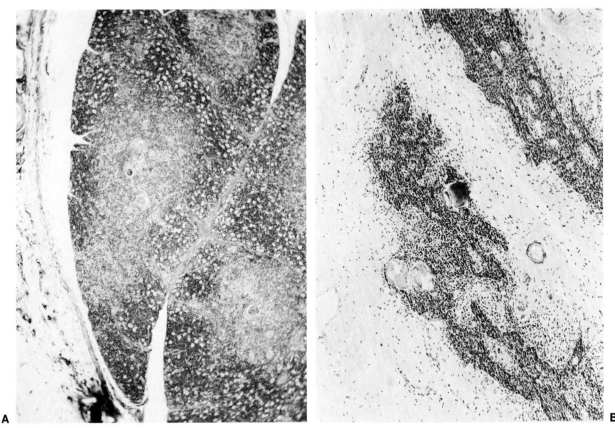

Figure 6-5   A, *Photomicrograph of normal thymus gland showing the cortex* (outer part) *composed of numerous small lymphocytes. The medullary portion contains Hassall's corpuscles of squamous epithelium, which produces thymosin, a hormone that maintains T cell function.* **B,** *Photomicrograph of thymus from child with immunodeficiency. The lymphocytes are nearly absent, only connective tissue remains.*

susceptible to bacterial infections. Lifelong gammaglobulin injections (containing antibodies) are required to maintain and protect these children.

The most common immune deficiency is a *selective deficiency of IgA*, which occurs in 1 out of 400 persons. Individuals with IgA immunodeficiency can occasionally develop chronic respiratory infections (chronic sinusitis, for example). They lack the immune defense provided by IgA antibodies, which inactivate microorganisms attempting to invade the respiratory tract. It should be noted that most persons with IgA deficiency have no recognizable symptoms. Subtle *selective T cell deficiencies* can also occur (Fig. 6-6). The child whose atrophic thymus is shown in Figure 6-5,B had an X-linked recessive inherited T-lymphocyte deficiency to the

Epstein-Barr virus. About 50% of the boys in his family died of infectious mononucleosis, which is caused by this virus. Otherwise, the boys were able to defend against many other infectious agents.

Secondary Immunodeficiencies

Acquired (secondary) *immunodeficiencies* occur *much more frequently* than primary immunodeficiency. A temporary acquired immunodeficiency results from many factors that suppress immune responses. Profound immunodeficiency is seen in *malnourished* persons. Individuals receiving *cortisone* or other *cytotoxic drugs* or *extensive radiotherapy*, victims of extensive *burns* or *malignancy*, or persons immunosuppressed for transplantation acquire im-

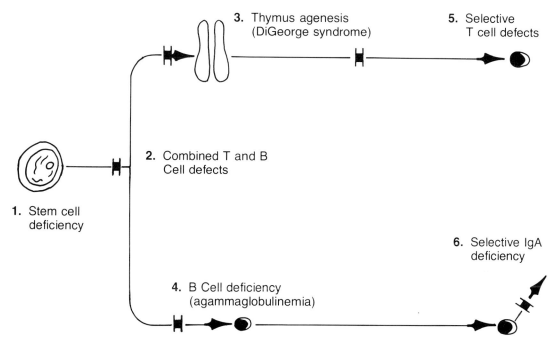

3. Thymus agenesis
(DiGeorge syndrome)

5. Selective
T cell defects

2. Combined T and B
Cell defects

1. Stem cell
deficiency

6. Selective IgA
deficiency

4. B Cell deficiency
(agammaglobulinemia)

Figure 6-6   *Primary immunodeficiency diseases. The blocks in the development of the immune system are shown by the interrupted lines at various stages in the development of the immune system.*

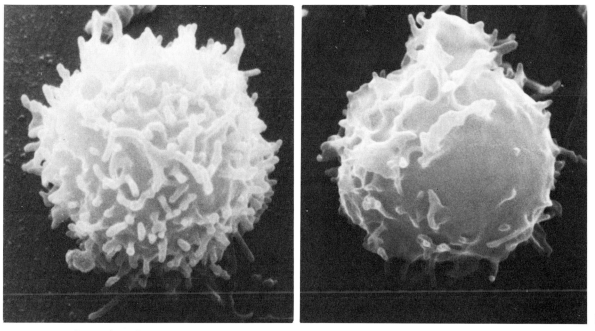

A   B

Figure 6-7   *Scanning electron photomicrograph of normal lymphocyte showing stubby microvilli* (left) *and abnormal lymphocyte from a boy with agammaglobulinemia showing bald spots and ruffles rather than microvilli on the surface of his lymphocyte* (right). × 10,000. *The patient had the X-linked lymphoproliferative syndrome discovered by the author. (Courtesy Dr. Gary Schneider.)*

munodeficiencies. Persons with either primary or acquired immunodeficiency disorders are more likely to become infected by microorganisms and develop cancer (see Chapter 7, Infectious Diseases, and Chapter 8, Neoplasia).

Mechanisms of Immunity

To illustrate how an immune response occurs, we will now discuss the events transpiring during tetanus vaccination (Fig. 6-8). When *antigens* such as tetanus toxoid are introduced into the body for the purpose of providing active specific immunization (vaccination), the following events occur: The tetanus bacilli antigens injected into the skin are transported by lymphatic vessels to regional lymph nodes. There the antigens are processed and concentrated nearly one thousand–fold in the macrophages. The superconcentrated (processed) antigens of the vaccine are then received by antibody receptors on B-lymphocytes. The stimulated B-lymphocytes, after a latency period (usually about a day or two), divide and proliferate to form new B-lymphocytes, which are sensitized and responsive to tetanus antigens. The new clone of B cells differentiate (mature) into plasma cells. These cells produce antibodies within days of the *primary exposure*. The antibody immune response to antigen reacts specifically with the tetanus antigen (Figs. 6-8 and 6-9). Memory cells and antibodies produced against the tetanus antigens persist in circulation and await invading tetanus bacilli. The puncture wound of a contaminated rusty nail, for example, may occur years following vaccination, yet protection persists because of the memory cells.

Following sensitization to an antigen, memory lymphocytes persist for prolonged periods and can be called into service again if challenged by the tetanus antigens. A rapid recall and heightening of B cell immunity is known as the anamnestic response (Fig. 6-9). When a person is reexposed to an antigen, the memory B-lymphocytes respond rapidly and differentiate into plasma cells that produce potent antibodies. The latent period for antigenic exposure to antibody response is shorter in a second-

ary response than during the initial primary sensitization to the antigen—booster vaccinations with tetanus toxoid are very effective because of the anamnestic response. Tetanus antitoxin is also given to victims of puncture wounds to provide *passive immunity* in case the patient has never been immunized (Fig. 6-10).

Vaccinations against polio, measles, rubella, and other viruses and BCG for prevention of tuberculosis result in development of both T- and B-lymphocyte-mediated immunity. Delayed-type hypersensitivity immune response (cell-mediated immunity) mediated by T-lymphocytes, which protect against intracellular microbes and cancer, are discussed later in this chapter.

Amplification of the Immune Responses

Both humoral and cell-mediated immunity can *amplify* (expand) their response or potency by recruiting other combatants into the struggle for immunologic defense against invasion by "foreign" living substance. The *T-lymphocyte*, which provides CMI, amplifies its potency by releasing various substances, termed *lymphokines*, which activate macrophages and other cells to assist in eliminating intracellular microbes, cancer cells, and organ transplants. *Humoral* immunity is amplified by three mechanisms: (1) *activation of serum complement*, (2) *recruiting of neutrophils*, and (3) *opsonization*, or coating, of microbes by antibodies that render the microbes palatable to phagocytic cells—the neutrophils and macrophages.

Serum Complement Amplification

Serum complement amplifies and gives humoral immunity the ability to burst cellular membranes of bacteria and other foreign agents. Complement consists of a dozen interacting, circulating enzymes that when activated, bind with antigens and antibodies to form *immune complexes*. Activated complement recruits neutrophils by a process called chemotaxis, or neutrotaxis, which induces acute inflammation. Neutrophils invade sites where antigens-antibody-complement immune complexes are

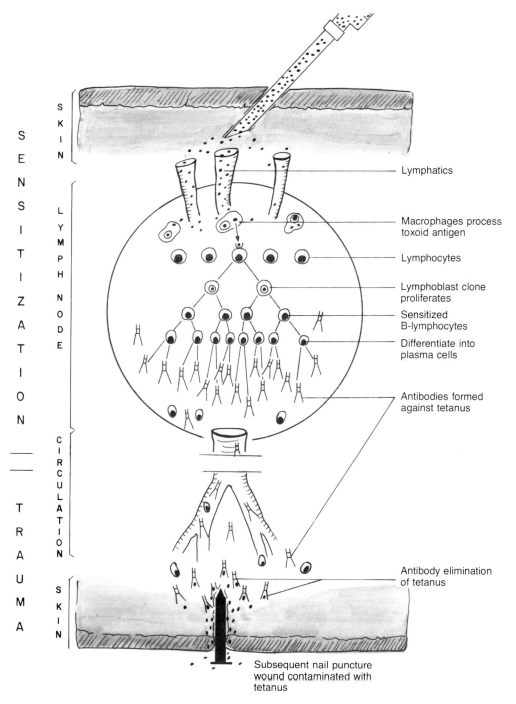

S
E
N
S
I
T
I
Z
A
T
I
O
N
—
T
R
A
U
M
A

S K I N

L Y M P H   N O D E

C I R C U L A T I O N

S K I N

Lymphatics

Macrophages process toxoid antigen

Lymphocytes

Lymphoblast clone proliferates

Sensitized B-lymphocytes

Differentiate into plasma cells

Antibodies formed against tetanus

Antibody elimination of tetanus

Subsequent nail puncture wound contaminated with tetanus

Figure 6-8   *Mechanisms of sensitization and memory obtained during vaccination for tetanus. The top portion shows the primary immune response to tetanus toxoid and the bottom shows antibodies reacting at a later time against tetanus bacilli.*

present. The lysosomal enzymes in the neutrophils spill into the site and digest microbes and the nearby cells.

Serum complement, together with certain antibodies (IgM and IgG class), is effective in killing bacteria. Complement binds with antibodies and antigens of the surface of a bacteria; complement then punches holes in the cell wall of bacteria or in other cells containing antigens reacting with IgM and IgG antibodies.

Chemotaxis and infiltration of tissues by neutrophils in response to complexes may cause damage. Enzymes released by the infiltrating neutrophils digest blood vessel walls. For instance, the kidneys are often damaged in this manner when immune complexes are deposited in the glomeruli.

Opsonization Amplification

On combination with antigen, IgG antibodies bind to specific sites on the surface of neutrophils and macrophages. For example, bacteria are eliminated when they become coated with antibody and become *opsonized* (Fig. 6-11). The bacteria thereby become palatable or "tasty for the phagocytes" and will adhere to phagocytic cells; the adherence facilitates the engulfment and subsequent digestion of the microbes.

With the foregoing as a briefing on basic immunology, we can now consider hypersensitivity disorders or clinical immunology. Virtually all organs of the body can be injured when the immune system "gets out of control." In subsequent chapters, the varied impact of hypersensitivity disorders will become obvious.

Hypersensitivity Disorders

Diseases of hypersensitivity usually are characterized by injury of tissues from reacting antigens, lymphocytes, macrophages, neutrophils, antibodies, or complement. *Hypersensitivity reactions* are classified into four groups: (1) immediate, or anaphylactic-type, sensitivity; (2) cytotoxic-type hypersensitivity; (3) complex-mediated hypersensitivity; and (4) cell-mediated, or delayed-type, hypersensitivity. The hypersensitivity reactions are summarized in Table 6-1.

Immediate or Anaphylactic-type Hypersensitivity

Antibodies of the IgE class are responsible for the sudden (usually within 30 minutes of exposure to antigen) events observed in immediate hypersen-

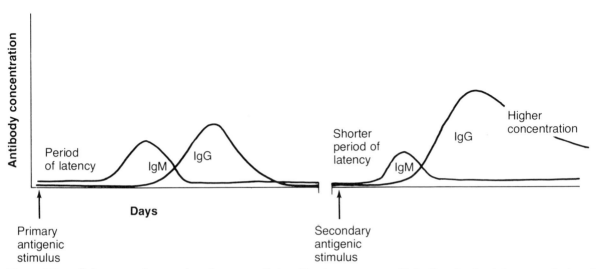

Figure 6-9   *Primary and secondary (anamnestic) antibody responses. Note the shorter latency period and greater antibody response following the second exposure to antigen.*

allergies to food, pollen, and other organic dusts and chemicals.

Asthma   Many individuals with asthma (50%) have IgE antibodies against a specific allergen and an increased concentration of IgE in their serum. The IgE antibodies coat mast cells, which contain *histamine* and other compounds that act on blood vessels (vasoactive compounds). Histamine is released by mast cells when allergins combine with IgE antibodies on the surface of mast cells. Histamine provokes smooth muscle in bronchioles to constrict and stimulates mucous secretion, causing the airways to become blocked. Asthmatic patients have difficulty exhaling because airways are constricted.

Their bronchi show hyperplastic mucous glands, and some contain plugs of mucus (Fig. 6-12). In addition, the smooth muscles surrounding the bronchi are thickened, as is the basement membrane beneath the bronchial epithelium.

Curiously, in some persons with asthma, no immunologic explanation is possible. Psychic inputs are important; for example, a severe asthmatic attack has been provoked by the viewing of a paper rose in a person allergic to roses. Exercise can also induce asthma in some persons.

In many asthmatic individuals, hypersensitivity to allergens can be identified by injecting antigens into skin. Those with allergies develop a raised, red, itchy, disc-shaped, edematous plaque at the site of injection with an allergen within minutes (immediate hypersensitivity).

Treatment is aimed at decreasing the hyperactive immune response by inhaling theophylline chromylin sodium or corticosteroids. In severe cases, adrenalin is injected intravenously to reverse the constriction of the bronchial airways. After the acute asthmatic attack has subsided, gradual desensitization of the patient to the allergen may be attempted.

Fatal Systemic Anaphylaxis   Systemic anaphylaxis is a dreaded medical emergency. A prerequisite is that the individual be previously sensitized to an antigen, for instance, penicillin. The combination of antigen with antibody (IgE) on mast cells

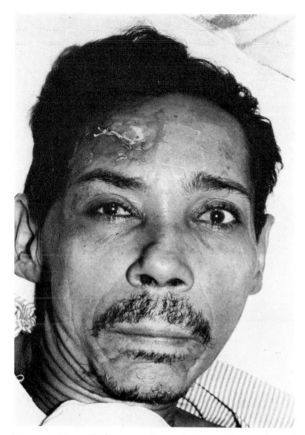

Figure 6-10   *This man shows tetany of muscles of his right neck. He was hit in the head with a rusty nail which contained the tetanus bacillum. He had not been immunized, but prompt administration of tetanus antitoxin saved his life.*

sitivity responses. Antibodies of the IgE class are excessively produced by susceptible *atopic* persons in response to an allergen, such as ragweed pollen; drugs, such as penicillin and aspirin; animal dander; food; and other organic dusts. Oftentimes allergies (atopy) are inherited. *Anaphylaxis* can be local. Hives, an example of anaphylaxis, are one of the most common manifestations of hypersensitivity disorders. Systemic anaphylaxis is more vexing than local anaphylaxis. The immediate hypersensitivity response in asthma, systemic anaphylaxis, causes profound respiratory impairment when the bronchial airways constrict. Immediate hypersensitivity is the immunologic mechanism causing most

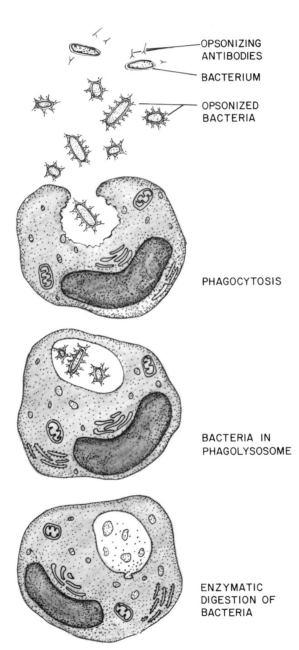

OPSONIZING ANTIBODIES

BACTERIUM

OPSONIZED BACTERIA

PHAGOCYTOSIS

BACTERIA IN PHAGOLYSOSOME

ENZYMATIC DIGESTION OF BACTERIA

Figure 6-11   *Opsonization of bacteria and phagocytosis. Antibodies coat the surface of the bacteria and the phagocytes readily adhere to the antibody-coated microbes and phagocytize them.*

and the sudden release of histamine from tissue mast cells may cause the entire capillary network and venules to leak plasma fluid and the smooth muscles of the bronchial tree to contract vigorously. Mast cells explode releasing histamine when the allergen (antigen) combines with the IgE antibody coating the mast cells. During anaphylaxis, a person experiences *reactions induced by histamine:* itching of the scalp, tongue, and throat; flushing of skin; and difficulty in breathing within minutes following exposure to the allergen (antigen).

Obstruction of airways is caused by bronchoconstriction, and circulatory collapse may suddenly ensue because plasma leaks from the blood vessels into the lungs. The venules leak plasma because histamine causes endothelial cells to separate (see Chapter 5, Inflammation and Repair). The circulatory collapse can be reversed by administering fluids and epinephrine (Adrenalin) and by placing the person in the "shock" position (supine with the head lower than the feet).

A diagnosis of systemic anaphylaxis cannot be solely established by the nonspecific findings seen at autopsy. The edema observed in the larynx and the disrupted lung tissue and hemorrhage are not specific for anaphylaxis. Hence, a clinical history of injection of a substance such as penicillin moments before collapse is necessary to make the diagnosis. Persons receiving injections of drugs such as penicillin are advised to remain seated for 30 minutes under medical supervision because life-threatening anaphylaxis can occur in sensitized persons.

Cytotoxic-type Hypersensitivity

Cytotoxic-type-hypersensitivity-induced injury results when complement binds to antibodies and antigens on the surface of cells (on erythrocytes, for example). The binding of antibody against antigen on erythrocytes and complement destroys the erythrocytes. Complement probably punches holes through the erythrocyte wall and causes the release of hemoglobin, and thus, *hemolysis* results. The concept of "autoimmune" hemolytic anemia and cytotoxic injury is further described in Chapter 11. Cytotoxic injury causes *inactivation* of certain hormones (insulin in some diabetic patients, for example) and blood-clotting factors in hemophilia.

Complex-mediated Hypersensitivity

Immune complexes composed of antigens, antibodies, and serum complement can circulate in persons with complex-mediated hypersensitivity and become trapped in capillaries (in the kidneys, skin, and joints). The immune complexes provoke an acute neutrophilic infiltration in the tissues, where they lodge and injury ensues. Many diseases of skin, blood vessels, kidneys, lungs, and the heart are caused by immune complex deposition. *Serum sickness*, an immune complex disease resulting from the injection of a foreign protein, such as horse serum, is the classical example of this type of hypersensitivity disease.

Table 6-1
Comparison of Hypersensitivity Disorders

Hypersensitivity	Examples	Time	Mechanism
Anaphylactic	Anaphylactic shock (bee sting, drugs)	1 to 15 minutes	Systemic vascular collapse from histamine, for example, released from IgE coated mast cells
	Cutaneous anaphylaxis (hives)	minutes	Local challenge and localized response
	Respiratory anaphylaxis (allergic rhinitis, asthma)	minutes	Low-dose continuous antigenic challenge releasing histamine
Cytotoxic antibody	Autoimmune hemolytic anemia, auto-antibodies against hormones, insulin, for example	minutes	Antibody reacts with antigen on cell (RBC) or to molecule (insulin)
Immune complex Arthus reaction (antibody excess)	Complexes in vessels of skin or organic dusts in lung	2 to 10 hours	Acute inflammatory response to Ag-Ab complex
Serum sickness (antigen excess)	Horse serum antitoxin Glomerulonephritis Lupus erythematosus Rheumatoid arthritis	Days after sensitization	Widespread deposition of Ag-Ab complexes in small vessels
Cell-mediated Response to intracellular infections	PPD skin test	24 to 72 hours	T-cell and macrophage infiltration
Graft rejection	Tumors/grafts	Days-months	T killer cells recognize foreign Ag

Serum Sickness   Serum sickness, an immune-complex disease, is characterized by fever, swollen lymph nodes, rash, and swollen joints in persons who have been injected with a large quantity of foreign protein, such as antisera to diphtheria raised in horses. The affected person raises antibodies against the horse proteins, and complexes of protein (antigen) and antibody circulate and lodge in capillaries (Fig. 6-13). The antigen-antibody-complement complexes and neutrophils become deposited in capillaries in the kidneys, skin, and joints. The inflammation and injury in these sites causes the symptoms of swelling, redness, pain, heat, and immobility.

Arthus Reaction   The Arthus reaction (Nicolas-Maurice Arthus, French physiologist, 1862–1945) is another example of a complex-mediated hypersensitivity reaction. An Arthus reaction appears within a few hours following exposure to an antigen in persons who already have a *high antibody concentration* to an antigen in their blood.

Clinically, the Arthus reaction is responsible for most cases of hypersensitivity pneumonitis. For instance, a pigeon breeder who has become sensitized to pigeon droppings has a high concentration of antibodies against the droppings and will experience fever and wheezing within a few hours after inhaling the pigeon dust. During the Arthus reaction, the alveoli (air spaces) in the person's lungs trap immune complexes composed of pigeon antigens, antibodies, and serum complement; neutrophils are also seen. The circulating antibodies react with the pigeon antigens, and complement and neutrophils infiltrate (by neutrotaxis), release lysosomal enzymes and injure the alveoli in response to the complement and immune complexes. Similar problems can arise in farmers or other workers inhaling other organic dusts (see Chapter 14).

Immunologic Renal Diseases   Hypersensitivity reactions are often responsible for immune injury to the kidneys. Acute *glomerulonephritis* (inflammation of glomeruli) is the most common form of immunologic injury in the kidneys. It can develop several weeks following a streptococcal sore throat. Antibodies to streptococcal antigens react with the

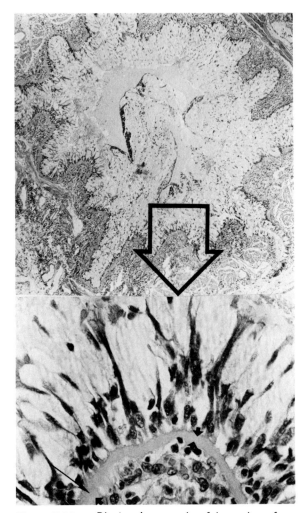

Figure 6-12   *Photomicrograph of bronchus from asthmatic patient showing contraction and mucous plug. The mucosa is thickened (large arrow) and the surrounding smooth muscle is hyperplastic. The lower photomicrograph demonstrates hypertrophy of goblet cells (the source of mucus) in the mucosa, a thickened basement membrane (small arrow), and lymphocytes infiltrating beneath the membrane.*

circulating streptococcal antigens and complement and the complexes become trapped in glomeruli. Probably by similar mechanisms, *rheumatic heart disease* develops following streptococcal infections. Also, individuals with *systemic lupus erythematosus (SLE)* develop immune complexes composed of antibody and their own DNA. The circulating

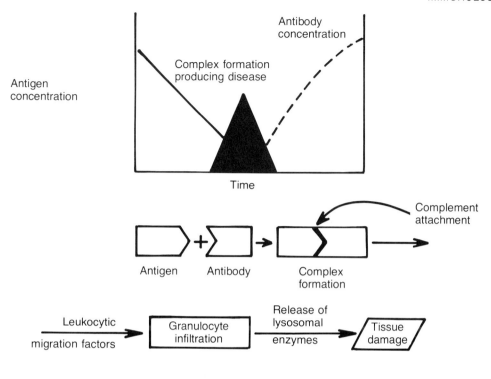

IMMUNE COMPLEX DISEASES

1. Serum sickness
2. Glomerulonephritis
3. Systemic lupus erythematosus
4. Autoimmune hemolysis

Figure 6-13   *Immune complex disease showing the formation of antibodies following the injection of horse serum. Immune complexes of antigen and antibody form at approximately ten days and give rise to the symptoms. Acute inflammation occurs when serum complement attracts granulocytes and invades and injures the tissues.*

complexes become deposited in the skin, synovia, and glomeruli and provoke inflammation and injury. In general, immune complex hypersensitivity is involved in autoimmune disorders.

Autoimmunity   The Nobel laureate Sir Mac-Farlane Burnet postulated that during the development of the embryo, self-antigens are recognized and that the embryo subsequently develops tolerance to itself; but tolerance can be broken when an antibody is formed against one's own antigens—*autoimmunity*. Antibodies against one's own tissues are detected in the serum of persons with autoimmune disorders.

The four most common autoimmune disorders are SLE, rheumatoid arthritis, rheumatic heart disease, and glomerulonephritis. Other organs including the thyroid, adrenals, and stomach can be damaged by autoimmune disorders. Rheumatoid arthritis and SLE are two of the most common autoimmune diseases. These diseases are also classified as rheumatic or collagen-vascular diseases because they involve blood vessels and connective tissues. Autoimmune disorders are frequently inherited.

Systemic Lupus Erythematosus   Systemic lupus erythematosus is a chronic inflammatory autoimmune disease of unknown etiology that affects many organs; that is, it is systemic. This chronic disease affects about 500,000 persons in the United States. It occurs ten times more commonly in young women than in men. Appearance of SLE depends on genetic and environmental factors: drugs, sunlight, and possibly viruses (all examples of environmental factors) induce SLE in genetically predisposed individuals. Hence the disease arises on an ecogenetic basis (see Chapter 1).

The *classical manifestations* of SLE include fever, rash, loss of hair, painful joints (arthritis), fatigue, and pleurisy (pain on deep breathing). Lesions frequently develop in the skin, especially on the face (Fig. 6-14), and in connective tissues throughout the body. Inflammation of the kidney and moist linings of the lungs and heart can occur, but many patients have limited SLE. The lesions in patients with SLE probably result from damage caused by autoantibodies circulating in the blood, which react with DNA in the nuclei of cells. Sunlight, drugs, or a virus initiate events leading to damage of nuclei of the DNA in cells; anti-DNA antibodies form against the damaged DNA.

Clinical laboratory tests for diagnosing SLE demonstrate antibodies against nuclear antigens or against DNA by examining a drop of blood. Immunofluorescence "sandwich" tests are used to demonstrate *anti-DNA antibodies* in the serum of SLE patients (Fig. 6-15). Over 95% of persons with SLE have antinuclear antibodies (ANA), but the tests are not specific; persons with other autoimmune diseases (rheumatoid arthritis, for example) may exhibit antinuclear or DNA antibodies. The *lupus erythematosus (LE) cell preparation* is more specific for SLE than the ANA test, but it is less sensitive. The LE cell preparation demonstrates antibodies against leukocytes. Thus a diagnosis of SLE is based on clinical, laboratory, and histopathologic findings.

The *skin lesions* in SLE are distinctive: a rash occurs on the bridge of the nose and on the cheeks in a butterfly distribution (Fig. 6-14). Keratin (the protein surface of skin) plugs the holes where hairs erupt from follicles and lymphocyes infiltrate the dermis. Immunofluorescence studies of skin from SLE victims reveal antibodies fixed to nuclei (DNA) of cells and the basement membrane.

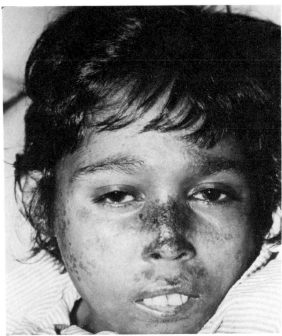

Figure 6-14 *Systemic lupus erythematosus. A rash with a butterfly distribution over the bridge of the nose displayed in this patient with lupus who was exposed to the tropical sun.*

Renal injury (glomerulonephritis) occurs in many SLE victims; the extent of renal involvement determines the patient's prognosis. Persons with severe involvement of the kidney frequently develop renal failure. The basement membrane of the glomerular capillaries are usually thickened, and necrosis may be seen. Complexes become trapped in the glomeruli, which are composed of antibodies to DNA and DNA and complement (Fig. 6-16). Neutrophils invade glomeruli because of chemotaxis. Patients with SLE are generally given aspirin to decrease the inflammatory response and to depress, to a limited extent, immunity. Cortisone is occasionally used to treat severe SLE.

Rheumatoid Arthritis *Rheumatoid arthritis (RA)* is another autoimmune disease of unknown etiology (see Chapter 20, Musculoskeletal Diseases). It affects chiefly the synovial lining of moveable joints. Early in RA, an acute inflammatory response can be seen within the synovial lining of joints. Edema, vascular engorgement, infiltration by neutrophils,

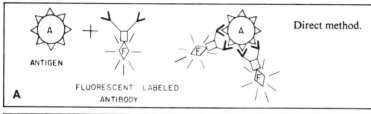
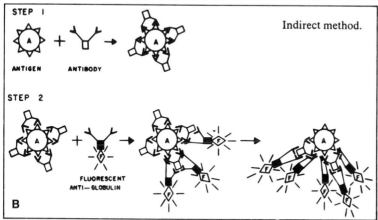
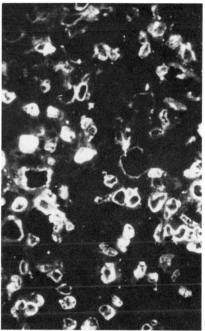

Figure 6-15   **A,** *Direct and,* **B,** *indirect immunofluorescence tests for demonstrating antigens in cells or tissues and antibodies in a patient's serum.* **C.** *Antinuclear antibodies demonstrated by indirect immunofluorescence. (From Nakamura, R. M. 1974.* Immunopathy. Clinical laboratory concepts and methods. *(Boston: Little, Brown, and Co.)*

and fibrin are seen in the synovium and joint space. Later, the synovial lining cells become hyperplastic, and there is an infiltration by lymphocytes and plasma cells.

Rheumatoid arthritis is considered an autoimmune disease because an autoantibody, *rheumatoid factor (RF)*, is usually present in the serum of individuals with rheumatoid arthritis. Rheumatoid factor is an IgM antibody directed against one's own immunoglobulin IgG. Complexes of RF become deposited in synovium and connective tissues (Fig. 6-13). The finding of rheumatoid factor in a patient's serum is not diagnostic of RA because it is commonly present in the sera of patients with SLE and other collagen-vascular diseases. Rheumatoid arthritis can progress to involve many joints and symmetrical joint involvement is common. Soft tissue swelling of the distal interphalangeal joints occurs early in the disease, and morning stiffness is noted. When the disease becomes advanced, the fingers become displaced toward the ulnar (medial) side of the hand (see diagram in Chapter 20). Subcutaneous rheumatoid nodules are rather common,

especially over the ulna, and occasionally, they develop in the eyes. Rarely, the eyeball ruptures.

The *inflammation* accompanying rheumatoid arthritis destroys the cartilage covering the surface of joints. In response to the inflammation, granulation tissue (pannus) forms and burrows into the underlying cartilage and bone (Fig. 6-17). The destruction of bone and cartilage also probably results from the inflammation; for example, the enzymes collagenase and hyaluronidase released by neutrophils destroy bone and cartilage. The bone melts (resorbs) and tendons, ligaments, and other supporting tissues become weak. The joints may eventually become deformed and unstable. For a discussion on prognosis and treatment of rheumatoid arthritis, see Chapter 20.

Cell-mediated Immunity (delayed-type hypersensitivity)

Cell-mediated immunity (CMI) is controlled by T-lymphocytes. An alternative name to CMI is *delayed-type hypersensitivity*. The response to antigen is delayed (occurs at approximately 48 hours). CMI defends against intracellular microorganisms and against malignant tumors. In addition, CMI is the immune response responsible for the rejection of transplanted organs. To illustrate the function of CMI in defending against intracellular microbes, we will discuss the CMI response against *Mycobacterium tuberculosis*.

Cell-mediated Immunity   Tubercle bacilli that have been inhaled travel from the lungs in lymphatic vessels to regional lymph nodes (Figs. 6-2 and 6-4). Here macrophages engulf, process, and concentrate the antigens of the bacilli. A few T-lymphocytes bearing receptors for tuberculosis antigens react with the bacillus and undergo multiplication. The newly formed sensitized T cells circulate back to the lungs, whereupon contact with antigens of the tubercle bacilli they release lymphokines, which induce the innocent bystander T-lymphocytes and macrophages to kill the bacilli. Enzymes in macrophages destroy the bacilli.

The hallmark of a vigorous CMI response to tubercle bacilli is the formation of a granuloma (Fig. 6-18). A *granuloma* is formed in the tissues from lymphocytes and macrophages; some macrophages fuse together forming Langhan's giant cells.

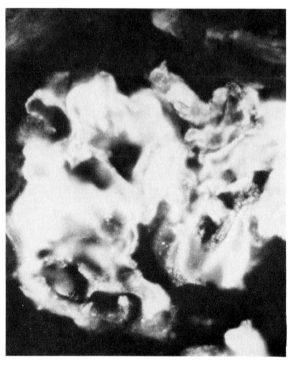

Figure 6-16   *Photomicrograph of immunofluorescence in the kidney. The glomerulus stains brightly because complement-DNA-antibody deposits (immune complex) are stained by direct immunofluorescence.*

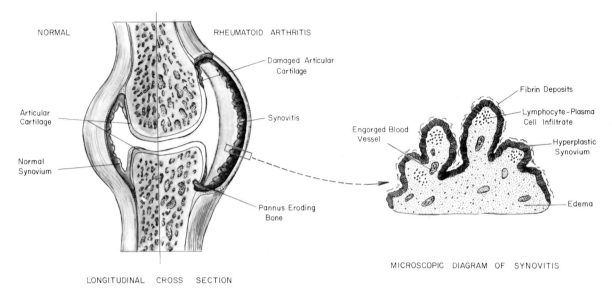

Figure 6-17   *Movable joint in rheumatoid arthritis illustrating inflammation and granulation tissue burrowing into the underlying cartilage.*

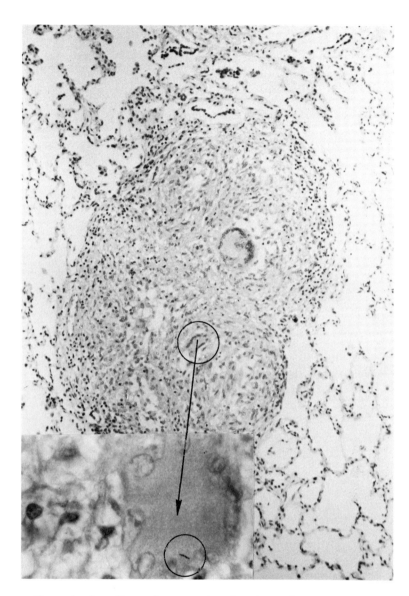

Figure 6-18   *Photomicrograph of granuloma caused by tuberculosis. Note the large multinucleated giant cell (Langhan's cell) surrounding macrophages and, toward the periphery, lymphocytes. The highly magnified inset shows a tubercle bacillus being digested by a Langhan's cell.*

Once the invading microorganism has been destroyed, memory cells persist for many years. A vigorous "recall" of the CMI response occurs when a sensitized person is reexposed to the bacillus. The tuberculin test, discussed earlier in this chapter, tests for the presence of memory cells (Fig. 6-19).

Consequences of Depressed Cell-mediated Immunity (CMI)   If a person has depression of their CMI, then reactivation of tuberculosis, which had remained dormant, can occur. Also, microbes normally kept in check by CMI can invade an im-

munosuppressed person (malnourished or immunosuppressed alcoholic, for example, as discussed in Chapter 7). Herpes simplex virus (normally only causes cold sores) and Candida (a common fungus) can disseminate throughout the body of immunosuppressed persons. Many factors suppress CMI and render the patient more susceptible to common infectious agents: corticosteroids, cytotoxic drugs used to treat malignancy, irradiation, aging, general anesthesia, viral infections, vaccinations, cutaneous burns, and pregnancy may induce immunosuppressive states. Inspection of the list reveals

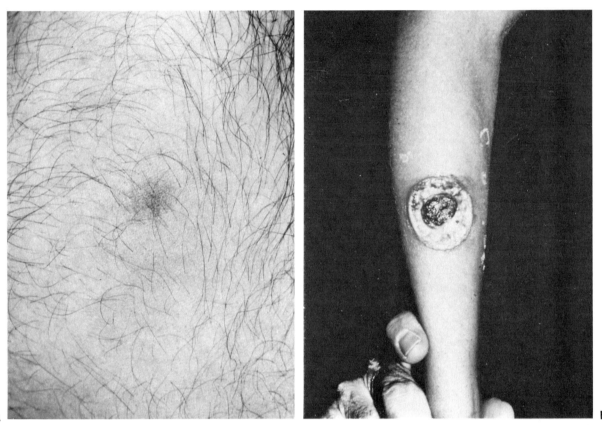

Figure 6-19   *Tuberculin-delayed hypersensitivity responses.* **A,** Normal *positive reactivity displaying red, firm (indurated), raised 1-cm diameter area.* **B,** *Marked positive reactivity leading to ulceration of injection site in a person with active tuberculosis and marked delayed hypersensitivity.*

that many hospitalized patients are immunosuppressed. Health professionals should try to prevent the occurrence of serious viral and fungal infections in these immunosuppressed patients by preventing the infection or detecting it at an early stage or by minimizing the patient's immunosuppression.

Transplantation Immunology

Rejection of organ transplants occurs from immunologic mechanisms chiefly mediated by T-lymphocytes. A transplanted kidney that has not been specifically matched for the appropriate *h*uman *le*ukocyte *a*ntigens (HLA) or *histocompatibility antigens* of the donor and recipient will be rejected within two weeks—a process called *first-set rejection.* Re-

jection can be prevented by matching the donor's and recipient's histocompatibility antigens and blood group antigens. At least 50 different HLA antigens are known, and thousands of combinations are possible.

HLA Tissue Typing

Testing for histocompatibility requires identification of antigens on lymphocytes of both the donor and recipient. The HLA antigens on the lymphocytes are present on all tissues of the body, including the kidney. Antigenic differences between people are usually present, except in identical twins.

Therefore, if the donor and recipient are not matched identically, the recipient's T-lymphocytes, which are chiefly responsible for the rejection of the graft, must be suppressed. Immunosuppressive drugs, such as cortisone or antilymphocyte serum, which destroy T-lymphocytes, are given. Virtually all renal transplants undergo at least one episode of rejection; renal allografts obtained from cadavers are more likely to be rejected than kidneys obtained from living HLA-matched donors.

Immune Rejection of Transplants

Immunorejection of transplants is classified according to the time of occurrence.

Acute rejection *Acute rejection* (first-set rejection) occurs within 10 to 14 days following grafting. Acute rejection invariably occurs in nonimmunosuppressed mismatched recipients. It is characterized pathologically by an infiltration of T-lymphocytes and macrophages between injured renal tubules.

Hyperacute Rejection *Hyperacute rejection* occurs in an individual who has been previously sensitized to antigens of the graft (second-set rejection). Prior sensitization or immunization can result from blood passing from a fetus to the mother during a pregnancy, from blood transfusions, or from previously transplanted kidneys. Such recipients have antibodies in the blood that react against the donor's antigens. When the graft is transplanted, these antibodies react against the antigens in the kidney graft. The antigen-antibody reaction occurring on the walls of blood vessels triggers coagulation of blood, and blood clots form in the arteries and block the blood supply to the kidney. Microscopic studies of the kidney reveal IgG and IgM antibodies and complement, which are responsible for hyperacute rejection within the walls of the injured blood vessels in the kidney. In addition, neutrophils infiltrate the vessels in response to the immune complexes and complement.

Chronic Rejection By contrast to the preceding types of rejection, *chronic rejection* results from scarring of the endothelial (intimal) cells lining the blood vessels. The immune response injures the intimal cells, and repair processes scar the vessel

wall and obstruct the blood channel. Renal tubules become small, or *atrophic,* due to a decreased blood supply. The blood supply is compressed because of the narrowing of the blood channel by the scar tissue. The renal function becomes impaired, and then renal dialysis is required to rid the body of toxic wastes.

Cancer Immunology

Immunologic Surveillance

T-lymphocytes provide *immunologic surveillance (IS)* against malignant tumors. The notion that IS protects us against cancer is based on the findings that cancer cells contain *tumor antigens* that stimulate the CMI response of the person to the cancer cells. Newly sensitized killer T-lymphocytes then eliminate the cancer cells.

Important clinical observations indicate that IS prevents us from being overcome by cancer. In at least 300 instances, individuals with cancer in organs such as adrenals, kidney, placenta, or skin have undergone spontaneous regression without treatment. Secondly, individuals with tumors infiltrated intensively by lymphocytes live longer than those without this immune response. Extracts of cancer antigens injected into the skin of cancer patients reveal CMI responses, indicating an immune reaction to the cancer. Children who have primary immunodeficiency diseases develop cancer 1000 times more frequently than do children with normal immunity. Adults who have acquired immunodeficiency (renal transplant recipients who are immunosuppressed) have an eightyfold increased occurrence of cancer.

With increasing age, CMI often becomes suppressed and cancer occurs more frequently. By 65 years of age, approximately 16% of persons will have developed cancer, and the frequency continues thereafter to dramatically increase with age. A breakdown in the IS probably permits cancer cells to sneak through and establish themselves. Attempts are now being made to increase the CMI of cancer patients by using immunotherapy. In addition to conventional surgery, irradiation, and drugs, various tumor and bacterial antigens (BCG, for example) are injected directly into the tumor or into malignant melanoma in the skin to enhance the patient's CMI.

Immunodiagnosis of Cancer

Newly developed immunologic methods for diagnosing malignancy have been made possible by detecting tumor-associated antigens produced by cancer and secreted in blood. Collectively, the antigens are known as *oncofetal antigens*. The tumor antigens are so-named because the same antigens are produced by both tumors and the fetus.

Fetal antigens are normally synthesized by fetal cells. During the postnatal period, a switching-off of synthesis of the fetal antigens occurs. When a cancer develops, the genes controlling synthesis of fetal antigens are switched-on. The cancer cells revert to a fetal-like state and produce the oncofetal antigens that are detectable in the patient's blood. The best known oncofetal antigens are *carcinoembryonic antigen* (CEA) and α-fetoprotein (AFP).

CEA is detectable in the blood of most patients with *colon cancer*, and *AFP* in patients with primary *liver cancer*. These tests are useful aids for diagnosing the cancer and for determining whether a cancer has been totally removed during surgery. CEA disappears from the patient's blood when colon cancer is completely removed by a surgical procedure. Likewise, AFP disappears from the blood when a liver cancer is totally resected. In the future, additional oncofetal antigens will probably be discovered and provide earlier diagnosis of cancer.

Summary

Basic immune mechanisms for recognizing and eliminating foreign invaders (microbes and cancer) have been discussed. The key attributes of specificity and persistence of memory of the immune response have been stressed. The clinical immunologic disorders arising from primary and secondary immunodeficiency are briefly outlined. Emphasis of the chapter focused on the four hypersensitivity responses responsible for most allergic disorders, anaphylaxis, cytotoxic, immune complex, and cell-mediated hypersensitivity responses. The mechanism whereby these responses cause disease were discussed and illustrated. Applications of new concepts of immunology which permit successful organ transplantation and immunodiagnosis of cancer make immunology the new frontier of medicine.

Bibliography

Eisen, H. N. 1974. *Immunology*. New York: Harper & Row, Publishers. An introduction to molecular and cellular principles of the immune system.

Fries, J. F., and Holman, H. R. 1975. *Systemic lupus erythematosus*. Philadelphia: W. B. Saunders Company. Clinical monograph of 199 pages.

Gel, P. G. H.; Coombs, R. R. A.; and Lachmann, R. J., 1975. *Clinical aspects of immunology*, ed. 3. Oxford: Blackwell Scientific Publishing. A standard reference textbook.

Good, R. A., and Fisher, D. W., eds. 1972. *Immunobiology*. Sunderland, Mass.: Sinauer Associates, Inc. The illustrations are superb.

Holborow, E. J. 1977. *An ABC of modern immunology*, ed. 3. Boston: Little, Brown and Company. Concise synopsis.

Nakamura, R. M. 1974. *Immunopathology*. Boston: Little, Brown and Company. Emphasizes laboratory studies employed for diagnosing immunologic disorders.

Nysather, J. O.; Katz, A. E.; and Lanth, J. L. 1976. The immune system. *Am. J. Nurs.* 76:1614–1628. Concise overview of theoretical and practical aspects of immunology.

Primer on the rheumatic diseases. 1973, ed. 7. New York: The Arthritis Foundation. Available gratis. Good classification and pathogenesis of rheumatic disorders.

Purtilo, D. T., and Connor, D. H. 1975. Fatal infections in protein–calorie malnourished children with thymolymphatic atrophy. *Arch. Dis. Child.* 50:149–152. Describes the immunopathology of this commonly acquired immunodeficiency disorder.

Purtilo, D. T. 1977. Opportunistic lymphomas in X-linked recessive immunodeficiency and lymphoproliferative syndromes. *Sem. Oncol.* 4:335–343. Discusses cancer in children with primary immunodeficiency.

Purtilo, D. T.; DeFlorio, D.; Hutt, L. M.; Bhawan, J.; Yang, J. P. S.; Otto, R.; and Edwards, W. 1977. Variable phenotypic expression of an X-linked recessive lymphoproliferative syndrome. *New Engl. J. Med.* 297: 1077–1081. Boys affected by this syndrome are immunodeficient to the Epstein-Barr virus and often die of infectious mononucleosis or malignant lymphoma.

Roitt, I. 1977. *Essential immunology*, ed. 3. Oxford: Blackwell Scientific Publishing. The single best reference for an introduction to immunology.

Stiehm, E. R., and Fulginiti, V. A. 1973. *Immunologic disorders in infants and children*. Philadelphia: W. B. Saunders Company. Describes the many special immunologic problems of children, immunodeficiency, for example.

Thaler, M. S.; Klausner, R. D.; and Cohen, H. J. 1977 *Medical immunology*. Philadelphia:J. B. Lippincott Co. Current, comprehensive, and clinically relevant textbook.

Williams, R. D. 1974. *Rheumatoid arthritis*. Philadelphia: W. B. Saunders Company. Clinical monograph of 268 pages.

CHAPTER 7

Infectious Diseases

Chapter Outline

Objectives

After reading this chapter you should be able to

List the major groups of biologic agents that can cause infectious diseases.

Discuss factors determining the severity of an infection.

List the four large groups of parasitic agents.

Describe five steps in the pathogenesis of infections.

Recognize the clinical features of an infectious disease in a patient.

List the events occurring as a virus infects a cell.

Define the terms incubation period, tropism, and Gram's stain.

List five pyogenic bacteria.

Describe impetigo.

Define the terms folliculitis, furuncle, and carbuncle.

Know the pathogenesis of acne.

Describe the etiology of the common cold.

List normal flora in the oropharynx.

Describe the pathogenesis of rheumatic fever and acute glomerulonephritis.

Name bacterium most commonly causing pneumonia.

List the findings required to diagnose pneumonia.

List five complications of pneumonia.

Compare primary and secondary tuberculosis.

Describe the cells of a granuloma.

Define the pathogenesis of miliary tuberculosis.

Know the tests employed for diagnosing tuberculosis.

Know factors predisposing to pyelonephritis.

List the common microbes that can infect the brain.

Describe the contribution of a lumbar puncture to diagnosis of central nervous system infections.

Define aseptic meningitis.

List the common etiologic agents of diarrhea.

Describe endotoxin: source, chemistry, and effect on a person with bacteremia.

Compare type A and type B viral hepatitis.

List five types of venereal disease.

Compare the three stages of syphilis as to: time of occurrence, lesions, and infectivity.

Describe how syphilis is diagnosed and treated.

Describe symptoms of gonorrhea.

List infectious agents that comprise the TORCH complex.

List clinical features of neonatal sepsis.

Describe the pathogenesis of toxoplasmosis.

Know the period of development at which most organs are formed.

Define the term opportunistic infection.

List common opportunistic infections.

Define the term nosocomial infection.

List conditions characterized by immunosuppression.

Know the major symptom heralding infection in a leukemic patient.

Name the most common opportunistic fungal infection.

List measures employed for preventing infections.

Describe how antibiotic sensitivity testing is done.

Know techniques commonly employed for diagnosing infectious diseases.

Describe other measures that should be taken, in addition to giving antibiotics, to cure a person of bacterial infections.

Introduction

The course of human history has been shaped to a great extent by the arbitrary forces of infectious diseases: smallpox, measles, influenza, typhoid fever, dysentery, malaria, plague, and cholera.* For example, the despotic dynasties in ancient Egypt were made possible by a peasantry debilitated by chronic (schistosomiasis) urinary bladder flukes. A mysterious disease called "the English sweats" broke up a crucial conference between Luther and Zwingli at Marburg in 1529 and, thus, sealed the split between the Lutherans and Calvinists. "Spanish smallpox" and not Spanish arms destroyed the Aztec and the Inca empires. Even rulers, such as "Bloody Mary" of England, were insane due to neurosyphilis.

Infectious diseases were by far the major cause of death in the United States early in this century. Test this assertion for yourself; ask your grandparents what their parents and uncles and aunts died of. Progressive improvements in sanitation and nutrition, the introduction of vaccination by Edward Jenner in 1796, and the discovery and use of penicillin by Fleming in the early 1940s caused a marked decrease in the frequency of fatal infectious diseases.

Infectious diseases persist in great numbers. According to a national health survey in 1976, approximately 50 million cases of acute infectious and parasitic diseases occurred in the United States, or

*McNeil, W. H. 1976. *Plagues and peoples.* New York: Doubleday Publishing Company.

about one in four persons were infected. The vast majority of human diseases of known etiology are produced by biologic agents such as (1) viruses, (2) rickettsia, (3) bacteria, (4) mycoplasma, (5) fungi, (6) protozoa, or (7) nematodes. Moreover, infectious diseases are more easily prevented and cured than any other major group of disorders.

"Medical progress" has played many tricks on us. For several decades, particularly in the last 20 years, there has been a decline in the prevalence of infectious diseases caused by certain highly pathogenic microorganisms, such as streptococci and staphylococci. This decline has been more than offset by a steady increase in the incidence of infections caused by microorganisms, previously considered to be less pathogenic. A *pathogenic* microbe is a species capable of causing disease when it infects.

Factors Determining Occurrence of Infectious Diseases

A dynamic struggle occurs constantly in our bodies between forces of microorganisms and the opposing defenses of each person (host). A simple equation for this process is

$$\text{Severity of infectious disease} = \frac{\text{Number of microbes} \times \text{Virulence}}{\text{Host defenses}}$$

Whether an infectious disease occurs or not and its severity depend on the three factors (Fig. 7-1): (1)

the *virulence* of the infecting microorganism, that is, the capabilities of the microorganism to invade the body and produce disease, (2) the *number of microorganisms* entering the body, and (3) the *host defenses*—the natural, physical, and chemical barriers and immune defenses preventing invasion. Infection is invariably the result of a failure of host defenses (see Chapter 6, Immunology). Infection is the result of defective defenses, and conversely, cure of the infection is the result of triumph of the host defenses.

Virulence and Number of Microbes

Bacteria and other organisms capable of multiplying in tissues vary greatly in their relationship to the body. Roughly, these parasites can be divided into the following four large groups: (1) *Symbiotic microbes* confer benefit on the host; for example, bacteria produce vitamin B_{12} in the ileum. (2) *Commensal microbes* have no deleterious effects on the "healthy" person. These microbes constitute "normal flora" (Table 7-1) and are recognized as potential pathogens of low virulence, for example, *Staphylococcus aureus* or *Escherichia coli*. (3) *Microbes of low pathogenicity* also constitute normal flora. And, (4) *highly pathogenic* microbes normally cause disease following infection, *Mycobacterium tuberculosis*, for example. Less than 1000 infectious agents in the millions of living organisms on our earth are pathogens (Table 7-2).

Before considering specific infectious diseases affecting certain organs of the body, we will discuss the pathogenesis and the clinical manifestations of infectious diseases.

Pathogenesis of Infection

The development of an infectious disease follows a consistent pattern: (1) the parasites *enter* the body through the skin, nasopharynx, lung, intestine, urethra, or other portals. (2) the organisms attach to the surface of cells, multiply, and establish a *local (primary) lesion*. (3) Next, they may *spread locally* along fascial planes or along tubular structures (bronchi or ureters, for example). (4) The next step is *systemic spread* via the circulating blood. Microbes invade tissues and lymphatics and are then carried via the thoracic lymphatic duct into the venous blood (*bacteremia*, for example, may ensue). (5) Via the blood stream, spread to other tissues can produce *distant or secondary lesions*. Depending on the specific characteristics of the microbe, other deleterious effects arise from *toxins* liberated by the organism, such as tetanus. Since certain organisms tend to infect specific sites (organs) the diagnosis of infectious diseases is approached as syndromes affecting given organs (Table 7-2).

Clinical Manifestations of Infections

The clinical manifestations of various infectious diseases are nonspecific; they can display manifestations of diseases of any other etiology. However, certain clinical features are highly suggestive of infection, including abrupt onset of fever, chills, myalgia (muscle pain), photophobia (sensitivity to light), pharyngitis, acute lymphadenomegaly (lymph node enlargement) and splenomegaly, gastrointestinal upset, and an increase in white blood count (leukocytosis) or, paradoxically, a decrease

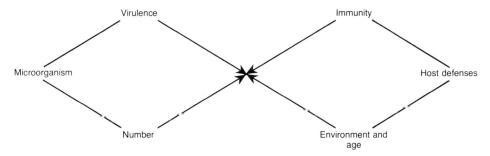

Figure 7-1 *Patient (host) and environmental factors which determine whether an infectious disease occurs and the severity of the infection.*

Table 7-1
*Normal Bacterial Flora**

Anatomic site	Microorganism	Range of incidence (percent)
Skin	*Staphylococcus epidermidis*	85–100
	S aureus (coagulase-positive)	5–25
	Streptococcus pyogenes (group A)	0–4
	Corynebacterium organisms	45–100
	Candida organisms	1–15
Nose and nasopharynx	*S aureus*	20–85
	S epidermidis	90
	Corynebacterium organisms	5–80
	S pneumoniae	0–17
	S pyogenes (group A)	0.1–5
	Neisseria catarrhalis	12
	Hemophilus influenzae	12
Oropharynx	*S aureus*	35–40
	S epidermidis	30–70
	Corynebacterium organisms	50–90
	S pyogenes (group A)	0–9
	S pneumoniae	0–50
	N meningitidis	0–15
	H influenzae	5–20
Stomach	Normally sterile (pH 2–3)	
Jejunum	A few nonpathogens	
	Candida albicans	20–40
Ileum	Small numbers of bacteria	
Colon	Enterobacteriaceae and scores of other microbes	10^{12} organisms/ per gram of stool
Kidneys and urinary bladder	Normally sterile	
Vagina and uterine cervix	Lactobacilli	50–75
	Clostridium organisms	15–30
	C albicans	30–50
	Trichomonas vaginalis	10–25

*Simplified from Youmans, G. P., Patterson, P., and Sommers, H. 1975. *The biologic and clinical basis of infectious diseases.* Philadelphia: W. B. Saunders Company. Tables 7-2 through 7-9, pages 85–94.

Table 7-2
*Infectious Disease Syndromes**

Site of infection	Common	Relatively common
Skin and subcutaneous tissue	*S aureus*	Group A streptococcus, *Candida* organisms, and superficial fungi
Sinusitis	*S aureus*	Group A streptococcus and *S pneumoniae*
Pharyngitis	Respiratory viruses, group A streptococcus	Gonococcus
Epiglottitis	*H influenzae*	
Otitis and mastoiditis	*S pneumoniae* and *H influenzae* (children)	*S aureus* and group A streptococcus
Pneumonitis	*S pneumoniae, Mycoplasma pneumoniae,* and *Mycobacterium tuberculosis*	*S aureus, Klebsiella* organisms, respiratory viruses
Empyema and lung abscess	*S aureus,* anaerobic streptococcus, and *bacteroides* organisms	*Klebsiella* organisms (abscess)
Bacterial endocarditis	*S viridans, Staphylococcus aureus,* and enterococcus	*S pneumoniae* and anaerobic streptococcus
Gastroenteritis	Salmonellae, and *Shigella* organisms	*S aureus, E coli* (infants), clostridia, Norwalk agent
Peritonitis, cholangitis, intra-abdominal abscess	*E coli,* enterococcus, and *Bacteroides* organisms	*Klebsiella-Enterobacteriaceae* organisms, *Proteus* species, anaerobic streptococcus
Urinary infection (cystitis and pyelonephritis)	*E coli, Klebsiella-Enterobacteriaceae* organisms, *Proteus* organisms, and *Klebsiella* organisms	*Pseudomonas*
Urethritis	Gonococcus	*Treponema pallidum*
Pelvic inflammatory disease	Gonococcus and *E coli*	*Klebsiella-Enterobacteriaceae* organisms, *Bacteroides,* anaerobic streptococcus, *Enterococcus* organisms
Bones (osteomyelitis)	*S aureus*	Salmonellae
Joints	*S aureus,* gonococcus, *S pneumoniae,* and *H influenzae*	Group A streptococci and *N meningitidis*
Meninges	*S pneumoniae, H influenzae* (children), *N meningitidis,* ECHO and mumps virus	*E coli, Klebsiella-Enterobacteriaceae* organisms, *Proteus* organisms, *Pseudomonas*

*From *Harrison's Principles of Internal Medicine,* ed. 7, by M. M. Wintrobe, et al. Copyright 1974 McGraw-Hill Book Company. Used with permission of McGraw-Hill Book Company.

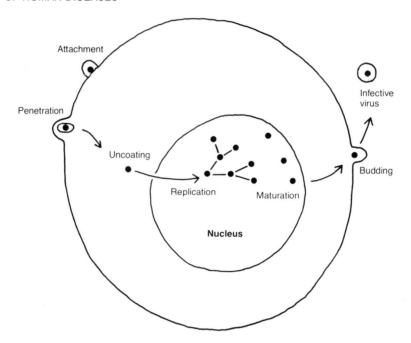

Figure 7-2   *Stages of viral infection of cells.*

in white blood count, called leukopenia. Leukopenia commonly occurs in viral infections.

Many specific infectious diseases can be recognized from information obtained by history, physical examination, and laboratory studies. The history focuses on past illnesses, predisposing factors such as alcoholism, familial disease, exposure to ill persons, contact with animals or insects, ingestion of contaminated food, type and order of onset of symptoms, residence, and travel.

Since viruses and bacteria are the two most common groups of infectious agents responsible for disease, a discussion of major aspects of these microbes follows. This discussion should provide you with a background for forthcoming descriptions of viral and bacterial infections affecting organs described in subsequent chapters.

Viral Infections

Viruses require living cells for growth; thus, they are *obligatory parasites* and are the smallest living organisms. Viruses have tropism, or they "zero in on" and infect specific cells. For instance, receptors are present on the tracheal lining cells for influenza virus and the B-lymphocytes have receptors for Epstein-Barr virus.

Five major events occur as viruses infect cells: (1) the virus becomes *attached* to receptors on the cell surface following invasion of the body. (2) It releases enzymes and *penetrates* into the cells. (3) Once within the cells, it becomes *uncoated*. (4) Thereafter, *replication* (multiplication) and (5) *maturation* and budding (*escape*) of the viruses from the cell ensues. The infection can then become established (Fig. 7-2) and spread to other cells or persons.

While the virus is infecting the cell, a battle erupts between the host's immune defenses (lymphocytes, macrophages, and antibodies—IgA, IgG, and IgM, for example) and the invading virus. Either the virus is eliminated by the immune system or, when the immune defense system fails, the virus persists and injures the host (Fig. 7-3). The cells harboring viruses can become injured when the immune response attacks the virus. Hence, lesions invariably occur while the immune response eliminates the virus.

Many common diseases of childhood, such as mumps, measles (rubeola), chickenpox (varicella), and German measles (rubella), are caused by viruses. The time from the initial contact with an infected individual to the appearance of disease is termed the *incubation period*. For the childhood viral infections, the incubation period is usually from 14 to 21 days. It is much shorter for the common cold (approximately 48 hours).

Clinically, viral infections generally cause fever, enlargement of lymph nodes, pharyngitis (soreness and redness of the oropharynx), and a rash. The rash probably results from an immune response; lymphocytes and macrophages infiltrate around the small blood vessels of the skin in an attempt to destroy viruses within cells. The virus can also, in some cases, enter the epidermis.

Bacterial Infections

Pathogenic bacteria, in contrast with viruses, are mostly free-living organisms that thrive in the human body. The tissues and fluids of the body provide a nicely packaged source of warm nutrients for supporting the growth of bacteria. Bacteria *attach* to epithelial tissues, as do viruses. How bacteria attach to surfaces is unknown, but it is well known that specific bacteria infect rather specific sites in the body, and hence, the phenomenon of *tropism* for tissues and organs prevails as in viral infections. Each bacterium seems to have an ecologic niche.

The lesions caused by bacteria result chiefly from two mechanisms: (1) Many bacteria elaborate substances. The substances can be *enzymes* that digest tissues (streptococci can elaborate collagenase and hyaluronidase, for example), or they can produce *toxins* (*E coli* can produce endotoxin, which induces fever, and can trigger coagulation of blood, for example). (2) The host *inflammatory responses* to bacteria can itself injure tissues. For instance, in acute inflammatory responses to staphylococci, the neutrophils migrating to the area liberate lysosomal enzymes that digest tissues (see Chapter 5, Inflammation and Repair of Tissue).

Bacteria are classified in many ways. One convenient classification is based on the staining characteristics of bacteria by the *Gram's stain*. Bacteria grown in culture media or taken from body fluids (sputum, for example) are smeared on glass microscope slides, Gram's stain is applied, and the slide is examined with a microscope. Bacteria staining purple are termed *gram-positive bacteria* (Fig. 7-4), and those staining pink are termed *Gram-negative bacteria*. The difference in staining characteristics of bacteria arises from differences in the content of proteins and other chemicals in the bacterial cell wall. Also, bacteria are classified by their morphology: *spherical* (cocci), *rod-shaped* (bacilli), *spiral* (spirochete). All of the classifications are germane to the clinical setting and permit a description of bacterial infections. Another classification of bacterial infections is based on the inflammatory response they elicit in the host. A *granulomatous inflammatory* response is caused by tuberculosis and fungal infections. A *pyogenic bacterium* elicits a neu-

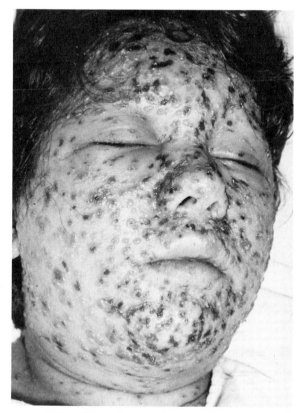

Figure 7-3 *Pustular chickenpox in a pregnant woman who succumbed to varicella pneumonia.*

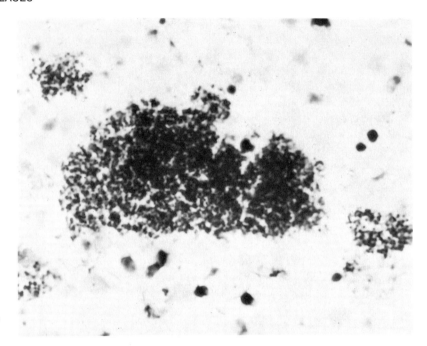

Figure 7-4   *Gram-positive staphylococci.*

trophilic inflammatory reaction (Fig. 7-5). The bacterium is said to be pyogenic, or pus producing. Pyogenic bacteria include *N meningitidis*, *N gonorrhoeae*, *H influenzae*, *S aureus*, *Streptococcus sp*, and *S pneumoniae*. All of these agents can be important pathogens.

The forthcoming discussion will concern infections in various anatomic sites (Table 7-2).

Cutaneous Infections

The skin is normally protected from infection by its high salinity, low pH, unsaturated fatty acids, lysozyme, and thick keratinized layers. Normal flora are constituted by corynebacteria, mycobacteria, and *S epidermidis* and *S aureus*. When the integrity of the skin is impaired from malnutrition, surgical or accidental wounds, or burns, invasion by bacterial infectious agents often ensues. Other patients with apparently normal host defenses can also become infected.

Group A streptococci, staphylococci, and *diphtheriae* are the most common bacteria infecting skin. Most *pyodermas* (skin infections by pyogenic bacteria) arise in preexisting wounds.

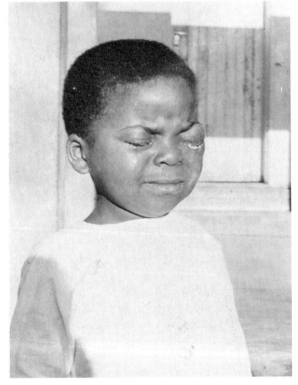

Figure 7-5   *Pyogenic infection of eye. The staphylococcal infection responded well to penicillin.*

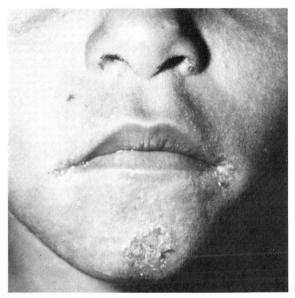

Figure 7-6   *Impetigo caused by staphylococci on the chin of a boy. The lesions at the corners of his mouth were probably caused by a riboflavin deficiency.*

Pyoderma

Impetigo, a type of pyoderma, occurs most commonly in pre-school-aged children (Fig. 7-6) during warm weather. Often insect bites become infected by staphylococci or streptococci. These infections seldom spread or cause systemic findings, such as fever. Treatment with soap, water, and penicillin readily leads to regression of the lesions.

Other staphylococcal infections can infect hair follicles causing *folliculitis*. In the beard area, this is termed *sycosis barbae*. *Pustular acne vulgaris* can also arise from a staphylococcal infection. An extensive and invasive staphylococcal infection of obstructed hair follicles with lesions in subcutaneous tissues is called a *furuncle*, or a *boil*. When boils are multiple, the condition is termed *furunculosis*. A *carbuncle* is another variant of folliculitis that occurs in the skin of the nape of the neck and upper back. Drainage by surgical incision as well as penicillin may be necessary for cure.

Acne vulgaris is the major disease affecting the sebaceous glands of the skin. It involves chiefly the face and, to a lesser degree, the back, neck, chest,

and shoulders. Noninflammatory papules are called *comedones* and may be open (blackheads) or closed (whiteheads). The blackheads can become inflamed or pustular. *C acne* is the bacterium responsible for breaking down lipid from the plugged sebaceous gland producing the inflammation. Acne vulgaris can be a serious problem in adolescent persons, and treatment is complex: tetracycline, Vitamin A, and ultraviolet light are mainstays of therapy.

Numerous other infectious agents invade the skin. Viruses, bacteria (leprosy, for example), and superficial (ringworm, for example) and deep fungi infect the skin. Some of these infectious agents are discussed in Chapter 19, Dermatology and Dermatopathology.

Respiratory Infections

The respiratory tract, including the sinuses, oropharynx, trachea, and bronchi, is protected by antibodies, epithelium, and leukocytes from invasion by microorganisms. Antibodies (IgA) and mucus react with microbes, and the microbes are either engulfed by leukocytes or are swept away from the lungs by the cilia of cells lining the respiratory tract.

The most common of the infectious diseases is the *common cold*, which causes discomfort and, on the average, causes each of us to lose one day of work each year. The viruses most often responsible for a "cold" are *rhinoviruses*. Among this group of viruses are more than 90 distinctive types. Our immunity only forms against one rhinovirus. Hence, another cold occurs from a different virus.

Children with the inherited disorder *cystic fibrosis* have thick mucus plugging their airways. Their respiratory cilia, IgA, and macrophages fail to remove staphylococci and pseudomonas bacteria, so these children develop frequent respiratory infections. Cigarette smokers invariably experience chronic bronchitis because cilia are damaged in the trachea and bronchi by the smoke and infection develops. Moreover, persons having immunodeficiency such as agammaglobulinemia are readily invaded by infectious agents in the respiratory tract.

Usually respiratory infections are divided into two groups: upper respiratory and lower respiratory infections.

Upper-respiratory Infections

The nose and nasopharynx contain many normal flora, the most common being *S aureus* and *S epidermidis* (Table 7-2). Like the nose, the oropharynx contains large numbers of staphylococci, α- and nonhemolytic streptococci, *H influenzae*, and *N meningitidis*. Of special importance is the finding that α-hemolytic streptococcus inhibits group A β-hemolytic streptococcus, pathogens causing *pharyngitis* ("strep throat").

Streptococcal Pharyngitis   The only accurate way a β-hemolytic streptococcal pharyngitis can be diagnosed is by throat culture. The inflammation seen in the pharynx and tonsils can be caused by numerous microbes. Serious complications can develop from "strep throat": *Abscesses* in the tonsils or cervical lymph nodes and *cellulitis*, wherein streptococci spread along fascial planes, can ensue. Before antibiotics were available, streptococci often spread to the brain; this may elicit meningitis.

Two very important systemic diseases can result from immunologic responses to group A β-hemolytic streptococcal pharyngitis: *acute glomerulonephritis* (AGN) and *acute rheumatic fever* (RF). These disorders appear at about ten days (AGN) and 18 days (RF) respectively following infection by streptococcus.

AGN is characterized by the abrupt onset of *proteinuria* (protein in urine), *hematuria* (blood in urine), *edema* of the face and legs, *hypertension* (high blood pressure), and renal function impairment. Culture of the patient's throat often reveals group A streptococcus and antibodies in serum against the bacterium. In children, the healing rate of AGN approaches 100%, whereas in adults, only about 90% heal; chronic renal failure can develop in 10% of the latter group. The strep throat, if active, is treated with penicillin, and the patient is given supportive care until the kidneys heal.

Rheumatic fever may be defined as a nonsuppurative, poststreptococcal, systemic, inflammatory process primarily involving connective tissue with major clinical manifestations reflecting injury to the heart, joints, and central nervous system.

Most often, RF strikes children from 5 to 14 years of age. Two to four weeks lapse between the onset of a strep throat and rheumatic fever. They develop a low-grade fever and signs and symptoms of inflammation of the joints, cardiovascular, and nervous systems (see Chapter 13). The disease can *recur* and cause further damage to the heart valves, leading to mitral stenosis (narrowing).

Hence, *prophylaxis* (prevention) of strep throats is important with respect to AGN and RF. Throat cultures are required to document the presence of the specific group—group A streptococcus—and then penicillin is given in adequate doses. Patients with RF are given continuous or intermittent penicillin for many years to prevent streptococcal infection and recurrence of RF.

Lower-respiratory Infections

The lungs inhale numerous pathogenic viruses, fungi, and bacteria that are eliminated efficiently by host defenses. Only two important pulmonary infections will be discussed here, pneumonia and tuberculosis. In contrast with upper-respiratory infections, the lower-respiratory infections are life-threatening.

Pneumonia   Bacterial pneumonia is caused by *S pneumoniae* (formerly called *Diplococcus*) in 90% of cases. Pneumonia is the sixth leading cause of death in the United States and one of the most common diseases requiring hospitalization. The disease is acquired by enhaling droplets containing microbes; these microbes are then spread along the bronchial tree. Infection of the lungs causes fever, chills, chest pains, shortness of breath, and cough and rust-colored sputum may be coughed up.

The *diagnosis* of pneumonia is made by clinical-history, physical examination, and laboratory studies. The sputum will contain numerous *S pneumoniae* diplococci within neutrophils as seen with Gram's stain. A culture of sputum will also identify and confirm the diagnosis. The chest X-ray reveals a cloudiness, or opacification, in one or more lobes of the lung.

The inflammatory reaction in pneumococcal *lobar pneumonia* (involves one lobe of lung) or *bronchopneumonia* (involving several lobes) occurs over a three-week period: The initial two days are characterized by an acute inflammatory response and the next two days by dilation of blood vessels (vascular engorgement) and a continuing neutrophilic inflammatory response. Days 5 to 8 result in further neutrophilic infiltration, and phagocytosis brings the bacterial growth in check. The lungs at the height of the inflammatory response are airless, heavy, and filled by inflammatory cells. The final two weeks of bronchopneumonia are characterized by a complete resolution of the pneumonia; engulfment of macrophages and removal of cellular debris lead to resolution of pneumonia.

The following serious complications of pneumonia may occur: (1) fluid accumulation in the chest cavity (*pleural effusion*), (2) *empyema* (pus in the thoracic cavity), (3) *bacteremia* (blood poisoning), and (4) on rare occasion, *meningitis* (inflammation of the covering of the brain) or (5) *endocarditis* (inflammation of the heart valves) develop. *S pneumococci* can also produce osteomyelitis (infection of bone).

S pneumococci is highly sensitive to penicillin. The mortality for patients with bronchopneumonia treated with penicillin is only 5%. However, pneumonia is seen to a variable extent at autopsy in many persons dying from chronic diseases. It can be the final "death blow" in a debilitated person.

Legionnaires' Disease   Legionnaires' disease is a type of pneumonia caused by a bacterium. It got its name and notoriety by striking 189 people, 29 fatally, who attended an American Legion convention in Philadelphia in July 1976. Patients showing signs of Legionnaires' disease experience malaise (fatigue), muscle aches, a slight headache, abdominal pain, rapidly rising fever and chest discomfort. Patients who have died of the disease have often been immunosuppressed by other chronic diseases. It is diagnosed by detecting antibodies in the patient's serum and is treated with antibiotics.

Tuberculosis   Tuberculosis is a disease caused by the tubercle bacillum, *M tuberculosis*. Tuberculosis formerly killed many young people in the United States; today, 30,000 new cases occur annually. It is a major cause of death in the developing world. This disease affects the lungs primarily, but the kidneys, brain, urogenital tracts, and bone can become infected also.

Pathogenesis of Primary Tuberculosis   Inhalation into the lungs of droplets containing tubercle bacilli elicits an acute inflammatory response by neutrophils in the bronchial mucosa. Following the acute inflammatory response, the bacilli drain from the lymphatics to the lymph nodes toward the center of the chest, and an immune response occurs (see Chapter 6, Immunology).

A *granulomatous immune response* develops in the infected lymph nodes and lymphocytes sensitized and reactive to the bacilli migrate in the lymphatic channels to the lung tissue and produce a granuloma. A *granuloma* is composed of macrophages, lymphocytes, and multinucleated giant cells (Langhans' cells). The "tubercule" bacillus is so named because it produces granulomas that resemble "tubercules" (small potatoes). A vigorous immune response limits the bacilli in the primary infection, and a scar is formed in the lymph node and in the site in the lung primarily infected.

Chest X-rays are taken routinely on admission to a hospital to look for the primary lesions of tuberculosis. The primary tuberculosis lesion appears as a calcified spot in the hilar lymph nodes and the upper portion of the lower lobe. This pathologic finding is termed the *Ghon complex*.

Secondary Tuberculosis   Reactivation tuberculosis, or secondary tuberculosis, occurs usually late in life. It results from reactivation of dormant bacilli that have been previously encased in fibrous tissue or by newly inhaled bacteria. Usually the immunity that develops in a primary infection of tuberculosis lasts throughout life. It is possible to test for immunity by using the *tuberculin test*, which indicates if an individual has been previously sensitized to tubercule bacilli. Purified protein derivative (PPD) of the bacillus are injected into the skin. If the individual has been previously sensitized to tuberculosis, memory lymphocytes will cause a cell-mediated immune response when coming into contact with the PPD. Redness and induration (a raised, red, firm disk-shaped area) of the skin occurring within 48 to 72 hours is typical of a positive tuberculin test. Individuals acquiring the secondary form of tuberculosis are often malnourished or chronic alcoholic individuals. *Miliary tuberculosis*, a severe form of secondary tuberculosis, can occur (Fig. 7-7) in a person with a weakened immunity. The bacilli and the inflammatory response may break through walls of blood vessels, disseminating bacilli into the blood stream and thus throughout the body. In countries where tuberculosis is prevalent, meningitis, renal destruction, osteomyelitis, and cervicitis are common complications of tuberculosis.

Diagnosis and Treatment   Tuberculosis is diagnosed by examining stained (Ziehl-Neelsen stain) sputum for the red, acid fast tubercle bacilli. In addition, the bacillus can be cultured on Löwenstein-Jensen media, a process requiring several weeks for growth. Treatment often requires the use of more than one drug. *Triple therapy* includes the use of streptomycin, isoniazid preparations (INH), and PAS. Combination therapy prevents the bacilli from becoming resistant to the chemotherapy. Because a few tubercle bacilli persist in the body, we do not speak of a "cure" but state that the tuberculosis is "arrested."

Urinary Tract Infections

Approximately, one-half of serious Gram-negative infections occur in the urinary tract, especially in persons with indwelling urinary catheters (a hollow tube is placed in urinary bladder for drainage) or in persons who have obstructed outlet channels for the flow of urine.

Cystitis

Cystitis, an infection and inflammation of the urinary bladder, is common in women. *Honeymoon cystitis*, a special form, occurs when *E coli* is introduced into the bladder during intercourse. Cystitis causes pain on micturition and can be diagnosed by observing leukocytes and by culturing bacteria in

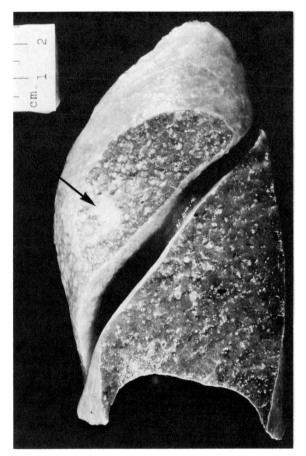

Figure 7-7   *Miliary tuberculosis. The lungs are speckled by numerous miliary granulomas* (arrow).

the urine. Gantrasin, a sulfa drug, is used as treatment.

Pyelonephritis

Pyelonephritis is an infectious disease of the kidneys resulting from bacterial infection that ascends from an infected bladder (see Chapter 17, Urology and Renal Medicine). It usually occurs secondary to obstruction of the outlet of urine flow. Women who are pregnant and men with enlarged prostate glands are apt to develop pyelonephritis. The renal tissue can be destroyed by the acute inflammatory response as microabscesses form in response to bacteria. *E coli* is the most common cause of pyelonephritis; however, *Proteus* and *Pseudomonas* are other common culprits. Persons with multiple sclerosis or with spinal cord injury often suffer dysfunction of the bladder, and urine flow becomes slowed (static); thus, they are subject to urinary tract infections. Persons who form stones in their urinary tracts (*urolithiasis*) have urinary stasis and also often get pyelonephritis.

Diagnosis   Individuals with pyelonephritis suffer with back pain, fever, chills, nausea, and loss of appetite. They may also experience burning on urination, and their urine will be cloudy. Tapping the individual on the back over the area of the kidney often elicits pain. Examination of the urine reveals pus (neutrophils) and numerous bacteria. A culture reveals microorganisms numbering greater than 100,000 colonies/mm³ of urine.

Antibiotic sensitivity testing determines which antibiotic would be ideal. Bacteria cultured from a patient's urine, blood, or throat are streaked on an agar culture plate. Paper disks impregnated with antibiotics are placed in the agar. The antibiotics diffuse into the agar and inhibit the growth of bacteria (Fig. 7-8). The antibiotic with the largest zone of inhibition of growth is thus used to treat the bacterial infection.

Central Nervous System Infections

The brain, its meningeal covering, and the cerebrospinal fluid (CSF) bathing the central nervous system (CNS) are normally sterile. The following three groups of infectious agents can infect the CNS: bacteria, viruses, and agents provoking granulomatous inflammation—tuberculosis and *Cryptococcus*.

Most infections of the CNS involve the meninges. Thus, typical expressions of *meningitis* occur, including fever, headache, nuchal rigidity (stiffness of neck), and altered CNS function.

Acute Bacterial Infections

Acute bacterial infections of the CNS are divisible into *focal abscesses* or *diffuse processes*, meningitis, for example. Both of these infections result from

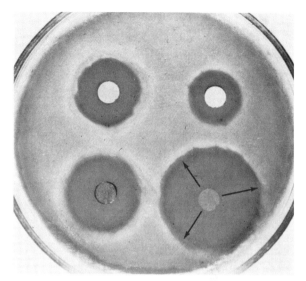

Figure 7-8   *Antibiotic sensitivity testing. The antibiotic with the largest zone of inhibition of growth of bacteria* (arrow) *was chosen for treatment because the bacterium was most sensitive to it.*

(1) direct invasion of nervous tissue of the subarachnoid space by bacteria or (2) "seeding" of the CNS by microbes from the blood stream.

Brain abscesses often develop following traumatic head injury or some direct extension of bacterial infections from adjacent structures; examples include osteomyelitis (infection of bone) of the skull, acute mastoiditis, sinusitis, or fractures. Fractures involving the cribriform plate are important sites for bacterial invasion from the nose.

Invasion of the CNS by bacteria secondary to bacteremia from primary infection in other organs is the most common cause of bacterial CNS infections. Primary infections of the skin, lungs, and gastrointestinal tract are the most common sources. A wide variety of microorganisms infect the CNS. For unknown reasons, specific types of microbes infect patients of a certain age (Table 7-3).

The diagnosis of meningitis is made by clinical history, physical findings, and a *lumbar puncture*. A lumbar puncture is a procedure wherein a needle is introduced in the lumbar region and CSF is withdrawn in a syringe and examined (see Chapter 21). With acute bacterial meningitis, numerous neutrophils can be seen in the CSF and a Gram stain reveals bacteria. A culture is taken, and the sensitivity to antibiotics is measured. Based on the Gram stain and culture, it is possible to prescribe an appropriate antibiotic. Usually ampicillin is given and occasionally chloramphenicol is also given.

Prior to the discovery of antibiotics, the mortality of meningitis approached 100%. Cures are the rule today. In a person who succumbs to menin-gitis, a white-yellow coating of pus is seen in the meninges and the brain is swollen (Fig. 7-9).

Viral Meningitis and Encephalitis

Viral diseases of the CNS are divided into specific categories, meningitis and encephalitis, for example, on the basis of clinical symptoms and signs

Table 7-3

*Classification of Infections of the Central Nervous System**

Type of infection and specific examples		Pathogenesis	Most frequent causative microorganisms
Acute bacterial infections	Abscesses: brain epidural subdural	Metastatic** (lung, intestinal tract, skin, paranasal sinuses) or direct invasion (trauma or ENT, neuro-orthopedic surgery)	Peptostreptococcus *Bacteroides* sp. Staphylocci Group A or D streptococcus
	Meningitis: Infants (2 months)	Metastatic (intestinal tract) or direct invasion (birth canal)	*E coli* Group B streptococcus
	Children (2 months to 5 years)	Metastatic (oropharynx); rarely direct invasion	*H influenzae,* type b *S pneumoniae* *N meningitidis*
	Adults	*Metastatic (oropharynx); rarely direct invasion*	*S pneumoniae* *N meningitidis* (*H influenzae* occasionally in adults)
	All ages	Direct invasion secondary to head trauma (old or recent), congenital neuromalformations, neurodiagnostic procedures, and neuro-orthopedic surgery	Staphylocci Group A streptococcus *S pneumoniae* *P aeruginosa*
Granulomatous meningitis	Tuberculous meningitis	Metastatic (lung)	*M tuberculosis*
	Cryptococcal meningitis	Metastatic (lung)	*C neoformans*
Acute viral infections	Aseptic meningitis	Metastatic (intestinal tract or oropharynx)	Enteroviruses Mumps virus ECHO virus
	Viral encephalitis	Metastatic (intestinal tract) or arthropod vector feeding	Mumps virus Herpes virus Enteroviruses Arboviruses

*From Youmans, G. P., et al. 1975. *The biologic and clinical basis of infectious diseases.* Philadelphia: W. B. Saunders Company.

**The term *metastatic* is commonly employed to denote hematogenous spread of microorganisms to the central nervous system, that is, in association with bacteremia, fungemia, or viremia.

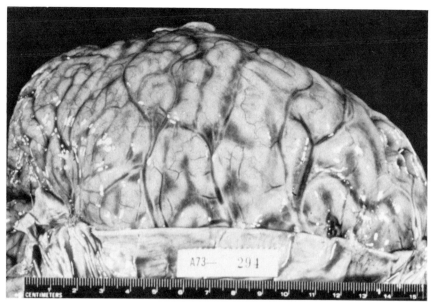

Figure 7-9   *Meningitis. The meninges overlying the cerebrum is filled with gray pus.*

reflecting involvement of a specific anatomic site. All of the viruses affecting the CNS, except rabies, can cause both syndromes of meningitis and encephalitis.

By definition, *viral meningitis* results when the inflammatory process is limited primarily to the coverings of the brain and spinal cord and is associated with stiff neck, headache, and fatigue. By contrast, the term *encephalitis* is used when the inflammatory process clearly involves brain tissue. Clinical signs and symptoms of cerebral dysfunction ensue: altered consciousness, disordered thought processes and behavior, or seizures. The most frequently occurring viral agents are listed in Table 7-3

The diagnosis of viral meningoencephalitis is occasionally difficult. A typical clinical picture and a lumbar puncture is required to achieve a diagnosis. The CSF in viral meningitis, in contrast to that in bacterial meningitis, will usually show only some lymphocytes. Moreover, bacterial cultures will not grow microorganisms, and hence, viral meningitis is termed *aseptic meningitis*. A specific viral etiologic agent can occasionally be isolated in tissue culture, and acute and convalescent (taken

about 12 days later) sera often reveal a rise in antibody concentration against the causative viral agent.

Treatment of viral meningitis is symptomatic. Only rarely will viral meningitis cause death. Also some viruses slowly cause damage to the brain, the slow viruses (see Chapter 4.)

Gastrointestinal Infections

The gastrointestinal tract contains an amazing number of bacteria. Approximately 10% of the dry weight of feces is composed of bacteria, predominantly bacilli. The common pathogens of the gut are also bacilli, *E coli*, *Salmonella sp*, and *Shigella sp*; all of these pathogens produce enteritis (inflammation of the intestine). In tropical countries, parasitic worms (nematodes), including hookworm, round worm, and others, produce extensive anemia and chronic gastrointestinal disease. These parasites can infect persons who travel to the tropics, in Puerto Rico, and in some areas of the southern United States. Amebiasis, caused by the protozoan *Entamoeba histolytica*, ulcerates the mucosa of the colon and rectum in persons who eat contaminated food. Occasionally, amoeba may disseminate to the liver and brain and produce abscesses.

Diarrhea

On a world-wide basis, cholera (*Vibrio cholerae*), *E coli*, *S typhosa* and *Shigella sp* (all gram-negative bacteria) frequently cause diarrhea, profound dehydration, and death. These bacteria are responsible for the diarrhea, which is unpopularly termed "Montezuma's revenge" or the "Aztec two step," experienced by travelers to Central and South America. Infants are vulnerable to these infections and they can die from dehydration caused by diarrhea because their fluid volume is small.

These gram-negative microbes invade the mucosa of the large and small intestines and elicit an acute inflammatory response (gastroenteritis); septicemia can also occur. The mucosa of cholera victims becomes so necrotic that it sloughs as "rice water" (the flakes of mucosa appear as grains of rice in the watery stool). Copious amounts of fluids and minerals (electrolytes K^+, Na^+, Cl^-, HCO^{-3}) are lost from the inflamed intestinal tract. The patient becomes febrile, weak, and dehydrated. Replacement of the fluids and electrolytes and antibiotics are given to restore health.

In addition to the gram-negative bacteria, several viruses can cause infectious gastroenteritis. The *Norwalk agent*, for instance, causes low-grade fever and diarrhea, vomiting, abdominal cramps, headache, and weakness. No specific treatment is available for viral infections (see Chapter 15, Gastroenterology).

Gram-negative Bacteremia

A major complication of primary gram-negative bacterial infections of the gastrointestinal and genitourinary tracts is the seeding of these agents into the blood stream. Bacteremia causes fever and weakness and can cause cardiovascular collapse. Approximately 100,000 persons die each year in the United States from gram-negative bacteremia. Most of these victims are predisposed to infection by se-

vere, debilitating, acute or chronic diseases that impair inflammatory, immune and healing responses.

The fever and other toxic signs arise from a substance called *endotoxin*, which is produced by gram-negative bacteria. Endotoxin is a complex molecule composed of lipopolysaccharides. It can trigger intravascular coagulation and cause necrosis in many organs; hence, a gram-negative bacteremia can be lethal (see Chapter 11, Hematology).

Viral Hepatitis

Viral hepatitis has been present since antiquity. But it was not until World War II that it was realized that this disease was a commonplace entity, and only during the last decade have we recognized the viruses that cause hepatitis.

Characteristically, persons with hepatitis experience a low-grade fever, loss of appetite, and lethargy. Persons with hepatitis also note that their skin and eyes have "turned yellow." Concurrently, they report that their urine has turned a dark color.

The development of immunologic methods for the identification of the etiologic agents has taught us that there are two major types of hepatitis (Table 7-4). The pathology of hepatitis is described in Chapter 16.

Viral hepatitis, type A, is spread by the fecal-oral route through person-to-person spread or by way of food or water. Hence, hepatitis virus A is found in areas having unsanitary conditions.

Viral hepatitis, type B, is transmitted chiefly via parenteral routes (blood and contaminated needles). Less frequently it is transmitted orally. Blumberg discovered the Australia antigen in 1965 in the blood of an Australian aborigine, and hence, the virus is also called the "Australia antigen." It is recognized that about 0.5% of all persons in the United States are chronic carriers of the virus. This is why blood banks screen donors for the virus. Moreover, only about 1 in 20 infected persons become symptomatic.

Type B viral hepatitis can be a major threat to patients and persons working in hemodialysis or transplantation centers. Also medical technologists can easily become infected by working with in-

Table 7-4
Viral Hepatitis

	Hepatitis Virus A	Hepatitis Virus B
Synonyms	Infectious hepatitis	Serum hepatitis
	Epidemic jaundice	Homologous serum jaundice
Etiology	Virus, type A	Virus, type B
Setting	Poor sanitation and crowding	Transfusion and contaminated needles, syringes, and surgical instruments
Incubation period	Average 1 month (2–5 weeks)	Average 3 months (2–16 weeks)
Immunity after recovery	To hepatitis virus A only	To hepatitis virus B only
Spread	Primarily by fecal-oral route	Primarily by blood injection, occasionally by inoculation
Duration of infectivity	*Stool:* 2–3 weeks before jaundice and 2–3 weeks after onset of jaundice	*Stool:* consider it infectious as long as blood is infectious
	Blood: 2 weeks before jaundice; 1 week after jaundice	*Blood:* variable, usually prolonged, 4–6 weeks, sometimes indefinitely, and hence, they cannot donate blood
Clinical picture	*Onset:* abrupt	*Onset:* slow and insidious
	Severity: usually not too severe (severity increases with age)	*Severity:* generally more severe with longer period of illness and jaundice
	Case fatality: 1–2 per 1000	*Case fatality:* 3–37 per 1000
Use of gamma globulin	*Effective:* minimizes symptoms	Standard gammaglobulin may be effective in decreasing symptoms
	Dosage: 1–2 ml/lb lasts 4–6 weeks and 5–6 ml/lb lasts 6–8 months	
Laboratory diagnosis by hepatitis associated antigen (HAA) test	Negative	*Positive:* acute-chronic hepatitis virus B *or* an asymptomatic carrier can have the viral antigen or antibody to the viral antigen
		Negative: antigen may have disappeared before symptoms appeared

fected blood. Precautions are thus used for preventing transmission of this virus. Gammaglobulin injection (containing antibodies against the virus) may decrease the severity of the hepatitis following injection of the virus.

In general, hepatitis virus B is more virulent than hepatitis virus A. Both can cause acute hepatitis and damage hepatocytes. A few patients may gradually develop chronic active hepatitis, and rarely, cirrhosis of the liver may ensue. Unfortunately, we thought we could identify all of the viruses causing hepatitis, but recently large groups of unclassifiable viruses which cause hepatitis have been discovered.

Venereal Diseases

A variety of diseases are termed *venereal diseases* because they are sexually transmitted (Table 7-5). These infectious agents are important since they cause discomfort and disability. Only syphilis will be discussed here. Gonorrhea, the other common

Table 7-5
Venereal Diseases

Disease	Microorganism	Clinical findings
Herpes genitalis	Herpes simplex, type II	Painful vesicles on genitalia
Chancroid	*H ducreyi*	Soft painful genital ulcer
Granuloma inguinale	Donovania or *Calymmatobacterium granulomatis*	Granulomatous lesions in inguinal regions
Condyloma acuminatum	Virus	Warty cauliflowerlike genital lesions
Gonorrhea	*N gonorrhoeae*	Discharge of pus from urethra and painful urination
Lymphogranuloma venereum	Virus	Swollen inguinal lymph glands
Syphilis	*T pallidum*	Painless genital ulcer (primary)

venereal disease, is discussed extensively in Chapter 18.

Syphilis

Syphilis, or *lues*, is an infectious disease caused by *T pallidum*. Except for congenital syphilis, it is transmitted almost entirely by direct, intimate contact with infectious lesions of early syphilis. These lesions contain the *T pallidum* spirochete. The spirochete penetrates the skin and, in *primary syphilis*, produces a *chancre* (ulceration) on the genitalia (Fig. 7-10). Primary syphilis occurs within a few days to two weeks following intercourse. Thereafter, if primary syphilis is not treated, secondary and tertiary stages of syphilis can ensue after variable periods of time.

A quiet (dormant) period persists for several weeks to months following healing of the chancre. *Secondary syphilis* ensues shortly thereafter and is characterized by a rash (Fig. 7-11). Individuals in the secondary stage remain infectious. A diagnosis can be made at this stage by detecting antibodies to syphilis in the serum or by examining scrapings of the skin for spirochetes (Fig. 7-12). The presence of antibodies in the patient's serum against the spirochete can be identified either by biologic tests (VDRL or Wassermann tests), which are lacking in precise specificity, or by a specific blood test, the *Treponema pallidum immobilization (TPI)* test, which can specifically detect the presence of syphilis. Another specific test is the fluorescence *Treponema pallidum* antibody test (FTA).

The most devastating form of syphilis is the *tertiary stage*. This stage occurs 10 to 20 years following the primary infection. The blood vessels of the cardiovascular system, especially of the ascending aorta and the cerebral cortex, are vulnerable. Fibrosis and a chronic inflammatory (cellular immune) response to spirochetes occurs in the aorta, an aneurysm (sac-shaped dilatation) of the ascending aorta may occur, and the coronary arteries may become obstructed by fibrosis.

Central nervous system involvement in tertiary syphilis can cause three lesions: (1) chronic meningitis, (2) destruction of the cerebral cortex, and (3) destruction of the dorsal columns of the spinal cord. Infected individuals may experience organic psychoses from the cerebral cortex lesions. These psychoses are characterized by delusions of grandeur. The involvement of the dorsal columns of the spinal cord by syphilis result in a disorder termed *tabes dorsalis*. Because patients lack sensation in their legs, they develop a slapping gait (tabes dorsalis syndrome). *Osteoarthritis* (a destructive joint disease) may develop in their knees and is termed *Charcot's joints*. A loss of sensation of the skin can result in ulcers in the feet (Fig. 7-13). The pathologic lesions of tertiary syphilis are not reversible. But syphilis in its primary and secondary stages is treatable by injections of penicillin, which will prevent the tertiary stage.

Gonorrhea

Neisseria gonorrheae is acquired through sexual contact. Gonorrhea may also be termed "the clap."

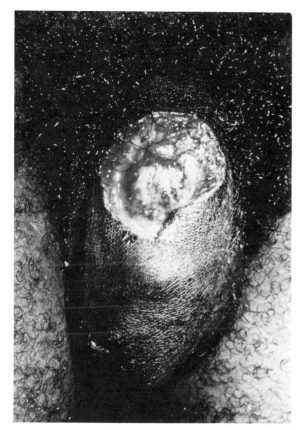

Figure 7-10   *Syphilis. Primary syphilitic ulcer chancre at the base of the penis.*

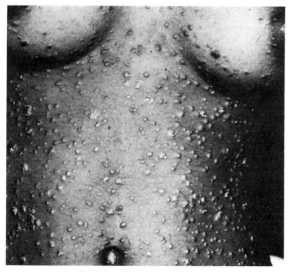

Figure 7-11   *Rash of secondary syphilis.*

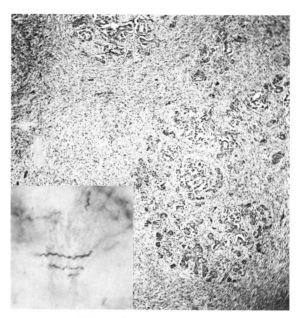

Figure 7-12   *Photomicrograph showing spirochetes of* T pallidum. *The pancreas has been destroyed by congenital syphilis (inset).*

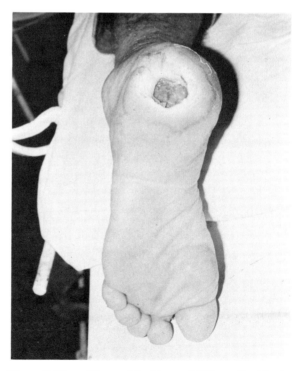

Figure 7-13   *Ulcer of foot in syphilitic patient lacking sensation in his feet.*

Gonorrhea produces acute inflammation (urethritis) of the passageway between the bladder and opening. Pus is seen at the opening of the urethra, and a burning sensation is experienced on urination. In women, the urethra, the cervix (cervicitis), and the uterine fallopian tubes (salpingitis) can become infected. Some women may be asymptomatic reservoirs of the infection. A serious complication of gonorrhea is the development of sterility from strictures of the reproductive ducts and abscesses in the pelvic organs (see Chapter 18, for a more thorough discussion of gonorrhea).

Infections of the Fetus

At various stages of life, persons are especially vulnerable to certain infectious diseases. Important age-dependent infections occur in the human fetus. Congenital infections of the fetus in utero can occur at any time from conception to birth. Congenital infections cause a profound impact, including death of the fetus, permanent disfiguring birth defects or mental retardation (see Chapter 3). Good prenatal care can prevent the infection.

The usual in utero infections can be easily remembered by the acronym TORCH complex, as shown in Table 7-6. The TORCH infectious agents affect approximately 1% to 5% of all newborns. Many of these diseases are preventable by antenatal care of the mother. For example, detection of syphilis in a pregnant mother enables treatment of the mother and fetus with penicillin.

Fetal Infection Syndrome

At birth, a newborn infected in utero has a characteristic syndrome: the infant will have a swollen liver and spleen, yellow discoloration (jaundice), and skin hemorrhages; will frequently be underweight; and may have defects in the central nervous system, eyes, viscera, and the heart. Examination of the infant's blood often reveals IgM antibodies against the agent responsible for the infection. Although the defects occurring in the brain are often irreversible, other birth defects, such as those occurring in the heart, can be corrected by cardiac surgery.

Toxoplasmosis is an infectious disease acquired by a pregnant woman eating inadequately cooked meat. This protozoan microorganism can traverse the placenta, enter the fetal circulation, and invade and damage the fetal brain. In contrast, *herpes simplex virus* can spread throughout the body of a newborn who lacks antibodies against it. Normally, the fetus is protected by maternal antibodies of the IgG class that pass through the placenta to the fetus. However, if the mother becomes infected late (final weeks) in pregnancy, time may be insufficient for the mother's body to form herpes simplex antibodies (Fig. 7-14). Subsequently, during the passage of the fetus through the birth canal, infection by the virus occurs. It is then possible for this infection to spread throughout the body, producing necrosis in many organs (Fig. 7-15).

The development of the organs of the fetus is nearly complete by 12 weeks following conception. Infections occurring later in pregnancy are less apt to produce malformations of organs than infections occurring when organs are developing. The time when the infection occurs is especially critical for *rubella*: 50% of babies infected by rubella in the initial three months in utero develop cataracts, impaired hearing, or other defects. Fortunately, measures are now available for preventing rubella birth defects by vaccinating the woman prior to pregnancy.

Because the fetus lacks prior exposure to infectious agents and has no acquired immunity, the newborn is also vulnerable to certain bacterial infectious agents. For instance, newborns are vulnerable to the colon bacillus *E coli* since they have not yet formed antibodies against it.

Table 7-6
The Torch Complex

Toxoplasma gondii
Other—syphilis, varicella, and other microbes
Rubella virus
Cytomegalovirus
Herpes simplex virus

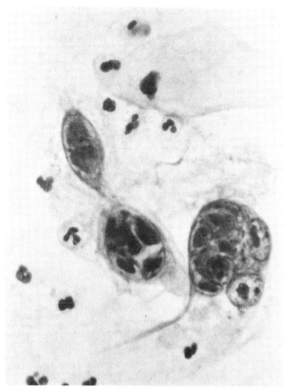

Figure 7-14   *Photomicrograph of pap smear of pregnant woman reveals multinucleated giant cells infected by herpes simplex virus.*

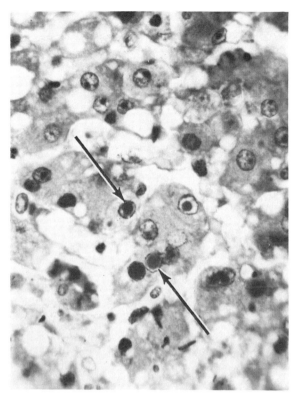

Figure 7-15   *Photomicrograph displaying hepatic necrosis in a newborn which was caused by herpes simplex. Viral inclusions are seen* (arrows).

Opportunistic Infections in Immunosuppressed Patients

The term *opportunistic infections* refers to infectious diseases that occur in persons whose protective immunity has been compromised. Oftentimes, the opportunistic infectious agent is an ordinary "garden variety" microbe that we ordinarily cope with. These organisms have low pathogenicity; that is, they do not usually cause disease. Many viruses, bacteria, fungi, protozoa, and nematodes can become opportunists in immunosuppressed persons. Some of the most common opportunistic infections are shown in Table 7-7.

Conditions that predispose persons to opportunistic infections have already been cited, malnutrition and alcoholism, for example. Modern medical progress, which offers remedies to prolong life, renders many patients susceptible to hospital-acquired (*nosocomial*) infections. Approximately 3% to 5% of all patients entering a hospital will develop

Table 7-7
Common Opportunistic Infectious Diseases in Immunosuppressed Patients

Viruses   Herpes simplex, chickenpox, and cytomegalovirus
Bacteria   Staphylococcus, *Pseudomonas* sp, and *E coli* and other Gram-negative rods
Protozoa   Pneumocystis carinii and *Toxoplasma gondii*
Fungi   *Candida,* sp and *Aspergillus* sp and Cryptococcus sp

*Legionnaires' pneumonia appears to be an opportunistic infection disease.

an infection as a result of that admission. The first dictum of medicine is "to do no harm." This dictum is often compromised by the therapy given to treat severe illness or desperate measures are required for dangerous diseases.

Many hospitalized patients have diseases characterized by immunosuppression (Table 7-8). These patients are vulnerable to opportunistic infections. Violation of the protective barrier of the skin by burns, trauma, or surgery permits invasion by organisms. The overuse and misuse of antibiotics and immunosuppressive drugs that destroy the immune response also render individuals susceptible to opportunistic infections. Chronic diseases, renal failure and cirrhosis of the liver, for example, also permit opportunistic infections to occur.

Severe malnutrition profoundly impairs immune defenses against viruses and tuberculosis. In many medical centers, persons with cancer constitute a large proportion of malnourished patients, and they easily become infected. Malnutrition, invasion of the lymphoid immune system by tumor, and therapies toxic to the immune system, such as irradiation and chemotherapy, prolong healing of wounds and predispose cancer patients to infections.

In addition, children with congenital immunodeficiencies are vulnerable to certain types of bacterial infections. For instance, children who lack antibodies (agammaglobulinemia, for example) are especially susceptible to pyogenic infectious agents. By contrast, infants lacking a thymus gland will be vulnerable to intracellular organisms, especially viruses, tuberculosis, and fungi (see Chapter 6, Immunology).

Table 7-8
*Conditions Associated with Immunosuppression**

Malignancy	Pregnancy
Excessive antibiotics	Burns
Diabetic acidosis	Postsurgical
Irradiation	Trauma
Cirrhosis	Transplant recipients
Immunodeficiency disease	Viral infections
Nutritional deficiency	
End-stage renal failure	

*Arranged for ease of memorization.

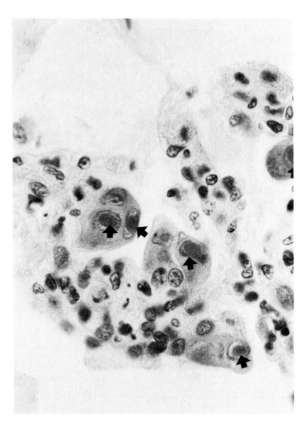

Figure 7-16   *Photomicrograph of cytomegaloviral pneumonia from renal transplant patient. Large viral inclusions are seen* (arrows).

Viral Opportunistic Infections

Opportunistic viral infections commonly encountered in immunosuppressed patients include herpes simplex, cytomegalovirus, chickenpox, and measles. For example, measles kills approximately 25% of the malnourished children who become infected. Individuals with malignancies, especially lymphomas or leukemias, are also highly vulnerable to this and other viral infections. Herpes simplex is the virus that causes common cold sores of the lips. In an immunosuppressed person, herpes simplex can disseminate throughout the body and produce necrosis.

Immunosuppressed renal transplant recipients and others being treated with a high dose of cortisone (for rheumatoid arthritis, for example) can develop life-threatening cytomegalovirus pneumonia (Fig. 7-16).

Bacterial Opportunistic Infections

Gram-negative bacterial opportunistic infections most often arise from an infected genitourinary tract or from the gastrointestinal tract. The prolonged use of indwelling urinary catheters permits infections with *E coli*. The infected patient may succumb to endotoxic shock and heart failure. Also, following surgical or obstetric procedures, there is a risk that patients may develop Gram-negative and other opportunistic infections.

A *fever* in a leukemic patient heralds a bacterial or fungal infection in approximately 85% of the cases. Alert health professionals should recognize this sign of an opportunistic infection so that treatment can be given. Both fungal and bacterial infections can be treated with specific drugs.

Fungal Opportunistic Infections

Fungi are troublesome to many immunosuppressed patients, especially in persons with leukemia. The most commonly occurring fungal infection is caused

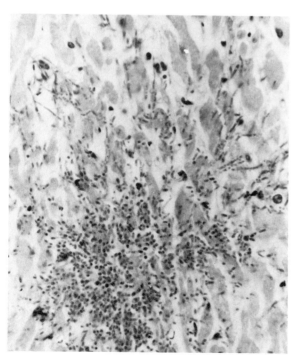

Figure 7-17 *Photomicrograph of the heart of a leukemic patient was invaded by* Candida *yeast organisms.*

by *C albicans*. This fungus is killed by antibodies and neutrophils. Since chemotherapy given to treat leukemia suppresses immunity and inflammatory responses, this fungal infectious agent often disseminates in the blood stream throughout the patient's body. Necrosis of vital organs, such as the heart, may ensue (Fig. 7-17).

To reiterate, the occurrence and severity of an infectious disease depend on three factors: (1) the immune capacity of the person, (2) the virulence of the microorganism, and (3) the number of microorganisms invading the person. Two important factors that influence the outcome of an infection are the stage of the infection at the time of the diagnosis (localized or systemic infection) and, secondly, the use of antimicrobial chemotherapeutic agents to arrest the growth of microbes.

Antimicrobial Treatment of Infectious Diseases

Prevention

An old proverb declares, "An ounce of prevention is worth a pound of cure." In quiet, unheralded ways, preventive medicine obviates infectious diseases. Adequate nutrition, sanitation, immunization, screening for infection with chest X-rays and skin testing, isolation of infected persons, the sterilization of food, and attention to aseptic technique and good hygiene are measures employed to prevent infectious diseases.

Diagnosis

Much has been said about techniques employed for the diagnosis of specific infectious diseases in this chapter. Clinical history, physical examination, X-ray studies, biopsy and, importantly, cultures of body surfaces, tissues, and fluids to isolate microbes are employed to diagnose infectious diseases. Specific chemotherapy can then be given for many infectious diseases. Viral infections are an exception to this rule.

The development of antimicrobial chemical agents in the 1930s provided potent weapons for controlling bacterial and fungal infections. The ability to predict a favorable clinical response to the use of an antimicrobial agent by in vitro measurement of the sensitivity of microbes to antibiotics has greatly advanced the response to therapy for infectious diseases.

Bacterial Sensitivity to Antimicrobial Agents

In vitro testing of an antibiotic's ability to inhibit the growth of bacteria in vitro permits the selection of effective antibiotics for treating the infected patient. Susceptibility testing is usually carried out by measuring a zone of inhibition of growth of a microorganism surrounding a paper disk impregnated with the antimicrobial agent (Fig. 7-8).

The choice of an antibiotic selected for treating the patient is based on the *therapeutic potential* and the *toxic potential* of the drug (on the bone marrow, kidney or liver, for example). Penicillin is nearly always the drug of choice for *S pneumoniae* and is nontoxic. By contrast, streptomycin is effective against *M tuberculosis* but can damage the eighth cranial nerve and cause deafness. Likewise, chloramphenicol is normally an excellent antibiotic, but it is toxic and can cause aplastic anemia (destroy bone marrow).

For antimicrobial therapy to be efficient and effective, the patient's immune system must be functioning. Factors or drugs that suppress immunity (for example, cortisone) should be reduced. Nutrition, too, should be optimal. Abscesses should be drained and dead infected tissues debrided (removed). Obstructed ducts (gallstones in bile duct or stones and strictures or tumors of the urinary tract, for example) should be removed or opened for proper drainage. All of these factors require attention or the drugs will not eliminate the "bugs."

Summary

The occurrence and severity of an infectious disease depends on a person's immunocompetence, the virulence of the microorganism, and the number of invading microorganisms. Specific infectious agents show a predilection for infecting certain persons and specific anatomic sites. Signs and symptoms of an infectious disease often include fever, tachycardia, leukocytosis, and discomfort.

Diagnosis of infectious diseases is frequently achieved by culturing body fluids or detecting antibodies against the infectious agent. A specific antibiotic can be given for bacterial infections following determination of antibiotic sensitivity testing. Antibiotics are not effective against viruses and hence viral illnesses are treated supportively with bed rest, fluids, etc.

Other measures important in treating infectious diseases include nutritional repletion, surgical drainage, and immunotherapy such as antitoxins and gammaglobulin. Prevention is possible by excellent sanitation, vaccination, adequate nutrition, and hygiene.

Bibliography

Alexander, J. W., and Good, R. A. 1970. *Immunobiology for surgeons*. Philadelphia: W. B. Saunders Company. Discusses infectious diseases in traumatized and postoperative patients.

Bailey, W. R., and Scott, E. G. 1970. *Diagnostic microbiology*, ed. 3. St. Louis: The C. V. Mosby Co. Standard diagnostic microbiology textbook.

Cohen, A. 1969. *Medical virology*. Oxford: Blackwell Scientific Publications, Ltd. Standard clinical virology textbook.

Davis, L. 1973. *Medical microbiology*, ed. 2. New York: Harper & Row, Publishers. Standard textbook.

Emmons, C. W., Binford, C., Utz, W. 1970. *Medical mycology*, ed. 2. Philadelphia: Lea & Febiger. The best reference for fungal infections. _____

Infectious control in the hospital. 1975. ed. 3. Chicago: American Hospital Association. Describes precautions established for infectious disease control.

Isler, C. 1975. Infection: Constant threat to perinatal life. *RN* August: 23–29. Describes intrauterine infections.

Krugman, S. 1976. Viral hepatitis; overview and historical perspective. Y. J. Biol. and Med. 49:199–203. Historical presentation on viral hepatitis.

Lurie, H. J., et al. 1970. Opportunistic infections of the lungs. Hum. Pathol. 1:233–257. A clinical and pathological review of opportunistic infections.

Meakins, J. L. 1975. Host defense mechanisms. *Can. J. Surg.* 18:259–268. Describes the interaction of factors determining infections.

Moffet, H. L. 1975. *Pediatric infectious diseases.* Philadelphia: J. B. Lippincott Company. The best current reference on childhood infections.

Nahias, A. J. 1975. The TORCH Complex. Hosp. Practice 9:65. Excellent summary of intrauterine infections of the fetus.

Purtilo, D. T., Connor, D. H. 1975. Fatal infections in protein-calorie malnourished children with thymolymphatic atrophy. Arch. Dis. Child. 50:149–152. Describes depressed immunity and fatal infections in malnutrition.

Purtilo, D. T. 1975. Fatal mycotic infections in pregnant women. *Am. J. Obstet. Gynecol.* 122:607–610. Describes fungal infections during pregnancy.

Remington, J. S. 1972. Compromised host. *Hosp. Practice* 7:59–64. Excellent illustrations and discussion about opportunistic infections.

Top, F. H., and Wehrle, P. F., Eds. 1972. *Communicable and infectious diseases*, ed. 7. St. Louis: The C. V. Mosby Co. A standard multi-authored reference textbook.

Youmans, G. P., Patterson, P., Sommers, H. 1975. *The biologic and clinical basis of infectious diseases.* Philadelphia: W. B. Saunders Company. By far the most clinical and readable reference of those available.

Youmans, J. B., Ed. 1964. Syphilis and other venereal diseases. *Med. Clin. North Am.* 48(3). Excellent discussion of pathogenesis depicted by numerous photographs.

CHAPTER 8

Neoplasia (oncology)

Chapter Outline

Objectives

After reading this chapter you should be able to

Define the terms neoplasm, tumor, benign, and malignant.

Describe the frequency of cancer as a cause of death and the relative frequency of
  cancer in various anatomic sites.

Understand the terminology used for describing neoplasms.

Define the term carcinoma-in-situ.

Understand why clinical staging is important for prognosis of cancer patients.

Describe the two major routes by which cancer cells spread.

List the three factors generally affecting prognosis of a patient with cancer.

List environmental agents that are carcinogenic.

Compare the relative importance of environmentally induced cancers and inherited cancers.

List examples of conditions that create a high risk for developing cancer in certain persons.

Describe and compare the mutation and oncogene hypotheses of carcinogenesis.

List the potential consequences of cancer.

Describe how metastases can reach the brain, liver, and lung.

Name the most common cause of death of cancer victims.

Describe measures that can be employed to prevent cancer.

List the cardinal signs of malignancy.

Describe the techniques used for diagnosing malignancies.

Describe the significance of a "frozen section" diagnosis of a breast mass.

Name the first line of treatment of most cancers.

List tumors usually sensitive to radiotherapy.

Describe two complications of radiotherapy.

Understand when chemotherapy is employed for treating cancer.

List the effects of chemotherapeutic agents on cancer cells.

Describe two major complications of chemotherapy.

Understand the objective of immunotherapy.

Introduction

Neoplasia is the most baffling complex of diseases confronting all multicellular animals. The term, neoplasia, is derived from the Greek "neos," "new," and "plasia," a molding. A *neoplasm*, literally means any growth of cells or tissue. However, a neoplasm generally refers to a focus of abnormal cells arising from one cell which has undergone an alteration of its genetic material. The new clone of cells has an inherited growth potential which is progressive and unlimited. Neoplasms can be classified as malignant or benign based upon their cytologic and histologic features, or on the anticipated clinical course (outlook or prognosis) of the patient. In general, the prognosis is good for benign neoplasms and bad for malignant neoplasms.

Malignant neoplasms manifest great autonomy, whereas benign neoplasms closely resemble normal tissues, especially in their rate of growth. The term tumor literally refers to any swelling, but it is often used interchangeably with cancer, especially by the laity. It is mandatory that the adjectives benign or malignant be used in referring to any tumor so the prognosis in any given case becomes more understandable.

Approximately 100 histologically distinct, malignant neoplasms can occur in human beings. Following arteriosclerotic heart disease and stroke, cancer is the third leading cause of death in the United States.* The number of new cases occurring in 1976 in various organs is depicted in Figure 8-1. Not shown are the estimated 300,000 new cases of skin cancer. Malignant melanoma, the most dreaded form of skin cancer, accounted for 9300 cases; approximately one half of these victims of melanoma will die of their malignancy.

Terminology

A *tumor* (neoplasm) is an abnormal mass of tissue which grows in excess, is uncoordinated with nor-

*19.5% of deaths in the United States during 1975 were caused by cancer.

mal tissues, and continues to grow beyond the cessation of the stimuli that originally evoked it. This definition applies to both malignant and benign tumors. No single characteristic is an absolute diagnostic criterion for malignancy; in evaluating a tumor for malignant or benignant potential, many factors must be considered. Some of these factors are listed in Table 8-1. Terms used to denote general types of tumors are listed in Table 8-2.

Additional factors affecting biological behavior of tumors include anatomic location; benign tumors when occurring in vital areas (like the heart or brain, for example) may kill an individual (Fig. 8-2) The size and ease with which the tumor can be removed, and the sensitivity of the tumor to irradiation and chemotherapeutic agents also determine prognoses.

Pathogenesis

The etiologic agents responsible for neoplasms are diverse. The marked variation in the frequency of occurrence of certain types of cancers in various

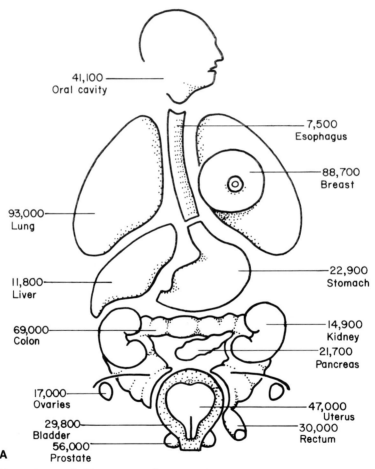

Figure 8-1   **A,** *New cases of cancer that occurred at various sites in 1976.* **B,** *Age-adjusted cancer death rates for selected sites, females, United States, 1930 to 1973.* **C,** *Age-adjusted cancer death rates for selected sites, males, United States, 1930 to 1973.* **B** and **C** were *standardized on the age distribution of the 1940 U.S. Census Population. (From* Ca—A Cancer Journal for Clinicians *26(1):18–19, 1976.)*

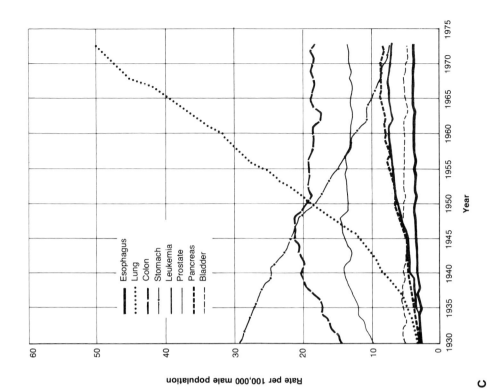

C

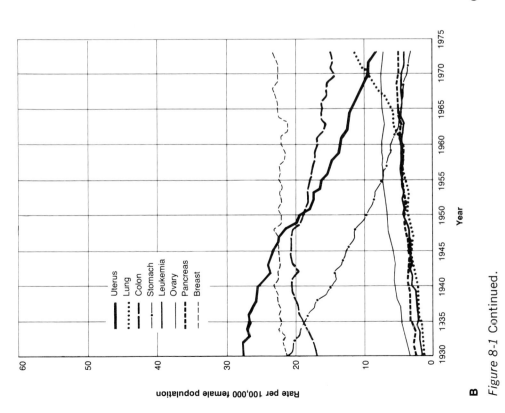

B

Figure 8-1 Continued.

Table 8-1
Comparison of Benign and Malignant Neoplasms

Characteristics	Benign	Malignant
Growth rate	Slow	Rapid
Mitoses	Few	Many
Nuclear chromatin	Normal	Increased
Capsule	Present	Absent
Local growth	Expansive	Invasive
Tissue destruction	Little	Much
Vessel invasion	None	Frequent
Metastases	None	Frequent

geographic areas implicates environmental agents as major causes of cancers. Genetic predisposition together with environmental agents (ecogenetic factors) are responsible for virtually all cancers. Cancer occurs predominantly in elderly persons; approximately 16% of adults develop a malignancy by age 70 years. In contrast, cancer occurs less commonly in young persons, but certain malignancies do occur with greater frequency in children and in young adults. Although cancer is rare in children, it is the most common cause of death in this age group.

The causes (etiology) of most malignancies are not known. However, initiating factors, or *carcinogens* (cancer generators) such as viruses, chemicals, or irradiation first provoke cells in a tissue to increase in number. We call this *hyperplasia*. Later, if the carcinogenic agent persists or other promoting carcinogenic agents affect the cells, they are pushed a step closer along a continuum towards malignancy. This next step, *carcinoma-in-situ* (CIS) can be later followed by a cancer whose cells invade underlying connective tissues, blood vessels, or lymphatics, and spread along these channels from the local primary lesion to distant sites in other parts of the body. Such secondary colonization we call *metastases*.

The process of carcinogenesis results in an apparent reversion back to a fetal-like state. The tumor cells fail to mature normally (differentiate). In three respects, cancer cells resemble fetal cells—the primitive cells (a) have a rapid growth rate, (b) remain immature, and (c) produce fetal proteins. Cancer cells differ from fetal tissues by their failure to discontinue their growth and mature.

Two steps in progression of developing carcinoma of the uterine cervix are depicted in Fig. 8-3. The use of a Papanicolaou (Pap) smear of the cervix can detect uterine cervical cancer early, or in a preneoplastic state, anywhere along the spectrum from hyperplasia to carcinoma-in-situ, to invasive carcinoma (Table 8-2). Carcinogenesis may often occur in persons who are exposed to carcinogens many times. But surprisingly it can take many years, even decades, for cancer to take hold.

Tumors are named according to the histologic type of tissue from which they arise. The Greek suffix "oma" denotes a tumor. Together with the prefix "sarc" we have sarcoma, a fleshy excrescence of tumor, indicating a malignant neoplasm. Sarcomas are usually highly malignant, proliferating connective tissue cells. Table 8-3 outlines a

Table 8-2
Terminology Associated with Neoplasms

Hyperplasia	Increased number of cells
Hypertrophy	Increased size of cells
Carcinoma	Malignant tumor of epithelium
Sarcoma	Malignant tumor of non-epithelial tissues
Adenoma	Benign tumor of glandular epithelium
Carcinoma in situ	Malignant epithelial tumor showing no invasion (limited to surface)
Metastasis	Discontinuous tumor spread from primary lesion to distant secondary site
Papilloma	Benign epithelial tumor growing outward from skin
Polyp	Tumor projecting outward from mucosal epithelial surfaces

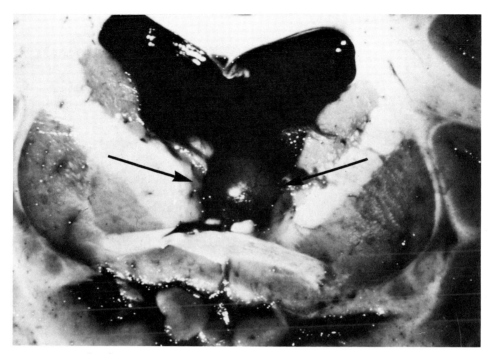

Figure 8-2   *Benign tumor* (arrows) *strategically compressing vital cardiorespiratory centers in the brainstem.*

classification of some benign and malignant tumor counterparts.

Prognosis

The prognosis (outcome) of a patient with cancer is based upon many factors, chiefly the *stage* of the tumor when it is discovered. The stage is determined by several factors: size, location, depth of invasion, and clinical findings. The earliest stage of tumor is designated stage 0 tumor, restricted to one small site (Fig. 8-4). In contrast, when invasion of surrounding tissues or distant spread (metastasis) of the tumor occurs, more advanced stages are designated (Fig. 8-5). When metastases occur the prognosis generally becomes bleak.

Carcinomas, malignancies of epithelium, spread by local invasion and they also mestastasize through lymphatic channels. In contrast, sarcomas usually spread through blood vessels. Tumors can also grow along nerves causing many cancer victims to experience pain. Our ability to predict the out-

comes of patients with various cancers is highly variable and depends first upon the histologic type of tumor. An approximate five year survival is usually possible for most malignancies. The *five-year survival* figure is based upon noting the number of persons who survive five years with similar tumors. For instance, approximately 60% of patients diagnosed as having breast cancer survive for five years. The prognosis becomes better or worse depending on: (a) *the size*, (b) *histologic type*, and (c) *stage* the tumor has attained when treatment is provided.

Etiology

Roughly 90% of malignancies are caused by carcinogenic agents in our environment. The lifestyle of a person determines to a great extent whether that person gets a certain type of cancer. Several examples underscore this point. Nuns virtually never get uterine cervical cancer; prostitutes frequently do. Thus, cervical cancer is thought to be transmitted as a venereal disease through intercourse.

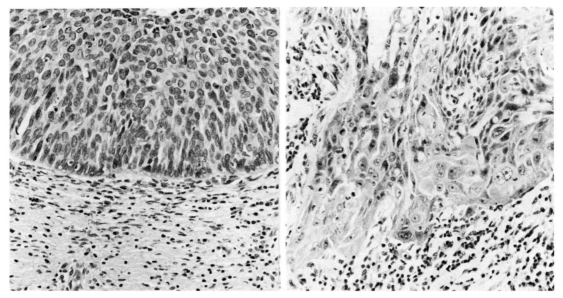

Figure 8-3 *Photomicrograph of the earliest malignant lesion, carcinoma in situ of the uterine cervix* (left) *can progress to invasive carcinoma* (right). × 200.

Table 8-3
Classification of Tumors

Tissue	Benign tumor	Malignant tumor
Connective tissue		
Adult fibrous tissue	Fibroma	Fibrosarcoma
Cartilage	Chondroma	Chondrosarcoma
Bone	Osteoma	Osteosarcoma
Fat	Lipoma	Liposarcoma
Muscle		
Smooth muscle	Leiomyoma	Leiomyosarcoma
Striated muscle	Rhabdomyoma	Rhabdomyosarcoma
Blood tissues		
Lymph vessels	Lymphangioma	Lymphangiosarcoma
Blood vessels	Hemangioma	Hemangiosarcoma
Lymphoid tissue	Infectious mononucleosis	Lymphosarcoma (lymphoma)
Bone marrow	Infectious mononucleosis	Leukemia
Neural tissue		
Nerve sheath	Neurilemmoma	Neurogenic sarcoma
Glial tissue	Gliosis	Glioma (malignant)
Epithelium		
Squamous epithelium	Papilloma	Squamous carcinoma
Glandular epithelium	Adenoma	Adenocarcinoma

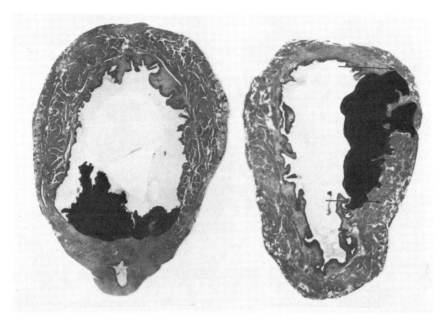

Figure 8-4   *Superficial bladder carcinoma projecting into bladder (exophytic) lumen* (left) *and invasive (endophytic) carcinoma* (right). × 1.

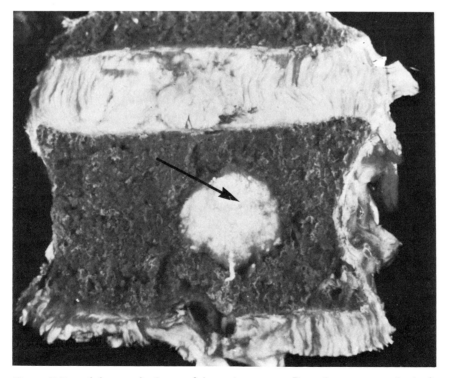

Figure 8-5   *Advanced stage of breast cancer. Breast cancer metastasis (white) has occurred in the spine.*

A recent, marked decline in the occurrence of cancer of the stomach in the United States suggests that a change in the way food is processed is probably responsible for this decline. By contrast, the sharp increase in carcinoma of the lung corresponds with the increase in cigarette smoking that has occurred since the 1930s. Lung cancer occurs predominantly in males; however, women have also recently shown a marked increase in both cigarette smoking and lung cancer.

The patient whose tumor is shown in Figure 8-6 worked during World War II packing asbestos around heating pipes. Thirty years later a lump appeared in her neck and dull pain in her chest disturbed her sleep. Asbestos is now known to cause mesothelioma, a tumor arising from mesothelial cells lining the thoracic or abdominal cavities. Attempts are being made to remove this carcinogen from our environment.

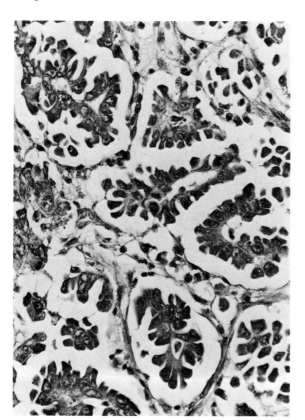

Figure 8-6 *Mesothelioma of the pleura (adenocarcinoma) of the lining of the thoracic cavity which developed in an asbestos worker.* × 400.

Table 8-4
Hereditary Cancer Syndromes

Hereditary neoplasms

Retinoblastoma (childhood cancer of eye)

Multiple endocrine adenomas (thyroid and parathyroid adenomas, for example)

Familial polyposis of colon

Preneoplastic conditions

Neurofibromatosis (may develop sarcomas of nerves)

Albinism (prone to squamous cell carcinoma, that is, sunlight induced.)

Immunodeficiency syndromes (5% to 10% develop lymphomas)

Genetic Susceptibility

Hereditary susceptibility to cancer appears to be a factor of minor importance in most cases of cancer. The *mutation theory of cancer* considers all carcinogens—chemicals, viruses, irradiation, etc.—to be *mutagens*. That is, carcinogens cause permanent heritable changes in the DNA comprising our genes. Furthermore, neoplasms can arise from one mutated cell and form a clone of cells having identical features. Usually the carcinogen strikes a *somatic cell* in the body, however, when *germ cells* (ovum or spermatozoa) are involved and undergo mutation, the mutant gene is passed on to offspring who may develop cancer. For instance, retinoblastoma, multiple endocrine tumors, and familial polyposis of the colon are inherited (Table 8-4). Patients with inherited (familial) cancer syndrome are more vulnerable to environmental carcinogens than normal persons.

Various other genetic conditions predispose certain individuals to malignancy. For instance, albinism is characterized by a lack of the pigment melanin. And the absence of protection against the carcinogenic rays of the sun by melanin renders albinos very susceptible to skin cancer. Roughly 1 in 100 individuals carry the recessive gene for albinism, whereas approximately 1 in 10,000 individuals in the United States develop albinism by having both recessive genes (see Chapter 9, Inherited Disorders). Skin cancer in albinos can be prevented by avoidance of direct sunlight.

Children with immunologic deficiency have a marked (1000 ×) increase in the occurrence of malignancy. They are especially prone to developing malignancies in lymph nodes and lymphoid tissues (lymphomas). Also, individuals who have undergone immunosuppression for transplantation of kidneys have a marked (80 ×) increase in malignancy. This increased occurrence of malignancy probably results from an immune deficiency—the protective effects of *immune surveillance* that normally eliminate foreign malignant cells is lacking (see Chapter 6, Immunology).

Viral Etiology

Despite the identification of numerous viruses that cause leukemia and lymphoma in chickens, mice, and rats, virus has not been definitely identified as a cause of cancer in human beings. The Epstein-Barr virus (EBV) has recently been shown to be the cause of infectious mononucleosis, a benign blood disease that occurs frequently during adolescence. EBV is probably also the cause of a malignant tumor of the jaw, Burkitt's lymphoma (see Chapter 11, Hematology, for discussion).

Oncogene Hypothesis

The oncogene theory of the cause of cancer suggests that certain RNA viruses (oncogenes) insert themselves within genetic DNA material of chromosomes (Fig. 8-7). These oncogenes could have entered the DNA of vertebrates eons ago and have been passed on to successive generations through germ cells as part of normal inheritance. The oncogenes are thought to be ordinarily suppressed, but various carcinogens, including viruses, can possibly derepress specific viral oncogenes enabling them to take over the function of the cells.

Environment

The occurrence of cancer of the nose and mouth in snuff users and the development of carcinoma of the skin of the scrotum of chimney sweeps in Victorian England are well known. Bladder cancer was also recognized over a century ago in aniline dye industry workers. A rare malignant tumor of the liver, angiosarcoma, has recently occurred at an astoundingly high rate among workers in the rubber and plastic industries. A chemical—vinyl chloride—present in over 1000 products used daily in homes is thought to be the carcinogenic agent responsible for the liver cancer. Numerous cancers caused by exposure to vinyl chloride will probably appear in the future.

Carcinogens present in our environment can contaminate our food. The high incidence of hepatocellular carcinoma in Africa is thought to be due to the ingestion of *aflatoxin*, a fungal toxin acquired by eating moldy, contaminated food. Studies have revealed that the highest levels of liver cancer are found in areas with the highest frequency of fungus contamination.

Cigarette smoking, mentioned earlier, has been established as a cause of cancer of lungs, larynx and mouth; it has also been associated with frequent occurrence of carcinoma of the urinary bladder.* The tars in cigarette smoke are carcinogenic in experimental animals.

Persons working with asbestos, arsenic, nickel, and uranium also experience high rates of lung cancer. And irradiation received from X-rays is, unfortunately, sometimes carcinogenic. For instance, children with previously irradiated thymus glands have developed carcinoma of the thyroid gland decades later. Also, radiologists and victims of Hiroshima and Nagasaki who were exposed to irradiation have a high incidence of leukemia.

Parasites, including Schistosoma, can probably give rise to malignancy. Urinary bladder carcinoma is common in Egypt near the Aswan dam where this parasite is present in water (Fig. 8-8). In addition, the author has studied a liver fluke of southeast China that is associated with carcinomas of the bile ducts.

Consequences of Cancer

Psychologic Consequences

Cancer can devastate some individuals and families psychologically, yet cause little physical harm: Many

---

*The Surgeon General reported in 1977 that 50% of bladder cancer is in men and that 30% of this cancer is caused by cigarette smoking.

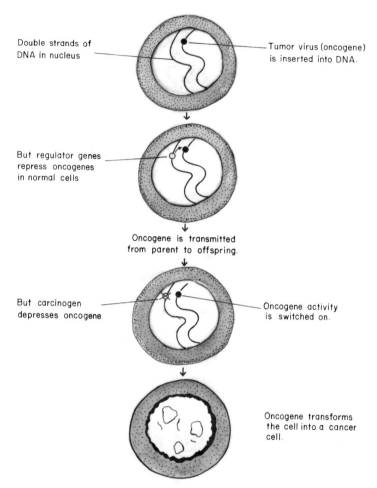

Double strands of DNA in nucleus

Tumor virus (oncogene) is inserted into DNA.

But regulator genes repress oncogenes in normal cells

Oncogene is transmitted from parent to offspring.

But carcinogen depresses oncogene

Oncogene activity is switched on.

Oncogene transforms the cell into a cancer cell.

Figure 8-7   *The oncogene hypothesis explains inherited predisposi-tion to cancer and the activation of oncogene virus by carcinogens.*

persons with cancer, because of early diagnosis and improved treatment, have a full life expectancy. While cure is not always possible, the lives of individuals can be prolonged and enjoyable, productive months or years may result from therapy. The patient and family members of victims of cancer should be dealt with honestly, and should usually be informed of the prognosis and efforts being made on their behalf.

Pain

The occurrence of pain in victims of cancer often results from obstruction of various tubes (esoph-

agus, intestinal tract, outlet of the urinary bladder, and so forth). Destruction of tissues and pressure resulting from expanding masses can also inflict pain. Infections are common complications; fever and discomfort can ensue. Fortunately, medication and neurosurgical procedures are available to relieve most pain.

Malnutrition

Cachexia (wasting) occurs in many cancer patients. They lose their appetite (anorexia), malabsorption can occur, and a depletion of protein production by the liver occasionally ensues. Such complica-

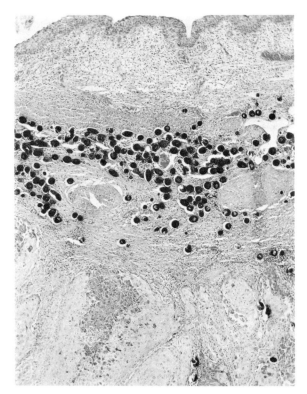

Figure 8-8 *Dark football-shaped eggs of the schistosome fluke are surrounded by invasive bladder carcinoma.* × 400.

tions are especially common in individuals who have malignancies of the gastrointestinal tract.

Neurologic and Hormonal Dysfunction

Neurologic complications such as numbness and tingling occur in many cancer patients because of vitamin deficiency arising from the effect of chemotherapeutic agents. Strangely, some cancer cells themselves may revert to a fetal-like state and begin acting like endocrine glands: Hormones may be produced and abnormalities in endocrine function may occur.

Metastasis

The dissemination of malignant tumor from the primary site of origin can destroy bone and also lead to severe pain. Such metastases can also cause

obstruction of various tubes or may spread to the brain. Commonly when malignancy arises in the colon, pancreas, or stomach, tumor cells metastasize via the portal vein and deposit in the liver. The lungs are also frequently affected by metastasis when blood vessels are invaded by a tumor. The tumor cells act as an embolus (dislodged clot circulating in the blood), which travels into the right side of the heart and from there is pumped through the pulmonary artery into the lungs. The metastatic tumor embolus is trapped and begins to grow.

Blood Disorders

Anemia (decreased amount of erythrocytes or red blood cells) is a common problem arising in patients with malignancy (see Chapter 11, Hematology). Anemia may be a sign of malignancy, especially when blood oozes or gushes from the surfaces of carcinomas of the uterus or the gastrointestinal tract. In addition, anemia can be caused by irradiation or the use of cytotoxic drugs. The same two factors can destroy production of blood platelets, which are important for clotting blood, and massive bleeding may ensue.

Causes of Death

Victims of cancer can die from cachexia (marked wasting) and bronchopneumonia. Hemorrhage, coagulation (thrombosis), and infections are the most common modes of demise. Less commonly, the primary or metastatic tumors impinge on the heart, airways, or brain and where vital functions become immediately impaired. Also, many patients with cancer die of diseases entirely unrelated to their cancer—heart attack or stroke, for example.

Prevention

Most cancers can be prevented by decreasing exposure to carcinogens. This can be done by stopping cigarette smoking and by increasing safety requirements in factories which produce or emit carcinogens into our environment. More rigorous testing and regulation of food additives which cause contamination by carcinogenic chemicals should be required.

Knowing that malignancies require a long incubation period from initial hyperplasia to frank invasion should motivate people to examine their own bodies and seek yearly medical checkups which could potentially lead to early diagnosis of cancer. All of us should be aware of the *cardinal signs of malignancy* (Table 8-5). Individuals who are predisposed to developing malignancy by inheritance should undergo medical examinations every six months. A proctoscopic examination (a long lighted hollow tube is inserted into the rectum and colon and the walls are inspected for cancer) should be performed yearly in all persons over 40 years of age. This procedure permits detection of both benign lesions such as polyps, and colorectal cancer, to be detected early (Fig. 8-9). Yearly pelvic examinations and Pap smears for carcinoma of the uterine cervix have proven their worth by resulting in a dramatic decline of invasive cervical cancer.

Diagnosis

The clinical diagnosis of malignancy, as in any disease, is based in part upon the clinical history of the patient. The cardinal signs of malignancy are especially important. A patient with a certain type of skin cancer might, in describing an increase in the size and pigmentation of a lesion, reveal features of a malignant melanoma. Increase in size of a lump, in the breast for instance, or the loss of weight or feeling of excessive fatigue and anemia

Table 8-5
Warning Signs of Cancer

1	Unusual bleeding or discharge from any site
2	A lump of thickening in any area, especially the breast
3	A sore that does not heal
4	A change in bowel or bladder habits
5	Hoarseness or persistent cough
6	Indigestion or difficulty in swallowing
7	Change in size or shape or appearance of a wart or mole
8	Unexplained weight loss

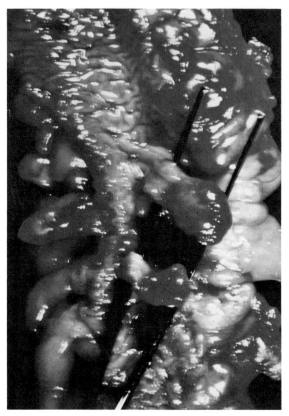

Figure 8-9 *Adenomatous polyps of the colon.*

should be thoroughly investigated. Often the pathologist will be asked to study the blood and tissues to offer a more definitive opinion. In addition to self-examination for breast cancer, screening by X-ray, xerography and mammography are of diagnostic value (Fig. 8-10).

Unfortunately the detection of lung cancer by X-ray examination of the lung is an insensitive method of detection; chest X-rays only detect well-developed, inoperable tumors. Barium sulfate, which is swallowed, outlines the contour of the gastrointestinal tract and permits malignancies to be visualized. Moreover, dyes detectable by X-ray can be injected into blood vessels aiding in the diagnosis of tumor.

Exfoliative Cytology

The microscopic examination of cells which have exfoliated (shed) or been scraped off (as in a Pap

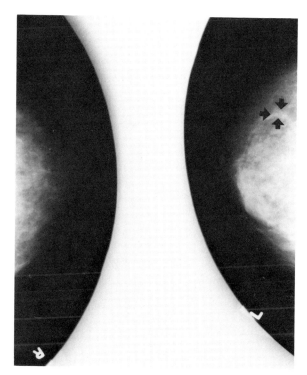

Figure 8-10 *A mammogram outlines breast cancer* (arrows).

smear) the surface of a tumor is valuable for detecting malignancy. Nearly all body surfaces can be examined for tumor cells by this technique—the mouth, and the intestinal, urogenital, and respiratory tracts (Fig. 8-11).

Biochemical Diagnosis

Recently immunologists have discovered that patients with cancer possess fetal antigens (oncofetal antigens), which are produced by the tumors and secreted into blood or urine. *Alpha-fetoprotein (AFP)*, for example, is produced by fetal liver and hepatocarcinomas. AFP can be detected in the blood of patients with liver cancer.

Likewise, colon carcinomas secrete an oncofetal antigen, *carcinoembryonic antigen (CEA)* Detection of CEA in the patient's serum can assist in diagnosis and in determining whether surgical resection has been successful. When a colon carcinoma has been entirely removed, CEA, if formerly present, should disappear from the patient's blood. Con-

versely, persistence of the tumor is signaled by persistence of CEA in the patient's blood.

Biopsy

A biopsy specimen of tissue can be obtained by introducing a needle through the skin. Needle biopsies of masses can often obviate the need for an open exploratory surgical procedure (Fig. 8-12). In addition, metastasis can occasionally be detected in bone marrow by aspiration samples.

A "frozen section" diagnosis of a biopsy may be requested by a surgeon in the case, for instance, of a breast lump. While the patient is anesthetized the surgeon excises the lump and the pathologist examines and freezes the specimen, cuts and stains it, examines the slide in a microscope, and based upon the frozen section diagnosis the surgeon either closes the wound (when the tumor is benign), or removes the breast (when the tumor is malignant).

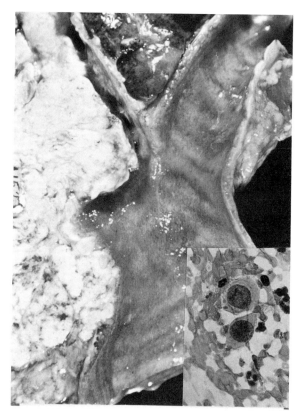

Figure 8-11   *A Pap smear revealed this tumor (inset, × 400) from a lung cancer.*

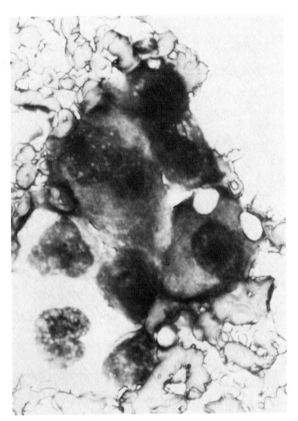

Figure 8-12 *A needle biopsy of bone marrow revealed this dark nest of metastatic liver cancer cells. × 300.*

The use of tubes, such as the bronchoscope, proctoscope, and cystoscope, permit the direct visualization of tumors. Through these tubes a portion of a tumor can be excised for microscopic evaluation. A pathologist may thus make a diagnosis and plans for proper therapy can be initiated.

Treatment

Surgery

Surgical removal of malignancies is the first line of treatment, but if metastases have already occurred, the chances of curing the patient by surgery alone are remote. Only localized lesions of the skin and tumors in their early stages of development are surgically curable. But surgical procedures can relieve pain, bypass obstructed ducts, or improve the patient's nutrition by insertion of a feeding gastrostomy tube. This type of procedure is termed *palliative surgery*. A major contribution made by surgons in the treatment of cancer is that of removing an adequate piece of tissue to permit a pathologist to establish the diagnosis. Sir William Osler said, "The three best forms of treatment are diagnosis, Diagnosis, DIAGNOSIS."

Radiotherapy

Ionizing irradiation is the best type of therapy for many victims of cancer. Ionization of compounds in the tissues by the irradiation destroys tumor or tissue. The two types of ionizing radiation are electromagnetic (using X-rays and gamma rays) and particulate (using beta and alpha particles, neutrons, and pions). Particulate forms of irradiation are more deeply penetrating.

The lethal dose for most tumors and normal tissues is about 300 rads (a rad is the unit measure of absorbed radiation dose). Generally, cells that are rapidly dividing are more sensitive to irradiation; most malignant tumors fit this criterion. But irradiation also damages normal tissues and thus the dosage of irradiation must be divided into small fractions and be given daily over a period of several weeks. Normal tissues tend to regenerate between exposure to radiation, whereas the more radiosensitive tumor does not (see Chapter 4, Adaptation, Injury, and Death of Cells).

Radiotherapy is effective in treating Hodgkin's lymphoma, certain malignancies of gonads (male seminoma and female dysgerminoma), squamous carcinomas of the mouth and oropharynx, uterine carcinoma, and Wilms' tumor of children.

Often, irradiation is used in combination with surgery and chemotherapy. Preoperative irradiation is often given to shrink the size of a tumor to enable the surgeon to remove it. Also postoperative irradiation is commonly given to eliminate residual tumor. Radiotherapy is also used to reduce the severity of localized, but inoperable cancers. Unfortunately, the vast majority of the most common tumors (lung, breast, and colon cancer) respond poorly to irradiation.

Many complications can result from irradiation. Radiation sickness and the partial destruction of bone marrow are two frequent complications of radiotherapy (Fig. 8-13). Infections invade the irradiated, immunosuppressed person, whose bone marrow fails to produce white blood cells which normally defend against infectious agents. Radiation sickness is caused by damage to the intestinal mucosa; the person usually has temporary diarrhea and nausea. Longterm effects, such as fibrosis and scarring of vital structures such as the ureters following pelvic irradiation, may prove to be lethal effects of irradiation. Also, radiotherapy can induce radiation pneumonitis and fibrosis of the lungs may ensue.

Chemotherapy

Chemotherapeutic agents for the relief or cure of cancer have had a dramatic impact on prognosis. New drugs introduced during the last two decades have resulted in cures of placental tumors, testicular and Wilms' tumors and Hodgkin's disease (Table 8-6). In addition, palliation and prolongation of life have resulted from the use of various drugs and hormones for the treatment of prostatic and breast carcinomas and for certain leukemias.

As with irradiation, chemotherapy, while not selectively lethal to cancer cells, usually produces more extensive injury to cancer cells than to normal tissues. Presumably, cancer cells are more vulnerable because they have increased metabolism and growth rates. The cancers most responsive to chemotherapy are primitive, rapidly growing ma-

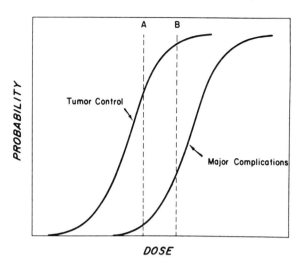

Figure 8-13 *Probabilities of achieving tumor control and development of major complications as a function of the radiation dose. A and B represent two different treatment programs. (Courtesy New England Journal of Medicine.)*

lignancies that frequently divide. Such tumors occur as uncommon forms of cancer. Common lung, breast, and colon cancers do not usually respond to chemotherapy or radiotherapy. But, the use of several drugs (combined chemotherapy) in treating women with breast cancer has recently resulted in a dramatic increase in their survival.

Chemotherapy Effects Formation of new deoxyribonucleic acid (DNA) and ribonucleic acid (RNA) is vital to the growth of new tumor cells. Effective cancer chemotherapy acts five ways to destroy tumor cells: (a) antimetabolite drugs block

Table 8-6
Cancers Responsive to Chemotherapy

Type of cancer	Useful drugs	Results
Placental (choriocarcinoma)	Methotrexate (nitrogen mustard)	70% cured
Wilms' cancer of kidney	Dactinomycin, surgery and radiotherapy	40% cured
Acute lymphoblastic leukemia of childhood	Prednisone, vincristine, methotrexate, etc.	90% remission 40% survive beyond five years
Prostate	Estrogen and castration	70% respond
Hodgkin's disease	Prednisone, vincristine, and radiotherapy	70% respond

the formation of DNA and inactivate vitamin folic acid; (b) certain other drugs bind with DNA and inactivate it; (c) other drugs may inhibit RNA and protein synthesis and impair the formation of new tumor cells; (d) mitosis (cell division) is inhibited by vincristine so the mitotic division of new leukemic cells is prevented and; (e) steroid hormones can suppress the growth of some cancers arising in tissues susceptible to hormonal suppression; as mentioned earlier, estrogen suppresses many prostatic and breast carcinomas.

Often a combination of several chemotherapeutic drugs works best to destroy cancers. Others are destroyed by using a combination of irradiation and drugs; Hodgkin's disease and Wilms' tumor respond favorably to this approach.

Complications of Chemotherapy   Depression of the bone marrow is the major common complication of chemotherapy. Growth of new bone marrow cells occurs at a rate comparable to many cancer cells and thus the bone marrow is vulnerable to injury. Hence, the patient's white blood count often becomes depressed (neutropenia) during chemotherapy and susceptibility to infectious diseases increases (see Chapter 7, Infectious Diseases). Likewise, the chemotherapeutic agents can be toxic to lymphocytes that provide immune defenses. An individual with a malignancy previously treated with surgery, irradiation, and chemotherapy, and who develops a fever, probably has a septicemia (infected blood stream). A blood culture is obtained to document this suspicion and if it is confirmed the patient is vigorously treated with antibiotics. In addition, the formation of blood platelets (small particles vital to blood clotting) is often depressed; thrombocytopenia results and then severe hemorrhage ensues. Transfusions of platelets, however, can prevent the hemorrhage.

Immunotherapy

Immunotherapy is the newest form of cancer therapy. It is aimed at increasing the immune defenses of the tumor-bearing person against malignancy. Neither surgery, irradiation nor chemotherapy are capable of eliminating all small clusters of metastatic cancer cells. Attempts, therefore, have been made to sensitize individuals against their own tumor cells to enhance their immune response against the tumor. Theoretically, the sensitized lymphocytes will then kill the few remaining tumor cells. Ethical considerations have thus far limited these experimental efforts to treatment of advanced metastatic cancer. Immunotherapy has been successful in the treatment of some cases of metastatic malignant melanoma of skin and lung cancer.

Summary

Over 100 different forms of cancer afflict human beings. These cancers are caused by exposure to carcinogens in our environment such as irradiation, chemical substances, and possibly viruses. Cancers probably arise from mutations induced by carcinogens and identical cells form a clone of tumor cells. The prognosis of cancer is based on the histologic type, location, and stage of the disease. Diagnosis of cancer is based on a clinical history of cardinal signs of cancer, radiologic and cytologic study, and biopsy. Death from cancer is often from bleeding or infectious disorders. Surgery is the mainstay of most cancer therapy, but chemotherapy and irradiation may either cure or palliate.

Bibliography

Allen, D. W., and Cole, P. 1972. Viruses and human cancer. *N. Engl. J. Med.* 286:70. Review article describing evidence for viral etiology of cancer.

Fialkow, P. J. 1974. The origin and development of human tumors with cell markers. *N. Engl. J. Med.* 291:26. Review article of efforts being made to detect cancer.

Fraumeni, J. F., Jr., ed. 1975. *Persons at high risk of cancer*. New York: Academic Press, Inc. Excellent description of inherited cancers and environmentally induced cancers.

Holland, J. R., and Frei, E., III., eds. 1973. *Cancer medicine*. Philadelphia: Lea & Febiger. The standard cancer textbook.

Irradiation-related thyroid cancer. 1977. U. S. Department of Health, Education, and Welfare. DHEW Publication No. (NIH) 1977–1120. Describes why and how persons exposed to prior cervical irradiation should be evaluated for possible thyroid cancer.

Kersey, J. H.; Spector, B; and Good, R. A. 1974. Cancer in children with primary immunodeficiency diseases. *J. Pediatr.* 84:263. Describes malignancies occurring in children who have immunodeficiency.

Klein, G. 1975. The Epstein-Barr virus and neoplasia. *N. Engl. J. Med.* 293:1353. The Epstein-Barr virus has been implicated as the cause of infectious mononucleosis and certain human cancers.

Prehn, R. T., and Prehen, L. M. 1975. Pathobiology of neoplasia: a teaching monograph. *Am. J. Pathol.* 80:529. Excellent review article on most aspects of cancer.

Preussmann, R. 1976. Chemical carcinogens in the human environment: problem and quantitative aspects. *Oncology* 33:51–77. Documents and discusses chemicals for which carcinogenicity to humans has been found or is suspected.

Purtilo, D. T., and Paquin, L. 1978. Genetics of cancer: impact of ecogenetics on oncogenesis. *Am. J. Pathol.*

In press. Discusses the interaction of nature and nurture in the oncogenesis of 235 inherited neoplastic syndromes.

Purtilo, D. T. 1976. Malignancies in the tropics. *Pathology of tropical and extraordinary diseases*, ed. C. Binford and D. Connor. American Registry of Pathology, Washington, DC. pp. 647–660. Describes the impact of environment on explaining variations in the frequency of cancers in different geographic areas.

Purtilo, D. T.; Yunis, E. J.; Kersey, J. H.; Hallgren, H.; and Fox, K. 1973. Alpha-fetoprotein: its use in diagnosis and prognosis. *Am. J. Clin. Pathol.* 59:295. Alpha-fetoprotein is detected in the serum of some patients with cancer and aids in diagnosis.

Uriel, J. 1976. Cancer, retrodifferentiation, and the myth of Faust. *Cancer Res.* 36:4269–4275. Cerebral discussion of hypothesis of reversion of cancer cells back to a fetal-like state.

Wynder, E. L., and Gori, G. B. 1977. Contribution of the environment to cancer incidence: an epidemiologic exercise. *J. Natl. Canc. Inst.* 58:825–832. Discusses the impact of cultural differences on the geographic variation of cancer incidence.

CHAPTER 9

Inherited Disorders

Chapter Outline

Objectives

After reading this chapter you should be able to

Categorize all diseases into three large groups with respect to relative genetic and environmental input.

Understand the relationship between heredity and environment in the pathogenesis of disease.

Describe the two major tools used for diagnosing genetic disorders.

List the three groups of genetic disease.

Define the terms chromosome, gene, locus, allele, genotype, and phenotype.

Describe the term mutation and list three factors causing it.

Describe a normal human karyotype.

Know the frequency of aneuploidy.

Describe the value of chromosomal banding technique compared to a regular karyotype technique.

Define the process of lyonization and the term Barr body.

Describe the genotype and phenotype of Turner's and Klinefelter's syndromes.

Define the term trisomy.

Describe Down's syndrome.

List three mechanisms whereby a chromosomal abnormality occurs.

List the major modes of Mendelian inheritance.

Know several Mendelian traits.

Analyze pedigrees and determine the mode of inheritance shown.

List several X-linked recessive traits.

Know the risks for offspring from patients with autosomal dominant and recessive traits.

Describe the concept of inborn error of metabolism.

Understand how PKU can damage a child and how it can be detected and treated.

Define the terms lysosome and sphingolipidosis.

Compare Gaucher's disease with Niemann-Pick disease.

Describe how polygenic (multifactorial) diseases are inherited.

List five examples of X-linked primary immunodeficiency diseases.

Describe the concept of disease susceptibility genes.

List examples of diseases inherited with certain HLA genotypes.

Describe the important information that should be communicated during genetic counseling.

Know the risk for offspring of parents with various types of inherited disorders.

Describe how amniocentesis is done and what information it can give.

Discuss one successful effort at biogenetic engineering.

Introduction

Robbins* has suggested that all human diseases might be grouped into three categories: (a) diseases almost *entirely environmentally* determined; (b) diseases almost *entirely genetically* determined; and (c) diseases in which *both* environmental factors and genetic factors interact to produce diseases.

It is clear that both inheritance and environmental experiences determine our health from conception to death. Genetic factors are largely unalterable throughout life, though they can and do interact with environmental factors, which constantly

*Robbins, S. L. 1974. *Pathologic basis of disease*. Philadelphia: W. B. Saunders Company.

change. That the impact of heredity on human disease can vary with environmental experiences is illustrated in an albino individual who has inherited an inability to produce melanin pigment—cancer of the skin develops in such a person only following excessive exposure to ultraviolet rays in sunlight (Fig. 9-1).

The role of genetic disorders in causing human disease is immense. Over 2300 inherited traits have been described thus far in human beings. Many of these traits produce only trivial disorders (certain abnormal hemoglobins, for example), but others produce tragic conditions like Down's syndrome (mongolism) (Table 9-1).

Geneticists use two major tools for detecting genetic disorders: (a) *chromosomal or karyotypic analysis (cytogenetics)*, and (b) *biochemical analysis* of blood, urine, and cells. Biochemists can identify enzyme deficiencies or excessive biological compounds in blood or tissues which signal inherited metabolic disorders.

Genetic disorders can be classified into three groups: (a) *chromosome disorders*, (b) *Mendelian or single-gene disorders*, and (c) *multifactorial or polygenic disorders*. Following a discussion of normal chromosomes, the first two types of genetic disorders will be discussed and illustrated.

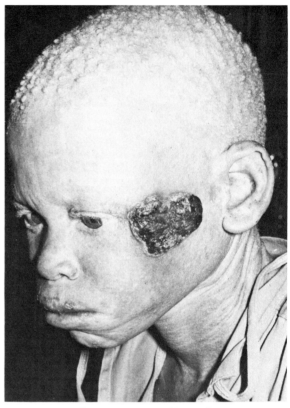

Figure 9-1 *A squamous cell carcinoma has resulted from exposure to sunlight in this albino boy with an autosomal recessive disorder.*

Genes and Chromosomes

Chromosomes can be seen in dividing cells as rod-shaped organelles composed of a double helix of DNA arranged in a series of individual units of hereditary material called *genes* (there are approximately 100,000 genes in one cell). Each gene has a precise location on a chromosome called a *locus*.

Table 9-1
Inherited Disorders

Autosomal dominant	Autosomal recessive	Sex-linked recessive
Achondroplastic dwarfism	Albinism	Hemophilias A and B
Renal disease with deafness	Cystic fibrosis	X-linked lymphoproliferative syndrome
Medullary thyroid cancer	Cretinism (familial)	
Neurofibromatosis	Niemann-Pick disease	G-6PD deficiency
Hemorrhagic telangiectasia	Tay-Sachs disease	Duchenne muscular dystrophy
Colorectal polyposis	Phenylketonuria	Progressive spinal muscular atrophy (Werdnig-Hoffman disease)
	Galactosemia	Color blindness
	Sickle cell anemia	Various immunodeficiencies

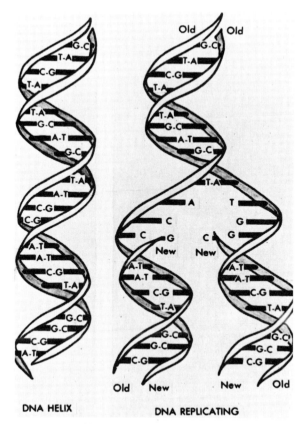

Figure 9-2   *The double helix of DNA. (From: Nora, J. J., and Fraser, F. C.,* Medical Genetics: Principles and Practice, *1974. Philadelphia, Lea & Febiger.)*

Chromosomes are paired; the corresponding genes on a pair of chromosomes at a given locus which can determine alternate forms of the same characteristics are termed *alleles* (Fig. 9-2).

Genes are the individual units of inheritance that determine the manufacture of single proteins. This small unit of DNA functions to produce polypeptide building blocks, which combine with other peptides to produce proteins. Many hormones, all enzymes, and the membranes of cells are proteins. Each gene contributes one product important in the composition of the body.

The *genotype* of an individual is his or her genetic composition, usually with reference to a particular locus; the *phenotype* refers to the expression of any gene in physical, biochemical, or physiological traits. For example, a person may have inherited the two genes required to result in blue eyes (they have a genotype for blue eyes). The actual presence or physical expression of blue eyes in a person is the phenotype. A person's phenotype is what can be observed and measured. The genotype is his genetic constitution.

Mutations

A *mutation* is a permanent hereditary alteration in the genetic material. This genetic alteration of the DNA of genes within chromosomes can result from various environmental agents: viruses, irradiation, or chemicals. Individual mutations are rare events, occurring in only 1 in 10,000 to 1 in 1,000,000 genes per generation of humans. The conditions new mutations cause, then, are also rare. Mutations cannot be identified even by high resolution microscopic techniques; they require special biochemical studies to be identified. The defects arising from mutations range from trivial to lethal. For instance, sickle cell disease is potentially a lethal disease which arises from a mutation of the gene that controls the synthesis of a peptide which forms hemoglobin (see Chaper 11, Hematology). The mutant gene produces sickle hemoglobin rather than normal hemoglobin.

Normal Chromosomes

Although human chromosomes were recognized in cells a century ago, it was not until 1956 that the correct number of chromosomes in humans was identified as 46, occurring in 23 pairs. The *karyotype* (number and appearance of chromosomes) of cultured blood cells of a normal person is assessed by microscopic examination of the appearance and number of chromosomes within a cell in mitosis (Fig. 9-3).

Cells of humans normally contain 22 pairs of *autosomes* and one pair of *sex chromosomes*. In standard notation a normal male is designated 46 XY, having a total of 46 chromosomes, the pair of sex chromosomes consisting of one X and one Y. A normal female is designated 46 XX.

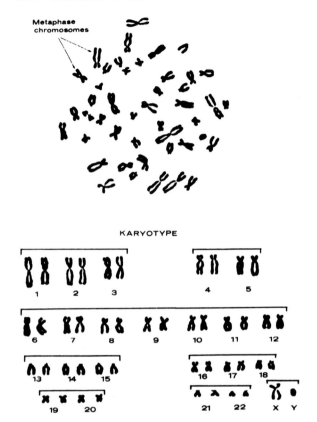

Figure 9-3   *Normal karyotye. 46 chromosomes (23 pairs) including 2 sex and 44 autosome chromosomes. The upper portion shows chromosomes in a mitotic figure and the lower part shows the groups of chromosomes.*

The individual autosomes are numbered 1 to 22 according to their size and shape. Identical pairs of autosomes contain complementary pairs of genes (alleles).

Chromosome Errors

Abnormal Karyotype

Approximately one in 200 newborns have abnormal karyotypes with respect to either the number or appearance of the 46 chromosomes. The frequency of abnormal karyotypes in spontaneous abortuses is 100 times greater; 20% of spontaneous abortuses show chromosomal abnormalities. In human beings the characteristic *diploid* number of chromosomes (in somatic cells) is 46 and the characteristic *haploid* number (in the egg and sperm) is 23. Conception returns the fertilized egg to 46 chromosomes. A person with normal chromosomes is *euploid* and those having an abnormal number are *aneuploid*.

Structural Changes

During mitosis, the replicated chromosomes are divided into two identical diploid cells. During meiosis, division of gametes leads to haploid cells, each of which contains only one example of the pair. During metaphase, while homologous chromosomes lie next to each other, the waving, flapping arms of adjacent chromosomal strands can get tangled with each other and errors can occur during separation.

Crossing Over   Chromosomes often break and reassemble. Segments of adjacent homologous strands break off, exchange position, and reattach to the opposite chromosome pair. Before the cells separate, the chromosome strands reassemble in the new haploid cell. This process of exchange and reassembly is called *crossing over*. It occurs frequently when gametes (ovum or sperm) undergo meiosis and genetic material is reapportioned into new combinations.

Deletion   Sometimes breakage is not followed by complete exchange and repair. A segment breaks off but does not reattach to a chromosome and the segment is lost to future generations of cells. The remaining chromosome has undergone *deletion*, loss of genetic material from a chromosome which continues independent existence minus the deleted fragment.

Translocation   If a fragment breaks off a chromosome and attaches to another chromosome, the process is called *translocation*. The resulting chromosomes have unbalanced amounts of genetic material and are unable to undergo meiosis. If symmetrical segments of chromosomal material exchange, the result is balanced translocation. This abnormality can perpetuate itself through meiosis and be transmitted to the next generation.

Nondisjunction   When mitosis or meiosis proceed normally, the offspring of a diploid cell have either 46 or 23 chromosomes, respectively. But sometimes accidents occur as the chromosomes separate. Instead of symmetrical division, both halves of a pair can migrate to one cell, leaving the other side with no representative at that particular pair. This asymmetrical division is called *nondisjunction*. The entire chromosome gets misplaced, and the daughter cells are abnormal forever. Approximately one half of chromosomal defects arise from abnormal numbers of sex chromosomes and the remaining half from autosomes.

If a diploid cell receives an extra member of one chromosome pair, the total number of chromosomes will be 47 instead of 46, and hence *aneuploidy* is present. The condition is called *trisomy* for the chromosome that has three representatives. A diploid cell lacking one chromosome of a pair will have only 45; this is called *monosomy* for the affected chromosome. In general, autosomal aneuploidy causes more severe alterations of phenotype than abnormalities of sex chromosomes. But altered growth, mental retardation, multiple birth defects, and death can result from sex or autosomal aneuploidy.

Mapping of Genes

Assigning genes to the X chromosome is relatively easy, but assigning location of genes in autosomes is difficult. Sometimes this is possible by detecting phenotypic peculiarities in persons with abnormal genes, and observing an associated phenotypic trait with the chromosome. Another technique employs cell cultures in which cells of different species are fused into genetic hybrids. Manipulating these hybrids and measuring their protein products of specific chromosomes has permitted the assignment of many traits to specific autosomes. Also, much information about relative positions of genes can be inferred from statistics on the frequency with which different traits remain associated during cell division. Genes on a chromosome can rearrange by crossing over. Genes that are very close to one another are unlikely to find themselves separated during crossing over, while those at opposite ends of

a segment cross over. The distance between genes, determined by the observed frequency of recombination of genes, is measured in centimorgan units.

Chromosomal Banding

The development of a new, high resolution *chromosomal banding technique* for identifying specific areas on a chromosome has revealed numerous sites on chromosomes responsible for many genetic abnormalities (Fig. 9-4). Banded chromosomes stretch out revealing smaller defects. In effect, the chromosome banding technique has enabled more precise localization and identification of chromosomal abnormalities. Many persons afflicted by birth defects who previously could not be identified as having chromosomal defects by ordinary karyotyping can now be shown to have defects in a specific band on an autosome. Such a finding enables investigators to further understand birth defects and their transmission.

Sex Chromosome Abnormalities

During the development of a female fetus, one X chromosome in each somatic cell becomes condensed and inactivated by a process termed *lyonization*. Through lyonization the amount of genetic material in somatic cells of males and females becomes approximately equal.

The condensed body of X chromatin, which can be seen in cells of females, is termed the *Barr body* (Fig. 9-5). The sex of an individual can be determined by staining a scraping of squamous cells from buccal mucosa of the mouth. The presence of Barr bodies in the nuclei indicates a female karyotype; their absence indicates a male karyotype.

During the formation of germ cells, an excessive or deficient number of sex chromosomes can arise from nondisjunction of the 46 chromosomes. For example, when a person has received only 22 autosomes and no sex chromosomes from one parent and 22 autosomes and an X chromosome from the other parent, her karyotype will be 45, XO.

Turner's syndrome (with gonadal dysgenesis) results from a 45, XO karyotype. A missing X chro-

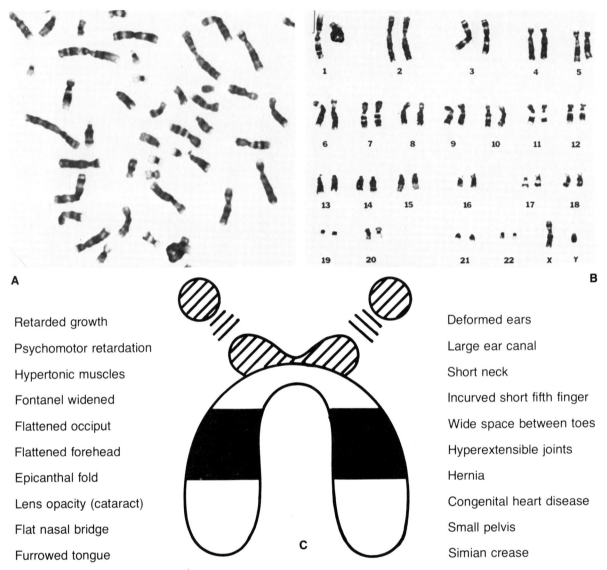

Retarded growth

Psychomotor retardation

Hypertonic muscles

Fontanel widened

Flattened occiput

Flattened forehead

Epicanthal fold

Lens opacity (cataract)

Flat nasal bridge

Furrowed tongue

Deformed ears

Large ear canal

Short neck

Incurved short fifth finger

Wide space between toes

Hyperextensible joints

Hernia

Congenital heart disease

Small pelvis

Simian crease

Figure 9-4   **A** and **B,** Banding. **C,** Chromosome No. 21. The bands are thought to be associated with various defects.

mosome occurs in approximately one in 2000 females and in about 20% of all spontaneous abortions. The affected individuals usually have short stature, webbing of the neck, internal abnormalities such as narrowing (coarctation) of the aorta, and amenorrhea (lack of menstruation) (Fig. 9-6). The lack of menses occurs together with a failure to develop ovaries. In Turner's syndrome the ovaries are replaced by fibrous streaks (a type of go-

nadal dysgenesis) that are devoid of ova (see Chapter 3, Development and Birth Defects). Many persons with Turner's syndrome can have a mixture or mosaic of normal 46 XX and 45 XO cells.

Multi-X female births occur approximately once in every 1000. Multi X females have an excessive number of X chromosomes (47 XXX or 48 XXXX, etc.) Persons bearing extra X chromosomes may be sterile and mentally retarded; the greater num-

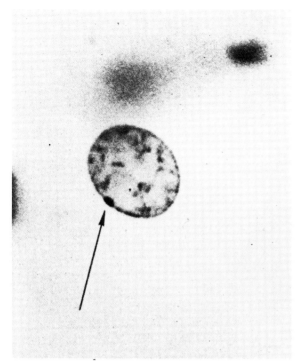

Figure 9-5 *Barr body. Condensed X chromosome (arrow) in epithelial cell.*

ber of X chromosomes present, generally the greater the mental retardation.

True hermaphrodites (both sexes in one) are rare. This results from a genetic mosaic of 46 XX and 47 XY combinations in various cells of the body. True hermaphrodites have both ovarian and testicular tissue.

Klinefelter's syndrome results in a male with a karyotype of 47 XXY. This syndrome occurs in approximately one in every 500 males. A female distribution of hair, small prostate and testes, increased breast size (gynecomastia), and elongation of the body (feminine body type) characterize this syndrome. Men with this type of gonadal dysgenesis have a thirty-three-fold increased chance of developing breast cancer compared to normal males.

Autosomal Abnormalities

Autosomal chromosome disorders often cause disfiguring abnormalities because most of these large

chromosomes contain many more genes than sex chromosomes. Autosomal abnormalities can result from *partial deletions* (for example, loss of chromosomal arm) or *translocation* of chromosomal arm to another chromosome. But the most serious autosomal abnormality arises from *aneuploidy*, the state of having other than the usual number of chromosomes, as in trisomy 21 (Down's syndrome).

Down's Syndrome

The most common and best known of the trisomies is *Down's syndrome* (trisomy 21). It occurs approximately once in every 2000 pregnancies in women in their early 20s, whereas the rate rises to one in ev-

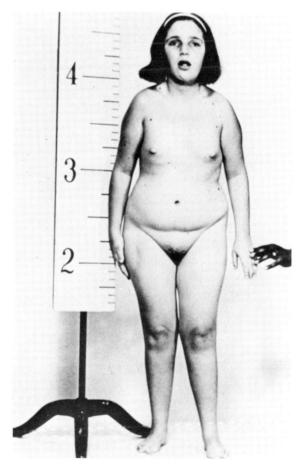

Figure 9-6 *Phenotype of Turner's syndrome 45, XO. (Published with permission of the American Journal of Human Genetics.)*

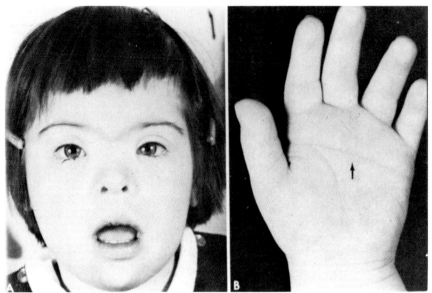

Figure 9-7 *Phenotype of Down's syndrome 47, XX (trisomy 21). (From Bartalos, M., and Baramki, T. A. 1967.* Medical Cytogenetics. *© 1967. The Williams & Wilkins Co., Baltimore.)*

ery 60 births in women aged 45. It is unknown whether aging men are also responsible for children with Down's syndrome.

Trisomy 21 arises from nondisjunction of chromosomes, a karyotype of 47 XX, 21+ is seen. Typically, affected individuals have folds in the skin of their upper eyelids (creating a Mongoloid appearance), coarseness of the tongue and skin, and I.Q. between 25 and 50 (Fig. 9-7). They generally are affectionate and can be taught to do simple tasks. In addition, a transverse simian (apelike) crease crosses their palms and short fifth fingers are also common.

Birth defects of the heart and genitourinary tract are present in most persons with Down's syndrome.* Hence, nearly 50% of children with Down's syndrome die by age 2 because of heart failure, renal failure or pneumonia. The multiple

*A medical ethics question currently receiving much attention is: To what extent should life-supporting measures be provided to these patients? See "Limited Resources in the Land of Plenty," *Essays for Professional Helpers. Some Psychosocial and Ethical Considerations,* Ruth B. Purtilo, Charles B. Slack Inc., Thorofare, N.J. 1975. pp. 109–120.

defects seen in Trisomy 21 are thought to result from the increased dose (50%) of an enzyme from the extra chromosome 21, which is toxic to developing cells.

Mendelian, Single Gene, Disorders

Hippocrates observed that blue eyes and baldness ran in families. But not until the end of the last century did the Austrian botanist, Gregor Mendel, explain the basis for inherited traits. By *Mendelian laws* and by simple analysis of *pedigree* (family trees) we are able to predict the inheritance of many genetic traits.

To date, 2336 Mendelian phenotypes have been described. Of these, 1218 are *autosomal dominant* traits which require only one (heterozygote) gene for the phenotypic expression; 947 are *autosomal recessive* traits which require the presence of two recessive genes on the two alleles (homozygote) for the phenotypic expression; and 171 are X-linked, almost all X-linked recessive (Table 9-2).

The notations used in pedigree analysis in genetics are shown in Figure 9-8 and Table 9-1 lists

Table 9-2

Numbers of Mendelian Traits Described in Successive Editions of McKusick's Mendelian Inheritance in Man

	Edition			
Trait	First–1966	Second–1968	Third–1971	Fourth–1975
Autosomal dominant	269 (568)*	344 (449)	415 (528)	583 (635)
Autosomal recessive	237 (294)	280 (349)	365 (418)	466 (481)
X-linked	68 (51)	68 (55)	86 (64)	93 (78)
Total	574 (913)	692 (853)	866 (1010)	1142 (1194)
Combined total	1487	1545	1876	2336

*Numbers in parenthesis refer to additional catalog entries that are not completely proven to be Mendelian or to represent a locus separate from another.

a few important inherited diseases. Genetic traits are inherited either as an autosomal or sex-linked dominant or recessive. The mode of inheritance of Mendelian traits is illustrated in Figure 9-9.

The long arms of chromosomes are termed q and short arms p. Loss of genetic material is designated − and extra material +. Hence much information can be expressed succinctly; for example, a karyotype of 14q+ means the long arms of chromosome number 14 have extra material.

X-Linked Traits

Genetic traits inherited on the female X chromosome are termed X-linked (or sex-linked) traits. X-linked traits are much easier to recognize than autosomal traits because they occur only in males and females are carriers. The X chromosome carries approximately 1000 genes, whereas the Y chromosome carries only a few traits: determination of maleness and some other questionable and trivial traits, such as hairy ears. The pairing of genes on complementary chromosomes determines that recessive X-linked traits will not be expressed in females because a dominant, complementary-paired gene suppresses the recessive trait.

X-Linked Traits and Diseases

Approximately 171 X-linked recessive traits have been observed. A female must possess two (homozygous) recessive genes to express an X-linked

genetic trait, but a male carrying only one (heterozygous) X-linked recessive gene can display an X-linked genetic trait.

The pedigree shown in Figure 9-10 represents a family the author studied. Try to figure out the mode of inheritance. Note that approximately 50% of the boys were affected with this blood disorder (X-linked recessive lymphoproliferative syndrome) and 50% of the girls were carriers.

Many diseases of the blood, including both hemophilia A and B, result from X-linked transmission (Table 9-2). Hemophilia is characterized by a severe deficiency of a blood clotting factor and boys affected by this disease can experience severe hemorrhage (see Chapter 11, Hematology).

Autosomal Diseases

More than 95% of inherited disorders occur from autosomal dominant or recessive traits. The frequency of the traits is proportional to the amount of genetic information carried on the autosomes. Autosomes comprise 95% of DNA and sex chromosomes comprise 5% of DNA.

Autosomal Dominant Inheritance

As shown in the pedigrees displayed in Figure 9-9, a *dominant gene* produces an effect in virtually every individual who inherits it, irrespective of the state of the other allele. The phenotypic expression of the trait may require exposure to an environmental

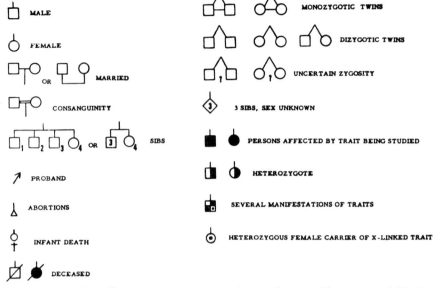

Figure 9-8 *Notations commonly used in pedigrees. (Courtesy of W. B. Saunders Co.)*

agent, be demonstrated only at a certain age, or may be suppressed. Hence, the *penetrance* of the phenotypic expression of the genotype is not always 100%.

The transmission of an autosomal dominant inherited disease in a family is passed directly from generation to generation. Each individual who inherits the gene will probably have the disease. Likewise, affected individuals usually have an affected parent. Sporadic cases arise from a new mutation when the family history fails to reveal transmission.

An affected person who marries a normal person will pass on the mutant gene to 50% of his or her children. Unaffected relatives of affected persons will not have affected offspring. All of these facts about autosomal dominant inheritance are important in assessing the chances of a disease occurring in offspring of relatives—facts needed for genetic counseling.

Autosomal Recessive Inheritance

A recessive deleterious gene only produces its disease in the homozygote, so affected individuals must receive one mutant gene from each parent, both of whom are heterozygous. Autosomal recessive traits do not pass directly from parent to child; hence the folklore that "inherited diseases skip a generation." The chances of two parents being heterozygous for a mutant allele are increased if the parents are related; rare autosomal recessive inherited diseases arise more frequently from consanguineous parents.

In summary, in autosomal recessive disorders: (a) the disease is seldom seen in the parents; (b) the sibs of an affected child have a one in four chance of being affected (Fig. 9-9); and (c) the parents are more likely to be related than are parents of normal persons.

Inborn Errors of Metabolism

Inborn (inherited) errors of biochemistry (metabolism) arise from a mutant gene and often cause a *specific enzyme deficiency* (Fig. 9-11). These errors are the most common and important category of genetic diseases arising from mutant autosomal genes.

In general, when a mutant gene results in an enzyme deficiency, one of two deleterious events occurs: (a) a deficient protein structure (for example,

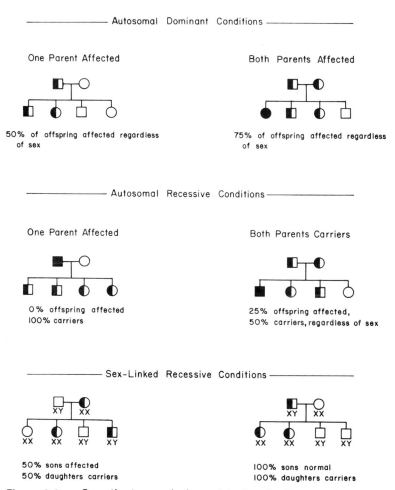

Figure 9-9   *Genetic transmission of traits. Pedigrees displaying mendelian autosomal dominant, autosomal recessive, and X-linked traits.*

sickle hemoglobin), or (b) an accumulation of a toxic chemical in the blood and tissues (for example, galactosemia). A few examples of important autosomal inborn errors of metabolism follow. These diseases, while rare, have a profound impact on the patient; and often occur in many persons in the same family.

Phenylketonuria

Phenylketonuria (PKU) is an inborn error of metabolism that is transmitted as an autosomal recessive trait. Phenylalanine hydrogenase is deficient and thus phenylalanine metabolites accumulate in

the blood and brain of the affected person and severe mental retardation can ensue.

The child affected by PKU generally has light skin, blond hair, and is progressively mentally retarded. The disease can be detected easily by examining the urine for phenylpyruvic acid. Early detection (at birth) and keeping the infant on a diet free of phenylalanine can prevent toxicity and severe mental retardation.

Galactosemia

Another autosomal recessive inborn error of metabolism, *galactosemia*, results from an absence of

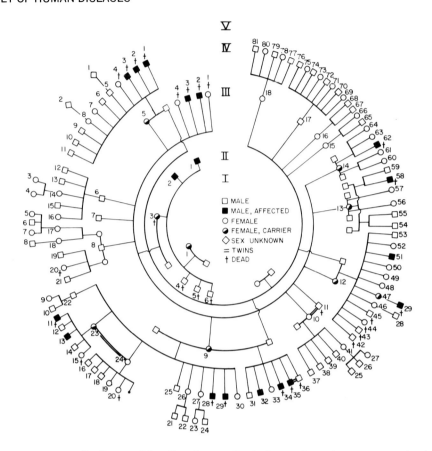

Figure 9-10   *Pedigree of family whose affected members have succumbed to infectious mononucleosis or lymphoma. The pedigree appears complicated because three brothers of one family married three sisters of an unrelated family.*

an enzyme (galactose–1–phosphate uridyl transferase) which normally digests galactose. The lactose of milk is composed of galactose and glucose. Infants with galactosemia suffer from mental retardation, cataracts, and cirrhosis of the liver because undigested galactose accumulates in the blood and damages these organs. As with PKU, the early detection of this inborn error of metabolism (by biochemical genetic testing) can prevent injury from occurring by placing the child on a diet free of galactose.

Glycogenoses

Disorders of glycogen metabolism (glycogen is carbohydrate stored in muscle and liver) are respon-

sible for at least seven rare fetal genetic disorders, the *glycogenoses*. When an essential enzyme, α-glucosidase, which metabolizes glycogen, is missing, glycogen accumulates in the heart and muscles. These deposits severely impair the neuromuscular system.

Lysosomal Storage Diseases

The concept of inherited lysosomal disease was developed in 1965 by Hers. *Lysosomes* are membrane-bound intracytoplasmic sacs that contain hydrolytic enzymes that degrade proteins, carbohydrates, and nucleic acids. Vacuoles containing cellular components to be degraded (glycogen) and

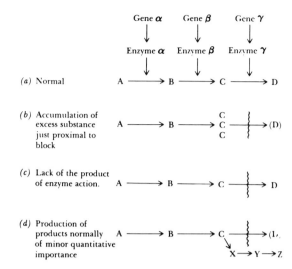

	Gene α	Gene β	Gene γ

$$Enzyme\ \alpha \quad Enzyme\ \beta \quad Enzyme\ \gamma$$

(a) Normal

$$A \longrightarrow B \longrightarrow C \longrightarrow D$$

(b) Accumulation of excess substance just proximal to block

$$A \longrightarrow B \longrightarrow \begin{matrix} C \\ C \\ C \end{matrix} \nrightarrow (D)$$

(c) Lack of the product of enzyme action.

$$A \longrightarrow B \longrightarrow C \nrightarrow D$$

(d) Production of products normally of minor quantitative importance

$$A \longrightarrow B \longrightarrow C \nrightarrow (D)$$
$$X \longrightarrow Y \longrightarrow Z$$

Figure 9-11 *Typical inborn error of metabolism. The absence of enzyme β results in an accumluation of substance A and a lack of substance B in the body. (Victor A. McKusick, HUMAN GENETICS, 2nd edition, © 1969, pp. 69, 100. Reprinted by permission of Prentice-Hall, Inc., Englewood Cliffs, New Jersey.)*

foreign materials engulfed by the cell, fuse with the *primary lysosomes* to form *secondary lysosomes* and the materials are normally digested.

More than 25 genetic diseases occur from autosomal deficiencies of lysosomal enzymes. In many of these diseases the secondary lysosome becomes engorged with material that it would ordinarily degrade. Examples of inherited lysosomal defects causing certain lipid storage diseases are presented.

Sphingolipidoses

In addition to cholesterol, phospholipids, and proteins, membranes of cells contain sphingolipids. The sphingolipids are normally hydrolysed by lysosomes and hence, certain inherited lysosomal deficiencies result in accumulation of sphingolipids in cells.

In *Gaucher's disease* damaging glycosphingolipid accumulates in phagocytic cells of the spleen, liver, and bone marrow (Fig. 9-12). Infantile, childhood, and adult forms of Gaucher's disease occur because of lysosomal enzyme deficiency of glucocerebrosidase. Massive hepatosplenomegaly (enlargement of

liver and spleen) and fatal hemorrhage develop because the lipid-packed macrophages crowd out cells that form blood platelets. In addition, neutrophils are not formed in bone marrow (neutropenia results), thus persons in whom this occurs are rendered vulnerable to infectious diseases.

Another sphingolipidosis, *Niemann-Pick disease*, results from lysosomal enzyme deficiency (sphingomyelinase) and leads to an excessive deposition of cholesterol and sphingomyelin in macrophages of liver, spleen, and lymph nodes. Children affected by this disease die within a few years, usually with brain involvement and severe wasting.

Tay-Sachs disease is another autosomal recessive disease and is common in Ashkenazi (European) Jewish children. It is caused by a hexosaminidase deficiency and is rapidly fatal because of an accumulation of gangliosides in neurons of the brain.

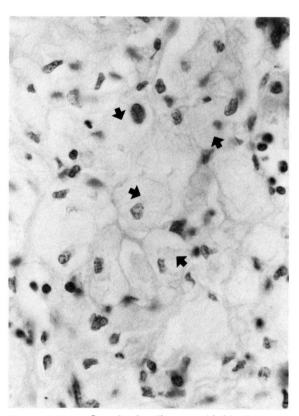

Figure 9-12 *Gaucher's disease. Lipids (glycosphingolipid) distend phagocytes in the liver* (arrows).

Fortunately, the carrier state can be identified accurately. If both parents are found to be carriers, there is a 1-in-4 risk of producing an affected child in each pregnancy.

Polygenic Inheritance

Polygenic (multifactorial) inheritance arises from a combination of two or more genes acting together to produce a serious defect. Multifactorial disorders tend to cluster in certain families but do not show the clear-cut pedigree patterns of single-gene traits as described and illustrated in this chapter.

The polygenic mode of inheritance probably underlies the genetic predisposition to the common disorders of human beings, especially disorders where both the genotype and the environment contribute. The largest segment of genetic abnormality or disease falls into polygenic multifactorial inheritance and approximately 10% to 20% of the general population is affected.

Examples

Examples of polygenic inherited disorders include cleft lip, congenital hip dislocation, congenital heart defects, cancer, manic-depressive psychosis, schizophrenia, hypertension and some forms of diabetes mellitus. The complexity involved in identifying the many factors acting concertedly in multifactorial-induced disorders has hampered our understanding of the inheritance of many diseases.

Inherited Immunologic Diseases

Primary Immunodeficiency

Almost all primary immunodeficiency diseases are inherited (see Chapter 6, Immunology). For example, five diseases have X-linked recessive inheritance: (a) combined immunodeficiency; (b) agammaglobulinemia; (c) Wiscott-Aldrich immunodeficiency; (d) immunodeficiency with increased IgM; and (e) the X-linked recessive lymphoproliferative syndrome. Other immunodeficiencies having autosomal recessive inheritance such as ataxia-telangiectasia, although rare, occur rather commonly in consanguineous matings. These rare disorders when encountered in one child can lead to the identification of many other affected relatives.

Disease Susceptibility Genes

The uniqueness we possess as individuals arises in part from our histocompatibility leukocyte antigens (HLA). The HLA system is the basis for histocompatibility matching of donors and recipients for organ transplantation (see Chapter 6, Immunology). Recipients possessing different HLA from donors will reject the transplanted organ. The HLA system helps protect us from foreign invaders (microbes, for example).

Demonstration of HLA-associated susceptibility to diseases (and to etiologic agents) has been an important spin-off from HLA research. Persons having certain HLA types react inappropriately to viruses, toxins, and even their own tissues. For example, leukemia and lymphoma commonly occur in persons with a specific HLA genotype. Similarly, the author has discovered that families with HLA A1 B8 genes frequently have rheumatoid arthritis, and a variety of other autoimmune diseases.

Genetic Counseling

Objectives

Genetic counseling is a communication process which deals with the occurrence or the risk of occurrence of genetic disorder in a family. This process involves an attempt to help an individual or family to: (a) comprehend the medical facts, including the diagnosis, the probable cause of the disorder, and the available management; (b) appreciate the way heredity contributes to the disorder and the risks of recurrence in specified relatives; (c) understand the options for dealing with the risks of recurrence; (d) choose the course of action which seems appropriate in view of the risks and family goals; (e) make the best possible adjustment to the disorder and the affected family member.

The diagnosis of genetic diseases like those described in this chapter is achieved by examining the patient and by obtaining a family pedigree. Laboratory tests such as karyotypic analysis and biochemical studies of fluids and cells of a person also aid in the diagnosis of a genetic disorder.

The patient and the family should be told, according to their specific inheritance patterns, the following risks of future occurrence of disorders: (a) low recurrence risks (2% to 5%) with many polygenic multifactorial disorders; (b) high recurrence (25%) for autosomal recessive disorders like cystic fibrosis, sickle cell anemia, Tay-Sachs disease; (c) for autosomal dominant afflictions 50% of progeny of affected persons will become affected; and (d) for X-linked recessive conditions like hemophilia 50% of females will become carriers and 50% of males produced by carriers will be afflicted.

For cousins contemplating marriage the risk of having a child with a recessive inherited disease will be increased one hundred–fold, but in absolute terms the risk is small—in the order of 1%.

With increasing maternal age, the risk of having trisomy 21 (Down's syndrome) increases twentyfold when the mother is aged 45 as compared to aged 20. The risk of recurrence in subsequent pregnancies is 3% to 5%. The risk can be determined for many disorders by antenatal detection by amniocentesis.

Amniocentesis

It is possible to diagnose some genetic disorders before birth by *amniocentesis*, a process whereby amniotic fluid is drawn through a needle from the amniotic sac in the uterus. Epithelial cells sloughed from the skin of the fetus can be withdrawn and stained for Barr bodies (condensed female chromosome). It is thus possible to detect males (whose cells lack Barr bodies) having a 50% chance of an X-linked disease in a carrier mother. Based upon the findings from amniocentesis, a therapeutic abortion can be contemplated. In addition, blood cells drawn from the fetus in utero can be placed in culture and assessed for inborn errors of metabolism by measuring the concentration of specific biochemicals, or karyotyped.

Most inherited disorders are not treatable; amniocentesis and therapeutic abortion offer an option for those parents who do not wish to give birth to a defective child and prepares parents for caring for a defective child should they choose to retain the fetus.

Therapy

Biogenetic engineering is a new field that attempts to replace enzymes or cells missing from persons with inborn errors of metabolism. For example, the glucocerebrosidase lacking in patients with Gaucher's disease has been extracted from human placental tissue and administered successfully to patients. Enzyme replacement therapy is promising and may offer relief from some genetic disorders. Secondly, restoration of immunity is possible in some children with inherited immunodeficiency by *transplanting* a thymus gland or bone marrow.

Summary

Many diseases have important genetic components and most diseases result from an interplay between nature (inheritance) and nurture (environment). Genes, the hereditary units of life, are subject to mutation by irradiation, viruses, or chemicals.

The altered genes can be passed to offspring by Mendelian inheritance, including autosomal dominant or recessive and X-linked modes. The inheritance pattern can be determined by analyzing a pedigree. Genetic disorders are diagnosed by three major methods: (a) pedigree analysis, (b) karyotype, and (c) biochemical analysis of bodily fluids or tissues.

About 95% of inherited disorders arise from autosomal mutations. X-linked disorders are easy to recognize because only males are affected whereas females who carry the mutant gene are protected. Abnormal numbers of autosomes and sex chromosomes produce profound anatomical defects. By contrast, one-gene defects produce metabolic inborn errors of metabolism which can cause widespread systemic effects because of the accumulation of toxic materials.

Biogenetic engineering by enzyme replacement or organ transplantation offers hope for many persons afflicted by inherited disorders. Alternatively, antenatal detection of inherited defects is possible in some cases by analyzing amniotic fluid obtained by amniocentesis.

Bibliography

Brady, R. O. 1976. Biochemical genetics in neurology. *Arch. Neurol.* 33:145. Describes the enzymes missing in many inherited inborn errors of metabolism that affect the brain.

Borgaonker, D. S.; Lacassie, Y. E.; and Stoll, C. 1976. Usefulness of chromosome catalog in delineating new syndromes. *Birth Defects* 12:87–95. Describes how new genetic sydromes can be recognized.

Childs, B. 1975. Genetic screening. *Ann. Rev. of Genetics* 9:67–89. A summary of genetically determined disorders for which screening and/or antenatal diagnosis is feasible.

Erbe, R. A. 1976. Current concepts in genetics. *N. Engl. J. Med.* 294:381, 430, 596, and 706. A lucid summary of genetics.

Fraumeni, J. F., Jr. 1975. *Persons at high risk of cancer.* New York: Academic Press, Inc. Excellent description of inherited cancers and environmentally induced cancers.

Fraser, F. C. 1971. Genetic counseling. *Hosp. Practice,* January, p. 49. Describes an approach to genetic counseling.

Hamerton, J. L., et al. 1975. A cytogenetic survey of 14,069 newborn infants. *Clin. Genet.* 8:223. Describes the common chromosomal abnormalities seen in a large population.

Kolodny, E. H. 1976. Lysosomal storage diseases. *N. Engl. J. Med.* 294:1217. The mechanisms responsible for lysosomal storage diseases are outlined.

Kushnick, T. 1976. When to refer to the geneticist. *J. Am. Med. Assoc.* 235:623. A practical guide to determining whether genetic counseling is needed.

Levin, H. 1971. *Clinical cytogenetics.* Boston: Little, Brown and Company. Describes the clinical findings and karyotypes of chromosomal abnormalities.

Lynch, H. T. ed. 1975. *Cancer genetics.* Springfield: Charles C Thomas, Publisher. Describes the inheritance of various cancers.

Martin, G. M., and Hoehn, H. 1974. Genetics and human disease. *Hum. Pathol.* 5:387. Provides an excellent overview of ecogenetics.

McKusick, V. A., and Clairborne, R. 1973. *Medical genetics.* New York: Hospital Practice Publishing Company. Comprehensive, well-written, beautifully illustrated articles on the principles of genetics, clinical syndromes, and biochemistry.

McKusick, V. A. 1975. The growth and development of human genetics. *Hum. Genet.* 27:261. A personal summary by the leading human geneticist in the United States.

McKusick, V. A. 1975. *Mendelian inheritance of man,* ed. 4. Baltimore: The Johns Hopkins University Press. Catalogs of autosomal dominant, autosomal recessive, and X-linked phenotypes. Lists all inherited traits and gives a brief synopsis of references for many inherited disorders.

Nora, J. J., and Fraser, F. C. 1974. *Medical genetics: principles and practice.* Philadelphia: Lea & Febiger. A standard textbook.

Purtilo, D. T. 1976. Pathogenesis and phenotypes of an X-linked recessive syndrome. *Lancet* ii:882–885. Describes the syndrome shown in Figure 9–10.

Purtilo, D. T., and Paquin, L. Genetics of cancer. A review. *Am. J. Pathol.* In press. Reviews and summarizes mutation and inheritance in cancer. Lists of all inherited cancers are provided.

Roberts, F. J. A. 1973. *An introduction to medical genetics,* ed. 6. London: Oxford University Press. An excellent introductory textbook.

Watson, J. D. 1976. *Molecular biology of the gene,* ed. 3. Menlo Park, California: W. A. Benjamin, Inc. The definitive textbook on molecular aspects of genes by the codiscoverer of the double helix of DNA.

Nutritional Diseases

Chapter Outline

Objectives

After reading this chapter you should be able to

List the four major food groups.

List the essential nutrients (or at least know where to find a list of them).

Discuss the body's capacity for storing energy reserves.

List factors that can impair nutrition.

Draw up a scheme classifying nutritional disorders.

Define the terms goiter, beriberi, pellagra, rickets, and scurvy and name the nutritional deficiency responsible for each.

Define and compare kwashiorkor and marasmus.

Describe the appearance of a child with kwashiorkor.

Discuss the impact of malnutrition on cerebral development.

Describe what happens to the pancreas in protein-calorie malnutrition (PCM).

List the acquired immunodeficiencies associated with PCM.

Know the frequency of PCM in hospitalized patients in the United States.

Describe the typical appearance of children with rickets.

Compare the etiology and pathology of rickets and osteomalacia.

Compare the etiology and pathology of rickets with scurvy.

Know why hemorrhage occurs in persons with scurvy.

Describe the two types of beriberi.

Discuss the etiology and clinical findings regarding pellagra.

Know what causes, cures, and prevents endemic goiter.

Define the term obesity.

List three major organs damaged by ethanol and frequent causes of death from alcoholism.

Describe the clinical findings seen in hypervitaminosis A.

List the sites where calcium can be deposited in hypervitaminosis D.

Introduction

Nutrients are required for growth and maintenance of all the metabolic processes. Essential nutritional requirements can be satisfied by ingesting four groups of foods: (a) dairy products; (b) meats or high protein foods such as eggs, beans, peas, or nuts; (c) vegetables and fruits; and (d) cereals and breads. Specific nutritional requirements are now discussed.

Essential Nutrients

Essential nutrients are molecules which the body does not synthesize itself. When these molecules are lacking, nutritional deficiency disease results. Of the thousands of molecules involved in human metabolism, only 47 are essential to life. Groups of these substances include: (a) *essential minerals* (elements); (b) *vitamins*; (c) *proteins*; (d) *carbohydrates*; and (e) *lipids*. The essential minerals for maintenance of normal functions are Na, K, Ca, Mg, P, Cl, S, C, H, O, and N. Many of these elements compose vital structures of proteins, carbohydrates, and lipids. In addition, Fe, Zn, Cu, Mn, Co, I, Cr, Ni, V, Sn, Mo, Se, and F are needed in small (trace) quantities. They are vital for enzymatic and hormonal function and for building hemoglobin and other molecules.

The essential water soluble vitamins are thiamine, riboflavin, the vitamin B_6 group, niacin, folacin, pantothenic acid, cobalamin, biotin, and ascorbic acid (vitamin C). The fat soluble vitamins are A, D, E, and K. Essential fatty acids—linoleic and arachodonic acids—are also required in the diet.

Eight essential amino acids provide the building blocks for protein: lysine, threonine, leucine, isoleucine, methionine, tryptophan, valine, and phenylalanine. Growing children also require histidine. All persons require water.

Storage of Nutrients

The human body can store nutrients for varying periods of time so temporary deprivation of essential nutrients will not necessarily result in acute malnutrition. For example, glycogen stored in the liver and skeletal muscle will maintain metabolism for 13 hours without drawing on other reserves. Body fat stores thousands of calories and is preferentially used as a source of energy during deprivation (Fig. 10-1). Elements such as iron are stored in the bone marrow and vitamin B_{12} is stored in the liver. All these storage reserves equip us to withstand temporary deprivation of food without ill effects.

Malnutrition

Causes

Adequate nutrition requires: (a) intake of food; (b) mastication (chewing) of food; (c) digestion; (d) absorption of nutrients in the intestine; (e) transport or distribution of nutrients in the blood stream; and (f) uptake and utilization of nutrients by cells.

A defect or abnormal functioning anywhere along this nutritional chain can result in malnutrition (bad nutrition), which usually is undernutrition.

Disturbed intake of food can occur from altered psychological states such as psychosis, neurosis, alcoholism, and food faddism. Inabilities to chew, swallow, or retain food in the stomach impair intake.

Defective digestion is caused by a failure to produce digestive juices. Hydrochloric acid, pepsin, intrinsic factor (for absorbing vitamin B_{12}), pancreatic enzymes (lipase, trypsin, and amylase for digesting fat, protein, and carbohydrates) and bile (for absorbing fat soluble vitamins A, D, E, and K) are all essential for digestion.

Malabsorption can result from an absence of digestive juices or from inflammatory or metabolic diseases of the gastrointestinal tract. Persons who

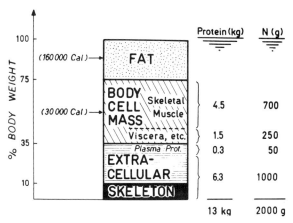

Figure 10-1   *Reserves of energy in the body of a typical 70-kg man. (From Fischer, J. E. 1976. Total parenteral nutrition. Boston: Little, Brown and Company.)*

have had their intestines removed will have some malabsorption for obvious reasons.

Transport of nutrients to the liver can be impaired by inflammatory diseases like hepatitis or cirrhosis. Cirrhosis, in particular, impairs the flow of blood into the liver, which then fails to synthesize proteins. Also various proteins (for example, lipoprotein) that carry lipids can be lacking and lead to metabolic nutritional defects.

Impaired utilization of nutrients can also result in malnutrition. For example, in diabetes mellitus the lack of insulin impairs the utilization of glucose by cells (see Chapter 12, Endocrine and Metabolic Disorders).

Finally, malnutrition can be caused by *protein-losing enteropathy*, which results in excretion of proteins from the gut. Likewise, diarrhea from infection or other inflammatory diseases of the intestines (enteritis) also causes excretion of protein and malnutrition can ensue.

Classification

Diseases of malnutrition are often closely related to socioeconomic conditions. The "haves" often suffer from excessive intake of food and obesity results; the "have-nots" lack food and suffer from undernutrition. (See Table 10-1.)

Excessive intake of nutrients results in *obesity* (excessive storage of fat), or toxicity to organs can

Table 10-1

Classification of Malnutrition

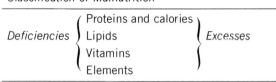

occur from *hypervitaminosis* (ingestion of an excess of one or more vitamins). The common nutritional deficiency syndromes listed in Table 10-2 occur predominantly in developing countries, but they also occur in the United States.

Several nutritional deficiencies can often occur at the same time in a patient (for example, deficiency of vitamins A and D, folate, and protein). It is often difficult to isolate a single malnutritional deficiency. Administering one single nutrient to a malnourished individual may aggravate coexisting deficiencies of other nutrients by increasing metabolism and depleting marginal reserves of nutrients the person has stored.

In this chapter emphasis focuses upon frequent and preventable nutritional deficiencies including *endemic goiter* (iodine deficiency); *beriberi* (thiamine deficiency); *pellagra* (niacin deficiency); *rickets* (vitamin D deficiency); and *scurvy* (vitamin C deficiency). Folic acid and iron deficiencies cause nutritional anemias and are discussed in Chapter 11, Hematology.

Another very important form of malnutrition, *protein-calorie malnutrition (PCM)* is stressed in this chapter because, on a worldwide basis, it is the predominant form of malnutrition. The World Health Organization estimates that approximately 300 million of 700 million preschool-aged children in developing countries are malnourished. The malnutrition makes the children vulnerable to infectious diseases. Deaths due to malnutrition and

Table 10-2

Common Nutritional Deficiency Syndromes

Deficiency	Clinical and pathologic findings
Protein-calorie malnutrition	Apathy or irritability and decreased brain size; hypopigmented skin and sparse easily pluckable hair; dermatitis and "flaky paint" skin; generalized edema and enlargement of liver; atrophy of other organs and tissues; lymphoid, pancreas, and intestinal mucosa; high mortality to infectious diseases
Vitamin A	Dryness (xerosis) of eyes and night blindness; keratin plugging of hair follicles
Thiamine (beriberi)	Weakness of legs and tingling sensation in extremities; cardiac enlargement and heart failure; Wernicke's syndrome (confusion and incoordination)
Niacin (pellagra)	Diarrhea, dermatitis, and dementia (madness); cracking of lips and atrophy of lining of tongue
Vitamin C (scurvy)	Spongy bleeding gums and cutaneous hemorrhage; poor wound healing (poor collagen and osteoid formation)
Vitamin D (rickets)	Rosary beading of ribs, bowing of legs, and enlargement of epiphyses; poor maturation of cartilage and failure of calcification of new bone; deformities of chest and skull in children; osteomalacia (softening of bone in adults)
Iodine	Goiter (enlargement of thyroid gland)*
Iron	Iron deficiency anemia
Folate	Folate deficiency anemia

*Nutritional anemias of iron and folate and vitamin B_{12} deficiencies (see Chapter 11, Hematology)

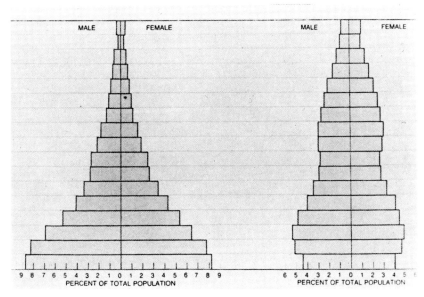

Figure 10-2 *Census profiles for a developing country* (left) *and for a developed nation* (right). *Many children in developing countries die before ten years of age from malnutrition and infections. (From Freedman, R., and Berelson, B.* The Human Population. *Copyright © 1974 by Scientific American, Inc. All rights reserved.)*

infections are common in children in developing countries (Fig. 10-2).

Protein-calorie Malnutrition

Kwashiorkor is a syndrome afflicting young children that results from a deficient protein intake despite an adequate caloric intake. The diets of children with this syndrome are essentially devoid of protein and consist chiefly of starchy foods like polished rice. The word "kwashiorkor" literally translated from the Ga language of Gold Coast, Africa means "one-two," or the disease which occurs when a child is displaced from the mother's breast by a new offspring.

An infant with kwashiorkor manifests edema (swelling), sparse, silky, reddish-brown hair, hypopigmented skin, infections, and a fretful or apathetic disposition (Fig. 10-3). These deprived children are immobile because they lack energy-

producing protein, hence the disease is sometimes called protein-energy malnutrition.

Marasmus, another form of nutritional deprivation, results from a total decrease of proteins and calories. It is distinguishable from kwashiorkor by the absence of edema. Marasmus can also occur from chronic debilitating disease or inborn errors of metabolism (Fig. 10-4) which prevent cells from effectively utilizing nutrients.

Pathology

All organs of the body are affected by PCM. The brain normally achieves 80% of its development by age 2. Children victimized by PCM have small brains, and studies suggest that children with PCM are prevented from reaching their full intellectual capacity. Since millions of persons in the world have suffered or are suffering from PCM, the impact of this form of malnutrition on intelligence and human potential is enormous.

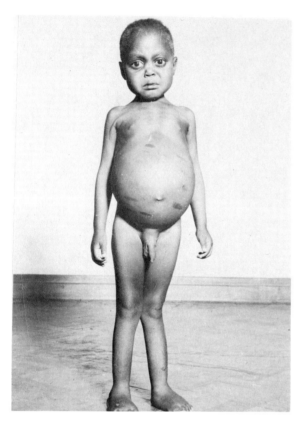

Figure 10-3   *Kwashiorkor. This 3-year-old boy manifests classical kwashiorkor, sparse reddened hair, extensive edema of the lower extremities, ascites, dermatitis, hypopigmentation of the skin, and anxiety. The markings on the abdomen were made by a native "practitioner."*

Skin on the legs of children with kwashiorkor is often thickened and scaly, it has a "flaky paint" appearance. Fluid accumulates in the skin (edema) and in the abdominal cavity (ascites), producing a protruding abdomen.

The pancreas is the first organ affected by PCM. As PCM persists and advances, the pancreas atrophies (withers) and the mucosa of the small intestine also atrophies (Fig. 10-5).

The liver becomes pale yellow because of anemia and fatty changes develop in the liver cells. When the fatty change is mild, only a slight amount of fat is present within hepatocytes; microscopically the liver looks like a chicken wire fence because fat is paradoxically abundant (Fig. 10-6).

The decreased production of enzymes by the pancreas and intestinal tract impairs digestion of fats, proteins, and carbohydrates. When children with advanced PCM are given whole milk they cannot digest it and develop diarrhea. They are only capable of sipping diluted skim milk for several days while new enzymes are produced in the pancreas and intestine. Only later can they digest more hearty food.

Immunodeficiency and Infection

Children with PCM invariably die if they are not given nutritional replenishment, and even when they are treated in hospitals nearly 40% die of infectious diseases. These children die because malnutrition causes immunodeficiency, which permits severe infections to develop (Table 10-3). The deficient host defenses are multiple: (a) defects of the tissues covering the surfaces of the body (e.g., skin and intestine) permit invasion by microbes; (b) phagocyte dysfunction (failure of granulocytes to migrate, ingest, and kill bacteria) occurs; (c) depressed cell-mediated immunity (CMI) occurs; and (d) low serum complement and failure to produce antibodies against certain bacteria occur (see Chapter 6, Immunology). Thus children with PCM are more than normally susceptible to the ill effects of ordinary infectious diseases. For example, measles kills approximately 25% of children who have kwashiorkor.

The *thymus* atrophies (decreases in function and size) to approximately 10% of its normal weight with kwashiorkor. The thymus gland and T lymphocytes help defend against intracellular viruses and bacteria such as tuberculosis (see Chapter 6). Virtually all lymphoid tissues atrophy and impaired immunity occurs (Fig. 10-7).

Protein-calorie Malnutrition in the United States

Approximately 25% of hospitalized adults in the United States have some degree of PCM—they often will have sustained at least a 20 lb weight loss within two months prior to hospitalization, and have low serum protein. Patients with intestinal

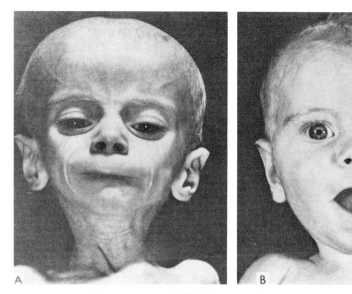

Figure 10-4   *Marasmus.* **A,** *This infant manifests marasmus resulting from excessive excretion of an amino acid (cystathionine).* **B,** *Massive doses of vitamin B₆ restored his nutrition within five months. (Reprinted by permission from the England Journal of Medicine, p. 722, 1967.)*

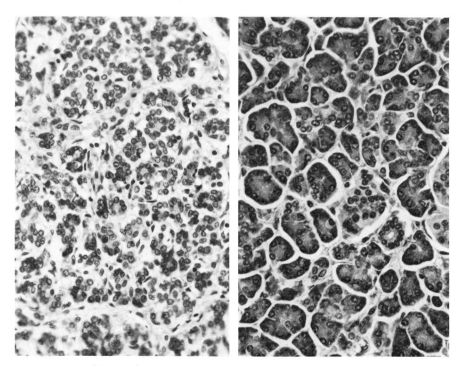

Figure 10-5   *Photomicrograph of pancreas from child dying from kwashiorkor* (left). *The glands are disorganized and small: enzyme granules are sparse. Compare with the plump enzyme-rich cells seen in the normal pancreas* (right).

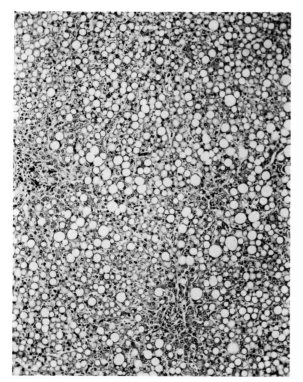

Figure 10-6 *Photomicrograph of fatty metamorphosis of the liver in protein-calorie malnutrition. Fat in hepatocytes gives the liver a chicken-wire fence appearance.*

diseases, psychoses, cancer, stroke, and chronic respiratory or renal failure often become malnourished. Also, malnourished individuals have poor healing of wounds, which can become readily infected by microorganisms that well-nourished persons can resist. Malnourished surgical patients require nutritional replenishment prior to surgery and good nutrition must be provided post-operatively.

Deficiency of Vitamin D (rickets)

Clinical Appearance

Rickets can cause marked deformities in growing children in bones of the skull, lower extremities, and chest. A classic deformity of rickets, the *rachitic rosary*, appears as bead-like swellings where the ribs fuse with the cartilage at the sternum (Fig. 10-8). The swelling results from a haphazard growth of cartilage at this juncture. The ends of other bones also become increased in thickness and the legs too can become deformed (Fig. 10-9). When rickets is extensive, marked deformities of the chest result which can impair respiration and cardiac function.

Table 10-3
Acquired Nutritional Deprivation Immunodeficiency

Humoral immunity

Serum complement decreased (hence, cannot kill Gram-negative bacteria)

Serum transferrin decreased (thus, lose this bacteriostatic defense)

Immunoglobulins actually *increased* during infection

Antibody forming capacity reduced (cannot mount antibodies against *Salmonella typhosa*)

Cellular immunity

Atrophic thymus and lymphoid organs. Increased vulnerability to intracellular microbes results in death from certain bacterial (tuberculosis, for example) and viral (measles, for example) infections

Phagocytes

Neutrophils fail to migrate, phagocytose, digest, and kill bacteria

Macrophages also fail to kill bacteria

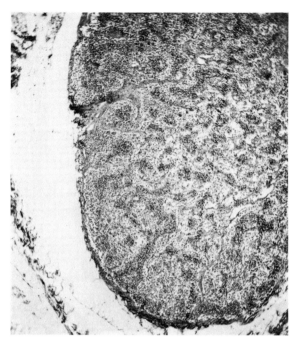

Figure 10-7 *Photomicrograph showing marked atrophy of a lymph node from a child who died from malnutrition and infection.*

Deficiency

Lack of vitamin D is responsible for rickets. This vitamin is present in dairy products like milk and is absorbed in the small intestine in bile. Activation of molecules of vitamin D by sunlight occurs in the skin, so children with a borderline deficiency of vitamin D can develop rickets when they are deprived of sunlight. Vitamin D is essential for the absorption of calcium and phosphorus from the intestine. If an individual has a decreased vitamin D intake, these minerals will not be absorbed and calcification of bones becomes impaired.

Pathology

Rickets is characterized by an *excessive proliferation (growth) of osteoid tissue*. This specialized connective tissue forms the framework for bone which eventually calcifies. In rachitic bones the cartilage cells grow in disorderly columns (Fig. 10-10). In-

adequate calcification of osteoid results and the bone spicules are weak and pliable; bowing of the legs occurs frequently in children with rickets whose weakened legs cannot support their body weight (Fig. 10-9).

Rickets can also occur as a result of obstruction of the bile duct. Malabsorption of vitamin D occurs when bile is not available in the intestine where it is necessary for the absorption of fat soluble vitamins A, D, E, and K.

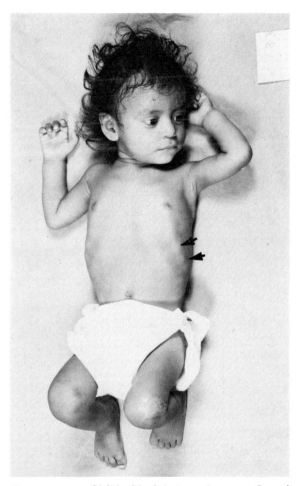

Figure 10-8 *Child with rickets and scurvy. Prominent "rachitic rosaries," which are characteristic of rickets, are noted (arrows) at the costochondral junction. Ecchymoses are present on her knees. Hemorrhage into the skin and bones is common in scurvy.*

Adults also can develop a form of rickets termed *osteomalacia* (bone softening). Persons with chronic rheumatoid arthritis and those lacking vitamin D, exposure to sunlight, and sufficient calcium can develop decalcified, soft, fragile bones. Fractures, especially compression fractures of the spine and hip fractures are serious complications of osteomalacia (see Chapter 20, Diseases of Muscles, Bones, and Joints).

Deficiency of Vitamin C (scurvy)

Clinical Appearance

Chronic alcoholics and senile elderly persons who live alone are prone to develop scurvy. The capillaries in scrobutic persons often rupture because the vessel walls are weak and hemorrhage into the gums and skin is common. In Figure 10-8 hemorrhage has occurred beneath the periosteum covering the child's femurs. Vitamin deficiencies are often multiple—this patient had both rickets and scurvy. The hemorrhage caused pain, which was relieved by flexing her knees.

Deficiency

Vitamin C is required for the formation of tissues derived from mesoderm, collagen, osteoid, dentin of teeth, and extracellular matrix substances (see Chapters 2 and 3). Vitamin C is required for the incorporation of an amino acid, tyrosine, into collagen. Collagen is the molecule which forms the fibrous component of teeth, bone, and connective tissue, and is an integral force in wound healing. Because vitamin C is vital to collagen formation, individuals with a deficiency of vitamin C have poor healing of all wounds.

Pathology

Scrobutic bone is adequately calcified, but the osteoid is inadequately formed. The scrobutic zone in bone shows fibroblasts that fail to produce collagen and osteoid. Consequently, bone spicules are irregular in shape, thin, and calcified but with no discernible osteoid (Fig. 10-11).

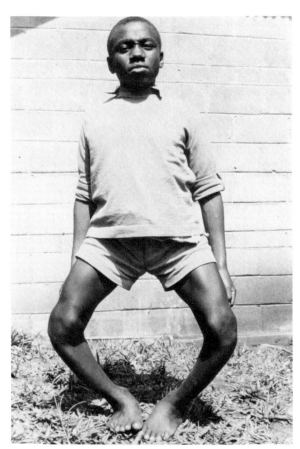

Figure 10-9 *Rickets bowing the legs of a deprived boy. (Courtesy Dr. Clitus Olson.)*

Deficiency of Thiamine (beriberi)

Thiamine (vitamin B_1) is vital to carbohydrate metabolism in the heart and central nervous system. Individuals suffering from beriberi, a deficiency of thiamine, have weakness, central nervous dysfunction, or cardiac failure. The nerves become demyelinated (lose their insulating sheath), impulses are not transmitted along the nerves, and difficulty in walking ensues (see Chapter 21, Neurology and Neuropathology). Two major clinical forms of thiamine deficiency occur.

Clinical Appearances

Cardiac Beriberi A person with cardiac beriberi has dilated blood vessels, a ruddy, warm, dry skin

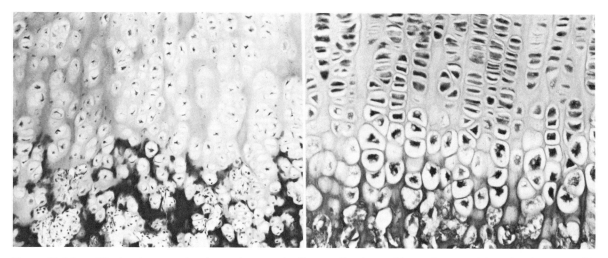

Figure 10-10   *Photomicrographs. Irregular saw-tooth growth plate of bone from a child with* rickets (left). *The chondrocytes (cartilage cells) have failed to grow in orderly columns (palisades). Compare with the straight columns of chondrocytes in a normal growth plate* (right).

and he or she has a massively enlarged heart. The myocardium becomes flabby and edema fluid separates the myocardial fibers. The heart is unable to pump blood adequately and heart failure can ensue.

Neuropsychiatric Disorders   Thiamine deficiency is most commonly seen in the United States in chronic alcoholics. Some thiamine deficient persons have *Wernicke's syndrome*, which consists of a triad of: (a) confusion; (b) ataxia (unstable gait); and (c) paralysis of eye movements.

Since the frequency of this deficiency is high in chronic alcoholic patients, they are generally treated with intravenous fluids containing high concentrations of thiamine and other vitamins. The signs of vitamin deficiency are frequently reversed within a few weeks. Even with treatment, however, the mortality rate of these patients is about 15%. At autopsy, focal degeneration and hemorrhage are found in the brain substance surrounding the ventricles and within the nuclei of the cranial nerves which supply the extraocular eye muscles (this latter finding explains the paralysis of eye movements).

Deficiency of Niacin (pellagra)

Pellagra was once a major problem in the southern United States and remains a problem in persons

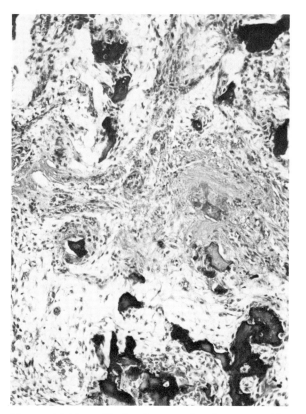

Figure 10-11   *Photomicrograph of scurvy. The bone spicules (black) are irregular, thin, and calcified. Fibroblasts proliferated in a disorganized manner; no collagen is seen.*

subsisting on a diet predominantly of corn. Individuals suffering from pellagra commonly experience "the three ds": dermatitis, diarrhea, and dementia (insanity). The skin of pellagra victims becomes scaly, thickened, and has alternating patches of hyper- and hypopigmentation (dark and light pigmented areas). Changes in the skin are prominent in areas exposed to the sun such as the back of the hands and neck. The tongue often becomes dry and swollen and the lips are cracked along the borders. The intestinal mucosa becomes atrophic and dementia results from degeneration of neurons in the brain. These pathological changes are reversible by nutritional replenishment.

A summary of common nutritional deficiency syndromes is presented in Table 10-2.

Deficiency of Iodine (endemic goiter)

Enlargement of the thyroid (goiter) often results from an inadequate intake of iodine. Persons living in the interior of continents (Great Lakes region of the United States, India, and Switzerland) in the past developed endemic goiter (endemic refers to the frequent occurrence of a disease in a particular geographical region). The ingestion of iodized salt in only one to two parts per million now prevents goiter in these regions.

Goiter occurs most commonly in females. The goiterous thyroid can be huge (Fig. 10-12). Pathological examination reveals a brittle, gelatinous, and sometimes fibrotic gland. The goiter may obstruct the trachea; thyroidectomy may be necessary to open the airway or the gland may be removed for cosmetic reasons. In the early stages of goiter, iodine administration will reverse the process. Surgical removal is required in later stages, when the thyroid gland becomes fibrotic and calcified.

Obesity

Obesity is the single most prevalent nutritional disorder in the United States. About 30% of adult Americans and probably 10% of children are obese.

Obesity is characterized by a weight more than 15 to 20% above the "ideal" as defined by life insurance weight-height tables. Overweight persons, in general, have increased mortality. Obesity tends to occur in socioeconomically deprived persons and females are more likely to become obese than males.

Etiology

Obesity occurs when the number of calories ingested exceeds those burned, producing a surplus that must be stored. Fat is the storage form for unused energy. Triglycerides, consisting of fatty acids linked with glycerol, are the reversible storage compound that fills adipose cells. Many circumstances can produce excess of intake over utilization. Obesity is sometimes categorized as *endogenous* or *exogenous*. Endogenous means that some identifiable physiologic abnormality produces the energy imbalance, while exogenous means that the individual eats more food than needed, without abnormal metabolism.

Pathology

Pathologically, obesity simply consists of adipose cells distended by fat. In some obese persons, fat may infiltrate organs (the heart or pancreas), but invasion of organs by fat does not generally alter the function of the organs. Obese persons are predisposed to diabetes and arteriosclerosis. Other problems of overweight persons include gall bladder disease, gout, degenerative arthritis, varicose veins, and skin disorders.

One pathophysiologic cause of obesity is a maladjustment of the "appestat" in the hypothalamus of the brain, which controls appetite. The causes for maladjustment in the appestat are complex, but probably result partially from abnormalities in cultural behavioral factors. Endocrine dysfunction of the thyroid, adrenals, and gonads is rarely responsible for obesity.

Treatment

Correction of obesity is by cutting calories. Intestinal bypass procedures to prevent absorption of

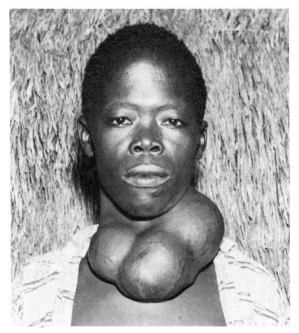

Figure 10-12   *Endemic goiter in a man from the Republic of Zaire. The thyroid is markedly enlarged. (Armed Forces Institute of Pathology Negative No. 69-3574.)*

food and wiring of the jaws are extreme measures used for treating obesity. In general, correction of obesity is difficult to attain. Episodic weight gain and loss is common and only about 10% of serious dieters achieve permanent weight reduction.

Nutritional Impact of Alcoholism

Acute alcoholic intoxication and chronic alcoholism are pervasive problems of immense importance. Sorrow, accidents, disease, and death are byproducts of this problem. Repeated, excessive alcohol intake imposes burdens on society and inflicts a spectrum of diseases on the consumer. Digestive organs, especially the liver, pancreas, and brain are damaged.

Metabolism

Alcohol enters the blood stream rapidly from the stomach and proximal small intestine. Via the portal vein it enters the liver and enzymes convert it into acetaldehyde and smaller fragments which burn to generate energy. The alcohol increases blood levels of lactic acid and mobilizes free fatty acids. Meanwhile, the liver is diverted from synthesizing important serum proteins such as blood clotting factors and fat begins to accumulate in the liver.

Toxicity

Hotly debated is the issue of whether alcohol can itself be toxic to cells or if undernutrition is required concurrently to damage the liver, brain, pancreas, bone marrow, and other organs. The weight of evidence is swinging in favor of the view that alcohol per se is toxic. However, chronic alcoholic individuals often do not eat normal diets. Hence they suffer from multiple vitamin and protein deficiencies.

Pathology

Amazingly, only about 10% of "heavy" consumers of ethanol develop serious liver disease in the form of alcoholic cirrhosis (See Chapter 16, Diseases of the Liver and Pancreas). But many alcoholics suffer from fatty liver, alcoholic hepatitis and acute and chronic pancreatitis often stem from drinking.

Death from chronic alcoholism can occur from overdose or complications arising from hepatic insufficiency. *Fatal hemorrhage* is common because cirrhotic livers fail to produce blood clotting factors, cause increased blood pressure in distended blood vessels in the inflamed esophagus and stomach, and the alcohol depresses blood platelets needed to prevent hemorrhage. Moreover, the liver fails to detoxify nitrogenous compounds and *hepatic coma* can develop.

Chronic alcoholism *damages* both the *central and peripheral nervous systems*. For example, *Wernicke's syndrome* results from vitamin B_1 (thiamine) deficiency. The syndrome partially resolves when vitamin B_1 is given. Cerebellar degeneration can also result from alcoholism, but it is not amenable to vitamin therapy. Peripheral nerves show dysfunction in many alcohol abusers. Tingling, burning sensations, and impaired motor functions are often found. Again, multiple vitamin therapy can partially correct this problem.

Hypervitaminosis

As with ethanol, excessive ingestion of vitamins can cause nutritional disorders termed hypervitaminosis. Acute or chronic toxicity results from excessive vitamins, especially vitamins A and D.

Acute hypervitaminosis A can occur in infants who swallow many tablets (300,000 International Units in a dozen or more tablets). They manifest nausea, vomiting, drowsiness, and bulging of the soft spot (fontanel) of their head. The latter results from cerebral edema which swells the brain and pushes the cerebrum between the bones of the skull. In hypervitaminosis A of long-standing, pruritus (itching), and loss of appetite occur. The affected children fail to gain weight, are irritable, and have tender swollen extremities. These abnormalities are reversible when the children are given normal amounts of vitamins.

Hypervitaminosis D results from an excessive ingestion of vitamin D. Vitamin D assists in the absorption of calcium from the intestine—excessive vitamin D intake causes excessive absorption of calcium into the blood. Neuromuscular dysfunction including hypotonia (floppiness), anorexia, irritability, constipation, pallor, or excessive thirst and urination can occur due to the increased concentration of calcium in the serum. Calcium deposited in the lungs, heart, stomach, and kidney can produce irreparable damage (Fig. 10-13). Well-intentioned but overzealous parents can harm their children by "pushing vitamin pills."

Summary

Malnutrition stems from excess or deficient utilization of nutrients: defects in the nutritional chain can cause undernutrition, overconsumption results in obesity, alcoholism induces diseases, as does hypervitaminosis. Decreased intake of protein and calories in children impairs growth and neurological development and renders them vulnerable to fatal infectious diseases.

Vitamin deficiencies cause arrest in development or abnormalities in structure and function in various organs. For example, vitamin D deficiency causes decreased calcification of growing bones and

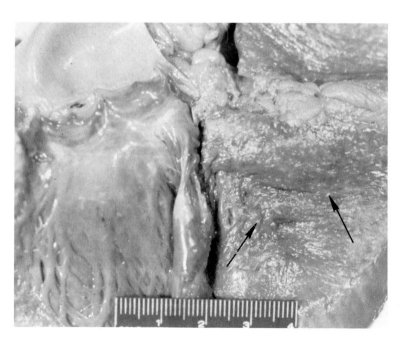

Figure 10-13 *Photomicrograph of heart. Hypervitaminosis D caused deposition of calcium (arrows on white calcium deposits). The heart failed.*

rickets ensues. Vitamin C deficiency causes scurvy; and impaired collagen synthesis results in poor wound healing, capillary fragility, and brittle bones. Other vitamin deficiencies affect cardiovascular and nervous systems.

Obesity is the number one nutritional problem in the United States and results from overconsumption of calories. The recent report that arteriosclerosis (which has been linked to improper diet) is now declining in incidence is gratifying. A decline in consumption of butter, animal fat, eggs, and sugar and other factors implicated in enhanced atherogenesis is thought to be responsible for the reverse in incidence of arteriosclerosis. Widespread ingestion of bran has become more popular; in the past American diets have been lacking in fiber, a major component of bran. Finally, many of us realize the importance of a daily exercise program for physical fitness.

Alcoholism has major sociologic and pathophysiologic effects on many people. The liver, brain, and pancreas are damaged by both the primary toxic impact of ethanol and from nutritional deficiencies (protein and vitamins). Excessive intake of vitamins can also be toxic.

Bibliography

Editorial: Nutrition in the Third World. 1973. *Ann. Intern. Med.* 78:296. Provides an overview on this topic.

Follis, R.H., Jr. 1958. *Deficiency diseases.* Springfield: Charles C Thomas, Publisher. A standard old, but good, reference of the pathology of malnutrition.

Gordon, J.E., and Scrimshaw, N.S. 1970. Infectious diseases in the malnourished. *Med. Clin. North Am.* 54:1495. Describes the problems with infectious diseases in malnourished children.

Guthrie, H.A. 1977. Concept of nutritious food. *J. Am. Diet. Assoc.* 71:14–19. A practical guide to optimal nutritional requirements.

Hegsted, D.M. 1977. Priorities in nutrition in the United States. *J. Am. Diet. Assoc.* 71:9–13. Presents perspectives and relative importance of various nutritional problems in the United States.

Kretchmer, N. 1977. Lactose and lactase. *Sci. Am.* 227:1–10. Discusses the inheritance and pathophysiology of lactase deficiency in people throughout the world.

Lieber, C.S. 1976. The metabolism of alcohol. *Scientific Amer.* 234:25–33. A comprehensive review by a leading worker in this field of the pathophysiologic effect of alcohol on the body.

Mann, G.V. 1974. The influence of obesity on health. *New Engl. J. Med.* 291:178–185 and 266–232. A dispassionate compilation of what is known about the true medical significance of obesity.

Purtilo, D.T. 1976. Nutritional deficiency diseases. In *Pathology of tropical and extraordinary diseases*, eds. C. Binford and D. Connor. Armed Forces Institute of Pathology, Washington, pp. 635–646. Pictorial summary of nutritional deficiency diseases.

Purtilo, D.T., and Connor, D.H. 1975. Fatal infections in protein-calorie malnourished children with thymolympathic atrophy. *Arch. Dis. Child.* 50:149. Discusses infections occurring in malnourished children.

Rimm, A.A.; Werner, L.H.; Van Yserloo, B.; and Bernstein, R.A. 1975. Relationships of obesity and disease in 73,532 weight-conscious women. *Pub. Health. Rep.* 90:44–51.

Rogers, S.; Goss, A.; Goldney, R.; Thomas, D.; Wise, P.; Burnet, R.; Philips, P.; Kimber, C.; and Harding, P. 1977. Jaw wiring in treatment of obesity. *Lancet* i:1221–1224. Desperate but effective in the temporary control of obesity.

Trowell, H.D.; Davies, J.N.P.; and Dean, R.F.A. 1954. *Kwashiorkor.* London: Edward Arnold Publishers, Ltd. An old but thorough description of this disease.

Vahlquist, B. 1975. A two-century perspective of some major nutritional deficiency diseases in childhood. *Acta Paediatr. Scand.* 64:161–167.

Vitale, J.J. 1974. Deficiency diseases. In *Pathologic basis of disease*, ed. S.L. Robbins, pp. 475–508. Philadelphia: W.B. Saunders Co. Provides a concise summary of nutritional deficiency diseases.

Vitale, J.J., and Good, R.A. 1974. Nutrition and immunology. *Clin. Nutr.* 27:623–628. The entire issue is devoted to this topic.

Williams, R., and Davis, M. 1977. Nutrition: effects of alcohol. *Proc. Ro. Soc. Med.* 70:333–336. Describes the impact of alcoholic abuse on the liver and the associated mortality.

CHAPTER 11

Hematology

Chapter Outline

Objectives

After reading this chapter you should be able to

List and describe the formed elements of blood.

Describe the three subspecialities of hematology.

List hematopoietic organs.

Describe the function and source of erythropoietin.

List the nutrients essential for erythropoiesis.

Describe the formation and destruction of erythrocytes.

Understand the terms describing abnormal shapes and sizes of erythrocytes.

List the normal values for erythrocytes, leukocytes and platelets.

List the normal values of an adult white blood cell differential count.

Define anemia.

Describe signs and symptoms of anemia.

List the three factors responsible for anemias.

Compare the size of iron deficiency anemia and vitamin B_{12} anemia.

Understand the pathogenesis of pernicious anemia.

Describe why erythrocytes are destroyed in the spleen in hereditary spherocytosis.

Define and give an example of a hemoglobinopathy.

Compare the inheritance of sickle trait and sickle disease.

Describe the metabolic defect in sickle hemoglobin.

Compare the racial groups affected by sickle disease and thalassemia.

Compare the inheritance of sickle disease, hereditary spherocytosis, thalassemia, and
    glucose–6 phosphate dehydrogenase deficiency.

Understand the basis for immune hemolytic anemia.

Describe the antiglobulin test and its use.

Know the pathogenesis, diagnosis and treatment for hemolytic disease of the newborn
    (HDN).

Compare the sites of injury in utero and following birth in HDN.

Define aplastic anemia and list several causes.

List the blood cells affected by polycythemia vera.

Define the terms leukopenia, leukocytosis, and leukemoid reaction.

Describe the etiologic agent of infectious mononucleosis.

Know the predominant origin of atypical lymphocytes in infectious mononucleosis.

Define and compare lymphoma and leukemia.

List the factors thought to be responsible for leukemia and lymphoma.

List the clinical findings in leukemia.

Classify leukemia.

Understand how leukemia is diagnosed.

List the complications and prognosis of leukemia.

Describe the treatment given for leukemia.

Define the term multiple myeloma.

List the diseases that can mimic lymphoma.

Classify lymphomas.

Define Hodgkin's disease and describe the significance of Sternberg-Reed cells.

Compare the prognosis of lymphomas.

Describe the four clinical stages of lymphoma.

Describe how patients with lymphomas are staged.

Compare the effects of radiotherapy and chemotherapy for lymphomas.

Compare the prognosis of nodular versus diffuse involvement by lymphomas.

Define hemostasis.

List the four factors providing hemostasis.

Compare primary and secondary hemostasis.

List the four components of the plasma coagulation system.

Compare the intrinsic and extrinsic pathways of activation of clotting.

Name the factor activated in the common final pathway of clotting.

List common causes of acquired plasma clotting disorders.

Define and compare petechiae, purpura, and ecchymoses.

List drugs and conditions associated with increased plasma clotting.

Compare hemophilia A, hemophilia B and von Willebrand's syndrome in terms of their inheritance and deficient clotting factors.

Define the term thrombocytopenia.

Describe the treatment for autoimmune thrombocytopenia purpura.

Understand the impact of aspirin on platelet function.

Define the term immunohematology.

Know what Landsteiner and Weiner discovered.

Understand blood grouping for ABO groups.

Describe how a cross match is performed.

List blood components and indications for their use.

Introduction

Hematology is defined as the study of blood. The *blood* consists of two major components: *plasma*, a pale yellow or gray-yellow fluid; and *formed elements*, red blood cells (RBC or erythrocytes), white blood cells (WBC or leukocytes) and platelets (thrombocytes) (Fig. 11-1). Blood is the circulating tissue of the body; the fluid and its formed elements circulate through the heart, arteries, capillaries, and veins. This chapter concentrates on disorders of the blood.

The *erythrocytes* carry oxygen to tissues and remove carbon dioxide from them. *Leukocytes* act in inflammatory and immune responses. The plasma carries antibodies and nutrients to tissues and wastes from tissues, and coagulation factors in plasma together with *platelets*, control the clotting of blood.

Primary hematologic diseases are uncommon, but hematologic manifestations secondary to other diseases are common. Three major subspecialties of hematology have evolved during this century for coping with hematologic disorders: (a) *Morphologic and clinical hematology* developed about 1900 when good microscopes became available. It is concerned chiefly with the study of the form and function of the formed elements of blood. (b) *Coagulation* of blood did not evolve until about 1935 because coagulation studies require access to specialized laboratory tests and knowledge about bleeding and clotting disorders. (c) *Blood banking* evolved during World War II. The advent of refrigeration permitted controlled storage of blood. The blood bank offers the patient both diagnostic and therapeutic blood transfusion services. The special emphasis of blood banking is on the ability to replace blood components missing in patients with hematologic disorders—components like blood clotting factors, plasma proteins, erythrocytes, leukocytes, and platelets. We will discuss these topics in this order.

Blood Composition And Formation

The total blood volume in an adult is about 6 liters or about 7.5% of the body weight. Approximately 45% of blood is composed of formed elements:

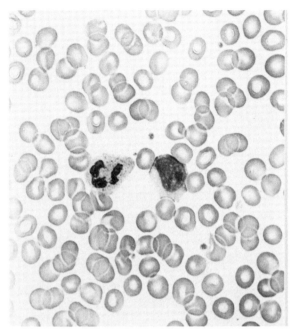

Figure 11-1 *Photomicrograph of peripheral blood smear showing leukocytes (largest cells), erythrocytes, and platelets.*

erythrocytes, leukocytes, and platelets. The remaining 55% of the blood is the fluid portion, which is called plasma. Approximately 90% of plasma is water. The remaining 10% is composed of proteins (albumin, immunoglobulin and other globulins, and fibrinogen), carbohydrates, vitamins, hormones, enzymes, lipids, and salts.

The *hematopoietic system* is composed of the circulating blood, the bone marrow, the spleen, the thymus, and the lymph nodes, supplemented by the reticuloendothelial (capable of engulfing or phagocytosing particles) cells lining blood sinuses and found in most organs of the body (see Chapter 2, Normal Cells, Tissues, and Organs). The term, *hematopoiesis* means the formation of blood.

Blood cells must go through stages of development in the same way a human being matures during development. In a healthy person, only mature adult cells are seen in the blood, whereas immature and abnormal cells can be seen in persons with many diseases. The student must be able to first recognize the normal blood cells before trying to comprehend abnormal cells.

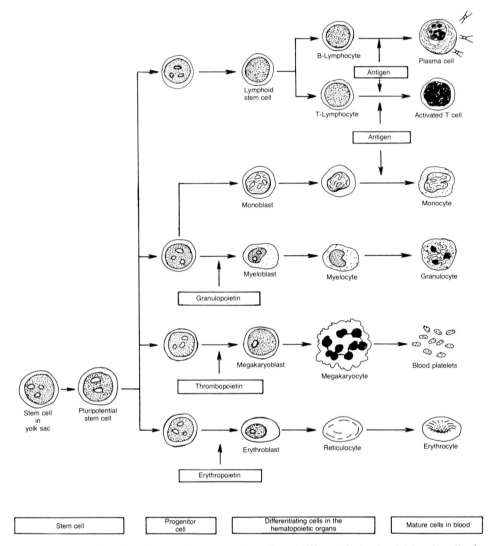

Figure 11-2 *The development and maturation (differentiation) of blood cells in hematopoietic organs.*

In the human embryo, hematopoiesis begins within two weeks following conception. Initially, primitive *stem cells* arise in blood islands within the yolk sac of the embryo (Fig. 11-2). Later, hematopoiesis takes place at different times in the liver, spleen, thymus, lymph nodes, and bone marrow. At birth, and continuing during life, hematopoiesis is confined to the bone marrow.

Red bone marrow is located in the flat bones of the skull, clavicle, sternum, ribs, pelvis, long bones of the extremities, and vertebrae (Fig. 11-3). In

adults, the bone marrow mass (see Chapter 2) is equivalent in size to that of the largest organs—the liver and brain. In total, the bone marrow weighs approximately 1200 gm.

Control of Hematopoiesis

Erythrocyte, leukocyte, and platelet production are all thought to be controlled by hormones and feedback mechanisms which maintain an ideal number of cells (Fig. 11-2). Without these control mecha-

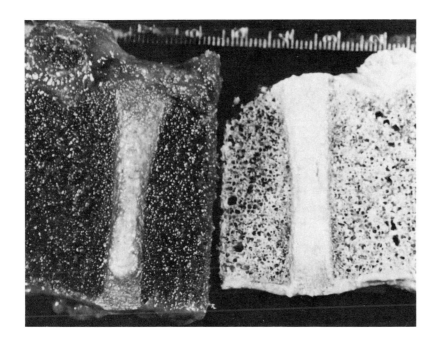

Figure 11-3 *Active red bone marrow* (left) *from patient recovering from hemorrhage and inactive pale bone marrow* (right) *in vertebrae from a patient with normal blood.*

nisms, blood cells would proliferate until the blood vessels became clogged with cells. The number of individual blood cells is probably controlled by specific hormones. Erythropoietin definitely governs erythrocyte production, thrombopoietin probably governs platelet production, and leukopoietin theoretically governs granulocyte production.

Erythropoiesis, for example, is governed by the oxygen concentration in the kidneys. The kidneys produce a hormone, *erythropoietin*, in response to lowered oxygen concentration in the blood. Erythropoietin is released from the kidneys and stimulates bone marrow stem cells to produce new erythrocytes. Production of erythrocytes is also limited by the availability of essential nutrients—iron, protein, folate, and vitamins B_{12} and B_6. Deficiency of any one of these essential nutrients results in a nutritional deficiency anemia.

Erythrocytes

The formation of erythrocytes is shown in Figure 11-2 and destruction in Figure 11-4. Normally five days are required to produce new erythrocytes from stem cell to mature erythrocyte. They live approximately 120 days in the blood stream. The spleen

is the "graveyard" of erythrocytes since it filters aged erythrocytes; passing through the spleen and in the liver, damaged erythrocytes are engulfed by reticuloendothelial cells. Hemoglobin is converted by the liver to bilirubin. In the liver, bilirubin is combined with two molecules of glucuronide. Bilirubin-diglucuronide is thus formed and can then be excreted in bile which is passed via the bile duct into the duodenum and eliminated in the feces from the body. Bacteria residing in the intestines convert the bilirubin into urobiliogen, which is partially absorbed by the intestine and then excreted in the urine.

During maturation in the bone marrow, nuclei of erythroblasts are extruded and biconcave shaped discs result. Thus erythrocytes are no longer true cells because they have no nuclei. The biconcave shape provides maximal surface area for O_2 and CO_2 exchange. Moreover, the erythrocyte membrane is flexible and enables the cells to squeeze through the splenic vascular filter which may have openings as small as 3μ in diameter.

Abnormal Erythrocytes

Ordinarily, erythrocytes are approximately 7μ in diameter and 90 cuμ in volume. The terminology

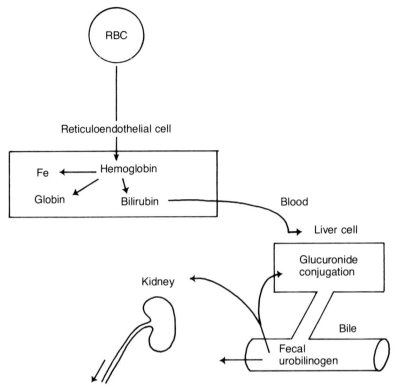

Figure 11-4   *Destruction of erythrocytes by reticuloendothelial cells in liver and spleen. Bilirubin is formed from hemoglobin and is subsequently detoxified (conjugated) in the liver cell with glucuronide and passes out the bile. It is converted into urobilinogen and excreted in the feces, primarily, and in the urine.*

used for abnormal erythrocytes provides shorthand definitions for various pathologic disorders. For instance, variations in erythrocyte size are described by the term *anisocytosis*, while variations in shape are described by the term *poikilocytosis*. Small erythrocytes lacking sufficient hemoglobin are pale, and are called *hypochromatic*. Microscopic examination of a stained blood smear is the method used for identifying erythrocytes seen in various anemias. For example, in iron deficiency anemia, hypochromic, microcytic erythrocytes (Fig. 11-5), are usually seen on a blood smear.

Normal Values

Normally there are 15 gm of hemoglobin/dl of blood, and approximately five million erythro-cytes/μl. When blood is centrifuged to obtain the *hematocrit* (volume percentage of erythrocytes), approximately 45% consists of packed red blood cells, 1% of WBCs and platelets, and the remaining 54% is composed of plasma (Fig. 11-6). The main difference between blood plasma and serum is that serum lacks fibrinogen which is utilized when blood forms a fibrin clot.

Leukocytes

Lymphocytes, monocytes, and granulocytes appear white when blood is observed in the fresh state (Fig. 11-2). For that reason they are called leukocytes or white blood cells (WBC). Normally, 4000 to 10,000 WBCs/μl are found in the blood. The

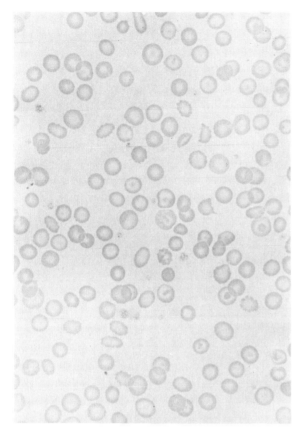

Figure 11-5 *Photomicrograph showing iron deficiency anemia. Note the small erythrocytes having pale centers; this indicates a lack of hemoglobin (hypochromic microcytic anemia).*

granulocytes generally measure approximately 10μ to 14μ in diameter—almost twice the size of erythrocytes. Blood contains three major groups of WBCs: lymphoid cells (lymphocytes, plasma cells), monocytes, and granulocytes. Granulocytes (neutrophils, eosinophils, and basophils) are named by the staining characteristics of their granules. The polymorphonuclear neutrophil (PMN) has two to five nuclear lobes and cytoplasmic granules which stain neutral (pale lilac) with Wright's stain. Eosinophils contain coarse, red-orange granules and have two to three nuclear lobes. Basophils have large, coarse, purple granules surrounding bilobed nuclei (Fig. 11-7).

Lymphocytes comprise above 50% of the circulating WBCs in children up until age 8. Thereafter

they make up from 20% to 40% of the WBCs. The nuclei of lymphocytes are single, round, and stain purple. A narrow rim of cytoplasm surrounds nuclei of lymphocytes which can measure from 9μ to 18μ in diameter. Occasionally plasma cells which have an eccentrically placed nucleus can be seen in the blood. Monocytes together with lymphocytes are also termed mononuclear leukocytes because they have one nucleus per cell. Monocytes are the largest circulating blood cells and have irregular shaped nuclei and cytoplasm. Macrophages are monocytes that have migrated into tissues and which have become activated by foreign substances such as bacteria. Thus a monocyte can be stimulated to become a macrophage (see Chapter 6, Immunology).

Granulocytes provide inflammatory responses (see Chapter 5) and defend the body against infectious agents (see Chapter 7) by phagocytosing bacteria or other infectious agents. Both neutrophils and monocytes have marked phagocytic capacities. Granulocytes are produced in the bone marrow by myeloblasts (Fig. 11-2). Approximately two to five days are required for their maturation, but their lifespan in the circulating blood is only a few hours.

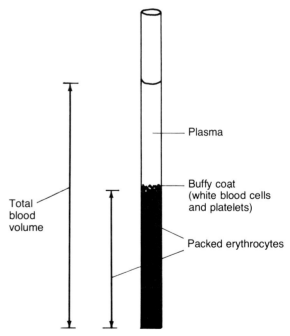

Plasma

Buffy coat (white blood cells and platelets)

Total blood volume

Packed erythrocytes

Figure 11-6 *Constituents of blood and measurement of hematocrit (% of packed erythrocytes).*

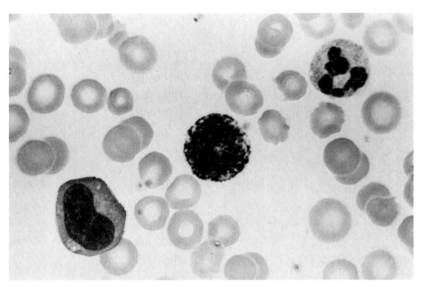

Figure 11-7   *Leukocytes in peripheral blood, neutrophil* (top right), *basophil* (center), *and lymphocyte* (left center).

A differential white blood count is often done to determine whether a person has an infection or leukemia. A differential count of 100 WBCs in an adult normally shows neutrophils numbering 60% to 70%, lymphocytes 20% to 40%, monocytes 4% to 8%, eosinophils 2% to 6%, and basophils 0% to 1%. When the number of leukocytes is below 4000/μl, *leukopenia* is present and when they exceed about 10,000/μl *leukocytosis* is present. A person with leukemia can have leukopenia (but with many immature leukocytic forms), or leukocytosis (with abnormal leukocytes), whereas a person with acute appendicitis usually shows leukocytosis with normal appearing leukocytes.

Platelets

Measuring 2μ to 4μ in diameter, platelets are the smallest of the formed elements in blood (Fig. 11-1). Normally platelets number between 150,000 and 400,000/cu mm, and are formed from megakaryocytes in bone marrow. Platelets are important in the blood clotting mechanism; they form hemostatic plugs in small ruptured blood vessels. They survive for approximately eight to ten days in circulation.

Thrombocytosis occurs when platelets number above 500,000/μl. When they number below 125,000/μl, thrombocytopenia is observed. When platelets number 50,000/μl or less, hemorrhage is likely to occur; in contrast, at levels above 600,000/μl thrombosis (clotting) may develop.

Anemia

Anemia results when insufficient hemoglobin is available to provide an individual's requirements for oxygen. Anemia can result from many causes, for instance, sudden loss of blood can produce anemia. A person can tolerate a gradual loss of blood (excessive menstrual blood loss for example), whereas a sudden loss (hemorrhage from duodenal ulcer) of as little as 500 ml can cause death. Tissues deprived of blood become anoxic (lack O_2) and shock may develop. In contrast, a gradual loss of blood can be compensated for by increased bone marrow production of RBCs. In adults a maximum of 50 ml of blood can be produced by the bone marrow (Fig. 11-3) each day.

An anemic person shows pallor of the skin, mucous membranes, and conjuctiva. Heart and respiratory rates usually increase to compensate for the anemia. Cardiac and respiratory compensation begin when the hemoglobin level declines to one-half of normal.

With rare exceptions, diseases of red cells themselves are manifested by a loss of plasticity of the cells. Plasticity is vital to movement of the erythrocyte through the capillaries and splenic filter. Plasticity abnormalities underlie hereditary spherocytosis (membrane defect) and sickle cell disease (hemoglobin defect). Both diseases result in a loss of plasticity of erythrocytes.

Anemias are usually classified on the basis of erythrocyte appearance (morphology), or etiology (cause) of the disease (Table 11-1). Most anemias are due to one of three factors: (a) loss of red cells, (b) increased red cell destruction (hemolysis), or (c) decreased production of red cells.

Anemias can also be classified by the morphology (staining quality which reveals hemoglobin content) and determination of the size of the erythrocyte as microcytic, normocytic, or macrocytic. Microcytes occur when the volume of erythrocytes is less than 87 cuμ and macrocytes occur when the volume exceeds 103 cuμ. Often small erythrocytes will also lack hemoglobin; they are thus classified as both microcytic and hypochromic (Fig. 11-5). Other types of anemia are discussed in the following several pages.

Nutritional Deficiency Anemias

Iron Deficiency Anemia

Iron deficiency anemia results from depletion of iron which is normally stored in the bone marrow. Often anemia can be detected just by a routine blood smear (Fig. 11-5). Blood smear examination of the blood is usually required by hospital rules for every hospitalized patient. Examination of bone marrow of an iron deficient person reveals inadequate iron stores. The serum of an iron deficient person also contains decreased amounts of iron. Bone marrow examination is not done commonly for iron deficiency anemia.

Iron deficiency anemia may result from a diet lacking iron. Elderly people who live on tea and biscuits, infants on a milk diet alone, or food faddists can develop iron deficiency anemia. A balanced diet of red meat, eggs, fruits, and vegetables will easily provide the 1 mg minimum daily requirement of iron. During pregnancy, however, 4 mg/day are needed since the fetus takes approximately 1 gm of iron from its mother. Repeated pregnancies in which iron intake is not increased invariably result in iron deficiency anemia in a woman.

A common cause of iron deficiency anemia is blood loss due to chronic bleeding, often from excessive menstruation. Gastrointestinal hemorrhage due to peptic ulcers, colonic carcinoma, hookworm, or hemorrhoids can also result in iron deficiency anemia (see Chapter 15, Gastrointestinal Disorders).

Iron deficiency anemia must be treated by correcting the condition responsible for blood loss. Iron tablets are also often given. The appearance of increased reticulocytes (young erythrocytes) in the peripheral blood signals a successful response to iron therapy.

Vitamin B$_{12}$ Deficiency Anemia

Macrocytic anemias generally result from insufficient intake of either folic acid or vitamin B$_{12}$. DNA synthesis is impaired when these vitamins are lacking and more cytoplasmic protein (RNA) is synthesized than DNA. The erythrocytes released into the peripheral blood are large (macrocytic). In addition, the neutrophils have an increased number of nuclear lobes. In fact, hyperlobulated neutrophils are often the first sign of macrocytic anemia.

Vitamin B$_{12}$ is obtained in meat and is also produced by bacteria in the intestines. A substance called intrinsic factor (IF) is required for the absorption of B$_{12}$ by the intestines. Intrinsic factor is produced by the parietal cells of the stomach. A special form of macrocytic anemia, *pernicious anemia* (PA), is caused by an inadequate secretion of IF or from autoantibodies in the patient's serum that inactivate IF.

For unknown reasons, patients with pernicious anemia are usually elderly Scandinavians with blue eyes and gray hair. In addition, they may have smooth red tongues and lemon-colored skin. They can have evidence of heart failure if the anemia is profound. Since vitamin B_{12} is also necessary for the formation of myelin, an insulation-like material that surrounds nerves; demyelination of nerve fibers within the spinal cord can also result from vitamin B_{12} deficiency (see Chapter 21, Neurology and Neuropathology). The demyelination results in a loss of the ability to sense positioning of the legs in space. A slipping, sliding gait results from the inefficient transmission of nerve impulses through the demyelinated nerves in the spinal cord.

Following a diagnosis of PA, vitamin B_{12} must be administered intramuscularly for the remainder of the person's life. The diagnosis of PA can be established by measuring the concentration of vitamin B_{12} in the blood by radioimmunoassay, a highly sensitive technique that reveals a low con-

Table 11-1
Classification of Anemia

Morphologic classification

1 Macrocytic normochromic anemia (MCV 103 cuμ)
   A Deficiencies of vitamin B_{12}, folic acid
   B Associated with variety of diseases, cirrhosis and hemolytic anemia, for example
2 Normocytic normochromic anemia (MCV 87 to 103 cuμ)
   A Sudden loss of blood
   B Increased destruction: hemolytic anemias
   C Decreased production: hemoglobin red cell mass deficit
      (1) Chronic disease and malignancy
      (2) Toxic agents and bone marrow failure
   D Compensated hemolytic anemia, hemoglobinopathy and hereditary spherocytosis, for example
3 Microcytic normochromic anemia (MCV 60 to 87 cuμ)
   A Hemoglobin red cell mass deficit
      (1) Chronic disease and malignancy
      (2) Toxic agents
4 Microcytic hypochromic anemia (MCV 60 to 87 cuμ with low hemoglobin)
   A Iron-deficiency anemia
   B Chronic lead poisoning
   C Thalassemia
   D Miscellaneous

Etiologic classification of anemia

1 Acute or chronic loss of blood (from hemorrhage, for example)
2 Destruction of erythrocytes (mechanical or autoimmune hemolytic bases, for example)
3 Decreased production from nutritional deficiency (iron, B_{12}, or folic acid lack, for example)
4 Molecular defects in proteins (hereditary spherocytosis, thalassemia, sickle cell disease, and enzyme deficiencies, for example)
5 Miscellaneous (marrow failure such as aplastic anemia, leukemia, chronic inflammatory and malignant diseases, and endocrine diseases)

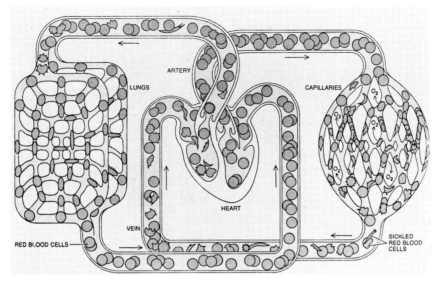

Figure 11-8   *Sickle cell anemia demonstrating the mechanism of formation in hypoxia and destruction of the sickle-shaped erythrocytes in the splenic filter. (From Ceraim, A., and Peterson, C. M. Cyanate and sickle-cell disease. Copyright © 1975 by Scientific American, Inc. All rights reserved.)*

centration of B_{12} in the blood of persons with PA. Moreover, the patient with PA fails to absorb radioactive vitamin B_{12}, confirming the diagnosis.

Folic Acid Deficiency

Deficient intake of folic acid in the diet also causes macrocytic anemia. This deficiency and the resulting macrocytic anemia are apt to occur in alcoholics. Pregnant women are also likely to develop folic acid deficiency. Remission of macrocytic anemia due to folic acid deficiency occurs within a few weeks following the oral administration of this nutrient.

Structural and Metabolic Defects of Erythrocytes

Premature destruction of erythrocytes by hemolysis may be due to either *extrinsic* (outside) or *intrinsic* (inside) abnormalities of the RBC. *Hemaglobinopathies* are caused by inherited intrinsic erythrocyte defects. In these conditions, an abnor-

mal hemoglobin is produced; changes in the shape of erythrocytes ensue. For example, in the hemoglobinopathy, called *sickle cell disease* (HbSS), amino acid valine is substituted for glutamic acid in the sixth position in the hemoglobin molecules. This small substitution causes the hemoglobin molecule to become rigid in hypoxic conditions; normal disc-shaped RBCs become "sickled" (Fig. 11-8).

In another disease, *hereditary spherocytosis*, the proteins in the erythrocyte membrane are abnormal and the erythrocytes become rigid spheres. The rigid spherocytes are subsequently easily destroyed in the spleen.

Physical trauma causes *extrinsic hemolytic anemia*. Prolonged walking or running, as occurs in some long distance runners, can induce "march" hemoglobinuria. Here, erythrocytes within the capillaries of the feet and joints become ruptured by trauma; hemoglobin is released into the plasma and excreted in urine. Mechanical heart valves can also mechanically destroy red cells as the erythrocytes pass over them.

Individuals with hemolytic anemia can become jaundiced due to the conversion of hemoglobin into bilirubin. Jaundice is a green-yellow discoloration of the skin that is seen when bilirubin levels exceed approximately 4 mg/dl. When hemolysis becomes so extensive that the liver is incapable of combining and detoxifying the bilirubin with glucuronide, jaundice results. Therefore, an increased bilirubin concentration in the serum can indicate hemolytic jaundice. Since RBCs are being destroyed, the bone marrow of patients with hemolytic anemia becomes very active (Fig. 11-3). Erythropoiesis is enhanced as the bone marrow attempts to replace hemolyzed erythrocytes, and many reticulocytes appear in the peripheral blood.

Hereditary Hemolytic Anemias

Hemoglobin has a molecular weight of 60,000 daltons and is composed of globin and heme. Hemoglobinopathies result from alterations (mutations) of genes which produce the globin portion of the hemoglobin. Over 200 different hemoglobinopathies have been described thus far. As described above for HbS, an amino acid substitution (valine for glutamic acid) results from the mutation of a gene and the subsequent change in the hemoglobin often deforms the erythrocytes.

Sickle Cell Disease

Sickle cell disease, an autosomal recessive disease, was discovered in the early 1900s when sickle-shaped erythrocytes were seen in the peripheral blood of an anemic black patient. Sickling occurs in the affected person at low O_2 levels; bubbling O_2 through the blood in vitro reverses the sickling.

Ordinarily, individuals with two genes for adult (A) hemoglobin and those with hemoglobin S genes can either be heterozygous (AS) or homozygous (SS); the former have sickle cell trait, the latter have sickle cell disease. The heterozygous individuals carrying the SA trait have approximately 20% to 40% of hemoglobin S; the remainder is hemoglobin A. Heterozygotes are usually asymptomatic; in fact, an individual with sickle trait won an Olympic track medal in 1972 in Mexico City where the altitude is 2300 meters. Sickle cell trait is probably the most common hemoglobinopathy in the United States. About 10% of American blacks have AS. The detection of heterozygotes by laboratory stud-

ies often calls for genetic counseling. If both parents are SA (heterozygous) they have a one in four chance of producing a homozygous child with SS.

Fortunately, less than 1% of American blacks have sickle disease (HbSS). This abnormal molecule of HbSS gels when deprived of O_2, distorting the cell into a rigid sickle shape. Sickled erythrocytes can "logjam" in capillaries in the spleen, liver, and elsewhere resulting in hemolysis, ischemia, infarction, and severe pain (Fig. 11-8). Sickle cell patients are also prone to develop ulcerations of the skin on their legs and are more susceptible to infections.

Thalassemia

Anemia from *thalassemia* results from a defect in the rate of hemoglobin chain production. The disease, inherited as an autosomal recessive, is prevalent in persons of Mediterranean ancestory (Italians and Greeks). In thalassemia, the hemoglobin chain form is structurally normal, but the rate of synthesis is diminished. After a normal birth, fetal hemoglobin (HbF) synthesis diminishes while adult hemoglobin (HbA) increases. When thalassemia occurs HbF synthesis continues and HbA is never synthesized in normal amounts.

Thalassemia major, or Cooley's anemia, is a homozygous condition generally appearing at birth. The most common physical symptoms are marked pallor and moderate splenic enlargement (splenomegaly). The growth of the child is retarded and mongoloid facial features and yellow skin may occur. Such children have profound anemia. By contrast the heterozygote condition, thalassemia minor, only shows mild anemia.

When individuals with thalassemia major are exposed to certain drugs, rigid hemoglobin inclusion bodies form on the surface of erythrocytes. These cells thus hemolyze when they pass through the splenic filter. No effective treatment is currently available for either thalassemia major or sickle cell anemia.

Hereditary Spherocytosis

Hereditary spherocytosis is inherited as an autosomal dominant, meaning the disease results when only one parent passes on the defective gene. It is the most common congenital hemolytic anemia in whites (1 in 5000 persons). A defect in the erythrocyte membrane causes the erythrocyte to assume a spherocytic shape. The spherocytes cannot fold while passing through the splenic filter and rapid hemolysis results. Splenectomy, removal of the spleen, enables the abnormal cells to remain in circulation, and the person can live a normal life. In this case, splenectomy does not cure the disease, but does relieve its effects.

Erythrocyte Enzyme Deficiencies

Enzyme deficiencies can also cause hemolytic anemias. For instance, *glucose-6-phosphate dehydrogenase deficiency (G-6-PD)* results in impaired metabolism of the erythrocyte. When affected individuals (10–12% of American blacks) receive certain oxidates or drugs, hemolysis results due to the formation of rigid Heinz bodies which cause fragmentation of the erythrocytes in the splenic filter. G-6-PD deficiency is transmitted as a sex-linked recessive disorder. Therefore, 50% of females may be carriers of the trait. Fifty percent of their sons can have the disease and 50% of their daughters can be asymptomatic carriers of the disease. The deficiency of G-6-PD can be detected by a simple laboratory test, and the patient is advised to avoid antimalarial and sulfa drugs.

Immune Hemolytic Anemias

Immune hemolytic anemias are acquired by individuals who develop specific cytotoxic antibodies *(autoantibodies)* to antigens on their own erythrocytes. The anemia thus is due to an extrinsic cause, the formation of an autoantibody. Each individual has a definite number of red blood cell antigens, such as A, B and Rh antigens. Ordinarily, persons do not form antibodies against their own antigens. However, some patients do develop autoantibodies for unknown reasons.

The antiglobulin, or Coombs' test is performed on the blood of a person thought to have antibodies coating the erythrocytes (Fig. 11-9). In the antiglobulin test, antibody-coated red cells agglutinate or clump when antiglobulin (antiantibody) is added.

Mismatched blood transfusion can result in a hemolytic transfusion reaction, while circulating antibodies in the recipient's blood react against the antigens on donor's erythrocytes. Massive intravascular hemolysis can result, hemoglobin is then released into the plasma. The greatest danger is impairment of renal function, since the hemoglobin can plug the renal tubules.

Hemolytic Disease of the Newborn

Hemolytic disease of the newborn (HDN) occurs in a newborn infant in whom a maternal antibody directed against an antigen on the infant's erythrocytes causes hemolytic anemia in the infant. Although other antigens can be involved, the most important antigen is RhD.

The pathogenesis of HDN involves sensitization of the mother by fetal erythrocyte antigens and the production of antibodies against the erythrocytes. Fetal erythrocytes enter the maternal circulation during most pregnancies. If the RhD antigen or other erythrocyte antigens are incompatible with the mother, antibodies may form against them. Usually two or more incompatible pregnancies are required to sensitize the mother sufficiently to cause hemolysis of fetal erythrocytes when the antibodies pass through the placenta from mother to fetus. Then, incompatibility between an RhD negative mother and an RhD positive fetus can result in HDN. The disease causes two major problems at two different times: (a) In utero the greatest danger is severe anemia in the fetus and (b) once born, the greatest danger is from elevated levels of bilirubin.

The mechanism responsible for HDN is illustrated in Fig. 11-10. Hemolysis occurs when maternal antibodies coat fetal red cells. Red cell destruction occurs, hemoglobin is released and converted into bilirubin, which is eliminated by the mother. Following birth, the hemolysis continues, and when the bilirubin reaches approximately 20 mg/dl, neurons in the basal ganglion of the brain are usually damaged and permanent brain damage such as cerebral palsy (spasticity) can result.

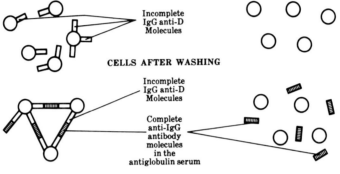

POSITIVE INDIRECT ANTIGLOBULIN TEST. ANTI-D PLUS D-POSITIVE CELLS

NEGATIVE INDIRECT ANTIGLOBULIN TEST. ANTI-D PLUS D-NEGATIVE CELLS

Incomplete IgG anti-D Molecules

Other IgG Molecules

INCUBATION STEP

Incomplete IgG anti-D Molecules

CELLS AFTER WASHING

Incomplete IgG anti-D Molecules

Complete anti-IgG antibody molecules in the antiglobulin serum

AGGLUTINATION FOLLOWING THE ADDITION OF ANTIGLOBULIN SERUM

Figure 11-9   *The antiglobulin test (Coombs' test). Antibodies coating the surface of erythrocytes agglutinate (clump) in the presence of antihuman globulin. This test is the basis for cross-matching blood for transfusion, for testing for autoimmune hemolytic anemia, or for detecting antibodies coating fetal red cells in "Rh babies." (From Lissett, P. 1970.* Applied blood group serology, *Spectra Biologicals Publications, Inc.)*

The probability of HDN can be detected prior to birth by typing and comparing the blood of the mother and father, and by doing a Coombs' test on the mother's blood to detect antibodies to the baby's erythrocyte antigens. At the time of birth, the Coombs' test can also be done on cells derived from umbilical cord blood.

The use of intrauterine fetal blood transfusion can potentially prevent fetal heart failure that occurs secondarily to profound hemolytic anemia. More commonly, exchange blood transfusions are performed on the baby following birth. Donor blood replaces most of the fetal blood including antibody-coated red cells, but more importantly, it removes toxic bilirubin.

Fortunately, Rh-immune globulin is now available for preventing Rh sensitization of the mother. Rh-immune globulin contains antibodies against the RhD factor and is given to RhD negative mothers shortly following an RhD positive birth. Rh-immune globulin prevents antibodies to RhD from

forming in the subsequent pregnancy. A woman's blood should be screened with an antiglobulin test for unexpected antibodies in all pregnancies, and even in spontaneous abortions which could also sensitize a mother.

When a woman is known to be Rh negative, her baby's blood should be typed for Rh factor. If the baby is Rh positive Rh-immune globulin is administered to the mother within 72 hours of delivery.

Aplastic Anemia

Aplastic anemia is characterized by a cessation of hematopoiesis. Pancytopenia results—a deficiency of all cell elements of the blood. A virtual absence of circulating erythrocytes, leukocytes, and platelets occurs. Blood transfusions must be given just to sustain life. Examination of the bone marrow usually reveals a marked decrease in number of all hematopoietic cells. Fat replaces the cellular ele-

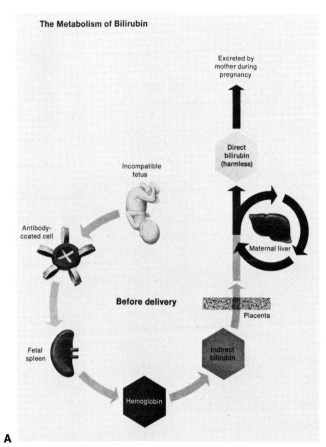

The Metabolism of Bilirubin

Excreted by mother during pregnancy

Direct bilirubin (harmless)

Incompatible fetus

Antibody-coated cell

Maternal liver

Before delivery

Placenta

Fetal spleen

Indirect bilirubin

Hemoglobin

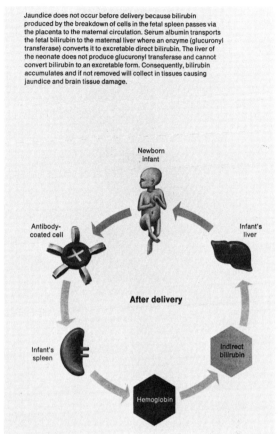

Jaundice does not occur before delivery because bilirubin produced by the breakdown of cells in the fetal spleen passes via the placenta to the maternal circulation. Serum albumin transports the fetal bilirubin to the maternal liver where an enzyme (glucuronyl transferase) converts it to excretable direct bilirubin. The liver of the neonate does not produce glucuronyl transferase and cannot convert bilirubin to an excretable form. Consequently, bilirubin accumulates and if not removed will collect in tissues causing jaundice and brain tissue damage.

Newborn infant

Antibody-coated cell

Infant's liver

After delivery

Infant's spleen

Indirect bilirubin

Hemoglobin

A   B

Figure 11-10 *Mechanism of sensitization and destruction of fetal erythrocytes in hemolytic disease of the newborn* **(A)** *before birth and* **(B)** *after birth. (From* Hemolytic disease of the newborn. *1968. Ortho Diagnostics.)*

ments in the bone marrow with only a few lymphocytes surviving.

Complications

Patients with aplastic anemia develop *infections* or *hemorrhage*. Neutropenia and thrombocytopenia precede the development of anemia because the life span of the neutrophils and platelets is much shorter (hours to days for neutrophils and platelets versus four months for erythrocytes).

Etiology

The cause of aplastic anemia is often unknown; however, certain drugs have been identified as causing aplastic anemia. For example, the antibiotic, chloramphenicol, usually causes only mild bone marrow suppression; however, severe aplastic anemia occasionally develops. Certain organic solvents such as benzene can induce aplastic anemia.

Transfusions of blood support those who show recovery from aplastic anemia. Transplantation of bone marrow is used (only available in large medical centers) to restore those failing to regenerate their bone marrow.

Polycythemia

Polycythemia is characterized by an excessive number of erythrocytes. It may arise as a physiologic response to hypoxia in some persons with chronic lung disease who oxygenate blood poorly. Also persons with congenital heart defects, or those living at very high altitudes, may acquire polycythemia.

Polycythemia vera is a special form of polycythemia that can progress to leukemia. In polycythemia vera, leukocytes, platelets, and erythrocytes all become increased in number with the hemoglobin increasing beyond 18 gm/100 liters. Thrombosis, due to sludging of blood, and thrombocytosis are common complications; paradoxically, hemorrhage often occurs. Later complications may include aplastic anemia with myelofibrosis (fibrosis of the bone marrow), or leukemia. Treatment of polycythemia vera is accomplished by bleeding (phlebotomy) or by the use of drugs that suppress activity in the bone marrow.

Disorders Of Leukocytes

Leukocytes include granulocytes, neutrophils, eosinophils, basophils: nongranulocytes— monocytes and lymphocytes. *Granulocytes* defend against infections and along with monocytes are active phagocytic cells. The cytoplasmic granules of granulocytes are rich in enzymes contained in lysosome sacs; they fuse with phagocytosed bacteria and the bacteria becomes inactivated by the enzymes (see Chapter 6, Immunology). Neutrophils are thus vital to defense against infections and serve a major function in acute inflammation (also see Chapter 5, Acute Inflammation and Repair). Indeed, neutrophils have been called "the first line of defense" in infections. Pathologically, neutrophils may fail to migrate to sites of inflammation and occasionally they become incapable of phagocytosis or of killing bacteria.

The term *leukopenia*, refers to a low WBC count (below approximately 4000/μl) in the blood. Often, viral infections induce leukopenia. Also, individuals with leukemia and those with malignancies treated with radiotherapy or chemotherapy often develop neutropenia or failure of bone marrow (aplastic anemia).

Leukocytosis occurs when WBCs are increased in number above 10,000/μl. Neutrophil predominance or *neutrophilia*, is often provoked by py-

Table 11-2
Conditions Associated with Leukocytosis*

Neutrophilia
Acute infections (especially pyogenic bacteria)
Toxic metabolic states and poisoning
Tissue necrosis (acute myocardial infarction)
Myelogenous leukemia

Eosinophilia
Allergic disorders (asthma and hayfever)
Parasitic infections
Chronic myelogenous leukemia and Hodgkin's disease

Lymphocytosis
Certain acute infections (infectious mononucleosis, whooping cough, mumps, measles)
Certain chronic infections (tuberculosis, hepatitis)
Lymphocytic leukemia

Monocytosis
Chronic infections (tuberculosis, endocarditis)
Hodgkin's disease
Monocytic leukemia

*Modified from Wintrobe, M. M. 1974. Clinical hematology, ed. 7. Philadelphia: Lea & Febiger. Tables 4-4 (p. 267), 4-7 (p. 273), 4-8 (p. 277), and 4-9 (p. 279).

ogenic (pus-producing streptococci, pneumococci, or staphylococci) bacteria. Many common diseases such as acute appendicitis, pneumonia, intoxication by chemicals, malignancy, acute rheumatic fever, and myocardial infarction provoke leukocytosis (Table 11-2). Extreme elevation of WBCs (approximately 50,000/μ1) is termed a *leukemoid reaction*.

Several infectious agents provoke *lymphocytosis* (increased number of circulating lymphocytes). Whooping cough, infectious mononucleosis and the disease caused by cytomegalovirus provoke numerous atypical appearing lymphocytes to appear in the blood (Fig. 11-11). Infectious mononucleosis is a common viral infection worthy of brief description.

Infectious Mononucleosis

Infectious mononucleosis (IM) is an acute leukemia or lymphoma-like illness caused by the Epstein-

Barr virus (EBV). It usually is self-limiting. IM has been called the "kissing disease" since the virus is transmitted in saliva. It strikes adolescents (Fig. 11-11) causing fever, sore throat, enlarged lymph glands, and fatigue. Examination of blood reveals atypical appearing lymphocytes and the serum contains heterophil and EBV antibodies.

The atypical lymphocytes seen in the blood (Fig. 11-11) of persons with IM are combatants in an immunological struggle. Epstein-Barr virus infects B-lymphocytes. T-lymphocytes and antibodies produced by plasma cells to combat EBV kill the infected B-lymphocytes. Most of the atypical lymphocytes seen in blood in IM after the first week are T-lymphocytes. The infected B-lymphocytes are eliminated (Fig.11-12).

Most persons (about 90%) who become infected by EBV never develop IM, instead they simply mount an effective immune response to EBV infected B-lymphocytes without ever becoming ill. The author has discovered a rare X-linked recessive immunodeficiency syndrome which results in fatal infectious mononucleosis or malignant lymphoma in affected boys. These boys lack the capacity to mount an antibody defense to EBV which triggers uncontrolled proliferation of B-lymphocytes. The

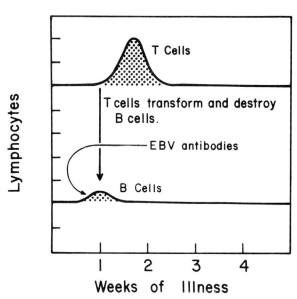

Figure 11-12   *Immune surveillance in infectious mononucleosis (IM). During the first week of IM B-lymphocytes infected by EBV proliferate and are seen in the blood. Thereafter, T-lymphocytes and antibodies against EBV kill the EBV-infected B-lymphocytes (Purtilo, D. T. 1976. Pathogenesis and phenotypes of an X-linked lymphoproliferative syndrome. Lancet ii: 882-885. Fig. 2, p. 883.)*

boys with the defective X chromosome die of IM or malignant lymphoma.

Leukemia And Lymphoma

Lymphoma is a malignancy of lymphoid tissues and *leukemia* is a malignancy resulting from an uncontrolled proliferation and accumulation of leukocytes.

How important are leukemias and lymphomas as causes of death? Leukemias and lymphomas are responsible for only 1% of all deaths from all causes. But approximately 10% of all deaths from cancer are caused by them. Moreover, they are the most common cause of death from malignancies in children, and cancer is a leading cause of death in this age group. By contrast, other malignancies tend to occur chiefly in elderly persons.

Leukemia was so named because leukemic blood when visualized in a test tube has a white tinge due to an excessive number of white cells. Leukemias are classified according to the type of WBC in-

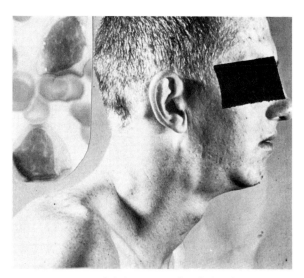

Figure 11-11   *Adolescent with infectious mononucleosis. He had enlarged lymph glands, fever, sore throat, and fatigue. Inset shows atypical lymphocytes that are seen in blood of infectious mononucleosis patients.*

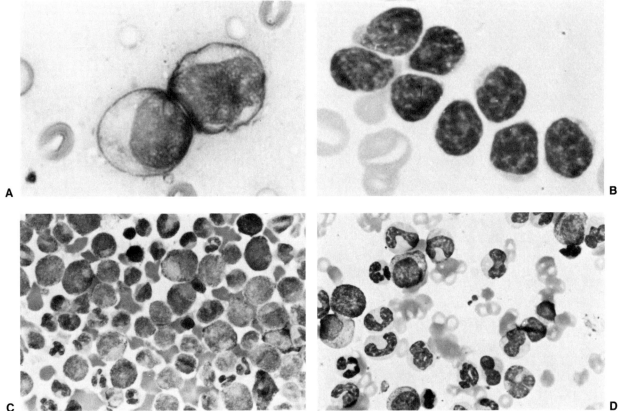

Figure 11-13   *Photomicrographs of representative leukemic blood cells*. **A,** *Acute lymphoblastic leukemia × 1200;* **B,** *chronic lymphocytic leukemia × 900;* **C,** *acute myeloblastic leukemia × 950; and* **D,** *chronic myelogenous (granulocytic) leukemia × 450.*

volved: *Myelogenous (granulocytic) leukemias* are derived from granulocytic precursors, while *lymphocytic leukemias* are derived from lymphoid cells. The adjectives, acute or chronic, originally implied the time that transpired from diagnosis to death. Cells of acute lymphocytic leukemia have more immature appearing WBCs, whereas mature WBCs are found in chronic leukemia. Representative leukemic blood cells are displayed in Fig. 11-13.

Surprisingly, leukemic cells may proliferate more slowly than normal leukocytes. A block in maturation of precursors appears to be the crux of the neoplastic problem; cells fail to mature and accumulate. Leukemic cells crowd out the normal stem cells of platelets, erythrocytes, and normal leukocytes in the bone marrow. Thus, while leukemic cells proliferate, normal white cells, red cells, and platelets decrease in number.

Etiology of Leukemia and Lymphoma

Virus   The etiology (cause) of leukemia and lymphoma is unknown. Studies have revealed that certain viruses cause leukemia in mice, rats, and cats. But no virus has thus far been identified as the cause of leukemia in human beings. Only one virus, EBV, is known which probably causes a malignancy of lymphoid tissue, lymphoma, in human beings. EBV, which causes infectious mononucleosis in the Western world, may cause *Burkitt's lymphoma*, a malignancy of lymphoid cells seen most often in African children (Fig. 11-14).

About 25 years ago an Irish missionary surgeon, Denis Burkitt, noted that many young children in Uganda had lymphomas involving their jaws. He also observed that these lymphomas occurred only in areas having a warm, moist climate where ma-

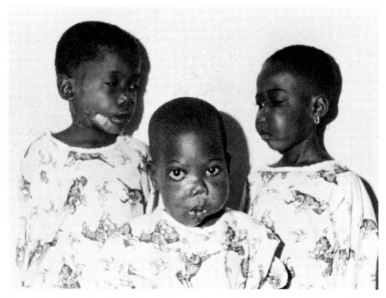

Figure 11-14   *Burkitt's lymphoma involving the jaw of three African children. (Courtesy Dr. Clitus Olson.)*

laria occurred. When the excised tumor was grown in tissue culture, the EBV was consistently found and when an extract of the tumor cells was injected into monkeys and apes, it induced a similar lymphoma.

Hence, many investigators conclude that EBV (which also causes infectious mononucleosis) is the etiologic agent of Burkitt's lymphoma. In an unknown way, EBV probably causes Burkitt's lymphoma in some African children and infectious mononucleosis in children living elsewhere. Our research on the X-linked recessive lymphoproliferative syndrome reveals that EBV can probably cause Burkitt's lymphoma or fatal infectious mononucleosis in brothers or male cousins who are immunodeficient to EBV.

Radiation   An increased incidence of acute leukemia and lymphomas has occurred in survivors of the atomic bombings of Hiroshima and Nagasaki; acute leukemia is also more frequent in radiologists and X-ray technicians. Irradiation induces mutation in chromosomes and can induce malignancy experimentally. Other persons with inherited abnormalities of their chromosomes, such as Down's syndrome, are prone to leukemia. These observa-

tions support the mutational theory of cancer (see Chapter 8).

Clinical Findings

The clinical and laboratory findings regarding leukemia are variable; anemia may be absent in chronic leukemia, but suddenly appear in acute leukemia. Likewise, numbers of circulating platelets vary in leukemia. Hemorrhage into skin and gums from decreased numbers of platelets may signal the onset of acute leukemia. Unusual infections associated with leukopenia often accompany leukemia, thus fever is often seen in leukemia. Enlarged lymph nodes (lymphadenomegaly) are often prominent with lymphocytic leukemia; in contrast, enlargement of the liver and spleen (hepatosplenomegaly) is characteristic of granulocytic leukemias (Fig. 11-15).

Classification and Age

Acute lymphoblastic leukemia occurs more commonly in childhood, while chronic lymphocytic leukemia commonly occurs in elderly persons (Table 11-3). Myelogenous leukemia of acute forms occurs

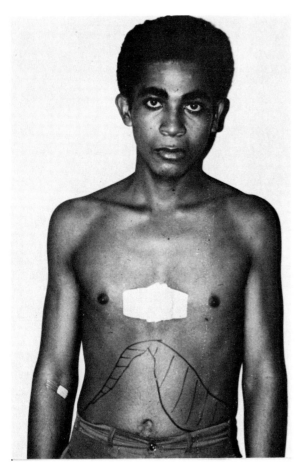

Figure 11-15 *Clinical findings of a young man with chronic granulocytic leukemia. The markings show enlargement of the liver and spleen* (left side); *he also is anemic (shown by pallor).*

in both children and adults and chronic myelogenous leukemia in adults.

Diagnosis

Examination of the peripheral blood of acute leukemia victims often reveals immature leukemic cells (Fig. 11-13). In contrast, with chronic leukemia victims an increased number of mature cells is noted. Diagnosis of leukemia is confirmed in an aspiration sample of bone marrow which is obtained through a needle inserted into the sternum, crest of the ilium, or tibia. Examination of bone marrow smears and sections usually establishes the diagnosis.

Complications

Leukemia patients develop complications because leukemia cells replace the normal precursors of white cells, red cells, and platelets. Leukemia cells are not effective disease fighters, thus infection is common in leukemia. Because platelets are reduced, hemorrhage occurs. Anemia results from a decrease in erythrocytes. Hemorrhage commonly ensues when platelets number less than $50,000/\mu l$. Platelet transfusion can prevent or stop hemorrhage. Moreover, treatment with cytotoxic drugs induces neutropenia and thrombocytopenia; hemorrhages or infections may again transpire. Thus, blood donors, blood bank technologists, and nurses work together to help sustain the leukemic patient.

When the WBCs drop below $1000/\mu l$, fatal "opportunistic" infections (See Chapter 7, Infectious Diseases) can occur. Infection is currently the major killer of leukemia patients. Candidiasis and aspergillosis are common fungal infections and *Pseudomonas* and *E coli* are the most troublesome bacterial infections in leukemic patients. Fever invariably signals infection in leukemia patients.

With increasing survival, new complications, namely infiltration of leukemic cells into the brain or the development of a second different malignancy occasionally ensue.

Treatment

During this decade the use of a combination of several new chemotherapeutic drugs has dramatically prolonged the lives of children with acute leukemia. One decade ago, virtually all children with acute lymphoblastic leukemia* died within two years; now many may attain remission.

Multiple Myeloma

Multiple myeloma is a *malignancy of plasma cells* (B lymphocytes) which occurs most frequently in elderly persons. Plasma cells are not usually seen in normal peripheral blood but may be present in

---

*Acute lymphocytic leukemia arises from T-lymphocytes in one-fifth of cases and this subtype continues to be associated with a grim prognosis.

multiple myeloma. Bone pain in the back or hip (Fig. 11-16) may be the initial complaint, since pain arises from pressure of malignant plasma cells on the nerves in the periosteum of the bone.

A *diagnosis* is achieved by identifying malignant plasma cells in the bone marrow. Malignant plasma cells arise from one clone of cells and produce increased levels of one antibody (immunoglobulin);

or a so-called monoclonal immunoglobulin spike is detected; however, this production occurs at the expense of normal antibody production.

Since the patient fails to produce effective antibodies, bacterial infections often end the lives of myeloma victims. Another serious complication of multiple myeloma is the development of *myeloma kidney*. Protein plugs the tubules and capillaries of

Table 11-3
Classification of Leukemia

| | Myelogenous leukemias | |
	Acute myeloblastic* (40%)	Chronic myelogenous (10%)
Age	Adults or children	Adults (under 50 years)
Onset	Acute	Insidious (gradual)
Symptoms	Fever, extreme fatigue, bleeding, sore throat	Fatigue, gastrointestinal disturbance, abdominal fullness, and hemorrhage
Physical	Pallor, petechial hemorrhage, splenomegaly and lymphadenomegaly	Massive splenic and hepatic enlargement with pallor
Blood	WBC variable to 100,000/μl or very low; platelets low	WBC 30,000 to 11,000,000/μl; platelets may be increased; "Philadelphia" chromosome
Myeloblasts	60% or greater with Auer rods	1 to 10%
Complications	Infection, hemorrhage	Blast crisis
Survival	Brief—days to months	Longer—months to years
	Lymphocytic leukemias	
	Acute (20%)	Chronic (30%)
Age	Children chiefly	Adults (over 50 years)
Onset	Acute	Insidious (gradual)
Symptoms	Pallor, petechial hemorrhages, enlarged lymph nodes, and fatigue	Often none or vague fatigue and pallor
Physical	Pallor, petechial hemorrhage, and enlarged lymph nodes and spleen	Enlarged spleen, liver, and lymph nodes; pallor
Blood	Accumulation of slowly dividing WBC 20,000 to 1,000,000/μl	WBC 10,000 to 100,000/μl or low
Lymphoblasts	60% or greater	Rare
Complications	Infection, hemorrhage, and meningeal infiltration	Infection and autoimmune hemolytic anemia
Survival	Months (untreated) or years (treated)	Years usually

*Myelomonocytic leukemia is virtually synonymous. All of the various types of myelogenous leukemias are sometimes grouped together as myeloproliferative disorders.

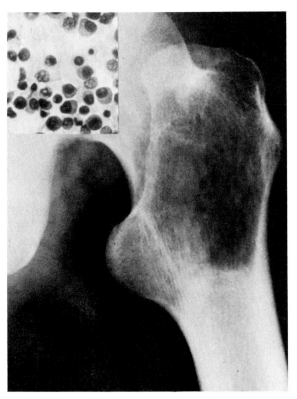

Figure 11-16   *X-ray of hip showing destructive lesions from multiple myeloma (darkened area of femur). The inset shows a photomicrograph of the malignant plasma cells seen in multiple myeloma ×300.*

the kidney, which leads to failure. The clinical course of myeloma is extremely variable. Survival ranges from weeks to many years, but in general, myeloma progresses rapidly. Certain drugs such as cyclophosphamide, are toxic to myeloma cells and may arrest the malignancy for a few months or years. Why some individuals respond to chemotherapy and others do not is unknown.

Lymphomas

The term *lymphoma* is used to describe those primary malignancies arising in the immune and reticuloendothelial lymphoid tissues. The vast majority of lymphomas arise from malignant B lymphocytes. The diagnosis is always made by microscopic examination of biopsy material. The precise histological type is important in determining prognosis and the type of therapy that will be instituted.

Differential Diagnosis

The *differential diagnosis* of *lymphoma* from *benign reactive lymphoproliferative disorders* is extremely important because obviously the treatment and prognoses are dissimilar. Enlargement of lymph nodes (lymphadenomegaly) can simply be an immune response to a skin infection. Careful screening of the patient reveals the skin infection or another focus of infection. Other infectious diseases commonly responsible for lymphadenomegaly include infectious mononucleosis, various viral and bacterial infections (usually associated with skin rashes) and toxoplasmosis. Characteristically, the benign lymphoproliferative disorders suddenly appear and disappear, whereas with lymphoma the lymphadenomegaly is chronic and progressive. Bacterial cultures and study of the patient's serum usually reveal antibodies against the infectious agents (for example, EBV and heterophil antibodies with infectious mononucleosis). Occasionally, a lymph node biopsy is taken to diagnose the benign disorder. By contrast, a lymph node biopsy must always be done to diagnose lymphoma.

Classification

A classification on which treatment is based is shown in Table 11-4. Lymphomas are classified into two large groups: (a) Hodgkin's disease lymphomas comprising approximately 40% of all lymphomas and (b) non-Hodgkin's lymphomas comprising the remaining 60% of lymphomas.

Hodgkin's Disease

Hodgkin's disease is a malignant lymphoma that tends to affect persons in two age groups with an early peak incidence at 15 to 35 years and a later peak after the age of 50 and hence has a bimodal age distribution.

Clinically, a person with Hodgkin's disease can have enlarged lymph nodes, fever, itching of the

Table 11-4
Classification of Lymphomas*

Type	Approximate percentage	Percentage of five-year survival
Hodgkin's disease (40%)		
Lymphocytic predominance	5	90
Nodular sclerosis	50	70
Mixed cellularity	40	35
Lymphocytic depletion	5	35
Non-Hodgkin's lymphoma (60%)		
Nodular lymphoma (with subtypes)	10	53
Lymphocytic lymphoma (well-differentiated)	35	25
Lymphoblastic lymphoma (poorly differentiated)	20	3
Histiocytic lymphoma	20	11
Undifferentiated stem-cell lymphoma	15	14

*From Aisenberg, A. C. 1973. Malignant lymphoma. N. Engl. J. Med. 288:883–890 from Table 2 (p. 886) and Table 3 (p. 888). Also non-Hodgkin's lymphomas are divided into nodular types having favorable prognoses and diffuse types having unfavorable prognoses. (Reprinted by permission from New England Journal of Medicine 288:883–890, 1973).

skin, and fatigue (Fig. 11-17). Hodgkin's disease usually begins in lymph nodes (usually in the neck), later other lymph nodes, the spleen, liver, and bone marrow can become involved.

Hodgkin's disease takes one of four histologic types (Table 11-4). The types are named according to the population of lymphocytes, histiocytes, and sclerotic connective tissue in the lymph nodes. The common biologic "thread" linking the four types is the presence of a distinctive tumor cell called the *Sternberg-Reed cell* (Fig. 11-18). Classically it is a large multinucleated or bilobed cell with the two halves of the cell being mirror images of each other. The nuclei have extremely large nucleoli giving the cell an "owl-eyed" effect.

Clinical Course   The clinical course of persons with Hodgkin's disease is dependent upon two closely related findings—the histologic type and the stage of the lymphoma. In general, the prognosis is more favorable with "nodular sclerosis" and "lymphocyte predominance" Hodgkin's disease. The extent of involvement of the body by the lymphoma at time of diagnosis is termed the clinical stage (Table 11-5). All of the staging classifications are designed to help decide whether it is

technically possible to irradiate all the known disease.

Following a diagnosis by examining a lymph node biopsy microscopically, the patient is thoroughly evaluated to determine the clinical stage. Procedures employed in staging include: (a) *lymphangiography*, where radiopaque dye is injected into

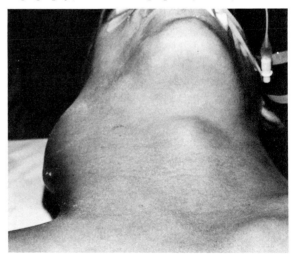

Figure 11-17   *Malignant lymphoma has caused marked enlargement of cervical lymph nodes. (Courtesy Dr. Wayne Silva.)*

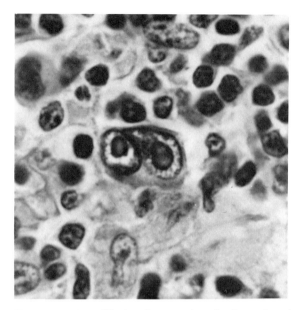

Figure 11-18   *Photomicrograph of giant Reed-Sternberg tumor cell of Hodgkin's disease. Note the large mirror-image nuclei and large nucleoli. (Courtesy Dr. Isao Katayama.)*

lymphatics in the feet and later the dye is observed in abnormal lymph nodes to see if they are enlarged (involved); (b) a *staging laparotomy*, where the abdominal cavity is opened and the spleen is removed and examined for tumor (Fig. 11-19) and enlarged lymph nodes observed in the lymphangiogram are removed for microscopic study; (c) *needle biopsy* specimens of both *bone marrow* and *liver* are taken for study to complete the clinical staging procedure. All stages are further classified by noting whether the patient has systemic symptoms of fever, night sweats, or cutaneous itching (pruritus). Stage A refers to asymptomatic patients and stage B to symptomatic patients. In general, more advanced stages (III and IV) are associated with the worst prognosis.

Treatment   The principles of treatment are easy to state and apply equally to the other lymphomas. Localized disease is treated with surgery and radiotherapy and generalized disease with chemotherapy. Radiation therapy is extremely effective in obliterating localized (stage I and II) Hodgkin's disease. Approximately 3500 to 4000 rads of irra-

diation are delivered during a four week period. In this situation a less than 5% recurrence rate is observed. By contrast, the five year chance of survival following radiotherapy in more advanced stages is much more discouraging. Only a 15% five year survival rate was noted, for instance, in symptomatic Stage III (III-B) patients after total nodal radiation.

Chemotherapy has been relegated to a palliative role in management of patients with all types of lymphoma (except for Burkitt's lymphoma). Among the drugs causing some improvement in the patient are alkylating drugs, vinblastine, procarbazine, bleomycin, BCNU, and prednisone.

Prognosis   With early diagnosis and vigorous treatment the outlook for patients with early stages of Hodgkin's disease is good. For instance, at Stanford University Medical Center, in a special study

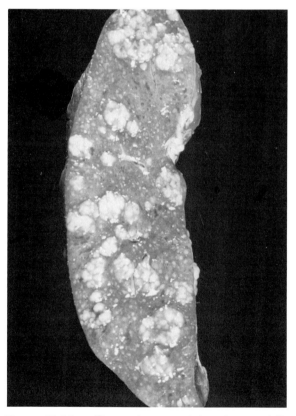

Figure 11-19   *The spleen contains large white lymphoma masses from a patient with Hodgkin's disease.*

of Hodgkin's disease, approximately 95% of selected patients were free of disease for five years after extensive radiation and are considered cured. Five year survival figures from Stanford are as follows: Stage I, 88%; Stage II, 66%; Stage III, 40%; and Stage IV, 20%.

Hodgkin's disease can spread (move from Stage I to Stage IV) and the histologic type can change to a more aggressive type (for example, lymphocyte predominance to lymphocyte depletion). Persons with advanced Hodgkin's disease show a depletion of lymphocytes and have a deficiency of T-lymphocyte function. Further rendering them vulnerable to viral, fungal, and bacterial infections is the immunosuppressive effect resulting from radiotherapy and chemotherapy. Persons succumbing to Hodgkin's disease often die from infectious diseases they are unable to defend against.

Non-Hodgkin's Lymphomas

Many of the clinical features described for Hodgkin's disease apply to all lymphomas. In general, persons with non-Hodgkin's lymphomas have an enlarged lymph node or spleen, fever, fatigue, anemia, or an infection.

Non-Hodgkin's lymphomas constitute approximately 60% of all lymphomas, and they are classified histologically by the pattern of distribution of the lymphoma in the lymph node as *nodular*

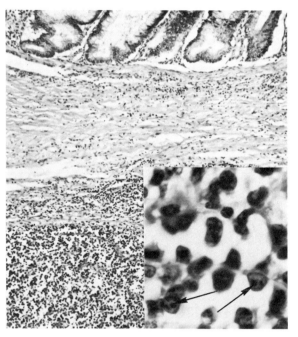

Figure 11-20   *Photomicrograph of lymphoblastic lymphoma. Note the tumor has invaded the muscular wall of the small intestine. The inset shows the immaturity of the lymphoblasts. Nucleoli are seen (arrows).*

(associated with a better prognosis) involvement or *diffuse* (associated with a worse prognosis) involvement (Table 11-4). They are classified cytologically by the predominant type of lymphoid cell forming the lymphoma. The clinical staging technique employed for Hodgkin's disease is used for all lymphomas (Table 11-5).

Lymphomas usually destroy the normal architecture of lymph nodes or the spleen. They can arise also in extranodal sites such as bones, liver, and intestines (Fig. 11-20).

The principles of treatment of non-Hodgkin's lymphoma are the same as for Hodgkin's disease, with radiotherapy for localized and chemotherapy for generalized disease. But there are two major differences. First, the behavior and prognosis vary with the histologic type of non-Hodgkin's lymphomas and second, the pattern of recurrence is not as predictable as in Hodgkin's disease. Prognoses are predicated upon the histologic type of lymphoma and the clinical stage.

Table 11-5
Clinical Stages of Hodgkin's Disease and Non-Hodgkin's Lymphoma*

Stage I	Disease limited to the lymph nodes of one anatomic region
Stage II	Disease in two or three regions on the same side of the diaphragm
Stage III	Disease on both sides of diaphragm but not extending beyond the lymph nodes, spleen, or oropharyngeal lymphoid tissue
Stage IV	Involvement of organs such as bone marrow, lung, liver, and gastrointestinal tract as well as hematopoietic tissues

*The letter A is added for asymptomatic patients and B for symptomatic patients.

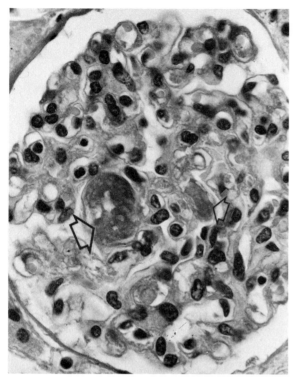

Figure 11-21 *Photomicrographs showing a fibrin blood clot in the glomeruli of kidney* (arrows). *Ten days later the fibrin clot had dissolved by fibrinolysis.*

Hemostasis and Coagulation

Hemostasis is the process which retains the blood within the circulatory system. When a blood vessel is injured, the hemostatic process repairs the leak and arrests the hemorrhage. This process probably evolved as fighting animals with hemorrhaging wounds developed the ability to form clots. Ironically, blood clotting has evolved beyond optimal benefit; hypercoagulability and consequent thromboses are now the major health problem in the United States.

In the following section the physiology and pathophysiology of hemostasis are considered. The vascular system, blood cells, and blood proteins provide hemostatic mechanisms to prevent both undesired hemorrhage and undesired clotting of blood. Hemostasis is specifically provided by: (a) the walls of capillaries and surrounding collagen; (b) blood platelets; (c) plasma clotting factors; and (d) a fibrinolytic system which prevents excessive coagulation. For example, blood clots (thrombi) form when clotting factors and platelets are activated to form fibrin (Fig. 11-21). Opposing fibrinolytic enzymes restore the blood flow to the tissues by lysing the clot.

Primary Hemostasis

Cessation of hemorrhage due to an incision in the skin occurs when arterioles at the edges of the wound suddenly constrict. Meanwhile, thrombi are formed by platelets which clump together and adhere to the injured wall to form a "primary hemostatic platelet plug" which inhibits further bleeding. Only platelets and trapped erythrocytes form the clot in primary hemostasis.

Secondary Hemostasis

In secondary hemostasis, plasma clotting factors circulating as inactive enzymes become activated and form fibrin. The fibrin forms a mesh which then traps platelets and erythrocytes to plug blood vessels. A fibrin clot requires more time to gel than a platelet clot. Fibrin deposition and entanglement with platelets is triggered by thrombin, an enzyme which converts fibrinogen to fibrin. Slow fibrinolysis of this clot begins and final repair to the injured site ensues.

Plasma Coagulation System

Thirteen (or more) coagulation factors participate in coagulation of plasma. A simplified scheme of the plasma coagulation cascade is illustrated in Fig. 11-22. Normally, plasma clotting factors (designated by Roman numerals in Figure 11-22) circulate in inactive forms; they become activated by substances released by injured tissues. Intrinsic and extrinsic pathways join in a final common cascade, triggering activated prothrombin to form thrombin, which in turn activates fibrinogen to form fibrin. The fibrin traps platelets and erythrocytes and a clot forms. A more detailed description of the process follows.

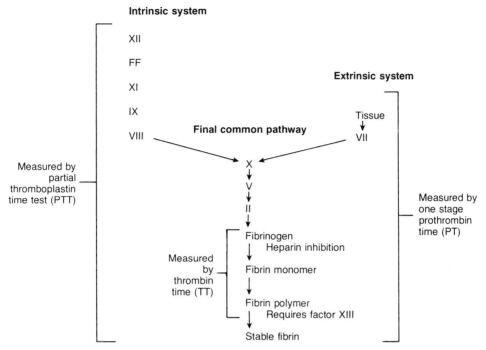

Figure 11-22   *Plasma coagulation cascade. The plasma-clotting factors become activated by tissue injury, which releases thromboplastin. A fibrin clot is the final result of the cascade. (Courtesy J. Roger Edson.)*

The concept of the plasma coagulation system (Fig. 11-22) that has evolved consists of four components: (a) *clottable protein and fibrin stabilizing factor* (fibrinogen, Factor XIII); (b) the *four vitamin K dependent factors*, all of which are enzymes (Factors II, VII, IX, and X); (c) *two rate regulating substances* that bind with enzymes but that have no enzymatic activity themselves (Factors V and VIII); and (d) the *contact system* (Factors XI, XII, and Fletcher Factor).

The terms intrinsic and extrinsic pathways have been applied to the plasma coagulation system. The *intrinsic pathway* is the cascade that begins with activation of Hageman Factor XII. It is called the intrinsic system because everything necessary for its activity is intrinsic to the blood itself. The *extrinsic pathway* begins with the activation of Factor VII by protein derived from damage to tissue—the protein being extrinsic to the blood itself. The intrinsic pathway including the contact system is long, whereas the extrinsic pathway is shorter. Both intrinsic and extrinsic pathways have a *final common*

pathway beginning with the activation of Factor X and ending with formation of a stable fibrin clot.

The concept of intrinsic and extrinsic pathways is artificial—both pathways provide normal hemostasis. The concept is useful because it explains readily what is measured by the common screening tests used for detecting defects in the plasma coagulation system, the one-stage prothrombin time, the partial thromboplastin time, and the thrombin time.

Bleeding Disorders

An etiologic classification of hemorrhage is shown in Table 11-6. The major causes of hemorrhage will be discussed.

Acquired Plasma-clotting Disorders

The plasma factors are presumed to be made principally or entirely in the liver and thus liver disease

Table 11-6
Etiologic Classification of Hemorrhage

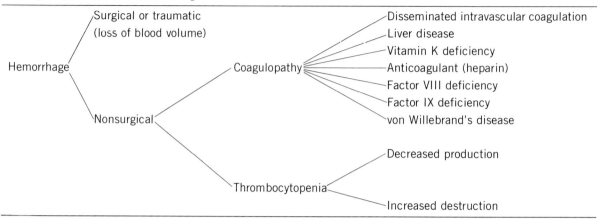

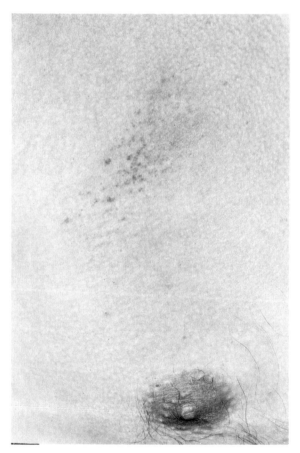

Figure 11-23 *Petechiae (pinpoint) hemorrhages and purpura from trauma.*

(for example, cirrhosis) is apt to result in hemorrhage because clotting factors are insufficiently produced. Factors II, VII, IX, and X require vitamin K for their synthesis. Therefore, obstruction of the common bile duct by a gallstone causes a deficiency of vitamin K since bile is required for this fat soluble vitamin to be absorbed into the intestine. The defect in clotting is reversed when vitamin K is injected directly into the patient or when fresh frozen plasma containing the clotting factors is transfused into the person.

Hemorrhage into the skin is a sign of failure of hemostasis. Three terms defined by the size of the hemorrhage spots in the skin are used: petechiae (pinpoint size), purpura (slightly larger), and ecchymoses (large) (Fig. 11-23).

Hemorrhage can develop when blood vessels are inflamed (vasculitis) or when the connective tissue surrounding blood vessels is weak, as in scurvy. Scurvy is a disease resulting from a deficiency of vitamin C, and purpura occurs because the connective tissue surrounding the capillaries is fragile (see Chapter 10, Nutritional Diseases).

Increased Plasma-clotting Factors

An increase in circulating plasma clotting factors can result in *hypercoagulability*. Epinephrine, cortisone, and estrogen in oral contraceptives, enhance synthesis and elevate levels of many clotting factors. Pregnant women, for instance, always have increased estrogen levels and blood factors, and thus their blood is hypercoagulable. The same occurs, to a lesser extent, in women using contraceptive pills. Thus, certain pregnant women or those using contraceptive pills may develop thrombosis.

The blood of patients with cancer also frequently becomes hypercoagulable; a tumor may undergo necrosis or release substances which trigger intravascular coagulation. This type of thrombosis is termed disseminated intravascular coagulation (DIC). Thrombosis is the second most common cause of death in cancer victims: DIC can also be triggered by the release of endotoxin from gram-negative bacteremias and factors from the necrotic infected tissue.

Inherited Plasma-clotting Disorders

Inherited deficiencies of blood clotting factors can cause alarming hemorrhage following minor injuries such as that of tooth extraction. Three inherited clotting deficiencies are relatively common, hemophilia A, hemophilia B, and von Willebrand's syndrome.

The trait for hemophilia is carried on the X chromosome and so is an X-linked recessive disorder (Fig. 11-24). The presence of the mutant X-linked gene in Queen Victoria and her male offspring shaped the course of European and Russian history during the nineteenth century.

There is a 50% chance that each child of a carrier will inherit the abnormal maternal X chromosome (see Chapter 9, Inherited Disorders). If that child is a male he will be a hemophiliac. If the child is a female she will be another carrier. The X-linked inheritance applies to both hemophilia A (Factor VIII deficiency) and hemophilia B (Factor IX deficiency).

Hemophilia A   Boys having a factor VIII activity of less than 5% have a classical *hemophilia A syndrome*. Generally, the lower the activity, the worse the bleeding tendency. The affected boys and, to a lesser extent, the female carriers bruise easily and have spontaneous nosebleeds. Provocation by injury, tonsilectomy, or extraction of a tooth can

prove fatal if replacement of factor VIII is not given by transfusion. The disease can cripple the boys since arthritis can develop following hemorrhage into the knee joints.

Hemophilia B   The inheritance and clinical findings are essentially identical in hemophilias A and B. Factor IX is missing in hemophilia B. To stop hemorrhage, fresh frozen blood plasma must be given.

Von Willebrand's Syndrome   Von Willebrand's syndrome is inherited as an autosomal dominant bleeding disorder. The major bleeding symptoms in affected persons are related to a platelet abnormality and in some, to a low level of Factor VIII. They hemorrhage excessively during menstruation. The abnormal platelet function in von Willebrand's syndrome is due to lack of a plasma cofactor closely associated with Factor VIII, hence transfusion of fresh plasma into a bleeding patient stops the hemorrhage and a paradoxical rise in Factor VIII ensues. The response to transfusion of plasma containing clotting factors is very transient in the three inherited bleeding disorders, thus repeated transfusions are often required.

Platelet Disorders

Thrombocytopenia

Hemorrhage frequently results from *thrombocytopenia*, especially when the platelets fall below $50,000/\mu l$. The major causes of thrombocytopenia include increased destruction and decreased production of platelets (for example, entrapment in spleen, autoimmunity, and malignancies). Transfusions of fresh platelets can prevent impending hemorrhage. At the other extreme, when platelets number above $600,000/\mu l$, thrombocytosis may cause thrombosis.*

Thrombocytopenia may also develop when antibodies are formed against one's own platelets (autoantibodies). This immunological disease,

*Thrombosis and embolism are discussed in Chapter 13.

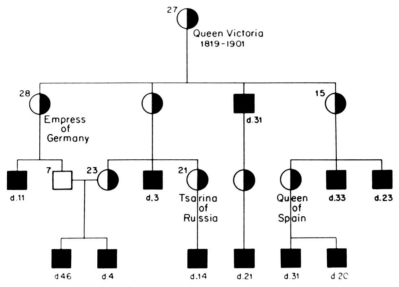

Figure 11-24   *X-linked recessive inheritance of hemophilia A in descendents of Queen Victoria. Fifty percent of her offspring inherited her mutant X-linked gene; 50% of women became carriers, and 50% of men were affected.*

autoimmune thrombocytopenia purpura, is usually caused by certain drugs, infectious agents, or unknown factors. It tends to be mild in children, but in adults can become chronic. Cortisone and other immunosuppressive drugs usually correct the condition, but splenectomy may be required to remove the splenic filter in difficult cases. Since platelets coated by antibody are destroyed in the spleen filter, splenectomy permits the platelets to have a more prolonged life span.

Thrombocytopathies

Both *inherited* and *acquired* inabilities of platelets to function *(thrombocytopathy)* occur. Of the drugs that impair platelet function, *aspirin* is the major culprit. Aspirin permanently damages platelets and is the cause of bleeding (for example, excessive menstrual hemorrhage is commonly caused by aspirin). The defect in platelet function lasts for up to ten days (the lifespan of the platelet). Fortunately, most antibiotics and narcotics do not impair platelet function and thus acetaminophen (Tylenol) or another analgesic is often substituted for aspirin.

Blood Banking

Our increasing capacity to successfully transfuse blood and components of blood has to a great extent made possible advances in the past three decades in cardiovascular and transplantation surgery, and has permitted patients with leukemia, lymphoma, or other malignancies to tolerate temporary suppression of their bone marrow by radiation and chemotherapy.

The study of blood groups and other erythrocyte antigens is termed *immunohematology*. Two major achievements have led to modern blood transfusion services. Karl Landsteiner at the turn of this century discovered the ABO blood group system, and A. S. Weiner discovered Rh blood factors in 1939. The discovery of anticoagulants such as heparin and coumarin and advances in refrigeration further facilitated blood transfusion services.

ABO Blood Groups

The antigens determining the four blood groups reside on the surface of erythrocytes and result from the expression of three genes: O, A, and B. The latter two are dominant to O. Only four phenotypes can be detected, but six occur: OO, AO, AA, BO, BB, and AB.

Depending on the person's blood group antigen on the erythrocyte, the reciprocal antibody (isohemagglutinin) is found in the plasma. For example, when the A antigen is present on the red cell, anti-B is present in the plasma (Table 11-7).

The information gained by blood grouping provides the basis for safely tranfusing blood. Technical aspects of blood grouping are described in books devoted to the subject. In general, persons with blood AB are "universal recipients" of all types of blood (since they lack anti-A and anti-B), and blood group O is a "universal donor" since the blood lacks blood group antigen. Hence, hemolytic transfusion reactions will not occur.

Other Erythrocyte Antigens

Earlier in the chapter we described the Rh antigens, especially RhD as related to hemolytic disease of the newborn. In addition to the ABO and Rh antigen systems, there are scores of other antigen systems on erythrocytes. In general, these antigens do not cause problems unless a person has been repeatedly transfused and has become sensitized (developed antibodies) to an antigen.

Cross Match

In addition to grouping blood of a donor and recipient, a procedure called compatibility, or "cross matching," testing is performed. Herein the erythrocytes of the donor are mixed with the serum of the recipient (*major cross match*) and the *minor cross match* consists of mixing the serum of the donor

with the erythrocytes of the recipient. The mixed serum and erythrocytes is incubated at 37C for 30 minutes and then it is inspected for agglutination (clumping). Agglutination of erythrocytes indicates an incompatible cross match. The blood should never be given to the incompatible patient or hemolysis of the blood can occur. One additional step is performed before concluding that blood is compatible. Following the incubation the erythrocytes are washed and the antiglobulin (Coombs') test is done (Fig. 11-9). The final step determines whether any antibodies are reacting against the erythrocytes of both donor and recipient that are not seen in the cross match. These important procedures virtually eliminate hemolytic transfusion reactions.

Recent advances in tissue typing (HLA—see Chapter 6) now permit HLA matching of blood of donors and recipients. Thus donors can be used repeatedly for patients with leukemia, for example, and no antibodies will form against the donor who is HLA matched.

Transfusion of Blood Components

There are only a few indications for ordering fresh whole blood (less than four hours old). The only components of fresh whole blood not present in ordinary banked blood (good for 21 days stored at 4C) are coagulation factors V, VII, and platelets. Hence, in most instances specific components are separated from fresh whole blood, stored, and individually given to meet specific clinical needs.

Selected blood component therapy conserves a valuable human resource: one donated unit (450 ml) can provide packed red blood cells; platelet suspensions and concentrates; leukocytes; fresh, frozen, or stored plasma; albumin; antihemophilic Factor VIII; rich cryoprecipitate;

Table 11-7
*Blood Groups and Antibodies**

Group	Antigens on erythrocytes	Antibodies in plasma	Incidence in the United States Blacks	Whites
O	None	Anti-A, Anti-B	48	45
A	A	Anti-B	27	41
B	B	Anti-A	21	10
AB	A and B	None	4	4

*Modified from Blood Group Antigens and Antibodies. Ortho Diagnostics. 1960.

Table 11-8
Indications for Transfusing Blood Components

Component	Indications
Whole blood	Acute blood loss in patient with shock
Packed red blood cells	Acute and chronic blood loss
Frozen red blood cells	For rare blood types
Concentrated leukocytes	Patients with leukopenia and bacterial infections
Platelet and rich plasma concentrate	Patients with thrombocytopenia
Plasma (stored)	Expansion of blood volume in shock
Fresh frozen plasma	Multiple clotting factor deficiency as in liver disease
Cryoprecipitate	Treating hemophilia and von Willebrand's syndrome
Gamma globulin	Agammaglobulinemic persons, prophylaxis against hepatitis
Albumin	Patient in shock or with burns
Rh_O (D) immune globulin	To prevent hemolytic disease of newborn

fibrinogen; gamma globulin; and Factor II-VII-IX-X concentrate.

The components are usually separated in plastic bags and centrifuged at various speeds. The plasma, platelets, WBCs, and RBCs layer in relatively discrete bands which can be separated. In major medical centers, a special machine called the cell separator is used for skimming platelets or WBCs from a donor's blood. Large numbers of platelets and WBCs can be obtained from one donor on a cell separator. Some of the specific indications for specific blood components are shown in Table 11-8.

The blood bank technologist also often assists in immunodiagnosis of various disorders, including hepatitis, by detecting hepatitis B virus antigen or antibody in a patient's serum. Also the technologist can usually identify the antibody responsible for an autoimmune hemolytic anemia. Moreover, tissue typing (histocompatibility testing) is often done in blood banks for transplantation of organs including bone marrow.

Summary

The blood is composed of formed elements (erythrocytes, leukocytes, and platelets) and plasma (clotting factors, immunoglobulins, albumin, and other biochemicals). Diseases of the blood result from quantitative (excesses or deficiencies) and qualita-

tive (hemoglobinopathies or aspirin-induced platelet dysfunction, for example) abnormalities of the formed elements. Likewise, excessive blood clotting factors can predispose to thrombosis and deficiencies of factors, to hemorrhage.

Malignancies of hematopoietic organs stem from uncontrolled proliferation and maturation of hematopoietic elements: leukemias; lymphomas; and myeloma. All three of these cancers can cause anemia and are associated with bleeding and opportunistic infections, especially following treatment by cytotoxic irradiation and chemotherapy.

The persons working in blood banks offer expertise to detect autoantibodies that cause hemolytic anemias and to provide fresh frozen plasma components and stored erythrocytes for correcting bleeding disorders and replenishing blood to anemic patients. Blood platelets and leukocytes are prepared to support cancer victims through periods of leukopenia and thrombocytopenia which occur from therapy. Finally, tissue typing offers a chance for HLA matching blood for transfusion or bone marrow and organ transplants for patients.

Bibliography

Aisenberg, A. C. 1973. Malignant lymphoma. *N. Engl. J. Med.* 288:883–890 and 939–941. Excellent review articles on lymphomas.

American Association of Blood Banks, *Technical methods and procedures of the American Association of Blood Banks*, ed. 6. Philadelphia: J. B. Lippincott Company. A how to do it manual with an excellent mix of the theory and techniques of blood banking.

Brown, B. 1976. *Hematology: principles and procedures*, ed. 2. Philadelphia: Lea & Febiger. The one best book for a clear presentation of most aspects of blood cells and coagulation.

Carter, R. L., and Penman, H. G., ed. 1969. *Infectious mononucleosis*. Oxford: Blackwell Scientific Pub. Monograph describing all aspects of this disease.

Cartwright, G. E. 1968. *Diagnostic laboratory hematology*, ed. 4. New York: Grune & Stratton, Inc. Techniques of laboratory tests are described.

Davidson, I., and Henry, J. 1974. *Clinical diagnosis by laboratory methods*, ed. 15. Philadelphia: W. B. Saunders Co. Standard textbook for medical technologists and clinical pathologists.

Diggs, L. W.; Sturm, D.; and Bell, A. 1970. *The morphology of human blood cells*. Abbott Laboratories, North Chicago, Illinois. Has beautiful colored photographs and drawings of blood cells.

Fairley, G. H., and Freeman, J. E. 1974. Treatment of lymphomas. *Br. Med. J.* 28: 761–765. Describes how and why radiotherapy and chemotherapy are used for treating lymphomas.

Gunz, F., et al. 1974. *Leukemia*, ed. 3. New York: Grune & Stratton. Describes all aspects of these diseases.

Ham, W. 1974. *Histology*, ed. 7. Philadelphia: Lippincott. Good section on blood formation.

Hillman, R. S., and Finch, C. A. 1974. *Red cell manual*, ed. 4. Philadelphia: F. A. Davis. Describes RBCs.

Hyun, B. H. 1975. *Practical hematology*. Philadelphia: W. B. Saunders Co. Concise (450 pages with Kodachrome slides) textbook for medical students and medical technology students.

Leavell, B. S., and Thorup, O. A. 1971. *Fundamentals of clinical hematology*. ed. 3, Philadelphia: W. B. Saunders Co. Good clinical and laboratory survey of hematology.

Lehmann, H., and Huntsman, R. G. 1973. *Man's hemoglobins*. ed. 2. Philadelphia: Lippincott. Describes the molecular basis for sickle cell disease and other hemoglobinopathies.

Miale, J. B. 1972. *Laboratory medicine—hematology*. ed. 4. St. Louis: The C. V. Mosby Co. Standard textbook with good section on hematology.

Mollison, R. L. 1972. *Blood transfusion in clinical medicine*. ed. 5. Blackwell Scientific Publishers. Very thorough discussion of clinical aspects of transfusion.

Nathan, D. G., and Oski, F. A. 1974. *Hematology of infancy and childhood*. Philadelphia: W. B. Saunders Co. Describes the special hematologic problems of infants and children.

Purtilo, D. T. 1976. Pathogenesis and phenotypes of an X-linked lymphoproliferative syndrome. *Lancet* ii 883–885. Describes hypothesis of inherited immunodeficiency to EBV in fatal infectious mononucleosis and malignant lymphoma.

Purtilo, D. T. 1977. Opportunistic lymphoma in X-linked recessive immunodeficiency and lymphoproliferative syndromes. *Seminars in Oncology* 4:335–343. The whole issue concerns lymphomas in children.

Purtilo, D. T. et al. 1977. Variable phenotypic expression of an X-linked recessive lymphoproliferative syndrome. *N. Engl. J. Med.* 297:1077–1081. This article describes inherited immunodeficiency to the Epstein-Barr virus and fatal infectious mononucleosis and malignant lymphoma in affected males.

Purtilo, D. T.; Paquin, L.; and Gindhart, T. 1978. Genetics of cancer: impact of ecogenetics on oncogenesis. *Am. J. Pathol.* In press. Describes how environmental agents can cause cancer in genetically predisposed persons.

Rapp, F., and Reed, C. L. 1977. The viral etiology of cancer. *Cancer* 40:419–429. Reviews the impact of genetics, age, hormones, immune competence, and stress on Epstein-Barr virus induction of lymphoma.

Rosen, F. S. 1977. Lymphoma, immunodeficiency, and the Epstein-Barr virus. *N. Engl. J. Med.* 297:1120–1121. Mechanisms of immune defense are defective in immunodeficient persons and they can therefore develop cancer from the Epstein-Barr virus.

Williams, W. J., et al. 1972. *Hematology*. New York: McGraw-Hill, Inc. A standard reference.

Wintrobe, M. M. 1974. *Clinical hematology*. ed. 7. Philadelphia: Lea & Febiger. The ultimate reference in hematology.

Zmijewski, C. M. 1972. *Immunohematology*, ed. 2. New York: Appleton-Century-Crofts. Concise, readable book on blood banking.

CHAPTER 12

Endocrine and Metabolic Disorders

Chapter Outline

Objectives

After you have read this chapter you should be able to

Define the term metabolism.

Compare exocrine and endocrine glands in their modes of secretion.

Describe how hormones function via the second messenger.

Describe mechanisms that control hormone levels in the blood.

Define the term radioimmunoassay.

List hormones produced by the adenohypophysis.

Name the target organs of trophic hormones of the adenohypophysis.

List two hormones produced by the neurohypophysis.

Describe the disease diabetes insipidus.

Understand the "margin of safety" of the pituitary gland.

List the sequence of changes occurring in panhypopituitarism.

Describe the two conditions arising from acidophilic adenomas of the pituitary gland.

List the three groups of hormones secreted by the adrenal cortex.

Describe Cushing's syndrome and its causes and cure.

Define the adrenogenital syndrome.

List the causes of adrenocortical insufficiency.

Describe Addison's disease.

Define the terms neuroblastoma and pheochromocytoma.

Define the term cretinism.

Compare the clinical pictures of hyperthyroidism and hypothyroidism.

Know what Hashimoto's thyroiditis is.

Understand the association between thyroid cancer and prior irradiation.

Describe the clinical findings of hyperparathyroidism.

Define the term tetany and give an example of one cause.

Define the term diabetes mellitus.

Compare juvenile diabetes with maturity-onset diabetes mellitus.

List three phases of diabetes mellitus.

Discuss the etiology of diabetes mellitus.

Discuss why diabetes mellitus is a syndrome rather than a disease.

List the three cell types of the islets and the hormones they produce.

Compare the finding of isletitis and hyalinization of islets of Langerhans.

List two functions of insulin.

Compare insulin coma with diabetic coma.

List organs likely to be damaged in diabetic patients.

Compare insulin and sulfonylurea therapy for diabetes.

List two broad categories of inborn errors of metabolism.

Describe the terms alpha$_1$ antitrypsin deficiency, and cystinosis.

Know the elements that are excessive in hemochromatosis and Wilson's disease.

Know the clinical findings regarding gout and its treatment.

Define the term xanthoma.

Introduction

Metabolism is the sum of the biochemical reactions occurring in living cells which provides energy and building blocks for vital functions necessary for making new protoplasm. Our metabolism is governed by our genes, diet, and the impact of hormones liberated by our endocrine glands. Endocrine and metabolic disorders are discussed together in this chapter because together they integrate physiologic processes.

Moreover, the nervous system, as well as the endocrine system, helps orchestrate and maintain metabolic processes (Fig. 12-1). The *endocrine glands* secrete hormones directly into the blood stream (the adrenal glands, for example, secrete cortisone into the adrenal vein*). By contrast, the *exocrine glands* secrete digestive fluids into ducts (such as the salivary and pancreatic glands). *Hormones* are composed of either *proteins* of small size (polypeptides like insulin), *amines* (like epinephrine or thyroxine), or *steroids* (like estrogen). The release of hormones by endocrine glands directly into the moving blood stream permits instantaneous action of the hormone at distant sites. At least 30 different hormones have been identified and many more are yet to be discovered. Hormones differ from enzymes and other catalysts (agents which act on metabolism) in that hormones themselves are metabolized, excreted in urine or bile, or inactivated in the liver.

Hormones can have a *general effect* on cells, as does the growth hormone, or thyroxine, which stimulate all cells to grow and produce energy. Other hormones have a *specific effect* on one *target cell*. For example, gonadotropic hormone acts only on gonads, stimulating growth and development.

Several endocrine glands (such as the parathyroid and pancreas) are free of control by the pituitary gland. They are instead controlled by *feedback mechanisms* which sense levels of chemicals such as calcium or glucose in the blood. Most other endocrine glands are "target glands" (thyroid, adrenals, and gonads) and are controlled by the pituitary gland (Fig. 12-1). Also, certain hormones produce opposite metabolic effects. For example, insulin lowers blood sugar and glucagon raises it.

How Hormones Act

The action of specific hormones on their target cells results because the *hormone* serves as a *primary messenger*. The hormone interacts specifically with a specific receptor (like a key and lock) on the membranes of the target cells. The receptor is associated with an enzyme, adenyl cyclase, which stimulates the formation of a *second messenger—cyclic AMP*. In a domino-like fashion the cyclic AMP changes the rate at which biochemical reactions occur in the target cell. For example, increased protein synthesis occurs (of thyroxine) when the primary messenger (thyrotropin) reacts with the receptor on thyroid follicle cells which interacts with the second messenger (cyclic AMP). The gland produces more thyroxine to meet the metabolic demands.

Often metabolic disorders are inherited. These disorders usually result from a missing enzyme which causes an excessive accumulation or an absence of a substance in cells (see Chapter 9). Endocrine disorders, on the other hand, may or may not be inherited. Endocrine disorders are usually discovered when the function of an endocrine gland increases (*hyperfunction*) or decreases (*hypofunction*). Hyperfunction of an endocrine gland usually results from *hyperplasia* of a gland, and hypofunction from destruction or atrophy of a gland. The defects in function of target glands such as the thyroid, gonads, and adrenals can result from defects in the pituitary gland or in the organ itself. Prior to considering these disorders we will briefly discuss some of the laboratory studies used for evaluating endocrine function.

Evaluation of Endocrine Function

Both the *physical* appearance of a patient and the *clinical history* offer clues to the source of the endocrine disorders. Often persons suffering from

---

*Jay Tepperman. 1973. *Metabolic and endocrine physiology*, ed. 3. Chicago: Year Book Medical Publishers, p. 1. Suggests the endocrine system is a wireless communications system in which messages are carried in the blood stream as highly specialized chemicals which interact with specialized target cells which have receptors for the hormones.

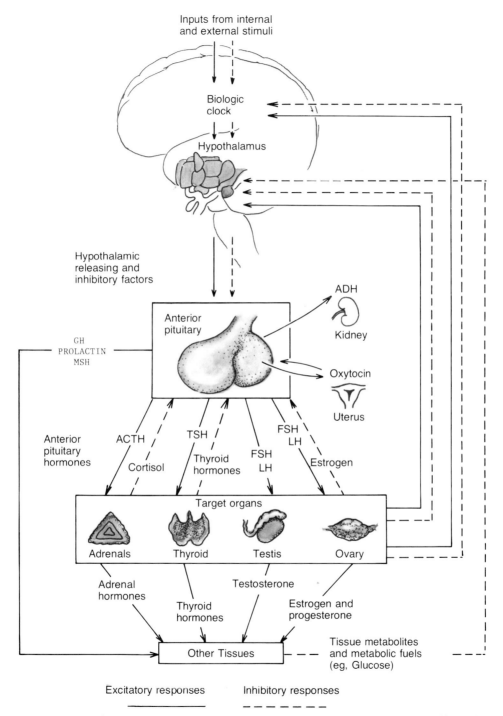

Figure 12-1 *Control of the endocrine system by the nervous system. Note the hypothalamus controls the pituitary through releasing and inhibiting factors. The anterior lobe of the pituitary gland then releases trophic hormones which act on target glands (thyroid, adrenals, and gonads).*

endocrine disorders undergo changes in their appearance or behavior. The endocrine abnormality can be diagnosed by measuring hormones or chemicals in the blood or urine. The modern day laboratory assessment of endocrine diseases depends upon *radioimmunoassay* (RIA) for accurate information regarding the concentration of hormones in blood and urine. RIA enables the detection of minute quantities of hormones; with RIA even 1×10^{-9} gm (one nanogram) of a hormone would be detectable in body fluids. Other laboratory studies such as X-ray, electrocardiogram, etc., assist in making diagnoses of endocrine disorders.

Pituitary Gland

We have learned during the past decade that the "master gland," the pituitary, also has a master. The pituitary gland is controlled by the *hypothalamus*. The hypothalamus is a part of the midbrain that supports the pituitary gland by a narrow stalk. Regulation of the secretion of hormones by the pituitary gland is exerted by the production and release of hypothalamic releasing or inhibiting hormones which act directly by inhibiting or stimulating the release of hormones by the pituitary (Fig. 12-1).

The pituitary gland lies in a saddle-shaped shell of bone in the base of the skull. In adults, the gland weighs approximately 0.5 gm, but doubles in weight during pregnancy. The pituitary gland is divided into *anterior* epithelial (adenohypophysis) and *posterior* (neurohypophysis) *lobes*. As the name implies the neurohypophysis is composed of neural tissues which extend downward from the hypothalamus.

Adenohypophysis

The anterior lobe is of epithelial origin and composed of three major types of cells—acidophils, basophils, and chromophobes. Approximately 50% of the cells are chromophobes, 35% acidophils, and the remaining 15% basophils. These cells produce one or more *tropic* (or stimulating) hormones (Fig. 12-1). Growth hormone (GH) is produced by acidophils, as is prolactin, a stimulating hormone of the mammary gland. Basophils are the major source of

thyrotropin, gonadotropin, melanin-stimulating hormone, and adrenal corticotropin (ACTH).

Sensor cells within the hypothalamus probably can detect or sense the concentrations of various hormones in the blood. This feedback mechanism is important for maintaining the proper concentration of hormones in the blood. When the concentration of a hormone is too low, the hypothalamus emits a releasing hormone which stimulates the tropic hormone in the adenohypophysis which, in turn, releases the appropriate tropic hormone.

The adrenals, thyroid, and gonads are target organs for tropic hormones which are released by the adenohypophysis. These hormones, adrenocorticotropic hormone (ACTH), thyroid stimulating hormone (TSH), luteinizing hormones (LH), and follicle stimulating hormone (FSH) respond to feedback mechanisms. The target organs have receptors on the surfaces of their cells which react with their individual tropic hormone.

Neurohypophysis

The neurohypophysis serves as a receiving center for hormones produced within the hypothalamus. For instance, *antidiuretic hormone (ADH)* and *oxytocin* are produced by specialized endocrine-neurons in the hypothalamus and the hormones slide down nerve fibers from the neurohypophyseal stalk to the neurohypophysis and in this site they are absorbed into the blood stream.

ADH is absorbed by the veins surrounding the neurohypophysis and carried in the blood to the **distal convoluted tubule of the kidneys where** it controls the reabsorption of 85% of the water in blood filtered by the kidneys. If the pituitary gland stalk is destroyed, *diabetes insipidus* occurs. In this syndrome, individuals experience extreme thirst because a massive outflow of urine occurs in the absence of ADH. The person must be treated by sniffing extracts of powdered human pituitary gland containing ADH.

Decreased Function

Infarction (necrosis) of the pituitary gland or any gland is a devastating condition. The pituitary can become infarcted due to cardiogenic shock from

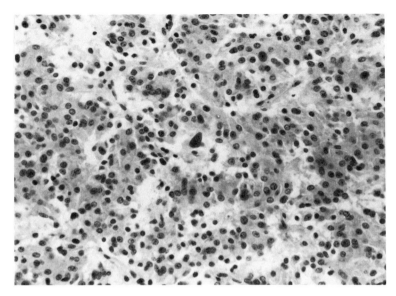

Figure 12-2 *Photomicrograph of acidophilic adenoma (producing growth hormone) of the anterior lobe of the pituitary. The patient suffered from acromegaly.* × 300.

hemorrhage during childbirth, or from intracranial hemorrhage. Destruction of more than 90% of the gland is necessary before pituitary function becomes severely impaired; a large margin of safety is reserved for maintaining the function of this vital gland. *Hypofunction* of the pituitary gland can be partial or total, the latter is termed "panhypopituitarism."

Marked destruction of the pituitary gland results in a progressive loss of hormonal function. First, gonadal hypofunction (such as amenorrhea or aspermia and loss of pubic and axillary hair) occurs; next, growth hormone becomes deficient; then deficiencies of thyrotropin, and finally adrenocorticotropin occurs. Deficiency of growth hormone alone is the most common cause of partial pituitary malfunctions and may result in dwarfism. Individuals suffering from panhypopituitarism, must, for the remaining years of their life, be given thyroxine, cortisone, growth hormone, and sex hormones to replace the deficient hormones.

Tumors

Two tumors, *adenoma* of the adenohypophysis and *craniopharyngioma*, cause endocrine dysfunction and visual impairment. The excessive production of growth hormone can result in *giantism*. When the hormone is produced in excessive quantities in an adult or following the fusion of boney growth plates,

acromegaly develops. Characteristic enlargement of the jaw ("lantern jaw"), results from an increased growth of the mandible and the fingers also become thickened.

Acromegaly and giantism often result from *acidophil adenomas* of the adenohypophysis (Fig. 12-2). Unfortunately, this benign tumor may produce pressure on the optic tracts that pass laterally to the gland, causing tunnel vision to occur. Such a symptom usually signifies a tumor in this site. The tumor can be seen in the skull X-ray film. Treatment involves surgical removal or irradiation of the tumor. Thereafter, the patient requires replacement of hormones (such as cortisone, sex hormones, thyroxine) for life.

The second most common type of pituitary tumor is *craniopharyngioma*. This tumor progressively enlarges from a nest of embryonic cells at the base of the skull. As with other pituitary tumors, progressive expansion of the tumor causes pressure on the nearby optic tracts and produces tunnel vision. Tumors of the pituitary can be surgically resected. Primary carcinomas of the pituitary gland are rare.

Adrenal Glands

The paired adrenal glands are located directly above the kidneys (suprarenal) and are triangular to crescent-shaped. At maturity they each weigh approx-

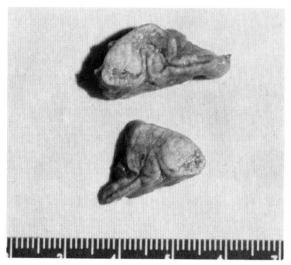

Figure 12-3 *Adrenal gland bisected. A small round cortical adenoma which was associated with hyperaldosteronism is displayed.*

imately 7 gm and are composed of a yellow cortex and a central gray medullary region. The adrenal cortex is controlled by ACTH from the pituitary, and the medulla by the sympathetic nervous system which, upon nervous stimulation, releases adrenalin.

Adrenal Cortex

The adrenal cortex is divided into three zones which produce salt, sugar, and sex hormones. The outermost zone is responsible for secretion of a hormone, aldosterone, which controls salt excretion by the kidneys. Excessive production of aldosterone usually results from an adenoma or hyperplasia of the adrenal cortex (Fig. 12-3) and rarely from carcinoma.

Hyperaldosteronism

A patient with hyperaldosteronism (Conn's syndrome) usually has muscle weakness, hypertension, excessive urination, and high sodium and low potassium serum levels. The muscle weakness is explained by potassium loss in urine. In addition, hypertension (high blood pressure) is common, and severe arteriosclerosis of the kidneys develops in longstanding cases. The blood of these patients contains ex-

cessive aldosterone, and injection of a dye into the adrenal arteries via a catheter enables the visualization of the adenoma in an X-ray. Surgical removal of the adenoma returns normal salt balance; the remaining normal adrenal is capable of sustaining normal adrenal function.

Cushing's Syndrome

The cells of the middle zone of the adrenal cortex produce hormones concerned with sugar metabolism (cortisol). *Cushing's syndrome* results from an excessive production of cortisol. This syndrome occurs (5% of cases) from a pituitary adenoma of basophil cells that secrete excessive ACTH. More frequently, hyperplasia of the adrenal cortex or an adenoma secreting cortisol produce hypercortisonism (Fig. 12-3).

Typically, an individual affected by Cushing's syndrome has a "moon" face and obesity of the trunk, but sparing of the distal limbs (Fig. 12-4). High blood sugar (hyperglycemia), hyper-

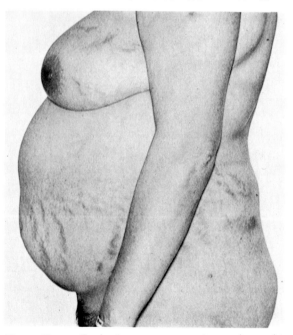

Figure 12-4 *Typical appearance of a patient with Cushing's syndrome. The patient has a "buffalo hump" on her back and truncal obesity with sparing of the limbs. Striae (stretch marks) are seen on her abdomen.*

tension, demineralization of the bones (osteoporosis), muscular weakness, hairiness (hirsutism), and psychological disturbances are commonly found. Surgical removal of a primary adrenal tumor or hyperplastic adrenal gland restores normal adrenal function. Cushing's syndrome can occur from prolonged administration of cortisol. In fact, iatrogenic (physician-induced) Cushing's syndrome is the most frequent cause of the syndrome. Gradual cessation of cortisol use returns the patient to normal.

Virilization (adrenogenital syndrome)

Male and female hormones are secreted by the cells of the inner layer of the adrenal cortex. When male hormones (androgens) are secreted excessively in a newborn female infant, masculinization occurs (*adrenogenital syndrome*). The female child's clitoris becomes enlarged, pseudohermaphroditism develops. In the male, precocious (early) puberty appears (enlargement of penis and appearance of pubic hair). This syndrome appears in several forms; some children have excessive loss of salt and others, chiefly hypertension.

Masculinization in both boys and girls results from six different inherited inborn errors of metabolism. The affected children have a deficiency of enzymes essential for the formation of cortisol. The lack of cortisol in the blood stimulates ACTH secretion by the pituitary, and the adrenals become hyperplastic and produce excessive quantities of androgens. Treatment of the adrenogenital syndrome involves administering cortisol and other drugs that shut off the ACTH synthesis, and the masculinization subsides.

Severe masculinization in women is usually caused by an adrenal cortical tumor. Surgical removal of the tumor reverses the process.

Adrenal Cortical Insufficiency

Insufficient adrenal gland function is either acute (immediate) or chronic (long term). *Acute adrenocorticosteroid insufficiency* can be caused by hemorrhagic destruction of the glands infected by *N meningitidis* as in the *Waterhouse-Friderichsen syndrome*. The adrenal glands, destroyed by hemorrhage, fail.

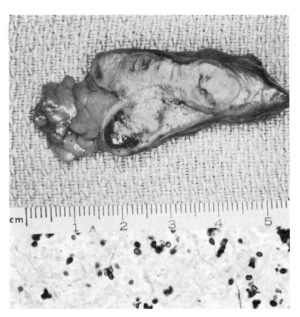

Figure 12-5   *Adrenal gland destroyed by histoplasmosis. The gland is necrotic and hemorrhagic (dark areas). The inset (below) shows histoplasma fungal organisms × 400. The patient suffered from Addison's disease.*

Acute adrenal insufficiency is characterized by sudden circulatory collapse (hypotension) and extensive hemorrhage into the skin, prostration, and cyanosis. The condition is treated with cortisol.

A second cause of acute adrenocorticoid deficiency is the rapid withdrawal of cortisone medication from patients being treated for rheumatoid arthritis. Chronic cortisone therapy causes the patient's adrenal gland to atrophy (the ACTH stimulation to the adrenal is decreased by the medication). Finally, the stress of surgical procedures can induce hypocortisonism.

Chronic adrenal insufficiency (Addison's disease) results from the gradual destruction of the adrenal glands. Over 90% of the cortex of the adrenal must be destroyed before obvious symptoms occur. *Addison's disease* is characterized by hyperpigmented skin, muscular weakness, loss of weight, and low blood pressure. Infectious diseases like histoplasmosis (Fig. 12-5) autoimmunity, and metastatic cancer of the adrenal glands are common causes of Addison's disease. A diagnosis is established by observing the clinical findings described above and

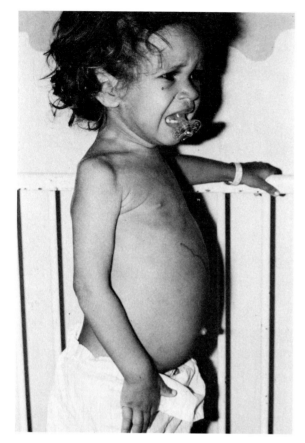

Figure 12-6 *This child suffered from neuroblastoma, a malignancy of the adrenal medulla. The tumor is distending the child's abdomen.*

by detecting low serum cortisol levels. Addison's disease can be easily treated by cortisol.

Adrenal Medulla

The adrenal medulla is composed of sympathetic nerves which end in ganglion cells. Within the adrenal medulla are stored packets of norepinephrine and epinephrine (adrenalin) which, upon release into the blood, mobilize the three "F" responses of fright, flight, and fight.

Neoplasms

Tumors are the major pathologic process involving the adrenal medulla. *Neuroblastoma* is a primitive malignancy of the adrenal medulla which occurs in infants and young children (Fig. 12-6). Ordinarily the tumor is located on one side; rarely are both sides involved. Usually, the mother detects the tumor while changing diapers or fondling her child.

The detection of catecholamine (precursors to adrenalin) in the urine of the infant confirms the diagnosis of neuroblastoma. Preoperative irradiation is usually given followed by surgery and chemotherapy. Unfortunately, the five year survival rate, even without evidence of metastasis, is only 30%. This rate of survival is low in contrast with another malignancy of childhood, Wilms' tumor of the kidney, which is cured in 70% of cases.

Pheochromocytoma is a benign adrenal medullary tumor of adults. It is bilateral in approximately 10% of cases and rarely malignant. Headache, sweating, palpitation, and hypertension result from the production and release of norepinephrine into the blood by the tumor. The tumor can be recognized with X-ray studies and by noting increased levels of norepinephrine in the blood.

The neural elements constituting the medulla can also become neoplastic; but *benign ganglioneuromas* and *ganglioneuroblastoma* rarely develop. The latter malignant tumor is often large and invades adjacent structures.

Thyroid Gland

The thyroid gland surrounds the trachea just below the larynx. It is bilobed, connected by a thin strand of tissue, and at maturity weighs approximately 20 gm. It is comprised of follicles filled with thyroglobulin. The follicle cells produce thyroglobulin and thyroxine, the major hormone of the thyroid. Between the follicle cells "C" cells reside. These produce thyrocalcitonin, a hormone capable of reducing calcium concentration in blood. Most of the common diseases of the thyroid gland arise from autoimmune disorders.

Hyperthyroidism

When excessive TSH or long-acting thyroid stimulating hormone (LATS) is produced, a goiter and hyperthyroidism may occur. LATS is an autoantibody that reacts with and stimulates the receptor for TSH on thyroid follicle cells, causing excessive production of thyroxine.

Typically, hyperthyroid patients are women aged 20 to 40, with diarrhea, weight loss, nervousness, heat intolerance, and an inability to sleep. Protrusion of the eyes (exophthalamos) is also a common sign. Emotional distress from the hyperthyroidism often leads to marital discord, and divorce occurs or is pending in many patients before diagnosis is made and treatment given.

Hyperthyroidism is treated by decreasing the production of thyroxine. This may be accomplished by removing the gland, but more commonly it is done nonsurgically by administering drugs which inhibit thyroxine production, the thiouracil drugs or radioactive iodine, which destroys the hyperplastic thyroid tissue. These modes of therapy can restore the patient to a normal (euthyroid) condition. Overtreatment, however, can result in abnormally decreased thyroid function or hypothyroidism.

Hypothyroidism

Hypothyroidism usually involves middle-aged individuals. Bloated faces; thickened, dry skin; sparse, coarse hair; muscular weakness; slow mentation; intolerance to cold; and a hoarse voice are common symptoms of hypothyroidism. Extreme hypothyroidism is termed *myxedema*. The disease may occur following the excessive administration of radioactive iodine or following the surgical removal of the thyroid. In addition, the gland can be destroyed by autoimmune diseases.

Typically, an individual with *myxedema* will have a low metabolic rate and a low thyroxine concentration in the serum. The administration of thyroxine results in the restoration of normal metabolism.

Cretinism

Cretinism is an extreme infantile form of hypothyroidism. It results when severe hypofunction of the thyroid occurs in newborn infants. This occurs in utero when the mother has severe hypothyroidism.

An infant with cretinism shows an enlarged thyroid (goiter) and tongue, thick, coarse skin, a protruding abdomen, flaccid muscles, and possibly permanent mental retardation. He or she may be unresponsive to thyroxine. Hypothyroidism can also result from an inability of the thyroid gland to concentrate iodine or form thyroxine from iodine.

Goiter

A goiter is an enlargement of the thyroid gland which can be due to an excessive stimulation of the gland by TSH or LATS. It may or may not be associated with thyroid dysfunction. The major cause of goiter is iodine deficiency which, on a worldwide basis, involves over 200 million individuals (See chapter 10, Nutritional Diseases). Goiterous thyroid glands may be nodular or diffusely enlarged. Correction is by iodine repletion when this element is deficient, but surgical removal may be required when extensive fibrosis and calcification occur.

Autoimmune Diseases

The thyroid can be damaged by infectious diseases, irradiation, or by autoimmune diseases (see Chapter 6, Immunology). The most common form of autoimmune thyroiditis is *Hashimoto's thyroiditis*. The gland becomes infiltrated by numerous plasma cells and lymphocytes and the patient's serum contains antibodies against the patient's own thyroglobulin. In thyroiditis, the gland is usually enlarged, and it can be atropic; later hypothyroidism can ensue.

Neoplasms

Adenomas consisting of an overgrowth of small glandular elements of the thyroid occur more commonly than carcinomas. The adenomas are generally encapsulated and rarely excrete excessive amounts of thyroxine.

Thyroid cancers are responsible for approximately one in every 200 cancer deaths and affect women more often than men. Papillary carcinomas comprise approximately 60% of thyroid carcinomas. Fortunately, they seldom metastasize beyond regional lymph nodes of the neck, so the prognosis is good. Other types of thyroid cancer have worse prognoses.

The cause of thyroid carcinomas is unknown, though a fairly large proportion of young adults who develop papillary carcinoma have had previous (15 to 20 years prior) irradiation to the neck or upper chest for skin disorders or to treat enlargement of the thymus or tonsils*. Treatment of thyroid cancer is either by surgical removal or by administration of radioactive iodine which destroys the tumor cells that use up iodine.

Parathyroid Glands

The four parathyroid glands weigh only 120 mg and are nestled within the substance of the thyroid gland. They produce parathormone, a hormone which maintains serum calcium and phosphorus concentrations. Parathormone acts upon bones causing resorption of calcium, and stimulates the renal tubules to excrete phosphorus.

Hyperparathyroidism

The clinical problems associated with hyperparathyroidism are easily remembered by the rhyme "stones, bones, groans, and moans." The hypercalcemia and hypophosphatemia associated with hyperparathyroidism produce bizzare psychological problems (psychic moans). The patients are prone to develop urolithiasis (stones) in the urinary tract. Parathormone induces thinning of bone due to resorption of calcium and pathological fractures (broken bones) can ensue. Finally, abdominal pain (groans) occurs from associated peptic ulcers. However, hyperparathyroidism is often asymptomatic and is detected accidentally by finding high serum calcium and low phosphorus concentrations on routine examination of the blood.

The major cause (80%) of primary hyperparathyroidism is adenoma of a parathyroid gland. Treatment is by surgical removal of the adenoma.

*A national campaign was launched in 1977 aimed at identifying thyroid cancer in the thousands of persons who received irradiation to the neck during childhood.

Secondary hyperparathyroidism results from chronic renal disease; the excessive loss of calcium in the urine stimulates the parathyroid glands to undergo hyperplasia. This occurs because the feedback mechanism which detects low serum calcium elicits growth of the gland. The resulting metabolic effects are identical to those of primary hyperparathyroidism.

Hypoparathyroidism

Hypoparathyroidism results from destruction or absence of the parathyroid gland. The most common cause of this disorder is the surgical removal of all of the parathyroid glands during thyroidectomy. These patients suffer from *tetany* (hyperexcitability of skeletal muscles with twitching) because of a low serum calcium. Treatment involves administration of parathormone and intravenous calcium.

Diabetes Mellitus

Over 200 million persons in the world are afflicted by diabetes mellitus. Following obesity and thyroid disorders, diabetes is the third most common endocrine-metabolic disorder. In the United States there are approximately two million persons suffering from diagnosed diabetes and an equal number with undiagnosed diabetes.

Diabetes mellitus is a chronic metabolic disease with widespread systemic effects. It is characterized by an elevation of blood glucose due to relative or absolute lack of insulin and with secondary alterations in lipid and protein metabolism. The major pathological change in diabetes is accelerated and early onset of arteriosclerosis, especially in the eyes, kidneys, and heart. Gangrene of the feet, arteriosclerotic heart disease, blindness, and uremia can be end results of diabetes mellitus.

Two major forms of diabetes occur. *Juvenile diabetes* occurs between birth and age 20, and *maturity onset diabetes* occurs in adults usually beyond age 40. Thus, diabetes mellitus appears at two periods when profound endocrinological changes are occurring—at puberty and menopause.

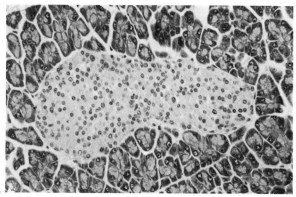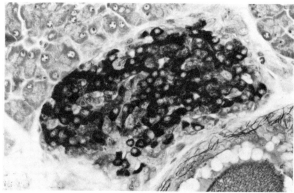

Figure 12-7   *Light microscopic photomicrographs of pancreatic islets from normal mouse injected with citrate buffer. The well-delineated islets are enmeshed in the surrounding acinar cells of the exocrine pancreas. Well-granulated beta cells stain intensely with aldehyde fuchsin (black in photograph) indicating an abundance of stored insulin.* **A,** *Hematoxylin and eosin,* × *144;* **B,** *aldehyde fuchsin,* × *222. (Courtesy Dr. Arthur A. Like and Science.)*

Diabetes often evolves through three phases. *Prediabetes* is undetectable by laboratory studies, but the person has an inherited predisposition to the disease. Prediabetes can only be speculated upon prospectively (in the future) or retrospectively (after the disease actually occurs). *Chemical (latent) diabetes* is characterized by an elevated blood sugar level in the glucose tolerance test, but only during the metabolic stresses of pregnancy, infections, or obesity do latent diabetics become overtly hyperglycemic. *Overt diabetes* is characterized by laboratory studies which reveal an elevated fasting blood glucose, glucose in urine, and abnormal metabolism. At first such diabetics may not have overt symptoms of diabetes; only later do the symptoms of overt, *decompensated diabetes* appear, such as excessive thirst, hunger, urination, and weakness.

Etiology

The cause of diabetes is unknown, but polygenic inheritance is likely in most cases (see Chapter 9, Inherited Disorders). Diabetes probably results from an interaction between genes, diet, and environmental agents which destroy the islet cells that produce insulin. *Viruses* (such as mumps or Coxsackie B virus) have been suggested as causal agents of diabetes. Also autoimmunity has been

suggested as a mechanism responsible for the disease. Diabetes mellitus (or at least hyperglycemia) results secondarily from other endocrinopathies like hyperthyroidism, acromegaly, and Cushing's syndrome. Also, chronic inflammatory lesions of the pancreas, as occur in chronic alcoholics, and in a metabolic disorder of iron metabolism called hemochromatosis, can cause the diabetes syndrome.

The pancreas is both an endocrine and exocrine gland. The islets of Langerhans number one million and are distributed throughout the pancreas; they comprise approximately 2% of the weight of the gland and weigh 1 gm in total. The islets are comprised of several cell types. *Beta cells* secrete *insulin* and *Alpha cells* secrete *glucagon*, a hormone that opposes the function of insulin (Fig. 12-7). A third cell, the *Delta cell*, secretes *gastrin*.

Pathology of Islets

Many different lesions occur in the islets of patients who have diabetes mellitus, but one-third show no lesions. In acute phases of diabetes, the islets are normal in number but enlarged.

Approximately 50% of diabetic individuals over age 50 years exhibit a decrease in number of islets, and degenerative fibrosis (hyalinization) of their islets occurs (Fig. 12-8). When children die of acute

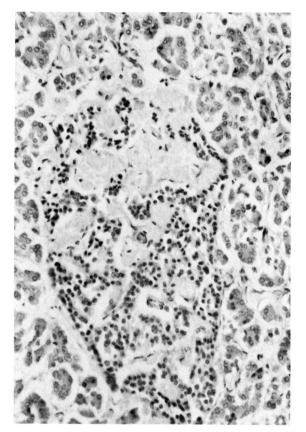

Figure 12-8 *Photomicrograph of islet of Langerhan's showing hyalinization of the beta cells from a woman with diabetes mellitus. × 450.*

juvenile diabetes mellitus, lymphocytes infiltrate into islets causing *insulinitis* or *isletitis*. This destructive immune response could be in response to a virus or an autoimmune reaction. Experimentally, diabetes and isletitis can be induced in mice with a drug, streptozoticin, which injures Beta cells (Fig. 12-9).

Action of Insulin

Insulin has two major functions. Glucose is transferred from the blood into fat and muscle cells by insulin (Fig. 12-10). This is a vital function because glucose is the body's primary fuel. Secondly, glucose activates metabolic processes in these cells. The systemic impact of insulin activity is increased use and storage of glucose, and retention and synthesis of fat and protein. Harmful alterations in carbohydrate, fat, and protein metabolism occur in diabetic patients because of deficient insulin and impaired entry of glucose into cells.

Just as the engine of an automobile uses internal combustion to convert the chemical bonds of gasoline to heat and mechanical force, animal cells use chemical bonds in food to produce energy. Most cells can metabolize several types of fuel (fat, protein, glucose). In contrast, the brain only metabolizes glucose. The inability of diabetics to use glucose results in the *catabolism* (breakdown) of protein

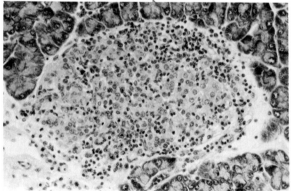

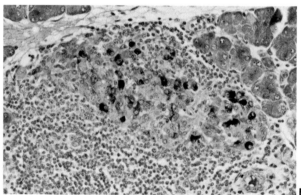

A   B

Figure 12-9   *Inflamed islets from mouse killed six days after receiving five injections of streptozotocin. The interior and periphery of the islets are permeated with large numbers of lymphocytes and macrophages, which distort the islet architecture and extend into the adjacent exocrine tissue. Substantial beta cell degranulation is evident, **B**, and caused hyperglycemia. **A**, Hematoxylin and eosin; and **B**, aldehyde fuchsin; both × 144. (Courtesy Dr. Arthur A. Like and Science. Coypright © by the American Association for the Advancement of Science.)*

is that the blood glucose concentration rises. In addition, the glucose derived from a meal cannot be used or stored in fat and muscle. When the blood glucose level rises above 150 mg/100 ml, the kidney tubules become incapable of reabsorbing it, glucose spills out into the urine causing glucosuria (glucose in urine) and increased frequency and volume of urination.

Some of the cardinal hallmarks of diabetes are hyperglycemia, decreased glucose tolerance, glycosuria, polyuria with loss of salts (especially sodium chloride), weight loss, thirst, and hunger. The symptoms of diabetes mellitus have been called the three *polys*: polyuria, polyphagia, and polydypsia (from excessive urination, eating, and thirst).

Acute Complications

Diabetic coma and *ketoacidosis* result when fatty acids are gradually catabolized (lipolysis) and the accumulation of ketoacids and ketone bodies (acetone) accumulate in the blood and tissues. Acetone is smelled on the breath of an individual suffering from ketoacidosis. The patient will have warm, dry skin, deep and rapid breathing, and be comatose. In addition, during this time the blood glucose level elevates above 400 mg/100 ml. The individual may be able to blow off the excessive acid (CO_2) by breathing deeply. The administration of insulin and intravenous fluids (sodium bicarbonate) rapidly corrects diabetic ketoacidosis. Severe diabetic coma is associated with an approximately 5% to 15% mortality rate.

Hypoglycemia (low blood glucose) may develop when the patient has taken too much insulin either by accident or design, because of a late meal, or because of strenuous, prolonged exercise. Sweating, hunger, tremor, and mental confusion occur when the blood glucose falls to between 40 and 50 mg/100 ml. If glucose is not given, coma will ensue. Injection of glucose intravenously promptly restores the blood glucose and consciousness. In addition to acute alterations and complications of altered blood sugar levels, a variety of chronic complications accompany long term diabetes. The effect of strict therapy in preventing complications is unclear.

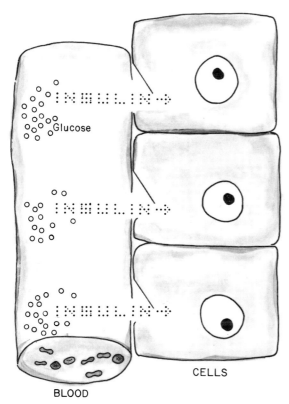

Figure 12-10 *Mechanism whereby insulin permits the entry of glucose into cells.*

in skeletal muscles as an alternative source of energy. The individual's muscles deteriorate, thus explaining the weakness and poor healing of wounds seen in diabetic patients. Also, fat is used excessively as a source of energy in these persons.

Ordinarily, insulin secretion by islet cells is regulated by the level of the blood sugar; a rise in blood sugar (glucose) stimulates insulin release. The granules containing insulin within the islet cells disappear as insulin is released, and the blood glucose level decreases as glucose moves into fat and muscle cells.

Insulin Deprivation

In overt diabetes, insulin activity is deficient. This may result from decrease in quantity, abnormality of activity or action, or inhibition of action of the insulin. The net effect when the insulin supply fails

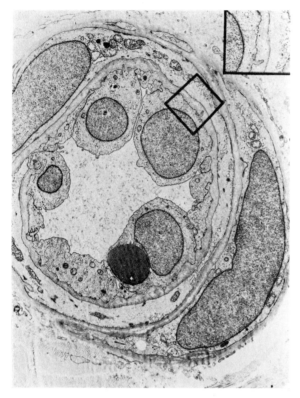

Figure 12-11 *Electron micrograph of cross-section of an arteriole from a person with diabetes mellitus. The inset displays a markedly thickened basement membrane characteristic of this disease. Magnification of inset × 12,000. (From Lin, J. 1975. Microcirculation in diabetes mellitus.* Human Pathology *6:89, W. B. Saunders Co.)*

Chronic Complications

The entire vascular tree in diabetics shows *severe vascular damage*. For example, arterioles, capillaries, and venules undergo marked thickening by a carbohydrate-rich substance (two- to threefold) of their basement membranes (Fig. 12-11). The vessels of the retina, eye, and kidneys are especially vulnerable. It is not known why the basement membrane thickens, but this pathologic change may be a basic component of this complex disease.

Persons who have diabetes for one or more decades may suffer from severe renal damage. The glomeruli often are obliterated by hyaline masses or the basement membranes are diffusely thick-

ened. Patients afflicted with diabetic glomerulosclerosis have proteinuria, edema, and hypertension. Renal failure and the resulting uremia may kill these patients, especially pregnant juvenile diabetics.

Prolonged hyperglycemia is often associated with damage to the eye. Cataracts form, but more significantly, microaneurysms occur. The small arterioles of the retina of the eye become ballooned (aneurysm) and subsequent hemorrhage into the retina and retinal detachment may cause blindness. In most instances, retinopathy and diabetic renal disease coexist.

Deaths in diabetic persons are due to arteriosclerotic cardiovascular disease such as stroke or heart attack in over 70% of this group (see Chapter 13, Cardiology). The vascular lesions consist of thickening of the capillary basement membranes and endothelial proliferation of small blood vessels and severe arteriosclerotic plaques in the coronary arteries. Because of inadequate circulation, the patients are especially prone to develop ulcerations and infections of the skin which are slow to heal; gangrene of the toes is a common problem in elderly diabetic persons. Also, diabetics are apt to develop infections of the urinary tract. The control of diabetes by diet and drugs does not seem to halt the relentless onslaught of vascular disease.

Therapy

Many cases of maturity onset diabetes can be controlled by a low calorie and low carbohydrate diet. Other patients may require a combination of diet and oral antidiabetic drugs. The oral sulfonylurea drugs such as tolbutamide stimulate the B cells to secrete insulin.

Metabolic Diseases

Metabolic disorders are responsible for many human diseases. Major inborn errors of metabolism (inherited metabolic defects) can be categorized into: (a) *disorders in amino acid or enzyme metabolism*, and (b) defects characterized by an *excessive accumulation of certain substances* in lysosomes in tissues (storage diseases). Metabolic or biochemical reactions require specific enzymes for the formation of new compounds (see Chapter 9, Inherited Disorders). Each enzyme is controlled by a gene. Mutant genes often result in the absence of their normal product and hence an enzyme is not produced and cellular and systemic abnormalities result.

Alpha₁ Antitrypsin Deficiency

A recent major breakthrough in understanding one cause of fibrosis of the lungs (emphysema) and liver (cirrhosis) was the discovery of alpha₁ antitrypsin deficiency. Persons lacking this enzyme have an accumulation of alpha₁ antitrypsin in their livers (Fig. 12-12), and the liver becomes fibrotic. The mechanism responsible for the damage in the brain and lung is unclear; one suggestion is that antitrypsin normally inactivates the enzyme trypsin, which is liberated from phagocytes in tissues. Absence of this protective mechanism could render the tissues vulnerable to injury by the enzymes.

Cystinosis

The absence in children of an enzyme which metabolizes the amino acid, cystine, results in an accumulation of cystine crystals in the kidneys. As the kidneys fail, the growth of the child is impaired. Many other metabolic defects result in a failure to metabolize carbohydrates, fats, or amino acids.

The so called storage diseases of glycogen and lipids result from an accumulation of these substances in the tissues (see Chapter 9, Inherited Disorders). Moreover, two major inborn errors of metabolism result from an excessive deposition of metals (iron and copper) in cells.

Hemochromatosis

Hemochromatosis is an inherited disorder characterized by an excessive accumulation of iron in the bone marrow, endocrine organs, and liver. The diseases can result genetically or on an acquired basis. The excess iron is associated with fibrosis of

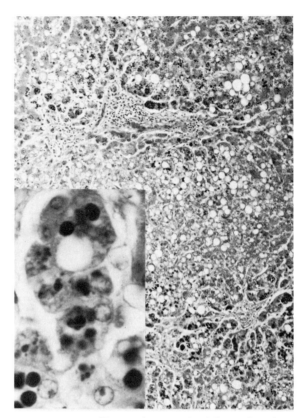

Figure 12-12   *Photomicrograph of liver of patient with alpha₁ antitrypsin deficiency. The black dots are alpha₁ antitrypsin globules that have become trapped within the liver cells. × 200. The inset displays them at a higher magnification × 450.*

the liver with cirrhosis resulting (Fig. 12-13). Deposition of iron in the heart may lead to heart failure. In addition, the endocrine glands become saturated with iron and hypofunction of the endocrine glands may occur (diabetes mellitus). The excessive iron is removed by phlebotomy (bleeding).

Wilson's Disease

Wilson's disease is an inherited metabolic disorder characterized by a deficiency in ceruloplasm which carries copper in the blood. Hence, an excessive deposition of copper occurs in the brain, liver and other organs. Typically, cirrhosis develops during childhood or early adulthood. The deposition of the copper in the brain may lead to severe neuro-

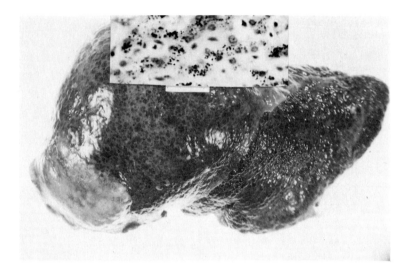

Figure 12-13 *Hemochromatosis of the liver. Note the black deposits of iron in the fibrotic liver. The light mass in the right lower lobe is a hepatocarcinoma. The inset shows particles of iron staining black. × 250. (Armed Forces Institute of Pathology, Negative No. 59-10494C.)*

logical symptoms including a flapping tremor, muscular rigidity, difficulty in speaking (dysarthria), and dementia (psychosis). The individuals have high serum, urinary, and tissue copper levels.

Penicillamine, a drug that binds copper, is given to children affected by Wilson's disease to prevent the deposition of copper in the brain and liver. Penicillamine must be given early in the course of the disease or irreversible hepatic and neurological changes occur.

Gout

Gout, another inherited (autosomal dominant) inborn error of metabolism, may cause severe arthritis and renal disease due to the deposition of urate crystals in tissues (Fig. 12-14). About 95% of gouty arthritis occurs in men of middle age. The affected joint is often acutely inflamed (swollen, hot, red, and painful to move).

A major complication of gout is the deposition of uric acid stones in the kidneys, which may result in renal failure. The crystals become precipitated in the synovium of the joints, and an acute inflammatory response leads to acute arthritis. This is especially apt to occur in the great toe at the tarsalmetatarsal joint. When uric acid is precipitated in subcutaneous tissues, the masses are called "tophi."

Colchicine, an inhibitor of mitosis, is used to treat gout. In addition, a drug which inhibits uric acid

synthesis, *allopurinol*, lowers the concentration of uric acid in the blood.

Hyperlipidemia

The role of high serum lipids (fats) in the pathogenesis of arteriosclerosis has been noted by many investigators during recent decades (see Chapter 13). The blood lipids of concern are cholesterol and triglycerides. These lipids are carried in the blood by lipoproteins. The term *hypertriglyceridemia* implies the presence of increased amounts of triglycerides in the patient's serum. The excess fat gives the serum a creamy, opalescent appearance. Individuals suffering from this problem develop deposits of fat in macrophages which form deposits (xanthomas) in their skin (Fig. 12-15). Some forms of hypertriglyceridemia can be caused by diets rich in carbohydrates.

Hypercholesterolemia may be familial. An abnormally high concentration of cholesterol is found in the serum of persons inheriting this disorder. A very serious tendency toward accelerated early arteriosclerosis may occur. The affected persons often develop xanthomas of the skin, especially of the upper eyelids, elbows, and knees (see Chapter 13).

The diagnosis of familial hypercholesteremia rests on the finding of cholesterol in the tissues and a marked elevation of the serum cholesterol. A change in diet, in some instances, lowers the serum cho-

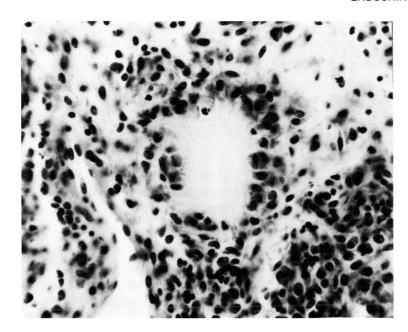

Figure 12-14   *Photomicrograph of tissue from a joint of a patient with gout; shows deposit (clear area) of uric acid crystals surrounded by inflammation (white blood cells). × 300.*

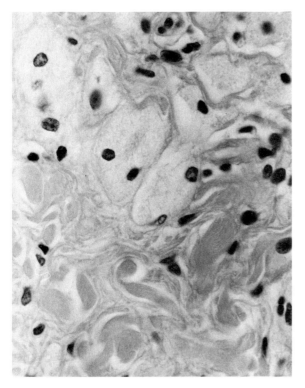

Figure 12-15   *Photomicrograph of xanthoma of skin. Note deposits of fat in foamy macrophages. × 450.*

lesterol level and certain drugs either decrease its synthesis or remove it from the blood. Numerous other metabolic disorders could be discussed at great length—see references for additional information.

Summary

Endocrine and metabolic disorders arise from defective function and regulation of the biochemistry of the body. Metabolic diseases often result from a mutation of a gene which causes a deficiency in an enzyme. Subsequently, abnormally high concentrations of toxic chemicals accumulate in tissues and can damage them.

Hormones are produced by endocrine glands, are secreted directly into blood, and cause target organs to undergo increased or decreased metabolic activity. Most endocrine disorders result from excessive (hyper) or decreased (hypo) function of an endocrine gland. Specific syndromes can be recognized clinically and diagnosed by detecting alterations in the hormone level in the blood.

Hyperfunction usually results from hyperplasia or adenomas in the endocrine gland. By contrast, hypofunction ensues from destruction or failure of stimulation of a target gland by the pituitary. Conditions of hyperfunction are treated by drugs or removing the gland (or part of it) surgically. Replacement therapy of a hormone (insulin, for example), is given for hypofunctioning endocrine glands.

Bibliography

Ezrin, C., et al., Eds. 1973. *Systemic endocrinology*. Hagerstown, Maryland: Harper & Row, Publishers. An excellent resource for discussion on clinical and pathophysiologic aspects of endocrinology.

Fink, D. 1977. Irradiation-related thyroid cancer. U.S. Dept. H. E. W. Public Health Service. D.H.E.W. Publication No. (NIH) 77–1120. This 27 page pamphlet describes measures being taken to detect irradiation-induced thyroid cancer.

Frohman, L. A. 1975. Neurotransmitters as regulators of endocrine function. *Hosp. Practice* 10:54–79. Describes the interplay between the hypothalamus and the endocrine glands.

Guyton, A. C. 1974. *Function of the human body*, ed. 4. Philadelphia: W. B. Saunders Co. An introductory chapter on endocrinology. A good source for the uninitiated student.

Lacy, P.E. 1975. Endocrine secretory mechanisms. *Am. J. Pathol.* 79:170–187. A molecular biological discussion of endocrinology.

Lin, J. H.; Duffy, J. L.; and Roginsky, M. D. 1975. Microcirculation in diabetes mellitus: a study of gingival biopsy. *Human Pathology* 6:97–112, 1975. Illustrates abnormalities in the microcirculation of diabetic patients.

Martin, G. M., and Hoehn, H. 1975. Genetic and human disease. *Hum. Pathol.* 5:387–405. Discusses the inheritance of diabetes and some metabolic diseases.

Passmann, J. M. 1976. Changing concepts of parathyroid pathology in primary hyperparathyroidism. *Lab. Med.* 7–10. An article devoted to the laboratory diagnosis of parathyroid diseases.

Rodman, G. P. 1975. Gout and other crystaline forms of arthritis. *Postgrad. Med.* 58:4–12. This article summarizes gout.

Sharp, H. L. 1971. Alpha$_1$ antitrypsin deficiency. *Hosp. Practice* 83–96. A well illustrated discussion of this inherited deficiency.

Tepperman, J. 1973. *Metabolic and endocrine physiology*, ed. 3. Chicago: Year Book Publishers. Concise (246 pages) and readable summary of pathophysiology of endocrine disease.

Thorn, G. W. 1974. General considerations and major syndromes of hormonal disorders. In *Principles of internal medicine*, eds. Wintrobe, M., et al., pp. 444–447. 7th ed. New York: McGraw Hill, Inc. A standard textbook of medicine.

CHAPTER 13

Cardiovascular Medicine

Chapter Outline

Objectives

After reading this chapter you should be able to

List in order of frequency the six major types of cardiac disease occurring in the United States.

Define the terms cardiology and arteriosclerosis.

List three variants of arteriosclerosis.

Describe the pathologic lesions of early and late arteriosclerosis in arterial walls.

List the risk factors for arteriosclerosis and name the four major ones.

List specific sites where arteriosclerosis are apt to occur.

Describe symptoms associated with arteriosclerosis induced by ischemia of the heart, brain, and legs.

List possible complications of arteriosclerosis.

Compare the chest pain in angina pectoris with that of acute myocardial infarction.

Describe two laboratory studies used for substantiating a diagnosis of acute myocardial infarction.

List three factors affecting the pathologic findings in acute myocardial infarction.

Describe the sequential gross and microscopic appearance of myocardial infarction at 12 hours, 24 hours, 48 hours, and about one week following onset.

List possible complications of acute MI.

Describe the etiologies of several types of shock.

Discuss the pathophysiologic basis of shock.

Know what period following an MI is most critical for survival; in other words, when do most patients with MI die?

Define the term aneurysm.

Know the American Heart Association's definition of hypertension.

Compare the etiologies of primary (essential) and secondary hypertension.

List causes of secondary hypertension.

Describe the pathophysiology of essential hypertension.

List the three organs most damaged by hypertension.

Know the two pathophysiologic adjustments made by the heart prior to development of congestive heart failure.

List the common causes of secondary hypertension.

Describe the drugs used for treating hypertension.

Define the term congestive heart failure (CHF).

List the three factors usually responsible for CHF.

Describe the signs and symptoms of CHF.

List three disorders that might lead to hypertension.

Describe the pathogenesis of pulmonary edema.

Know how pulmonary edema is treated.

List the four cardiac diseases having an infectious etiology.

Describe the pathogenesis of rheumatic heart disease.

List criteria used for diagnosing rheumatic fever.

Define the terms endocarditis, myocarditis and epicarditis.

List laboratory findings supporting a diagnosis of acute rheumatic fever.

List complications of rheumatic heart disease.

Describe the signs and symptoms of bacterial endocarditis.

Discuss factors or conditions that might lead to bacterial endocarditis.

List the bacteria most frequently causing endocarditis.

Describe possible complications accompanying bacterial endocarditis.

Discuss the prognosis for subacute and acute bacterial endocarditis.

List the three stages of syphilis.

Describe the major lesion caused by syphilis in the cardiovascular system.

List several viruses that can cause viral myocarditis.

Define the term thrombophlebitis.

Compare the clinical findings regarding superficial and deep thrombophlebitis.

List the three factors that can precipitate thrombophlebitis.

Describe how venous valvular incompetence can occur.

List complications that may accompany varicose veins.

List the three organs where arterial thrombosis and infarction cause deaths.

Describe the signs and symptoms of pulmonary embolism.

Compare treatments given for thrombophlebitis, varicose veins, and pulmonary embolism.

Describe measures that can be taken to prevent pulmonary embolism.

List the major cardiac emergencies.

Describe the ABCs of basic life support.

Introduction

Cardiovascular diseases account for more than one half of all deaths in the United States (almost all related to arteriosclerosis). The dramatic increase in incidence of arteriosclerotic coronary artery disease in this century is due largely to prolongation of life and life styles predisposing us to this disease.

The study of cardiovascular diseases is termed *cardiology*. Seven types of cardiac disease commonly affect people living in the United States:
1. Coronary arteriosclerotic heart disease (80% of all cardiac deaths)
2. Hypertensive heart disease (9%)
3. Rheumatic heart disease (2% to 3%)
4. Congenital heart disease (approximately 2%). See Chapter 3, Development and Birth Defects.
5. Bacterial endocarditis (1% to 2%)
6. Syphilitic heart disease (less than 1%)
7. Other types (4% to 6%)

Space will be devoted in this chapter according to the relative importance of the seven cardiac diseases listed above. The chapter focuses on arteriosclerosis—its etiology, pathogenesis, complications, and treatment.

Arteriosclerosis

To most people, the term arteriosclerosis means hardening of the arteries. Scientifically, it is a chronic disease of the arteries characterized by abnormal thickening and hardening of the vessel walls resulting in a loss of elasticity and narrowing of the channel of blood flow. Some degree of arteriosclerosis occurs in all individuals middle-aged or older. Three variants of arteriosclerosis are found: *Atherosclerosis*, a stage of arteriosclerosis, is characterized by the deposition of soft fatty substances and fibrosis within the intimal lining which narrows the channels of arteries (in this chapter the terms arteriosclerosis and atherosclerosis will be used interchangeably). *Medial calcific sclerosis* is characterized by calcification of the media of muscular arteries. The third variant, *arteriolosclerosis*, involves the arterioles (the smallest arteries). The arteriolosclerotic endothelium thickens to block the channel and the walls thicken and harden.

Normal Artery Wall

Normal elastic arteries (Fig. 13-1) consist of three distinct layers. The *intima*, or innermost layer (lamina), consists of a narrow region bounded on the lumenal (channel) side by a single continuous layer of endothelial cells and bounded peripherally by a sheet of elastic fibers perforated by holes called the *internal elastica lamina*. The *media*, or middle layer consists of smooth muscle surrounded by collagen, small elastic fibers, and mucopolysaccharides. The *adventitia*, or outermost layer, consists chiefly of fibroblasts and smooth muscle cells and is separated from the media by a discontinuous sheet of elastic tissue, the *external elastica lamina*.

Pathogenesis

Despite tremendous research efforts, the exact pathogenesis of arteriosclerosis is not fully understood. Three different types of lesions appear at various ages. The *fatty streak* consists of a focal accumulation of subintimal smooth muscle cells surrounded by lipid. The streaks are present in the aorta of every child by age 10. The *fibrous plaque* is an advancing atherosclerotic lesion (Fig. 13-2). It consists primarily of an accumulation of intimal lipid-laden smooth muscle cells. The third type of lesion, called the *complicated* lesion, is a fibrotic plaque complicated by hemorrhage, calcification, cell necrosis, or mural thrombosis (Fig. 13-3). This type of lesion is associated with occlusive disease —thrombosis, for example.

The *intima* is the layer of artery cells principally involved in atherosclerosis, although secondary changes are occasionally found in the media. Injury to the arterial endothelium causes *platelets* to im-

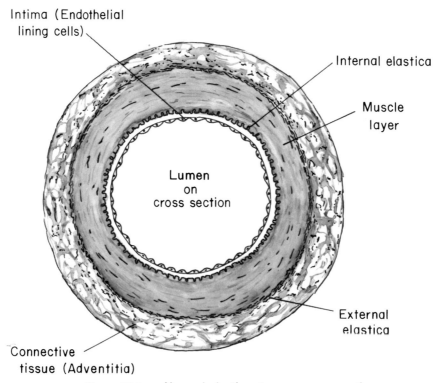

Figure 13-1   *Normal elastic artery on cross-section.*

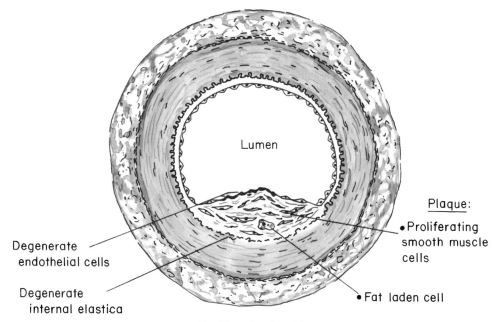

Figure 13-2   *Proliferative (early) atherosclerosis.*

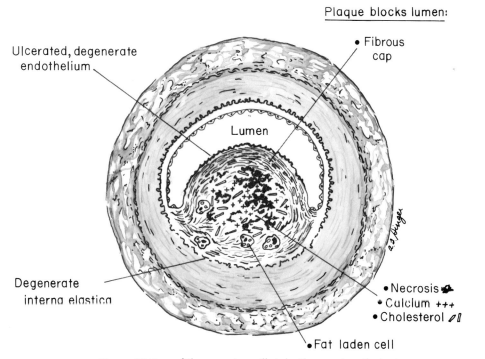

Figure 13-3   *Atheromatous (late) atherosclerotic lesion.*

mediately *adhere* to the intimal lining. This interruption in the intact endothelial barrier is followed not only by more platelet adherence but also by proliferation of smooth muscle cells.

Lipids from the plasma accumulate in macrophages and proliferating smooth muscle cells produce collagen, elastic fibers, and mucopolysaccharides. Together, the cells and lipids form an *atheromatous plaque* (Fig. 13-3). A fibrous cap gradually forms over the atheroma and necrosis ensues in the center of the plaque. Next, calcification begins. These processes result in marked narrowing of the lumen (channel) of the artery, which is eventually blocked. The condition can become complicated by hemorrhage within the plaque, or mural thrombosis can develop. When thrombosis occurs, necrosis (infarction) of the brain, heart, lung, toes, or other organs which lack an arterial blood supply ensues.

Risk Factors

The probability of occurrence of arteriosclerosis is associated with the presence of numerous risk factors listed in Table 13-1. The factors are listed in a mnemonic (remember "CAGED FEM HOPES") to assist you in recall. Inspection of the list reveals that many of the risk factors for arteriosclerosis are byproducts of our Western civilization.* Four of the factors stand out as severe risk factors: (a) elevated blood lipids, (b) obesity, (c) hypertension, and (d) cigarette smoking. When two or more risk factors are present, the risk of arteriosclerosis multiplies, and a dramatically increased frequency of the disorder is observed. Males are maximally vulnerable between the ages of 35 and 55, the so-called myocardial infarction-prone years. During this time in life the male:female incidence of myocardial infarction from coronary arteriosclerosis is 5:1. Beyond 55 years the ratio equalizes.

Inherited or *familial hypercholesterolemia* (FH) is a single gene mutation that produces both hyper-

*To the delight of epidemiologists the incidence of heart attack and stroke declined about 25% during the decade from 1963 to 1973. During this period, many persons, including myself, began to exercise regularly and eat less animal fat and butter.

Table 13-1
Multiple Risk Factors for Arteriosclerosis

Cigarette smoking*
Aged person
Gout
Elevated blood lipids* (hypercholesterol, triglycerides)
Diabetes mellitus
Family history
Ear lobe crease
Males
Hypertension*
Obesity*
Physical inactivity
Excessive stress (cardiac Type A personality)
Soft water

*Severe risk factors

cholesterolemia and arteriosclerosis. FH is an autosomal dominant disorder, occurring in 1 in 500 persons in the general population and in one in ten patients with myocardial infarction.

The universal feature of FH is elevation of a major cholesterol-carrying lipoprotein called low density lipoprotein (LDL). This lipoprotein normally functions to carry cholesterol from the liver and intestine to cells of the body. Cells normally have receptors for LDL and permit cholesterol to pass into them for use. The mutation for FH causes a deficiency of LDL receptor and thus cells are unable to receive and take up LDL and cholesterol. Consequently, the blood cholesterol is elevated and arteriosclerosis and myocardial infarction can ensue.

Homozygote FH patients (who have two mutant genes) have blood cholesterol above 600 mg/dl and sustain myocardial infarction at about age 15. Heterozygote FH patients (with one mutant gene) have cholesterol levels of about 400 mg/dl and sustain myocardial infarction at about age 45. By contrast, persons lacking the mutant gene have cholesterol below 200 mg/dl and are usually free of myocardial infarction. The importance of elevated blood cholesterol in the induction of arteriosclerosis in nonfamilial cases is poorly understood.

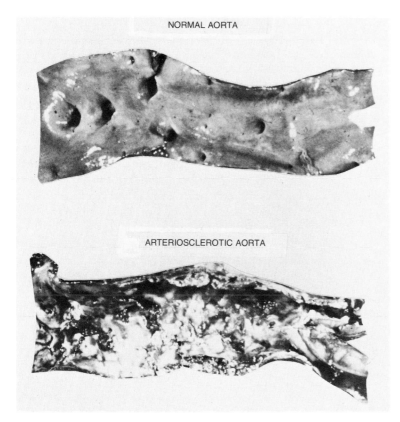

NORMAL AORTA

ARTERIOSCLEROTIC AORTA

Figure 13-4   *Normal aorta (upper) with smooth lining and openings where arteries branch. Only a few faint yellow atherosclerotic streaks are seen. By contrast, arteriosclerotic aorta (lower) has a rough lining and openings of arteries are nearly blocked.*

Areas Involved

The arterial tree is vulnerable where branching or tapering of arteries occurs. Severe atheromatous plaques develop in these sites possibly because a local suction or vacuum effect lifts the intima from the wall, injuring it as blood flows by when the heart contracts. Also, parts of the endothelial cells herniate (become displaced) into the subintimal region of the artery.

Arteriosclerosis occurs in many crucial areas: (a) in the coronary arteries (which supply the heart); (b) at the branching of the internal and external carotid arteries (which supply the brain); and (c) in the abdominal aorta where major arteries branch to supply the abdominal organs and lower extremities (Fig. 13-4).

Signs and Symptoms

The clinical signs and symptoms of arteriosclerosis are related to vascular insufficiency (ischemia) aris-

ing from a lack of oxygen (hypoxia) or ischemic injury to organs. The target organs (brain, heart, kidneys, feet) are damaged when the supply of oxygen is insufficient. For example, when the brain is subjected to brief periods of hypoxia, transient "blackout spells" result (see Chapter 21, Neurology and Neuropathology). Associated with the occurrence of these transient ischemic attacks is a loss of neurons in the brain and also of memory. When arteriosclerosis decreases the blood supply to the kidneys, toxic nitrogenous compounds build up in the blood. The accumulation of these compounds is referred to as azotemia (see Chapter 17, Urology and Renal Medicine). Coronary artery insufficiency leads to painful ischemia and injury to heart muscle (myocardial fibers).

The extremities, especially the legs and feet, can be seriously affected by arteriosclerosis. A symptom of arterial insufficiency in the legs is the sudden cramping of leg muscles upon walking (intermittent claudication). The pain results from the hypoxia and resulting ischemia in the exercised muscles. In addition, the affected individual often has dependent rubor (redness) of the legs when they are left to dangle over the edge of a bed or while standing. Severe complications of arterial insufficiency to the extremities are actual necrosis of tissues and gangrene (Fig. 13-5).

Complications

Complications of arteriosclerosis can cause misery, pain, and death. Progressive arterial narrowing (*stenosis*) can cause ischemia in organs by depriving them of circulating blood. Sudden *thrombosis* of an artery or *hemorrhage* into an arteriosclerotic plaque blocks the lumen causing total disruption of the blood flow to an organ. Another complication, *rupture* through the wall of an arteriosclerotic plaque, is a rare event except in small cerebral arteries.

The weakened arteriosclerotic wall can balloon outward forming an *aneurysm*. The thin walls of an aneurysm can *perforate* and blood can gush forth into body cavities. Another type of aneurysm, a *dissecting aneurysm*, occurs in arteriosclerotic aortas. Here, blood dissects beneath an arteriosclerotic plaque working downward between the muscular layers of the aorta. Arteries branching from the aorta to the gut and kidneys become blocked by the dissecting aneurysm and these organs undergo infarction. Immediate surgical intervention is generally required; the dissected aorta is sewn back together or a dacron graft is inserted to replace the dissected aorta.

Embolization of a thrombus from a plaque, another complication, blocks blood flow at a distal site. In embolization, a portion of thrombus breaks off and is carried in circulation as far as its size will allow and then it lodges, blocking the artery. Gangrene as shown in Figure 13-5 can result from embolization of a thrombus from the heart, aorta, or femoral arteries. It can also be caused by hemorrhage or thrombosis of an arteriosclerotic artery supplying the foot.

Coronary Artery Disease (Ischemic Heart Disease)

The term ischemic heart disease (coronary heart disease) refers to the cardiac disability, acute or

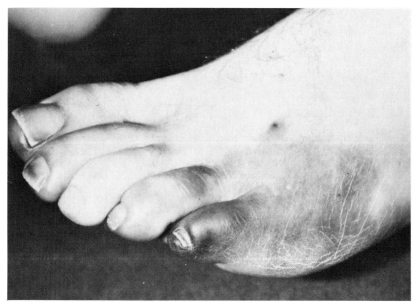

Figure 13-5   *Gangrene of toes arising from severe arteriosclerosis that caused ischemic necrosis.*

chronic, arising from reduction or arrest of blood supply to the myocardium in association with coronary arteriosclerosis. Coronary arteriosclerosis accounts for more than 99% of all ischemic heart disease. Pain in the chest upon physical exertion is a warning sign to persons with stenotic coronary arteries. Ischemic myocardial pain often occurs when the lumen of a coronary artery is narrowed to approximately 40% of the normal diameter.

Angina Pectoris

Angina pectoris is a clinical syndrome of ischemic heart disease signaled by a temporary sensation of pressure or a strangling sensation and/or acute pain beneath the sternum, which can radiate to the throat, neck, back, jaws, or arms. Angina is provoked variously by exertion, emotion, eating, or exposure to cold, and disappears upon removal of the exciting event or when nitroglycerine is given.

Invariably, moderate to severe arteriosclerosis of the coronary arteries is responsibe for angina pectoris. Although no infarction of myocardium is seen with angina pectoris, repeated attacks of increasing duration and severity can progress to a myocardial infarction (MI). The precise reason why angina pectoris occurs upon exertion is unknown; possibly the coronary arteries constrict and temporary ischemia results. Undoubtedly, exercise increases the demand for oxygen by the myocardium.

Myocardial Infarction

An MI generally develops from sudden blockage of all or some of the blood flow through the coronary arteries. (Myocardium can sustain anoxia for about 10 to 30 minutes; thereafter, myocardial necrosis usually ensues.) If the occlusion occurs gradually, collateral (alternate or detour) arteries provide circulation to the area normally supplied by the blocked vessel. Via collaterals, the myocardium is able to receive adequate oxygenation and nutrition. For decades it was thought that coronary occlusion preceded myocardial infarction, but evidence is accumulating to prove that in many instances coronary artery thrombosis actually occurs after infarction of the myocardium. However, moderate to severe coronary arteriosclerosis is present and reduced blood flow is responsible for the MI.

Clinical Findings

Typically, patients sustaining acute MI are middle-aged, obese, cigarette-smoking males. Upon moderate exertion or following a large meal, they experience a crushing, substernal pain. The pain often radiates from the heart down the left arm and is sustained for 30 minutes or more. The individual has great apprehension and sweating (diaphoresis) ensues. By contrast, the pain of angina pectoris is less severe, brief, and is brought on by exercise and relieved by rest.

Diagnosis

The typical clinical history described above, together with certain physical and specific laboratory findings substantiate a diagnosis of MI. Physical examination reveals a slightly elevated temperature (37.8 C), a rapid or irregular heart beat and cardiac shock may be noted. Signs of shock are a weak, rapid pulse, decreased blood pressure, and cold, clammy extremities. An electrocardiogram (EKG) usually reveals inversion of T waves and alteration of the S-T segment (Fig. 13-6). These findings reflect myocardial injury. The injured myocardium also releases enzymes into the circulation and these can be detected in the patient's serum (Fig. 13-6). In summary, the patient's clincal history, physical status, EKG, and laboratory studies document the presence and extent of MI.

Pathology

The pathologic state of the heart of a person dying of MI will depend upon: (a) the coronary artery blocked, (b) the size and location of the resulting MI, and (c) the length of time from the onset of MI to death. The right coronary artery supplies the bulk of the heart muscle (left ventricle and posterior interventricular septum) in 50% of persons. The right and left coronary arteries contribute equal

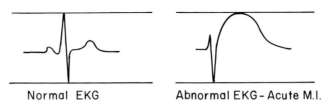

Normal EKG   Abnormal EKG – Acute M.I.

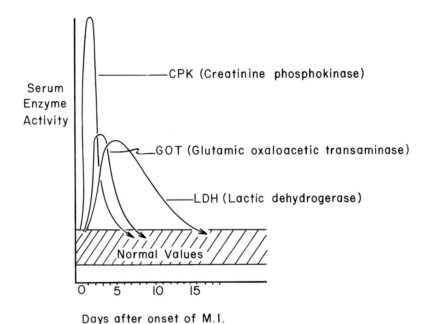

Figure 13-6   *Typical changes in the electrocardiogram (ECG) and elevated serum enzymes in a patient with myocardial infarction (MI).*

amounts of blood to the heart in 30% of persons, and 20% show left coronary artery predominance. Myocardial infarction usually occurs when the predominant artery is partially blocked, not when a nondominant artery is blocked. The location of the MI is most often in the posterior part of the left ventricle (Fig. 13-7).

The most severe arteriosclerosis is generally found in the coronary arteries 3 to 4 cm from their origin off the aorta. The left coronary artery is most often severely involved. *Coronary thrombosis* is found in less than 25% of cases of MI. In other cases, hemorrhage within an arteriosclerotic plaque blocks the lumen or severe coronary artery stenosis is responsible.

Sequential changes in the infarcted myocardium determined by examination at autopsy indicate when the MI occurred. Initially, the area of MI is pale (normally myocardium is red-brown), then it becomes gray-brown, and by the fourth day the central portion of the infarct becomes yellow-brown and soft and is rimmed by a red hemorrhagic border. Two weeks later, necrotic muscle is replaced by pink, vascularized scar tissue.

The microscopic appearance of the myocardium also varies with time. During the first 12 hours following MI the only change seen microscopically is elongated and wavy myocardial fibers ("chewing gum sign"), and some of the striations of the myocardial fibers disappear. At 12 to 24 hours, neu-

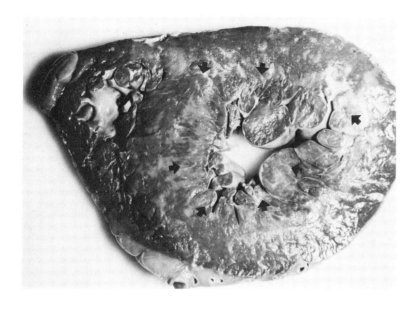

Figure 13-7   *Heart cut on cross-section with acute myocardial infarction. Gray mottled areas had infarcted* (arrows).

trophils infiltrate the necrotic myocardial fibers (Fig. 13-8). For several days thereafter, neutrophils and macrophages clean away the dead myocardium. By day 12, fibroblasts are seen producing collagen fibers to form a scar. Several months later, a well formed scar composed of collagen is seen. Persons who survive MI have scar tissue in their hearts for the rest of their lives.

Prognosis and Complications

Recognition of signs and symptoms of complications associated with acute MI can provide valuable prognostic information (Table 13-2). An individual sustaining an acute MI should not attempt to continue walking or working because the damaged heart can develop *arrhythmias* (irregular contractions) and cease to function. Heart failure ensues when infarcted heart muscle cannot pump the blood needed for walking. Of those dying of an acute MI, 85% die within 24 hours and most succumb to MI during the first few hours. They should be brought to an intensive coronary care unit where complications can be prevented and treated. An estimated 20% to 30% reduction in mortality has resulted from these units. Bed rest is prescribed and the individual is monitored with an EKG, pulse rate, blood pressure, and other studies to detect com-

plications. Morphine is given to relieve pain and oxygen is administered to assist in oxygenating the blood and myocardium.

Sudden death occurs in 25% of patients with MI due to arrhythmias that prevent proper pumping of blood by the heart. Improved management of arrhythmia is the significant treatment that can be offered to persons with MI. The arrhythmia of greatest concern is cardiac arrest or *asystole* (failure of the ventricle to contract). Signs of cardiac arrest include sudden loss of consciousness, absent pulses, ashen cyanosis, dilated pupils, and gasping or apnea (absence of breathing). Asystole is treated by closed chest cardiac massage, artificial ventilation, and electrical stimulation. The salvage rate of patients with asystole is low.

Shock

Shock occurs when cardiac output fails to satisfy the oxygen requirements of tissues. If cardiac pumping insufficiently circulates blood through the vascular system the disorder is termed *cardiogenic shock*. Likewise, blood circulation can become inadequate. Inadequate blood circulation may be caused by noncardiac disorders, such as blood loss or depletion of blood volume. With an acute drop in blood volume, the blood vessels are simply

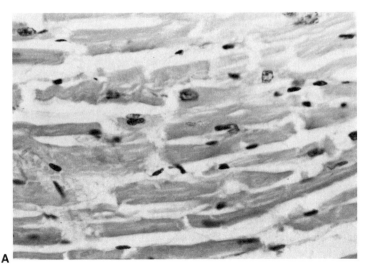

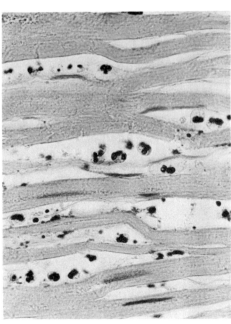

A

B

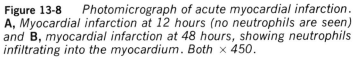

Figure 13-8   *Photomicrograph of acute myocardial infarction. A, Myocardial infarction at 12 hours (no neutrophils are seen) and B, myocardial infarction at 48 hours, showing neutrophils infiltrating into the myocardium. Both × 450.*

not filled. This is termed *hemorrhagic* or *hypovolemic shock*. The other type of shock is termed *vascular shock* (also called toxic or septic shock) and arises from marked vasodilatation. The vasodilatation can be caused, for example, by bacterial septicemia from *E coli* which releases endotoxin which is toxic to the venules.

Regardless of the etiology of shock, the pathophysiologic problem is inadequate perfusion of tissue with blood. Low cardiac output or shock is characterized by hypotension, oliguria (decreased urine output—less than 30 ml/hr in adult), cold and maybe clammy and cyanosed extremities, and impaired consciousness. At the conclusion of this chapter cardiovascular emergencies and their treatment are surveyed.

The impact of shock can be profound; it varies in different organs depending on the oxygen requirements of the organ. Only three to five minutes of cerebral ischemia can be tolerated before permanent brain damage sets in. The brain requires abundant oxygen and glucose, or neurons die. The myocardium can sustain ischemia for roughly ten to thirty minutes before the cells die. Kidneys, when deprived of blood supply for prolonged periods, undergo acute tubular necrosis. The liver and mucosal lining of the alimentary tract are also vulnerable to the impact of shock. To a lesser extent other organs are damaged by shock.

Congestive Heart Failure

Another major acute complication of MI is *congestive heart failure (CHF)*. Over one half of patients with MI develop CHF and in 30% it becomes moderately to extensively severe. Congestive heart failure can occur with cardiogenic shock—the individual will be hypotensive (systolic blood pressure of 80 mm Hg or lower) and will have cold, clammy, moist skin, cyanosis, and a decreased urine output.

Other Complications

Another complication is the formation, after several days to a couple of weeks, of a thrombus on the damaged wall of the myocardium (*mural thrombus*). Major problems arise when mural thrombi break off and embolize to the kidneys, spleen, extremities, or brain. For example, a cerebrovascular accident can suddenly occur in a person convalescing from an MI when embolization arises.

The myocardium can rupture at about six to eight days after MI because neutrophils and macrophages infiltrate the MI site and digest the dead

Table 13-2
Prognostic Classification of Acute Myocardial Infarction*

Class	Complication	Mortality†
I	No heart failure	8%
II	Mild to moderate heart failure	16%
III	Severe heart failure (pulmonary edema)	38%
IV	Cardiogenic shock	81%

*Modified from Killip, T. and Kimball, J. T. 1967. Treatment of myocardial infarction in a coronary care unit. *Am. J. Cardiol.* 20:457–464.
†Note that the mortality approximately doubles from one class to the next highest.

myocardial fibers; the wall of the injured heart becomes weak and fibroblasts have not yet formed a tough scar. When the heart ruptures, blood flows into and fills the pericardial sac. The blood pressure builds up in the pericardial sac when it is filled with blood and this obstructs the filling of the heart (cardiac tamponade). Heart failure rapidly occurs.

An *aneurysm*, a thin bulging of the infarcted myocardium, can occur and cause the heart to become an inefficient pump. Other individuals develop *post myocardial infarction syndrome* consisting of fever, chest pain, pericarditis, pleuritis, and pneumonitis. Acute MI can progressively extend into adjacent myocardium. Finally, the psychological impact of acute MI on a person should not be overlooked: A fearful person may become a "cardiac cripple." People can sustain "ego infarcts" as a result of life-threatening events and they often live in constant fear of having another MI. Table 13-3 summarizes the possible complications of MI (mnemonic—"AS PAP HEART").

Hypertensive Cardiovascular Disease

The American Heart Association has defined hypertension as blood pressure above 140/90 mm Hg. Approximately 15% of all adults in the United States are hypertensive by this criterion and 30% of persons above age 50 are hypertensive.

Hypertension is not a disease, but a sign of a disease. A pathologic constriction of the arterial tree elevates the blood pressure. Hypertension aggravates and accelerates atherogenesis and, therefore, complications in hypertensive individuals often arise because of arteriosclerosis.

Primary Hypertension

In 90% of patients hypertension has no identifiable cause and is categorized as primary (essential, idiopathic, benign) hypertension. Several observations suggest that heredity and environment are key factors in hypertension. Hypertension is more common in certain families and races. For instance, black persons have a higher incidence of hypertension than other races. Although hypertension occurs twice more frequently in females than in males, women tolerate it better, suffering fewer complications than do men. Stress is also a key factor in inducing hypertension. Hypertension is less common in countries with rural, low-stress life styles, and where diets are low in salt. Obesity and diabetes mellitus, to a lesser extent, are associated with hypertension.

Secondary Hypertension

Although in most persons (90%) with hypertension there is no identifiable cause, approximately 10%

Table 13-3
Complications of Myocardial Infarction

Asystole and death
Shock
Post MI syndrome
Arrhythmia
Psychological—"cardiac cripple"
Heart failure
Extension of infarction
Aneurysm
Rupture of heart (cardiac tamponade)
Thrombus formation with embolization

of cases have a definable cause. These causes are: (a) renal, (b) endocrine, and (c) coarctation (constriction of a segment) of aorta. Renal hypertension occurs either due to narrowing (stenosis) of one renal artery or damage to the renal tissue itself. The stenosis of the renal artery can be surgically corrected and reversal of renal hypertension generally occurs. But when kidneys are damaged by chronic infection or immune responses (such as chronic pyelonephritis or glomerulonephritis) the ensuing hypertension is not reversible except by renal transplantation.

Endocrine causes of hypertension result from either excessive thyroid activity (hyperthyroidism) or disorders of the adrenal glands. For example, when the adrenal glands are overproducing the hormone aldosterone (from an adenoma), sodium is retained by the kidneys. The sodium apparently causes arterioles to constrict and blood pressure rises. Another adrenal tumor, pheochromocytoma, produces epinephrine which constricts arterioles. Finally, Cushing's syndrome (hypercortisonism) causes hypertension (see Chapter 12, Endocrine and Metabolic Disorders). Virtually all hypertension caused by abnormalities of the adrenal glands is correctable by either resecting the adrenal tumor or by drugs which correct the hormonal dysfunction.

Coarctation (constriction) of the aorta is caused by a congenital fibrous constriction (stenosis) of the aorta just beyond the exit of the left subclavian artery from the aorta (see Chapter 3, Development and Birth Defects). Coarctation of the aorta causes hypertension only in arteries arising proximal to the constriction. Hence, blood pressure is increased in the arms, head, and neck but is normal in the abdominal cavity and lower extremities. (The blood pressure in the legs is weaker than in the arms.) This form of hypertension can be corrected surgically.

Pathophysiology

Hormonal Dysfunction   The pathophysiologic basis for vasoconstriction occurring in hypertension is shown in Figure 13-9. The renin-angioten-

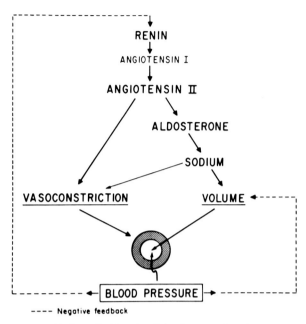

Figure 13-9   *Pathophysiologic mechanisms responsible for essential hypertension. (From Laragh, J. H.: Modern system for treating high blood pressure based on renin profiling and vasoconstriction-volume analysis: a primary role for beta blocking drugs such as propranolol. Am J Med 61:797, 1976.)*

sion-aldosterone hormone system regulates arterial blood pressure and sodium balance. *Renin*, an enzyme secreted by the kidney, reacts with *angiotensin I* in the blood and the latter is converted in the lung to *angiotensin II* which vasoconstricts the arteriovasculature, increasing the blood pressure. Many patients with primary hypertension will have raised renin levels which can be measured in their blood or urine.

Aldosterone, a hormone produced by adrenals, causes renal retention of sodium. This expands plasma volume, raising the blood pressure. Aldosterone levels may be variously raised in the blood of patients with primary hypertension. It is markedly elevated in cases of adenoma of the adrenal.

Organ Damage   Three organs are damaged by prolonged hypertension: (a) the heart, (b) the brain, and (c) the kidneys. If hypertension is not diagnosed and treated with antihypertensive drugs, the individual can "wear out" (cardiac failure), "blow

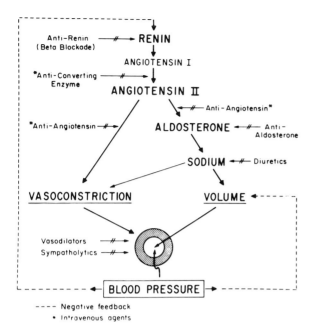

Figure 13-10 *Alternative approaches to medical (drugs) treatment of essential hypertension. (From Laragh, J. H.: Modern system for treating high blood pressure based on renin profiling and vasocontriction-volume analysis: a primary role for beta blocking drugs such as propranolol. Am J Med 61:797, 1976.)*

out" (cerebrovascular accident) or "run out" (renal failure).

Mild or moderate hypertension (95/100 to 100/165 mm Hg) can be tolerated for long periods (from one to four decades) before damage to the heart, kidneys, or brain occurs. Elevated blood pressure increases the workload on the myocardium. To compensate for the increased work, the myocardial fibers undergo hypertrophy (see Chapter 4, Adaptation, Injury, and Death of Cells). Further compensation for the increased workload occurs with elongation of the myocardial fibers (Starling's law). The elongated fibers contract more efficiently, but eventually the overburdened heart fails. Prolonged hypertension causes the heart weight to increase by from 25% to 100% above normal. The patient whose heart is shown in Figure 13-7 had hypertension (untreated) for 30 years and died of MI.

One-fourth of patients with hypertension die of congestive heart failure when their heart decompensates. An additional 10% die of direct effects of coronary heart disease. Multiple minute scars are seen within the heart muscle and acute myocardial infarction can develop. An additional 15% of patients die of cerebrovascular accidents; small blood vessels become damaged by the prolonged hypertension, and hemorrhage can ensue within the substance of the brain (see Chapter 21, Neurology and Neuropathology).

Arteriolosclerosis of the kidneys can complicate hypertension. Twenty percent of hypertensive patients die of renal failure from hypertension. A small number (roughly 5%) develop malignant hypertension. This severe form of hypertension occurs when the diastolic pressure reaches about 140-150 mm Hg. The pressure causes extensive necrosis of the arterioles and renal tissue, with renal failure resulting.

Treatment

Surgical The 10% of patients who have secondary hypertension usually require surgical treatment. By contrast, primary hypertension is treated with various drugs.

Medical (Drugs) There are presently about 50 antihypertensive drugs available in the United States. Depending on the cause, severity, and responsiveness of the patient, various drugs are used (Fig. 13-10).

Diuretic administration is the first step and the cornerstone of almost all antihypertensive therapy. Elimination of excess sodium (which reduces plasma volume) decreases the blood pressure of many patients.

If the patient is found to have elevated renin levels, an *antirenin drug* (propranolol hydrochloride) is usually given to prevent vasoconstriction. Other possible approaches with drugs which block sympathetic nerve impulses to the arterioles are illustrated in Figure 13-10.

Treatment of hypertension prolongs life by preventing the complications that can accompany this condition. The lowering of blood pressure by drugs reverses some arteriosclerotic lesions. In recent years, the number of individuals dying with congestive heart failure due to hypertensive heart disease has decreased dramatically due to successful treatment. Weight reduction reduces hyper tension.

Congestive Heart Failure

A serious consequence of most severe heart diseases is congestive heart failure (CHF, cardiac failure, or cardiac decompensation). This condition develops when the myocardium cannot pump blood at a rate necessary to meet the oxygen requirements of tissues. Cardiac failure generally arises from one of three factors: (a) decreased capacity of the myocardium to contract; (b) excessive blood pressure; or (c) excessive pumping of large volumes of blood by the heart.

Ordinarily, compensatory mechanisms like those described above (hypertrophy and elongation of myocardial fibers) develop whenever CHF begins to occur. When compensatory mechanisms fail, CHF ensues.

Signs and Symptoms

Shortness of breath (SOB, dyspnea) upon physical exertion is a common complaint of persons with CHF. Later, SOB is present even at rest. The individual with CHF has to sleep in a sitting position (orthopnea) to facilitate pumping of blood by the heart. When severe cyanosis occurs because oxygenation of blood is inadequate, the individual with CHF often has an enlarged liver and swollen ankles (Fig. 13-11). When cerebral hypoxia occurs the individual becomes irritable or drowsy; stupor and coma can be an end result of CHF.

By convention, heart failure is described as either left heart failure or right heart failure. The vast majority (about 95%) of CHF arises from failure of the left ventricle to deliver blood. Right heart failure occurs most often from left-sided CHF and occasionally due to pulmonary hypertension.

CHF is usually caused by: (a) coronary arteriosclerosis; (b) hypertension; or (c) heart valve disorders (such as rheumatic heart disease, calcific aortic stenosis, congenital heart disease, or bacterial endocarditis). With CHF, the left ventricle dilates and softens. A life-threatening complication of CHF is pulmonary edema.

Pulmonary Edema

Pulmonary edema is caused by excessive pressure of blood within the pulmonary capillary circulation. Normally, pressure in the capillaries in the lungs is about 7 mm of Hg and increases four-fold to approximately 29 mm of Hg during CHF. When the pressure reaches this magnitude, fluid exits from the capillaries and passes into alveoli. The fluid-filled alveoli cannot fill with air. The fluid becomes foamy as respiratory movements churn and mix air with the fluid.

Persons with pulmonary edema become cyanotic. The lungs can become so filled with pulmonary edema that foamy fluid may actually bubble from the patient's mouth. Fluid can pass into the pleural space (pleural effusion). In summary, symptoms of pulmonary edema include SOB, cyanosis, and marked apprehension. The urine output of the person is also often reduced.

Treatment When pulmonary edema has resulted from CHF, the condition is considered a medical emergency and requires immediate therapy. The blood volume must be rapidly decreased to ease the workload on the failing heart. Tourniquets are applied and periodically rotated on three of the four extremities to decrease the circulating blood volume the heart is required to pump. Digitalis is given to improve the efficiency of myocardium contraction, diuretics rid the body of excessive fluids, and O_2 is given under positive pressure by a respirator. When these measures are given sufficiently early, patients lives can be saved, otherwise they drown in their own fluids. The person loses up to 5 kg of fluid in a day while eliminating the edema.

Right-sided CHF

The major cause of right-sided CHF is not from primary problems in the lung, but from congestion of blood flow in the lungs secondary to left-sided CHF. Rarely, however, pure right-sided heart fail-

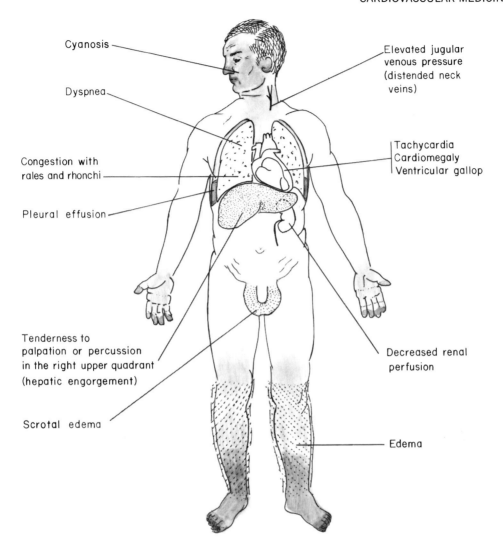

Cyanosis

Dyspnea

Congestion with
rales and rhonchi

Pleural effusion

Tenderness to
palpation or percussion
in the right upper quadrant
(hepatic engorgement)

Scrotal edema

Elevated jugular
venous pressure
(distended neck
veins)

Tachycardia
Cardiomegaly
Ventricular gallop

Decreased renal
perfusion

Edema

Figure 13-11   *Typical appearance of a patient with congestive heart failure.*

ure occurs from *cor pulmonale* arising from severe pulmonary disease or pulmonary artery abnormalities. The right ventricle must work excessively to push blood in vessels in the lung tissue. The right ventricle can dilate after first undergoing compensatory hypertrophy.

Right-sided CHF usually causes only minor pulmonary congestion and pulmonary edema, but marked engorgement of the veins in the liver and intestinal tract is sometimes seen. The hallmark of right-or left-sided CHF is the development of edema in gravity-dependent portions of the body such as the ankles. The edema, however, can become generalized (anasarca). The differential diagnosis of edema is described in Chapter 17, Urology and Renal Medicine.

Other Major Heart Diseases

We have mentioned that coronary heart disease accounts for 80% and hypertensive heart disease for

9% of cardiac deaths. Rheumatic heart disease, congenital heart disease, bacterial endocarditis, syphilitic heart disease, viral myocarditis and primary myocardial abnormalities (cardiomyopathy) account for the remaining 11% of cardiac deaths. Four major cardiac disorders have infectious etiologies: rheumatic heart disease, bacterial endocarditis, syphilitic heart disease, and viral myocarditis.

Rheumatic Heart Disease (RHD)

Acute RHD (rheumatic fever) results from an altered immune response to Group A Beta hemolytic streptococcus bacteria. Characteristically, the disease strikes children aged 4 to 8 about two weeks following a streptococcal pharyngitis. The onset can be abrupt, with fever, tachycardia, and painful swollen joints. Because other diseases may mimic rheumatic fever, diagnostic criteria have been established for rheumatic fever (Table 13-4). The clinical findings in patients with rheumatic fever are variable, so at least two major or one major and two minor criteria must be present.

The most feared lesion of rheumatic fever is carditis. The myocardium can become inflamed because antibodies to streptococci cross react with myocardial fibers and the smooth muscle in the intimal lining of blood vessels. This provokes an acute inflammatory response to neutrophils. Later, lymphocytes, plasma cells, and macrophages infiltrate the affected area.

Rheumatic carditis develops in about one half of patients with rheumatic fever. All three layers of the heart—endocardium, myocardium, and epicardium—can be inflamed (pancarditis). When the epicardium is inflamed (pericarditis) a friction rub is heard with a stethoscope.

When the endocardium is inflamed (endocarditis), the heart valves are also affected. In 50% of instances the mitral valve alone is inflamed; in the remaining cases both the mitral and aortic valves are simultaneously inflamed.

Complications When RHD endocarditis heals, severe deformities of the heart valves can remain. For example, the chordae tendineae can become shortened (Fig. 13-12) and the heart valves become

Table 13-4
Criteria for Diagnosis of Rheumatic Fever

Major	Minor
Carditis	Clinical history
Polyarthritis	Previous rheumatic fever
Choreiform movements	Pain in joints
Specific skin lesions	Fever

incompetent. Either stenosis (narrowing) of the outlet occurs (Fig. 13-13) or the valve fails to completely close. The turbulence caused by blood rushing through a deformed heart valve causes a heart murmur which can be heard with a stethoscope. The incompetent valve becomes inefficient in directing the flow of blood; the heart then works excessively to pump blood. CHF can arise as a complication of the incompetent or stenotic heart valve. CHF due to RHD usually develops in middle-aged individuals.

The deformed, scarred valve provides a site where bacteria from the blood can stick and begin growing on the valve. Thus, individuals who have had RHD are at increased risk for developing bacterial endocarditis. (Fig. 13-12).

Recurrence of RHD, with further damage to the heart, can develop years after an acute episode if the individual is reinfected with streptococci. Penicillin in maintenance doses is given for the rest of life to prevent such recurrences.

Replacement of defective heart valves with mechanical valves permits a person who has had RHD to have a normal life span. During the past two decades a greater than 90% decline in deaths due to RHD has occurred in the United States. Also a decline in incidence of acute RHD has occurred and this is attributed to a higher standard of living and better medical care.

Table 13-5
Laboratory Findings of Rheumatic Fever

Antibodies to streptococcus in serum
Positive throat cultures for Group A B streptococcus
Leukocytosis and documentation of inflammation
EKG abnormality
Raised erythrocyte sedimentation rate

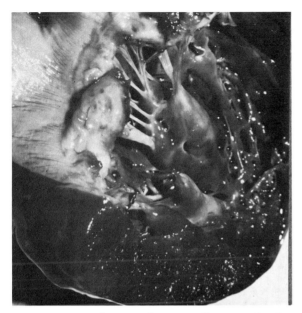

Figure 13-12   *Rheumatic heart disease affecting mitral valve. The chorda tendineae and valve were damaged by inflammation and repair. The valve was infected (bacterial endocarditis had occurred).*

Bacterial Endocarditis

Individuals with deformed heart valves from RHD or congenital heart failure (see Chapter 3, Development and Birth Defects, for discussion of CHD) are predisposed to developing bacterial infections. Clinically, a person with endocarditis shows signs of: (a) infection (fever, weakness, and leukocytosis); (b) a heart murmur that sounds different from day to day; and (c) embolization of bits of bacteria and heart valves to distant sites in the blood stream. These particles embolize to the brain causing stroke, or pass to the kidney causing pain and hematuria (bloody urine). Petechial hemorrhages in the skin, eyelids, or fingernails can also be seen from embolization. Embolization to the coronary arteries, although rare, can cause acute MI. If the process is extensive in the heart, or if the valve becomes incompetent, CHF ensues.

Pathogenesis   Malformed or damaged heart valves provide a surface upon which bacteria or even fungi can grow. Implantation of bacteria on a normal heart valve occurs, however, in 30% of

the cases where no previous valvular deformity is is found. Surprisingly, even brushing of teeth causes a transient bacteremia. Chewing of food and extraction of teeth also shower bacteria into the blood stream. Bacteria arising from the genitourinary tract also can infect the heart: Catheterizing a urinary bladder, cystoscopy, or the birth of a baby can also shower bacteria into the blood. Likewise, cardiac catheterization or intravenous therapy can infect deformed heart valves.

The bacterium most commonly responsible for acute bacterial endocarditis is *Staphylococcus aureus*. Other pyogenic organisms such as *D streptococcus*, *Haemophilus influenzae*, and *E coli* can be cultured. The persistent form, subacute bacterial endocarditis, is usually caused by *Streptococcus viridans*. A diagnosis of endocarditis is made by noting fever, changing heart murmur, and growth of bacteria in blood cultures.

Pathology   The heart valve (Fig. 13-12 and 13-13) affected by bacterial endocarditis is red and

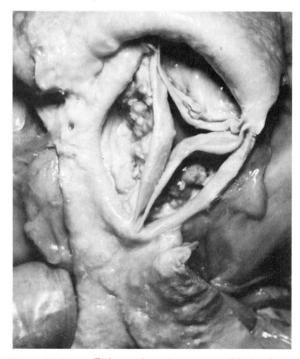

Figure 13-13   *This aortic valve was unable to close (incompetent and stenotic) because of injury from rheumatic heart disease.*

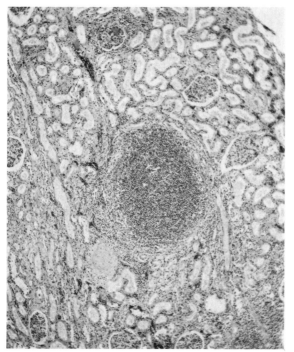

Figure 13-14 *Photomicrograph of kidney with microabscess (center), which occurred because of embolization of bacteria from the heart valve shown in Figure 13-12.*

thickened because thrombi form from fibrin, platelets, neutrophils, and bacteria. Within the nearby heart muscle, microabscesses may be seen arising from microemboli. Likewise, infarcts caused by embolization can occur in the spleen, liver, kidney (Fig. 13-14), and brain.

Prognosis and Treatment   The cure rate for the subacute form of endocarditis is approximately 90% but only 25% for the acute form. Acute bacterial endocarditis produces the most severe destruction of the heart valves, and heart failure in these cases is common. Treatment requires high concentrations of intravenous antibiotics. Surgical resection of the infected valves and insertion of artificial heart valves can save the person's life when antibiotic therapy fails.

Syphilitic Cardiovascular Disease

Details of the pathogenesis of syphilis were described in Chapter 7, Infectious Diseases. Only

features pertinent to the cardiovascular system are described here. Three stages of syphilis appear after several decades if treatment with penicillin is not given. The stages are primary syphilis (chancre), within one to two weeks; secondary syphilis (rash), within 9 to 90 days; and one to three decades later, tertiary syphilis (damage to the brain and aorta).

Tertiary syphilis can severely damage brain and spinal cord, and psychosis and neurological impairment result. Another target organ of tertiary syphilis is the ascending aorta. Here, the small blood vessels (vasa vasorum) nourishing the aorta become infected and chronic inflammation (aortitis) develops. The inflamed wall of the ascending aorta becomes fibrotic and weak, then dilates (aneurysm). The opening to the coronary arteries from the aorta can become blocked (stenotic) by the aortitis and MI may develop. The tertiary lesions of syphilis in the nervous and cardiovascular systems are irreversible. Prevention, early detection, and treatment of syphilis by penicillin effect the only means for coping with this disease.

Viral Myocarditis

A fourth, and rare, type of infectious heart disease is caused by viruses. The fetus is especially vulnerable to infection by coxsackievirus which can induce congenital heart disease (see Chapter 3, Development and Birth Defects). Other viruses, including rubella, Epstein-Barr virus, and influenza, can also cause myocarditis in persons of various ages. Virally infected myocardium becomes edematous and numerous lymphocytes infiltrate the heart. No definitive treatment is available for viral myocarditis. Some individuals with viral myocarditis succumb to CHF, but most spontaneously heal. Viral myocarditis is much less frequent a problem than are other types of heart disease, and no definitive treatment is available.

Thrombophlebitis

The assumption of a vertical posture by Homo sapiens has produced a pressure barrier of 100 mm of Hg in the veins of the legs. Veins carry blood to the heart under low pressure by the sucking action of respiration and pumping from contracting skeletal muscles. The skeletal muscle pump is especially important in moving blood against gravity in the lower extremities. It reduces the pressure from 100 mm Hg to 0 to 5 mm Hg.

Most veins in the lower extremities that are more than 2 mm in diameter are equipped with valves which prevent the backflow of blood within the vessel. These valves direct the flow of blood towards the heart. The veins become diseased because of increased venous pressure, injury, or infection.

Thrombophlebitis is the term used to describe inflammation in the wall of a vein. We will discuss the pathogenesis of thrombophlebitis and the complications of: (a) varicose veins, (b) thrombosis, and (c) pulmonary embolism.

Clinical Findings

Pain and swelling in an extremity (generally lower) are the cardinal signs of both superficial and deep thrombophlebitis. The symptoms and signs particular to superficial thrombophlebitis are the sudden development of throbbing pain in a circumscribed area of skin, erythema, localized subcutaneous swelling, and extreme tenderness (Fig. 13-15). A tender cord is often palpable, especially when thrombosis occurs in a superficial varicose vein.

The symptoms of localized deep thrombophlebitis can be progressive calf heaviness, swelling, and sudden aching pain on slight movement of calf muscles. A physical sign of phlebitis is Homans' sign—deep calf pain on dorsiflexion of the foot which stretches the inflamed veins in the muscle.

Etiology

Three factors can precipitate thrombophlebitis: (a) local changes in veins such as intimal damage; (b) venous stasis (stagnation of flow); and (c) increased blood coagulation. The most important factor predisposing an individual to thrombophlebitis is venous stasis. Patients immobilized in bed as a result of injuries, burns, infectious diseases, cancer, dehydration, shock, heart failure, myocardial infarction, anemia, obesity, pregnancy, or surgical procedures, are at high risk for developing throm-

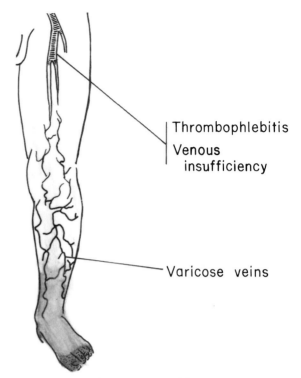

Figure 13-15   *Thrombophlebitis. A thrombus has formed in the common iliac and femoral vein. Dilated (varicose) veins are seen in the leg and the leg is swollen.*

bophlebitis and complicating pulmonary embolism. Such patients have both stasis of venous blood and increased coagulability of the blood.

Immobilization permits blood to pool (stasis) in the deep veins of the leg. Platelets then stick to injured, inflamed veins and a thrombus forms. The thrombus becomes firmly attached to the wall of the vein when fibroblasts and capillaries grow into the clot and "organize" it. If the clot does not become organized, the clot may embolize.

Complications

The major complications of thrombophlebitis are *varicose veins* (usually in superficial veins), *thrombosis,* or thrombosis with *pulmonary embolism* (usually arising from deep venous thrombophlebitis).

Varicose Veins   Varicose veins are the most common disorder presented to general surgeons.

About 20% of men and 40% of women over age 30 have them and beyond age 50, 40% of men and 60% of women are affected in the United States. The dilatation that characterizes varicose veins results from incompetency of the valves of the veins. Superficial veins of the greater saphenous system along the leg and thigh are vulnerable to valvular incompetence because they are not supported by skeletal muscles (Fig. 13-15).

Valvular incompetence results from two conditions (a) as a complication of thrombophlebitis, or (b) from increased abdominal pressure. The inflammation of thrombophlebitis causes the walls of the veins to become fibrotic, in turn causing the valves to fail to close off the flow of blood in veins away from the heart. Increased intraabdominal pressure is another mechanism that could be responsible for varicose veins (Fig. 13-16). This type of pressure is excessive in persons with varicose veins when they are compared to those with normal veins. Complications of varicose veins are common

—ulceration, hemorrhage, dermatitis, and inflammation occur in advanced cases. An *ulcer*, characteristically over the bony prominences at the ankles, is a chronic problem for many persons (Fig. 13-17). Almost invariably these ulcers appear directly over a varicose vein. The varicose ulcer is due to a poor blood supply in the skin overlying the bony prominences. Varicosities can also *rupture* and considerable hemorrhage occurs without warning. Varicose *dermatitis* gives the skin a leathery, scaly, red appearance. This itchy lesion is usually located on the lower third of the leg. Thrombophlebitis frequently occurs with varicose veins.

Thrombosis   A thrombus (blood clot) can complicate thrombophlebitis. A thrombus is composed of fibrin, platelets, and erythrocytes and blocks the flow of blood through a vessel. Thrombi either become lysed (dissolved) by fibrinolytic enzymes in the plasma or they become organized when fibroblasts and capillaries grow into them from the

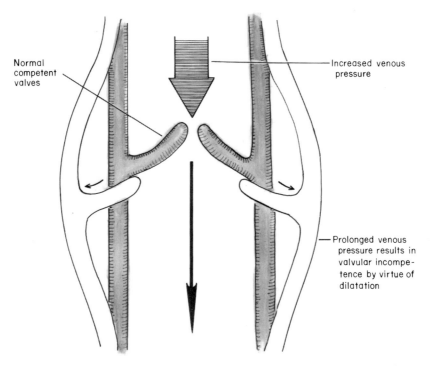

Normal competent valves

Increased venous pressure

Prolonged venous pressure results in valvular incompetence by virtue of dilatation

Figure 13-16   *Pathogenesis of varicose veins. Increased intraabdominal pressure dilates the vein and makes valves incompetent. Prior phlebitis may have also damaged the valves.*

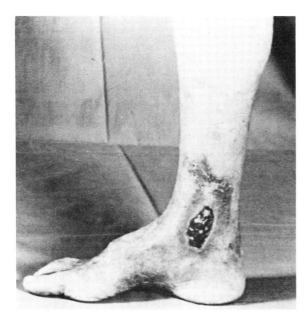

Figure 13-17   *Ulcer of ankle resulting from venous insufficiency in a person with thrombophlebitis. (Courtesy Medicom.)*

blood vessel wall. Following a thrombus, anoxia (absence of O_2) and necrosis (cell death) of tissues distal to the occluded vessel can occur.

Thrombosis is responsible for the majority of all deaths in the United States. The major types of thrombosis include: (a) coronary artery thrombosis with myocardial infarction; (b) cerebral arterial thrombosis or cerebral vascular hemorrhage and infarction; and (c) deep venous thrombosis with pulmonary embolism and infarction.

Pulmonary Embolism   Pulmonary embolism is the fourth leading cause of sudden death. Careful postmortem examinations reveal the incidence to be in excess of 25%. An *embolus* is a thrombus which becomes dislodged from one vessel and travels to another vessel where it becomes lodged, blocking the flow of blood. The most commonly occurring embolus starts as a thrombus in a vein deep in the leg. The thrombus breaks away from the vessel wall and travels through the inferior vena cava to the right ventricle, the pulmonary artery, and finally into the lung. There, pulmonary infarction can develop (Fig. 13-18).

The classical clinical findings for pulmonary embolus are: (a) sudden onset of constricting chest pain, (b) dyspnea (S.O.B.), (c) anxiety, (d) shock, and (e) cyanosis. Some patients with pulmonary embolus cough up bloody sputum (hemoptysis), have tachycardia (excessive rapidity in the beating of the heart), and tenderness of the chest wall. Shortness of breath, fever, and leukocytosis complete the clinical picture of pulmonary emboli. X-ray studies confirm the diagnosis of pulmonary embolus, with or without infarction.

When thrombosis occurs, collateral arteries can provide alternate routes for blood flow. Collaterals are prominent in the lungs of healthy young individuals, and hence pulmonary infarction seldom

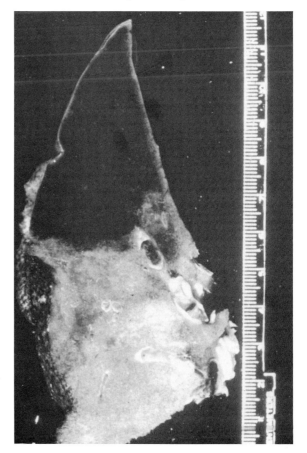

Figure 13-18   *Pulmonary infarction. The dark wedge-shaped area of lung has undergone infarction because a pulmonary embolus obstructed the proximal arterial blood supply.*

occurs during youth. By contrast, the first pulmonary embolus in elderly patients is fatal in 25% of cases when associated with CHF or emphysema.

Treatment of Thrombophlebitis and Complications

Treatment of superficial thrombophlebitis is with: (a) bedrest; (b) elevation of affected limb; and (c) administration of heparin. By contrast, thrombophlebitis involving deep leg veins is treated by wrapping elastic bandages from the toe to the groin and with immediate anticoagulation therapy (heparin).

Treatment of varicose veins includes: (a) elevation of the affected leg; (b) external compression with elastic stockings; or (c) surgical removal of the involved veins.

Surgery is the preferred method of treatment for symptomatic varicosities. The technique is called intraluminal stripping. The greater saphenous vein is ligated near the inguinal region, a "stripper" is introduced into the lumen of the vessel, and the entire vein is then pulled out through the intralumenal rod down to the dorsum of the foot.

Treatment of pulmonary embolus is directed at reducing the risk of thrombophlebitis by anticoagulating the patient with heparin. In some instances, the inferior vena cava may have to be tied off (ligated) to prevent additional pulmonary emboli. Also, the pulmonary embolus may be removed from the pulmonary artery (embolectomy).

Early ambulation after surgery is a simple, important measure effective in preventing thromboemboli. If ambulation is impossible, massage of the legs, leg exercises, and periodic deep breathing should be instituted.

Cardiovascular Emergencies

Emergency medicine has recently emerged as a medical specialty that focuses on the diagnosis and treatment of trauma and other emergencies. Cardiovascular emergencies lead the list of life-threatening disorders (Table 13-6). In this chapter and in other sections of this book I have discussed many

Table 13-6
Cardiovascular Emergencies

Cardiac arrest
Hemorrhage
Aneurysm, dissecting
Hypertensive crisis
Pulmonary edema
Anaphylaxis
Stroke
Shock

cardiovascular emergencies. Diagnosis and rapid administration of therapy can save the lives of patients afflicted by these disorders. In quick succession the clinician must make a differential diagnosis and determine the etiology, assess the magnitude of the problem to predict prognosis, and administer appropriate therapy.

Cardiopulmonary resuscitation (CPR) and emergency cardiac care provide basic life support until the victim recovers sufficiently to be transported or until more advanced life support (in an intensive cardiac care unit) is available. This includes the A-B-C steps of CPR:

A. Airway } artificial
B. Breathing } ventilation } cardiopulmonary resuscitation

C. Circulation } artificial } circulation

In case of collapsed or unconscious persons, the adequacy or absence of breathing and circulation must be determined immediately. If breathing alone is inadequate or absent, rescue breathing may be all that is necessary. If circulation is also absent, artificial circulation must be started in combination with rescue breathing. The methods used for CPR are described and illustrated in a pamphlet distributed by your local Heart Association or in JAMA 1974 227:833–868.

Shock is a common manifestation or pathophysiologic condition observed in patients with various cardiovascular emergencies. Hence our efforts at providing emergency therapy seek to correct shock and precipitating conditions.

Therapy for cardiovascular emergencies characterized by shock is aimed at improving perfusion of blood to tissues by placing the patient in the Trendelenberg (shock) position wherein the patient's lower extremities are elevated above the level of the head; fluid (blood or plasma if necessary) is given intravenously; oxygen is often provided; and various vasopressor (elevators of blood pressure) drugs are given. Meanwhile, efforts are made to identify the etiology of the shock and to return the patient to normal.

Summary

Cardiovascular diseases, especially arteriosclerosis and accompanying thrombosis and myocardial and cerebral infarctions, account for the majority of deaths in the United States. The technologic revolution has provided excessive rich foods and promoted indolence, sedentary living, obesity, hypercholesterolemia, stress, hypertension, and cigarette smoking. Excessive cardiovascular mortality results from these environmental or host factors which promote atherogenesis. The precise pathogenetic mechanisms of this disorder are unknown. The lumen of arteries are progressively narrowed by the deposition of lipid, calcium, and proliferating smooth muscle cells in the intima of arteries.

Decades of exposure to risk factors often lead to disorders of hypoxia arising from narrowed, arteriosclerotic blood vessels: angina pectoris (heart), transient ischemic attacks (brain), and intermittent claudication (legs). Much of modern hospital medicine focuses on the diagnosis and treatment of arteriosclerotic cardiovascular disease. Cardiovascular emergencies of acute myocardial, cerebral, or pulmonary infarctions and shock consume the energies and resources of emergency rooms and intensive care units. Also, efforts are made to evaluate the extent of ischemic cardiovascular disease and to develop methods of preventing them from occurring. Early arteriosclerotic disorders are often reversible by surgical operations which bypass the blocked artery. If the occlusive arteriosclerotic disease occurs suddenly and collateral blood supply is

inadequate, then infarction of myocardium, cerebrum, or feet may ensue.

Persons sustaining infarction of the heart, lungs, or brain may die immediately or various complications may occur depending on the size and location of the infarct, the collateral blood supply, and availability and prompt application of cardiopulmonary resuscitation. Survivors of major infarction are often left with permanent disability and are vulnerable to additional complications or recurrent infarction.

Bibliography

Baron, H. C. 1976. Valvular incompetence and varicose veins. *Hosp. Med.* April, 24. Describes and illustrates the role of defective valves in the pathogensis of varicose veins.

Brown, M. S., and Goldstein, J. L. 1975. Familial hypercholesterolemia: genetic, biochemical, and pathophysiologic considerations. *Adv. Intern. Med.* 20: 273–296. The title describes the content.

Burkett, D. T. 1976. *Varicose Veins Archives of Surgery* 111:1327–1332. The high prevalence of varicose veins in Western countries is attributed to fiber-depleted diets.

Degré, S. 1977. Therapeutic effects of physical training in coronary heart disease. *Cardiology* 62:206–217. Reviews the therapeutic effects of physical training for coronary heart disease from clinical, pathophysiologic, psychologic, and social points of view.

Editorial. 1976. Essential hypertension and psychosomatic research. *Psychosom. Med.* 38: 1. This editorial summarizes information concerning the contribution of psychological factors in hypertension.

Finnerty, F. A. 1975. The nurse's role in treating hypertension. *N. Engl. J. Med.* 293:93. Describes the contribution nurses make in treating this common disorder.

Galen, R. S. 1975. The enzyme diagnosis of myocardial infarction. *Hum. Pathol.* 6:141. Detection of enzyme elevation in the serum of patients with myocardial infarction is discussed.

Gordon, A. S., and Nobel, J. J., Eds. 1974. Standards for cardiopulmonary resuscitation (CPR) and emergency cardiac care (ECC). *J.A.M.A.* 227:833–868. This special article illustrates and describes how CPR and ECC are done.

Haller, J. A., 1967. *Deep thrombophlebitis pathophysiology and treatment*. Philadelphia: W. B. Saunders Company. The differential diagnosis and medical and surgical treatment of thrombophlebitis is discussed.

Hurst, J. W., Ed. 1974. *The heart*, ed. 3. New York: McGraw-Hill Book Company. A standard, comprehensive textbook.

Kannel, W. B. 1964. Risk factors in coronary heart disease. The Framingham Study. *Ann. Intern. Med.* 61:888. This classical study resulted in identifying many coronary risk factors.

Keys, A. 1975. Coronary heart disease: the global picture. *Atherosclerosis* 22:149–192. Dr. Keys has studied arteriosclerosis and the impact of diet on atherogenesis for decades. He reviews many etiological factors of atherosclerosis.

Laragh, J. H. 1976. Modern system for treating high blood pressure based on renin profiling and vasconstriction-volume analysis: a primary role for beta blocking drugs such as propranolol. *Am. J. Med.* 61:797. Describes the pathophysiologic basis of hypertension and therapy illustrated in Figure 13-9.

Lichstein, E. 1975. Evaluation of acute chest pain. *Hosp. Med.* July, p. 8–18. Pictorial summary of differential diagnosis of chest pains.

Martin, A., and Smee, W. O. 1976. Pressure changes in varicose veins. *Lancet* i:768. This article reports increased intra-abdominal pressure in patients with varicose veins.

Moore, M. E., Ed. 1976. Differential diagnosis and treatment. *Medical emergency manual*, Ed. 2. Baltimore: Williams and Williams Co. A concise and practical reference for major medical emergencies.

Mundth, E. D., and Austen, W. G. 1975. Surgical measures for coronary heart disease. *N. Engl. J. Med.* 293:75. Discusses coronary artery bypass graft procedures for coronary arteriosclerosis.

Murphy, G. E. 1960. Nature of rheumatic heart disease. *Medicine* (Balt.) 39:289. This classical article discusses clinical aspects of rheumatic heart disease.

Murphy, M. L. 1977. Treatment of chronic stable angina. *N. Engl. J. Med.* 297:621–627. Patients treated medically (drugs) and surgically (saphenous vein–bypass grafting) showed no difference in survival.

Reisin, E.; Silverberg, D. S.; Eliahou, H. E.; and Modan B. 1978. Effect of weight loss without salt restriction on the reduction of blood pressure in overweight hypertensive patients. *N. Engl. J. Med.* 298:1–6. Weight reduction reduces blood pressure significantly.

Roberts, W. C. 1971. The pathology of acute myocardial infarction. *Hosp. Pract.* 6:89. A well written summary of this topic.

Ross, R., and Glomset, J. A. 1976. The pathogenesis of atherosclerosis. *N. Engl. J. Med.* 295:369. A review article summarizing this subject.

Russel, R. 1975. How does blood pressure cause stroke? *Lancet* ii:1283. An hypothesis which attempts to explain mechanisms responsible for stroke with hypertension.

Sah, A. L.; Hartman, E. C.; and Aronson, S. M., Eds. 1976. *Guidelines for Stroke Care*. U. S. Department of Health, Education, and Welfare. A comprehensive monograph on the pathogenesis, pathology, diagnosis and treatment of patients with stroke. DHEW Pub. No. (HRA) 76–14017. Costs only $1.75.

Wilson, L. M. 1963. Pathology of fatal bacterial endocarditis. Ann. *Intern. Med.* 58:84. A classic article describing the pathology of endocarditis.

Wissler, R. W., and Geer, J. C. 1972. *The Pathogenesis of Arteriosclerosis*. Baltimore: The Williams & Wilkins Company. These two luminaries have summarized the theories of pathogenesis of arteriosclerosis.

CHAPTER 14

Pulmonary Medicine

Chapter Outline

Objectives

After reading this chapter you should be able to

Describe the protective mechanisms of the lung.

List the major groups of pulmonary disorders.

Define and describe the major signs and symptoms of respiratory disorders.

List the causes of dyspnea.

Know what questions pulmonary laboratory tests answer.

List laboratory studies commonly employed for studying respiratory disorders.

Describe the common birth defects in the respiratory tract.

Describe the typical clinical and pathological findings of respiratory distress syndrome of children.

Define the terms cystic fibrosis, antitrypsin deficiency, atelectasis, and pneumothorax.

Name the virus responsible for the common cold.

Describe why children frequently develop otitis media and adults do not.

Know why epiglottitis is a life-threatening disease in infants.

Define and compare tracheobronchitis and bronchiectasis.

Compare lobar pneumonia and bronchopneumonia.

Name the bacterium usually responsible for bronchopneumonia and the microbe causing "walking pneumonia."

Describe the clinical findings regarding viral pneumonia.

Understand why alcoholics develop pulmonary abscesses.

Compare primary and secondary tuberculosis.

Describe the immune response to the tubercle bacillus.

List four techniques used for diagnosing tuberculosis.

Describe the immunological basis for a positive tuberculin test.

List three drugs used for treating tuberculosis.

Describe the pathologic features of the lungs of asthmatics.

Describe the pathogenesis and etiology of chronic bronchitis.

Define the term pneumoconiosis and give three examples.

Know why organic dusts can damage the lung.

List the disease entities included in the chronic obstructive lung disease group.

Define the term emphysema.

List the signs and symptoms of pulmonary emphysema.

Describe the posture and appearance of a person with severe emphysema.

Compare panlobular and centrilobular emphysea.

Describe the laboratory abnormalities that document the presence and extent of emphysema.

Know the role of cigarette smoking in chronic bronchitis, emphysema, and lung cancer.

Describe the contribution of antitrypsin deficiency to emphysema.

List methods of treating emphysema.

Describe the typical findings of a person with laryngeal cancer.

Know how laryngeal cancer is diagnosed and treated.

Compare the survival of persons with intrinsic and extrinsic cancer of the larynx.

Describe the evidence linking cigarette smoking with lung cancer.

List four metals known to cause lung cancer.
List the signs and symptoms of lung cancer.
Know the systemic manifestations of lung cancer.
Describe how lung cancer is diagnosed.
List nonmalignant conditions that can mimic lung cancer.
List the histologic types of lung cancer and the frequency of their occurrence.
Describe the treatment and prognosis of lung cancer.

Introduction

The respiratory tract is lined with biologic barriers that both remove and prevent entry of injurious agents. Filtration begins in the nose, where particles larger than 10μ are efficiently removed by vibrissae. The airway is protected by the cough reflex, which allows excess secretions and foreign bodies in the trachea or major bronchi to be removed. Particles deposited between the posterior two-thirds of the nasal cavity to the terminal bronchioles land on airways lined by mucus-covered ciliated epithelium and are removed by mucociliary transportation mechanisms and swallowed or expectorated. Within the mucus, antibodies of the IgA class as well as cell-mediated immunity protect against infectious agents and dust. Finally, macrophages provide means for removal of inhaled particles from the lung. When these defense mechanisms are destroyed by various toxic environmental agents, a variety of respiratory tract diseases can ensue (Fig. 14-1). In this chapter the common pulmonary diseases with congenital-inherited; traumatic; infectious and inflammatory; occupational; or neoplastic bases are discussed.

Signs and Symptoms of Pulmonary Diseases

Coughing occurs when the nerves in the mucosal lining of the larynx, trachea or bronchi become irritated. The irritated nerves send messages to the brain, provoking an involuntary cough.

A cough is the most common symptom of acute respiratory disease. Nonproductive coughing means no fluid (sputum) is brought up; conversely, a productive cough produces secretions. *Hemoptysis* (bloody sputum) is the coughing up of blood. It can be caused by infectious diseases (bacterial pneumonia, tuberculosis); neoplasms (laryngeal and bronchogenic carcinomas); trauma; or cardiovascular diseases (pulmonary embolism with infarction or mitral valve narrowing with congestive heart failure).

Dyspnea (difficult breathing) is another common symptom of respiratory dysfunction. Common causes of dyspnea are shown in Fig. 14-2. *Cyanosis* is a blue discoloration of the skin and mucous membranes that results when blood is inadequately oxygenated. *Tachypnea* refers to an increased rate of respiration. *Wheezing* occurs upon expiration when bronchi and bronchioles are partially obstructed. Pain in the lungs usually originates from inflamed pleural surfaces. Pleuritic pain is a common symptom of pneumonia, infarction or neoplasia of the lung which irritates the walls of the chest or lungs.

Laboratory Assessment of Pulmonary Diseases

The clinical signs and symptoms of respiratory disorders result from many different etiologic agents and lesions of the lungs. Since the clinical findings are nonspecific, laboratory assessment of the patient is required to answer such questions as: Where is the lesion? How extensive is the disease? What is the etiologic agent? What therapy is needed? Is the patient improving or deteriorating with the prescribed therapy?

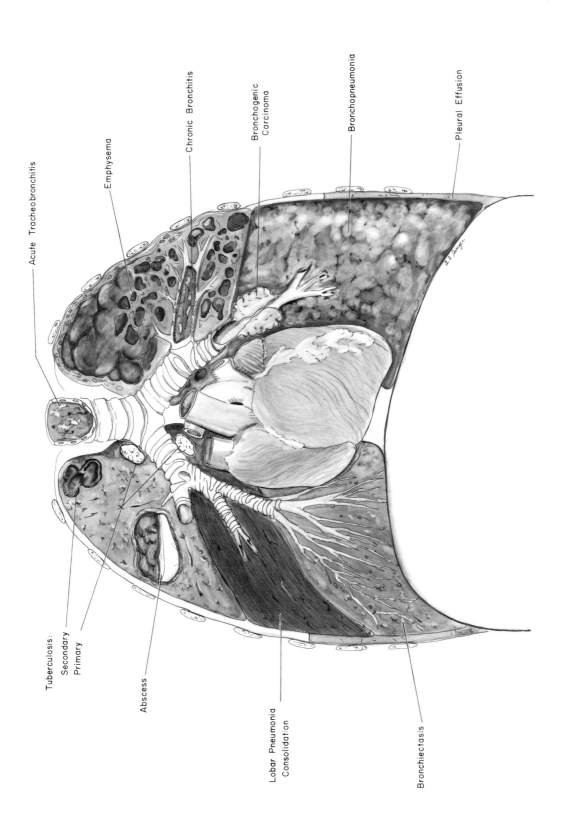

Acute Tracheobronchitis

Emphysema

Chronic Bronchitis

Bronchogenic Carcinoma

Bronchopneumonia

Pleural Effusion

Tuberculosis:
Secondary
Primary

Abscess

Lobar Pneumonia Consolidation

Bronchiectasis

Figure 14-1   *This composite diagram illustrates several common disorders of the lungs.*

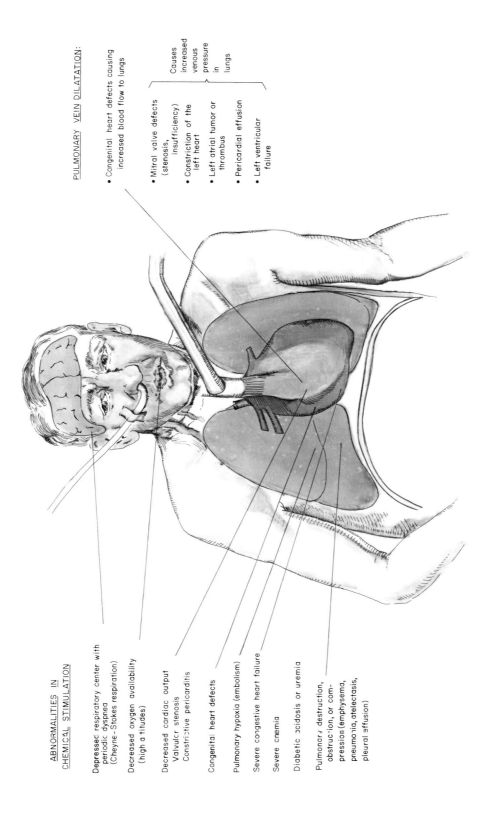

- Congenital heart defects causing increased blood flow to lungs

- Mitral valve defects (stenosis, insufficiency)
- Constriction of the left heart
- Left atrial tumor or thrombus
- Pericardial effusion
- Left ventricular failure

Causes increased venous pressure in lungs

ABNORMALITIES IN CHEMICAL STIMULATION

Depressed respiratory center with periodic dyspnea (Cheyne-Stokes respiration)

Decreased oxygen availability (high altitudes)

Decreased cardiac output
Valvular stenosis
Constrictive pericarditis

Congenital heart defects

Pulmonary hypoxia (embolism)

Severe congestive heart failure

Severe anemia

Diabetic acidosis or uremia

Pulmonary destruction, obstruction, or compression (emphysema, pneumonia, atelectasis, pleural effusion)

Figure 14-2   Causes of dyspnea. The differential diagnosis of lung diseases includes many disorders.

Laboratory studies commonly used for documenting the etiology and extent of pulmonary diseases are listed in Table 14-1.

Congenital and Inherited Disorders

Premature birth, inherited disorders and birth defects commonly cause problems in the respiratory tract of infants.

Birth Defects

Common congenital anomalies of the respiratory tract include the formation of an abnormal (fistulous) tract linking the trachea and esophagus (see Chapter 3, Development and Birth Defects). A *tracheoesophageal fistula* is characterized by a malformed upper esophagus which connects with the trachea. The following typical clinical picture signals this abnormality: During initial feeding an affected newborn regurgitates fluid through the mouth and nose, and fluid passes into the lungs through the fistulous opening. The stomach becomes distended with air as the baby tries to breathe and pneumonia ensues a day or two after the contaminated food passes into the lungs.

Another common congenital defect is *cysts* in the lungs. The cysts are usually associated with cysts of the kidneys, pancreas, and liver. A severely life-threatening condition is the absence (aplasia) of an entire lung or, less threatening, an undersized (hypoplastic) lung.

Prematurity

Not until beyond the twentieth week of gestation do the alveoli develop sufficiently to oxygenate

Table 14-1
Laboratory Study of Respiratory Disorders

Physical examination

X-ray
  Plain chest film
  Fluoroscopy to reveal movements of chest wall, diaphragm and lung
  Laminograms—body section films to define location of lesions such as tumors, cavities
  Bronchography—radio-opaque materials are placed in bronchial tree to demonstrate bronchiectasis
  Arteriography to demonstrate pulmonary emboli

Sputum—cellular composition, neutrophils, eosinophils
              —microorganisms—Gram stain, acid fast, wet mounts, silver stains cultures
              —other constituents—Charcot-Leyden crystals and Curschmann's spirals of asthma

Cytopathology: Pap smears of sputum and pleural fluid for tumor cells or infectious agents

Blood gases: P_{O_2}; P_{CO_2}, pH, oxygen saturation

Bronchoscopy: rigid tubes, fiber optic scopes to demonstrate foreign bodies or tumors

Scans: radio-labeled albumin delineates regional variation in blood supply, pulmonary embolus

Spirometry and other pulmonary function tests: most useful in determining the extent of functional impairment and its progression (for following the patient) Often less important in diagnosing the specific disease entity

Skin testing: for immune reactivity to infectious diseases

Biopsy: lung, scalene or mediastinal lymph nodes for cancer or infections

---

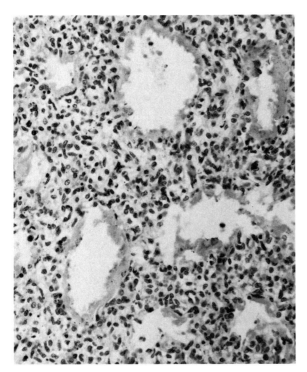

Figure 14-3   *Photomicrograph of lungs of neonate who died of respiratory distress syndrome. Thick hyaline membrane lines the air spaces.* × 450.

blood. Even postnatally the number of alveoli increases, continuing throughout infancy and childhood. Thus, extrauterine life before the twentieth week is nearly impossible. Premature birth and associated immaturity of lungs is a common cause of death.

Respiratory Distress Syndrome of the Newborn*

One disorder with a high mortality rate is *hyaline membrane disease* (respiratory distress syndrome of the newborn). This condition is responsible for about one-third of neonatal deaths. Especially vulnerable are infants delivered by cesarean section, premature male infants, and babies of both sexes born of diabetic mothers.

*Respiratory distress syndrome can also occur in adults from trauma shock, overhydration, and pneumonia (see reference by J.F. Tomashefski for a thorough discussion of this problem).

During the initial hours following birth the baby appears normal, but dyspnea occurs within 24 to 36 hours. This usually signals the presence of respiratory distress syndrome in a premature baby. Chest X-rays reveal an opaque, ground glass appearance in the lung.

Hyaline membrane disease probably results from a deficient production of *surfactant* fluid which acts as a detergent and bathes alveoli thereby preventing them from collapsing and permitting gases to pass normally through alveoli. When surfactant is lacking, *hyaline membranes* form (Fig. 14-3). The thick hyaline membrane coats the alveoli, blocking the passage of gases through the alveolar capillaries. The mortality rate is high because children with this disorder can asphyxiate or die of heart failure. The lungs at autopsy are heavy, airless, and sink in water. The babies may survive if their respiration is assisted for several days on a mechanical respirator. Such therapy may provide sufficient time to permit the lungs to mature and produce surfactant.

Inherited Pulmonary Disorders

Cystic Fibrosis   Cystic fibrosis is an autosomal recessive disorder causing approximately 1 death in 20 in infancy or childhood. Affected children have a unique hypersecretion of sodium chloride in their perspiration and this, together with chronic respiratory tract infections and destruction of secretory glands (liver, pancreas), leads to chronic debilitation and early (Fig. 14-6) death if pulmonary therapy and antibiotics are not given (see Chapter 7, Infectious Diseases).

α_1Antitrypsin Deficiency   This autosomal recessive disease can cause cirrhosis in homozygous children or emphysema in homozygous adults (see Chapter 9, Inherited Disorders). It is hypothesized that persons lacking α_1 antitrypsin are unable to inactivate the proteolytic enzyme, trypsin, when it is liberated from neutrophils and inflames the lungs. Trypsin liberated by neutrophils in inflamed lungs could then cause destruction of the alveolar septa, and emphysema would ensue.

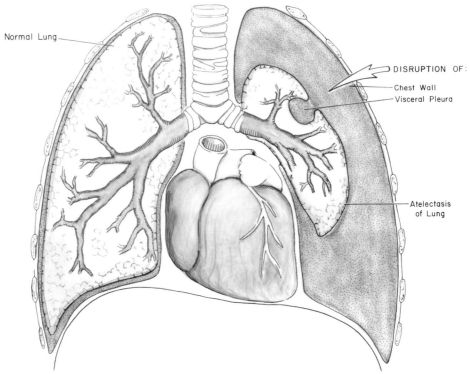

Normal Lung

DISRUPTION OF:
Chest Wall
Visceral Pleura

Atelectasis
of Lung

Figure 14-4   *Pneumothorax results when a hole is punched through the chest wall or lung surface. Air rushes into the vacuum. A "tension pneumothorax" results when the air cannot escape.*

Mechanical and Traumatic Injury

Atelectasis

A common problem in newborns is the mechanical collapse of the lungs (*atelectasis neonatorum*). It results from blockage of an airway or from a failure of the lung to expand properly. At autopsy the airless, collapsed, lungs are red-pink and sink in water. In older children and adults atelectasis is often due to compression of lung tissue by pleural fluid (hydrothorax or empyema) or by air (pneumothorax or atelectasis) which accumulates in a pleural cavity.

Pneumothorax

A tension pneumothorax occurs from a spontaneous rupture of the lung in young adults or from rupture of an emphysematous lung in older per-

sons. Also a wound, as occurs in a stabbing, can cause pneumothorax. Air enters the pleural cavity upon inspiration, but cannot escape. Gradually the lung collapses as the pleural cavity fills with air (Fig. 14-4). Reversal of atelectasis or pneumothorax is achieved by removing an obstruction of the airway, draining fluid, or aspirating the pleural cavity.

Inflammatory and Infectious Respiratory Diseases

Common Cold

Colds are caused by many different viruses, especially *rhinoviruses* (see Chapter 7, Infectious Diseases). Common colds occur repeatedly because the immunity we acquire for one virus does not protect us against other viruses. The viruses incite acute inflammation in the respiratory mucosa and cause mucus to flow, fever, and headache. No cure is available thus far, only symptomatic relief is possible with analgesics, fluids, and antihistamines. Sometimes serious complications such as otitis media, epiglottitis, and tracheobronchitis can arise in children.

Otitis Media

Bacterial infection of the middle ear (*otitis media*) causes earache and fever. The reason children are so susceptible to otitis media is that their Eustachian tubes (which normally equalize atmospheric pressure in the mouth and middle ear) can flush bacteria along a horizontal plane from the infected pharynx into the chamber of the middle ear. Drainage is further impaired because inflamed mucosa in the oropharynx blocks the opening for drainage of the Eustachian tubes. Bacteria then flourish and pass laterally from the pharynx into the middle ear. Otitis media should be diagnosed and treated because the infection can damage the hearing apparatus and can also spread to the brain. Otitis occurs less commonly in older children and adults because the Eustachian tubes pass upward from the oropharynx, and bacteria do not readily ascend into the middle ear.

Epiglottitis

A life-threatening complication of the common cold is infection of the epiglottis. A bacterium called *Haemophilus influenzae*, when infecting the epiglottis, elicits marked swelling and blockage of the airway opening. The opening of the glottis in children aged 2 or under is less than 1 cm in diameter; the infected, inflamed mucosa swells, blocks the airway, and suffocates the child.

Tracheobronchitis

The trachea, bronchi, and bronchioles can also become infected. The respective infections are termed *tracheobronchitis*, *bronchitis* and *bronchiolitis*. The cartilage in the airways of young children is normally soft and becomes even softer when the airway

is inflamed. An inflamed trachea can collapse, blocking passage of air. Bacterial infections usually respond rapidly to appropriate antibiotics.

Bronchiectasis

Bronchiectasis is a degenerative process caused by infection and inflammation that result in dilatation of bronchi. Immunodeficiency (Fig. 14-5), or cystic fibrosis (Fig. 14-6), or defective neutrophil function can predispose an individual to bronchiectasis. Persistent bronchitis can cause the walls of bronchi to dilate (bronchiectasis) and obstruction of the passageway by a mucous plug may lead to bronchiectasis (Fig. 14-4). Often bronchiectasis is accompanied by fever and a hacking cough that produces at least one-half cup of pus-streaked sputum daily. Bronchiectasis can be reversed in early stages by removing an obstructing mucous plug and in late stages by surgical resection of the affected lobe of the lung. However, when bronchiectasis becomes chronic it results in irreversible, extensive, cylindrical or saccular widening of bronchi. Such patients can also develop abscesses.

Pneumonia

Lobar and bronchopneumonia were previously described in Chapter 7, Infectious Diseases. Here, only major points will be reemphasized. The most common cause of bronchopneumonia is a bacterium, *Streptococcus pneumoniae*. Pneumonia involving one lobe is called *lobar pneumonia*. *Bronchopneumonia* differs from *lobar pneumonia* only by its having several lobes of the lung involved. Pneumonia causes chest pain, fever, coughing, and shortness of breath. Pain occurs in the chest wall during inspiration due to irritation of nerves in pleural surfaces that are inflamed.

Diagnosis and Treatment

Examination of the patient's sputum with a Gram stain reveals numerous neutrophils which have phagocytosed *S pneumoniae*. The chest X-ray shows whitening or opacification in areas affected by pneumonia (Fig. 14-7). With acute bronchopneu-

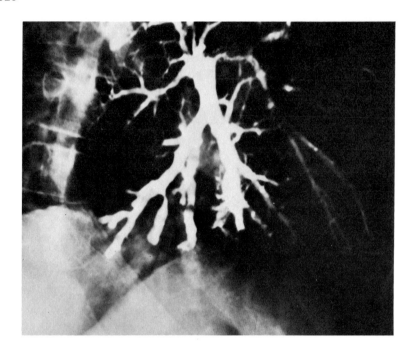

Figure 14-5   *X-ray bronchogram demonstrating dilated bronchial tree (bronchiectasis) in child with agammaglobulinemia and chronic bronchitis.*

monia the lung becomes white on the X-ray because alveoli and bronchi become filled with neutrophils and edema fluid. Penicillin efficiently cures this disease. The lungs usually heal completely following bronchopneumonia and pulmonary function is restored.

Nonbacterial Pneumonias

A variety of nonbacterial infectious agents cause pulmonary infections. Two major microorganisms are involved—viruses and a small, bacteria-like organism called mycoplasma. *Mycoplasma pneumoniae* causes "walking pneumonia" in young adults. Curiously, on X-ray examination the lungs appear to be extensively involved yet only fatigue and a persistent, nonproductive, cough trouble the patient. Mycoplasma pneumonia responds to tetracycline.

By contrast, viral pneumonias are unresponsive to antibiotics. The common viral pneumonias are caused by influenza, respiratory syncytial, rheo, and adeno viruses. On rare occasions, viruses of childhood, such as measles and chickenpox can produce fatal pneumonia in immunosuppressed

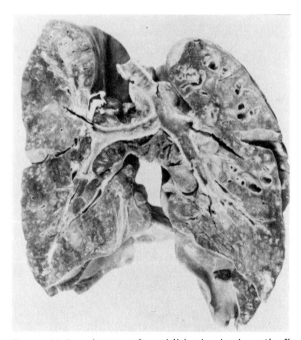

Figure 14-6   *Lungs of a child who had cystic fibrosis. Bronchopneumonia, bronchiectasis (dilated bronchioles), and abscesses have formed (From Kissane, John, M.: Pathology of infancy and childhood, ed. 2, St. Louis, 1975, The C. V. Mosby Co.)*

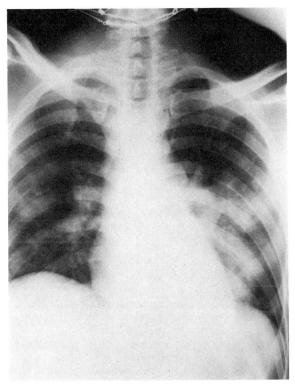

Figure 14-7 *Bronchopneumonia. This X-ray shows opacification (whiteness) in the affected lobes of the lung.*

persons with malignancy, malnutrition, and chronic debilitating diseases. Likewise, fungi may infect the lungs of immunosuppressed persons (see Chapter 7, Infectious Diseases).

Persons with viral pneumonia may be infected during an epidemic. Fever, aching muscles, headache, rash, and a dry, nonproductive cough are usually evident. No bacteria are seen in sputum. The inflammatory response consists mainly of macrophages and lymphocytes, and a few neutrophils are seen. These lymphoid cells are evidence of cell-mediated immunity. The lymphoid cells try to destroy the viruses which infect lung cells. The diagnosis is made by culturing the virus or by noting an increase in antibody concentration against the virus in the patient's serum drawn during acute illness and convalescence. The viral pneumonia subsides when the patient's immune responses eliminate the virus.

Pulmonary Abscesses

Abscesses of the lungs can be a complication of pneumonia or of bronchiectasis. Staphylococcal or anaerobic Gram-negative bacteria are most often responsible for abscesses (Fig. 14-4). Cavities or abscesses caused by staphylococcal pneumonia are rather common in young children.

Pulmonary abscesses form in adults who aspirate food into their lungs. Persons delerious due to alcoholism or other disorders (such as cerebrovascular accident) have impaired cough reflexes and thus they aspirate food containing bacteria into their lungs. Poor oral hygiene is often a contributing factor to the abscess. Since the abscesses occasionally respond poorly to antibiotics, surgical drainage may be required for cure. In spite of therapy, the mortality rate for pulmonary abscesses is 5%.

Tuberculosis

Tuberculosis (TBC) is an acute and/or chronic communicable disease caused by *Mycobacterium tuberculosis*. This disease was once the major cause of death in the United States; today, however, it ranks twentieth. Only 1 in 20 Americans who become infected by TBC develop clinical signs. Persons who have impaired immunity from debilitating disorders such as diabetes mellitus, malnutrition, or chronic alcoholism are especially vulnerable to TBC.

Two basic forms of TBC occur. Primary TBC occurs in children following initial contact with the bacillus. Usually small areas of fibrosis and calcification are seen in the lung and in a hilar lymph node (Ghon complex) which drains the infected lung (Fig. 14-8). Secondary TBC results from reinfection or reactivation of the primary infection. The latter form of tuberculosis is more common in adults than in children.

Primary Tuberculosis

Primary pulmonary tuberculosis occurs when an individual inhales tubercle bacilli in infected droplets coming from the lungs of another person. The inhaled bacilli are then engulfed by macrophages and neutrophils in the bronchioles and alveoli. Initially, an acute inflammatory response of neutrophils surround the bacilli in the alveoli and bronchioles. Next, bacilli drain into hilar lymph nodes where cell-mediated immunity (CMI) develops (see Chapter 6, Immunology). Subsequently, sensitized T lymphocytes react with the bacilli and release substances which activate macrophages. The latter cells engulf and destroy the bacteria and form tubercles. The center of the tubercles often become necrotic (look cheesy) or caseation necrosis occurs —following the engulfment and killing of the bacilli, calcium salt deposits and fibrous tissue grows and encases the bacilli. However, a few viable bacilli remain present for the life of the person. The TBC is therefore arrested, not cured, so reactivation can occur when immunity becomes depressed.

Secondary (Reactivation) Tuberculosis

Secondary tuberculosis is due to reactivation of bacilli that were encased in tubercles during primary infection. The secondary (reactivation) form of tuberculosis usually occurs in adults and produces extensive lesions that cavitate the upper portion of the lung (Fig. 14-9). In addition, the inflammatory response and organisms can erode into a vessel and organisms then spread in the blood stream throughout the body or lung. Numerous small foci of infection can be seen in organs seeded with TBC bacilli. These foci look like millet seeds and hence this type of TBC is termed *miliary* TBC.

Diagnosis

The diagnosis of tuberculosis is achieved by: (a) clinical history of cough, night sweats, and weight loss, (b) evaluating a chest X-ray film for characteristic tuberculous lesions (Fig. 14-9), (c) detecting the bacilli in stained smears of sputum, or (d) by culturing the sputum for growth of the bacillum. In addition, the patient's immune responses can be tested (tuberculin test) by injecting tuberculin antigens into the skin and noting whether the person mounts a vigorous cellular immune re-

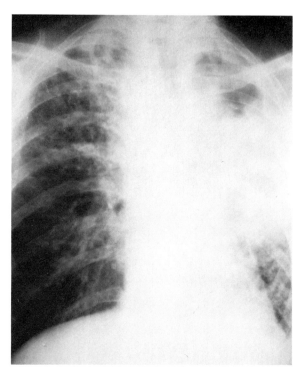

Figure 14-8   *Tuberculosis. The chest X-ray reveals severe infection in the left side.*

sponse. Positive swelling and redness at the site of injection after 48 hours indicates that a person has been exposed to bacilli and has mounted an immune response. The tuberculin test, however, does not tell us whether active infection is occurring. The *Tine test* is a commonly used type of tuberculin test.

Treatment

Treatment of tuberculosis is generally done with drugs such as Streptomycin, INH, and PAS. Commonly, the patient on antituberculosis drugs will feel well within a week and stop taking the drugs too soon, allowing a relapse to occur. Hence, the patient with tuberculosis should be kept under surveillance for 12 to 24 months and sputum should be examined periodically for tubercle bacilli. Also, malnutrition and alcoholism, if present, should be treated.

Individuals with a high risk for developing tuberculosis, especially persons working in hospitals, should be periodically skin tested for TBC. Those who convert from tuberculin negative to positive are often placed on antituberculosis therapy for one year. This precaution prevents severe tuberculosis. In Third World countries, where TBC is common, vaccination with BCG is given to many children.

Asthma

Asthma was discussed previously, in Chapter 6, Immunology. Only major aspects of the disorder are repeated here. In asthma, narrowing of the airways occurs in a sensitized (allergic) person in response to inhaled antigens. The bronchioles of asthmatic persons constrict when antigens like pollen react with IgE antibodies coating mast cells in the lung. Constriction of smooth muscles surrounding bronchioles ensues as histamine is released from the mast cells. Also, mucous plugs form and obstruct airways. Expiration of air is im-

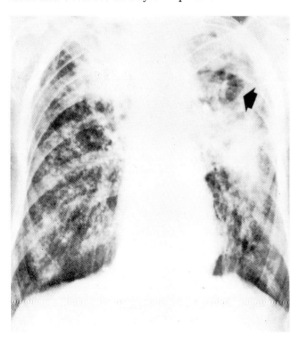

Figure 14-9 *Secondary tuberculosis has produced cavitation of the upper portion of this lung.*

paired and wheezing is heard. The process is usually reversible with inhalation of theophylline, corticosteroids, or injection of epinephrine, all of which dilate the bronchioles.

Chronic Bronchitis

Chronic bronchitis results from a chronic inflammatory process in the bronchi. The inflammation causes hyperplasia of mucous glands in the large bronchi and the mucus formed provokes coughing up of sputum. The strict definition of chronic bronchitis requires that the productive cough be present for three or more months during a period of not less than two successive years.

Clinical Findings

Persons with chronic bronchitis are sometimes called "pink puffers," whereas patients with emphysema are called "blue bloaters." Persons with chronic bronchitis can compensate for respiratory efficiency by hyperventilating ("puffing") and their skin is thus normally pink. In contrast, a decompensated patient with emphysema cannot oxygenate his or her blood and cyanosis ("blue bloating") ensues.

Etiology

The airways of a person with chronic bronchitis become obstructed and this interferes with the drainage of the bronchi; bacteria such as *Haemophilus influenzae* or *Streptococcus pneumoniae* can infect the mucosa of the bronchi (Fig. 14-1). The resulting chronic infection and inflammation of the small airways obstruct the flow of air. The bronchioles become plugged by mucous secretions and hypoxia ensues.

In many instances chronic bronchitis is attributable to cigarette smoking and, in industrial cities, atmospheric pollution. Sulfur dioxide (SO_2) especially aggravates the problem. Chronic bronchitis can be complicated by asthma, viral infections, and passive congestion of the lung associated with cardiac failure. Chronic bronchitis often precedes or occurs concurrently with emphysema.

Treatment

Chronic bronchitis is usually treated with moist vapors and antibiotics. The individual is urged to stop smoking cigarettes and to look for an environment where the quality of the air is pure.

Occupational Pulmonary Disorders

Many diseases of the lungs arise from the exposure of workers to various toxic substances that injure the lungs. These pulmonary disorders are called occupational or industrial diseases. They are also termed *pneumoconioses*, or diseases of the lungs caused by the habitual inhalation of irritant material or metallic particles. Types of pneumoconioses are named according to the type of dust the patient has inhaled. Eventually, most pneumoconioses lead to emphysema.

Silicosis

Silicosis is the best known pneumoconiosis. Persons especially vulnerable to silicosis work as sandstone blasters, pottery makers, and polishers of quartz and granite. Silicon dioxide is hazardous because it is dispersed into finely divided particles measuring less than 5μ in diameter. These fine, floating particles are inhaled into the lungs and produce inflammation. Gradually, fibrosis of the lungs occurs in response to the recurrent injury. Approximately 10 to 20 years of exposure are required before fibrotic lung disease or emphysema ensue. Silicosis is diagnosed by clinical history, physical examination, and X-ray findings.

Asbestosis

Asbestos, which has been discovered to be a carcinogen, was until recently, widely used for insulating and fireproofing. Approximately 25% of persons who live in urban areas show asbestos particles in their lungs. Old plumbers or miners of asbestos have a high incidence of lung cancer and pleura (mesotheliomas). The study of the relationship between asbestos and cigarette smoking in the etiology of lung cancer reveals that these two carcinogenic agents have a potentiating effect. When a person is exposed to these two agents the person is at much greater risk for developing cancer than if exposed to a single agent.

Anthracosis

Coal miners, after many years of exposure to carbon particles, often develop a condition called black lung disease or coal workers' pneumoconiosis. The patient often shows dyspnea, fever, and cough. The inhalation of the particles of coal containing silica induces injury and inflammation. The injured lung is repaired by fibrosis and the scars that form cause emphysema.

Irritant Gases

Examples of irritant gases are ammonia, chlorine, nitrogen dioxide (NO_2), and ozone. All of these agents are capable of inducing "chemical pneumonitis." Clinically, the workers exposed to these gases experience acute upper respiratory pain and tearing of the eyes immediately upon exposure. Exposure of a farmer to NO_2 in a silo can result in fatal pulmonary edema hours later.

Metal Fumes

Exposure to metallic fumes containing solid particles measuring between 0.2 and 1μ in diameter causes an influenza-like disease with cough, shivering, and fever. Cadmium, for instance, can cause acute pulmonary edema and toxic changes in the kidneys. Other heavy metals such as beryllium, lead, and zinc can also damage the lung.

Organic Dust Disease

Persons (most often farmers) working with moldy hay can develop an allergy (immune reaction) to the molds in the hay and develop a destructive immunologic reaction in the lung called "farmers

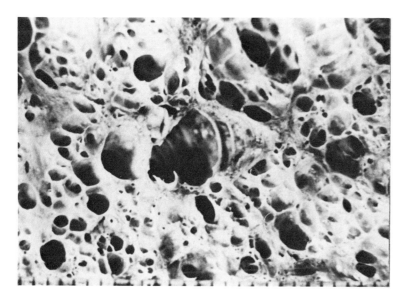

Figure 14-10 *Pulmonary emphysema. This slice of lung reveals dilated honeycomb cysts and fibrosis.*

lung." The lungs become inflamed and injured when the molds (antigens) inhaled into the lungs combine with antibodies in the patient's serum. Likewise, individuals handling and inhaling maple bark, mushrooms, compost, wheat, or wood pulp are subject to developing severe pulmonary allergies to the antigens in these organic dusts.

The author was once consulted about a 14-year-old boy who had developed respiratory insufficiency. Careful questioning of the boy and mother revealed that he had a pet dove in his bedroom. Our studies revealed that he had antibodies in his serum against the dove's droppings (feces) and intestinal mucosa. Inflammation occurred in his lungs because the boy had formed antibodies that reacted with antigens from the droppings inhaled into his lungs. Removal of the dove from the environment led to resolution of his antigen or organic dust-induced pneumonitis. Continuous exposure to organic dusts, gases, fumes, or particles can lead to transient or permanent inflammation and fibrosis of the lung.

Chronic Obstructive Lung Disease

Chronic obstructive lung disease (COLD) encompasses common pulmonary disorders which obstruct the flow of air through airways. This disorder is responsible for the major chronic pulmonary illnesses that afflict more than 4 million persons in the United States. Chronic obstructive lung disease includes pulmonary diseases discussed earlier, pneumoconioses, asthma, and chronic bronchitis.

Pulmonary Emphysema

Pulmonary emphysema is defined as a local or generalized condition of the lung marked by distention, progressive loss of elasticity, and eventual rupture of the alveoli (Fig. 14-10) and is accompanied by labored breathing, a husky cough, and labored heart action.

Emphysema is by far the most common type of chronic obstructive lung disease. It causes more major disability than any other pulmonary disorder; several million men in the United States are living restricted lives because of emphysema. Fewer women than men have emphysema. The disease typically occurs in cigarette smoking males past the age of 40.

Signs and Symptoms

The earliest symptom of emphysema is dyspnea upon physical exertion. A second common symptom is wheezing; when a person over the age of 40 wheezes, emphysema is likely. If the causal factors (such as cigarette smoking) are not removed, emphysema makes a person exhausted, thin, and unable to move more than a few feet without becoming hypoxic (oxygen deficient).

Characteristically, emphysematous individuals assume a posture that optimizes the intake of air (Fig. 14-2). Their lips are usually pursed on expiration to maximize ventilation and they hunch forward. Eventually they can suffer from failure of the right side of the heart (cor pulmonale) and respiratory acidosis can ensue. Acidosis occurs because excessive CO_2 accumulates in the blood. Mental vagueness, headache, twitching of fingers, and eventual deep cyanosis may occur.

Pathology

Two main types of emphysema are recognized— *panlobular* and *centrilobular* (Fig. 14-11). In panlobular emphysema alveolar dilatation and destruction occur in the peripheral portion of the lung and involve the whole primary lung lobule. In contrast, *centrilobular emphysema* results in dilatation of respiratory bronchioles and alveolar ducts in the central portion of lobules (Fig. 14-11). The most severe emphysematous involvement occurs at the apices or top of the lung. *Bullae*, which are large, air-filled sacs that measure up to several centimeters in diameter, can also be seen (Fig. 14-1). The exchange of gases in the alveoli becomes markedly impaired in both types of emphysema. The important pathologic features of emphysema are dilatation and destruction of alveoli with fibrosis and chronic inflammation. This pathologic process is not reversible.

Laboratory Evaluation

Characteristically, chest X-ray films reveal increased volume of the lungs. The anterior-posterior dimension of the chest increases and the diaphragm extends downward and becomes flattened to accomodate the enlarged emphysematous lungs. Also, tissue destruction and fibrosis can be seen in the X-ray. Pulmonary function tests document and

PANLOBULAR EMPHYSEMA

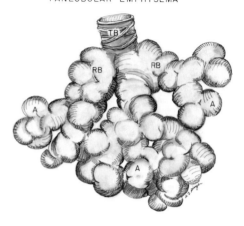

NORMAL LUNG

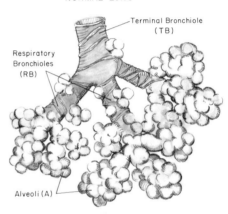

CENTRILOBULAR EMPHYSEMA

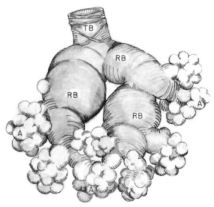

Figure 14-11 *Pulmonary emphysema.* Centrilobular emphysema *dilates respiratory bronchioles and* panlobular emphysema *dilates alveoli.*

quantify the extent of impairment of the lungs causing inability to exchange gases. Measurement of O_2 and CO_2 in arterial blood further quantifies the extent of pulmonary insufficiency. In summary, many of the tests listed in Table 14-1 are employed to evaluate the extent of the lung destruction.

Etiology

Cigarette smoking is definitely associated with an increased occurrence of both chronic bronchitis and pulmonary emphysema. Mortality increases with the smoking of cigarettes; Smokers have a 20 times greater chance of developing and dying of COLD than nonsmokers, and the incidence of chronic bronchitis ranges from 20% in heavy smokers to 5% in smokers who have quit.

Cigarette smoke damages the ciliated mucosal cells. Initially, smoke inhibits the movement of cilia in the mucosal lining cells of the airways. Also, macrophages become sluggish and fail to destroy bacteria. Later, the ciliary cells are replaced by squamous cells (by squamous metaplasia, for example), and the mucous glands increase in size. These pathologic findings of chronic bronchitis have been demonstrated in biopsy specimens taken from bronchi of supposedly healthy young cigarette smokers.

Air pollution is also an important etiologic factor in chronic bronchitis and emphysema; the incidence of COLD is highest in polluted urban areas. Individuals who smoke cigarettes, work in certain industries, and who live in urban areas have great danger of developing COLD.

Inherited susceptibility to emphysema has only been recognized during the past decade. A deficiency in an enzyme, α_1 *antitrypsin*, occurs in a few young individuals with emphysema. This enzyme can be detected in the blood of normal persons, whereas it is absent in the blood of persons with the inherited deficiency. The finding of low levels of α_1 antitrypsin should lead to screening of relatives. Persons deficient in this enzyme should be told about their increased risk of developing emphysema. They should not smoke cigarettes.

Treatment

Patients with emphysema should be made aware that their disease is not reversible. Prevention of emphysema by early diagnosis and modification of self-destructive behavior like cigarette smoking can be achieved in motivated persons. Emphysema is progressive if the patient persists in smoking cigarettes. Working and living in a highly polluted atmosphere is also detrimental. Antibiotics are helpful in those with concurrent chronic bronchitis. Other rehabilitative efforts such as breathing exercises improve the quality of life.

Breathing exercises have a threefold purpose since they: (a) help the patient to minimize the effort of ventilation and to breathe efficiently; (b) increase the strength, coordination, and efficiency of the muscles of respiration; and (c) reinforce the patient's determination to prevent progression of disease.

Some persons with emphysema require breathing assistance with oxygen and portable oxygen tanks are available for this purpose. The author recalls seeing a patient smoking a cigarette through his tracheostomy tube even though a mechanical respirator was required for his survival. These desperate measures are a high price to pay for abusing one's lungs.

Cancers of the Respiratory Tract

Cancers of the lip, mouth, nasopharynx, larynx, and lungs are common. They are especially common in smokers beyond the age of 50. Pipe smokers can develop cancers of the lip and mouth whereas cigarette smokers are apt to develop cancer anywhere in the respiratory tract.

Laryngeal Carcinoma

Carcinoma of the larynx is about ten times more common in men than in women; it appears at an average age of 60 and often as a complication of extensive cigarette smoking. Persistent hoarseness of the voice usually signals this form of cancer.

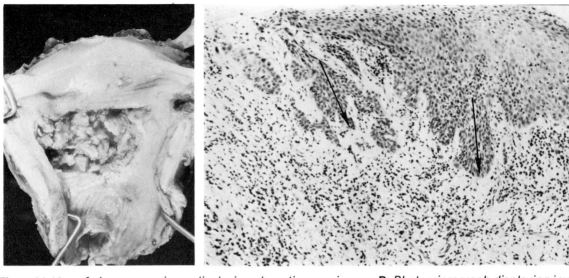

Figure 14-12   **A,** *Larynx specimen displaying ulcerating carcinoma;* **B,** *Photomicrograph displaying invading laryngeal carcinoma cells* (arrows).

Subsequently, worsening of the hoarseness, pain, coughing up of blood, and dyspnea can develop.

Diagnosis   A presumptive diagnosis of laryngeal carcinoma is made by studying a Pap smear of sputum. The next diagnostic step is to inspect the laryngeal lining through a bronchoscope; the tumor mass can be directly visualized and biopsied. (Fig. 14-12, A). If the individual has a squamous cell carcinoma, the neoplastic cells can be seen in a microscope (Fig. 14-12, B).

Differential Diagnosis   Not all hoarseness is caused by laryngeal cancer. Infection, a benign tumor, or a "singer's nodule," can also cause hoarseness. The latter occurs as an occupational hazard in persons such as singers, preachers, and politicians.★ A singer's nodule consists of a fibrous nodular swelling at the free edge of the vocal cord. The nodule can be removed and the individual's voice quality improves.

Treatment   Tumors that develop directly on the vocal folds are called *intrinsic* and constitute about

★During the height of the Vietnamese war President Johnson had a singer's nodule removed and his hoarseness disappeared.

70% of laryngeal cancers; those extending beyond the cords are *extrinsic*.

Treatment is aimed at complete eradication of primary, as well as metastatic, tumor. Radiation alone is used only for small cancers of the middle third of the cord. Total or partial laryngectomy is the treatment of choice for many cancers; preoperative radiation and extensive removal of lymph nodes is done by some physicians. Partial laryngectomy is preferred in some patients with cancer of the epiglottis and/or false vocal cords because it permits retention of normal speech without jeopardizing chances for cure.

The overall cure rate for laryngeal cancer is approximately 60%. For intrinsic cancer of the larynx it is around 90%, but extrinsic laryngeal cancer with metastasis has only a 30% cure rate. These tumors kill by direct extension associated with ulceration, infection, metastasis, obstruction, and pulmonary infections.

Lung Cancer

Never before has a specific malignancy reached epidemic proportions. Lung cancer has been accelerating in incidence during the past two decades in both sexes. Carcinoma of the lung affected approximately 93,000 Americans in 1976. Carcinoma of the lung is the number one killer from cancer in the United States. The peak incidence of lung cancer occurs in men of 50 to 60 years of age.

Etiology   Hard facts clearly implicate environmental factors rather than hereditary factors as the major causes of laryngeal and lung cancer. The undeniable link between lung cancer and cigarette smoking is recognized by everyone.

Cancers of the lip, mouth, oropharynx, larynx, lungs, and urinary bladder also occur chiefly in cigarette smokers. The author is convinced that cigarettes are carcinogenic. This has been clearly demonstrated to the author in Colombia, where he worked for Project HOPE. There, a nearby tribe smoked cigarettes with the lit end in their mouths. This old custom grew from an attempt to hide the cigarettes from the slave owners and also permitted the individuals to "enjoy the cigarettes to their utmost." But approximately 25% of these persons developed carcinoma at the base of their tongues where the cigarette ashes fell. Others developed "nicotine stomatitis" on their palates. The cigarette smoke, heat, and tar proved to be carcinogenic to the tongue. Virtually all patients with cancer of the mouth and of the respiratory tract are or were cigarette smokers.

A dose-response relationship exists between cigarette smoking and the development of lung cancer: The frequency of lung cancer is directly proportional to the number of cigarettes smoked per day multiplied by the total number of years of smoking. The "pack-years" give an accurate prognostication of the likelihood of developing lung cancer.

It is interesting to note that Mormons, whose religious convictions and practice forbid cigarette smoking, seldom develop lung cancer. It is also worth noting that persons who stop smoking have a lower incidence of cancer of the lung than those who persist smoking. Pathologic studies on cigarette smokers reveal widespread premalignant changes in the bronchial mucosa; the extent of these chages has a dose-response relationship to the extent of cigarette smoking. Finally, experimental studies in animals have revealed carcinogens in to-

bacco smoke. Carcinomas can be induced in laboratory animals by direct application of cigarette tar to the skin of rats or in lungs of animals that are taught to smoke cigarettes.

To a lesser extent, other environmental agents are carcinogenic. Miners of arsenic, uranium, nickel, and chromate, have an increased incidence of lung cancer.

The smoking of cigars and pipes is associated with a slightly increased risk of lung cancer; the risk is far less than in persons who smoke cigarettes. The long range impact of air pollution on lung cancer has not yet been determined.

Signs and Symptoms   Lung cancer most often originates in the mucosal lining of a primary or secondary bronchus and hence is termed *bronchogenic carcinoma*. The signs and symptoms of lung cancer stem from three mechanisms: (a) local extension of a tumor within the lung; (b) metastasis; or (c) by systemic effects related to metastasis or the production of hormones by a tumor.

Nonspecific findings related to malignancy including weight loss, anorexia, nausea, vomiting, and weakness are often seen in persons with lung cancer. Pain in the chest from damage to the pleura can signal metastases. Another sign of lung cancer is the coughing up of blood (*hemoptysis*). Hemorrhage occurs when the tumor becomes necrotic or ruptures into a blood vessel.

Distant metastases to any site in the body frequently occurs. The author recalls a patient who had an unusual metastasis: While eating his Thanksgiving turkey, the patient's tooth loosened due to a metastasis to the jaw. Common sites of metastases are lymph nodes, liver, adrenal glands, bone, and brain.

Numerous unusual systemic manifestations of lung cancer occur because lung cancers often secrete hormones. For example, adenocorticotropin hormone (ACTH) can be produced by a lung cancer. The ACTH produced by the tumor stimulates the adrenal glands to produce cortisone excessively. The individual then develops Cushing's syndrome (see Chapter 12, Endocrine and Metabolic Disorders). In addition, neuromuscular dysfunction such as loss of sensation, loss of coordination, and weak-

Table 14-2
Lung Cancers

Histologic type	*Approximate frequency (percent)*	*Parenchymal abnormality*	*Hilar lymph node involvement*	*Intrathoracic or extrapulmonary involvement*	*Comments*
Epidermoid (squamous cell) carcinoma	35–60	Central large or small ill-defined mass	Common	Pleural effusion	Grows by direct invasion Cavitation Obstructive pneumonia and collapse Late metastases
Small cell ("oat cell")	35	Hilar mass	Typical	Mediastinal widening	Grows by submucosal lymphatic extension Early metastases Obstructive pneumonia and collapse
Large cell anaplastic	5–15	Peripheral, large, ill-defined mass	Common	Occasional mediastinal mass	Very rapid growth Early lymphatic and hematogenous metastases Infrequent cavitation
Adenocarcinomas	15–20	Peripheral small or large, ill-defined mass	Uncommon	Uncommon	Early hematogenous metastases Rare cavitation, arises in scar
Bronchial adenoma (note: "benign")	5–10	Central, sharply marginated mass	Rare	Uncommon	Low-grade malignancy Infrequent metastases Bronchial obstruction Hemoptysis

ness often ensues. Clubbing of fingers or bulbous, club-shaped ends of fingers and toes can appear in patients with lung cancer. This abnormality could arise from production of growth hormone by the tumor.

Diagnosis   Individuals at high risk (chronic cigarette smokers and miners) for developing lung cancer and persons who have appropriate clinical findings should be thoroughly evaluated for lung cancer (Table 14-1). Traditional approaches to the diagnosis of lung cancer include X-ray, cytologic, and bronchoscopic examination. Unfortunately, X-ray examination proves to be too insensitive a technique for the early diagnosis of lung cancer; only large lung cancers which usually have already metastasized can be seen (Fig. 14-13). Curative surgical resection is impossible.

Cytologic examination of the patients sputum usually reveals bronchogenic carcinoma cells (Fig. 14-14) and can lead to an earlier diagnosis than can X-ray examination. Other major techniques for the diagnosis of lung cancer are bronchoscopy and biopsy. These methods enable the surgeon to directly view and biopsy the tumor. Often the biopsy reveals a nonmalignant process.

Many nonmalignant conditions such as adenomas and a variety of infectious agents produce round, opaque, tumor-like lesions that are detected in X-rays. These so-called "coin lesions" are caused by fungal infections that have healed and calcified. Tuberculosis also can mimic lung cancer.

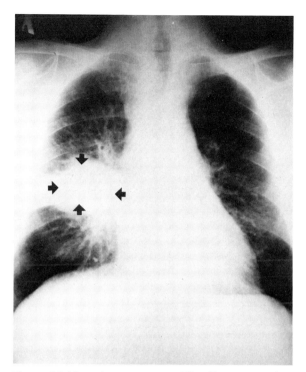

Figure 14-13   *Lung cancer. The X-ray reveals a large mass* (arrows).

Pathology   Most lung cancers protrude into and fill the lumen of the involved bronchus (Fig. 14-15) and can invade the bronchial wall and enter the lung tissue. Occasionally, small metastatic satellite tumors are seen around the large primary tumor. Metastases to the liver and other organs are common. Approximately 50% of lung tumors are *squamous cell (epidermoid) carcinomas*.

If bronchial mucosa near the tumor is studied, widespread premalignant changes can be seen throughout mucosa of the bronchi. This finding suggests that the cigarette smoke coats the entire bronchial tree with carcinogens and induces premalignant and malignant changes througout the airways.

Another common histologic type of lung cancer is small cell ("oat cell") cancer, which has an oat seed-like appearance. Large cell undifferentiated carcinomas and adenocarcinomas constitute the other lung cancers. Adenocarcinoma is the only type of lung cancer that is not associated with cig-arette smoking and it is as common in women as in men.

Treatment and Prognosis   In general, the prognosis for patients with lung cancer is poor. The overall five-year survival of all patients with lung cancer is approximately 5%. Regardless of treatment (surgery, radiotherapy, or chemotherapy) 80% of the patients die during the first year, and about 95% die within five years. Well differentiated squamous cell carcinomas are associated with the best prognosis, whereas "oat cell" carcinomas are highly malignant. Most of the tumors detected in a chest X-ray have already metastasized; removal of all the tumor becomes impossible. The average survival time from diagnosis to demise ranges between 5 and 14 months.

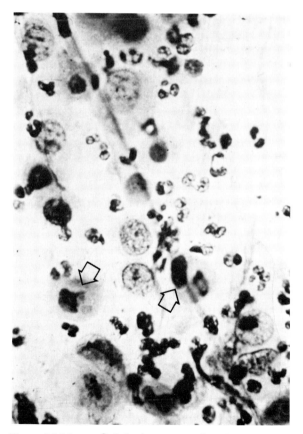

Figure 14-14   *Cytologic smear of sputum reveals bronchogenic carcinoma cells* (arrows).

The major cause of death from lung cancer is bacterial pneumonia caused by extension of the tumor into the bronchus and lung, which obstructs the flow away from the lungs of mucus containing bacteria. Metastases to the brain and vital organs and concurrent emphysema can cause cardiopulmonary failure and death.

Major gains in survival will occur only by preventing lung cancer and by achieving early diagnoses. Facts supporting this assertion are: (a) the resectability rate of small lung cancers (less than 4 cm in diameter) is 98%, and (b) the five-year survival for small bronchogenic carcinomas is 45%.

Summary

Pulmonary diseases cause frequent morbidity (common cold), marked chronic disability (emphysema, asthma, bronchiectasis), and frequent cancer mortality (carcinoma of lung). Diseases of the respiratory tract are second only to cardiovascular diseases in persons in the United States.

The airways are exposed to the environment and thus, when protective mechanisms fail or exposure to toxic environmental agents is excessive, then infectious, degenerative or neoplastic disorders ensue. Occupationally induced pulmonary disorders are now recognized as important preventable diseases. Likewise, lung cancer and emphysema could be prevented by the cessation of cigrette smoking.

Characteristic signs and symptoms are displayed in persons with respiratory disorders. Specific diagnosis requires laboratory evaluation by X-ray, pulmonary function tests, bacterial culture, or cytologic and biopsy evaluation. Treatment varies with the etiology, lesion, and extent of involvement. Infectious diseases are declining in frequency in the wake of improved living conditions, vaccination, and antibiotics. Meanwhile, pulmonary emphysema and lung cancer are increasing at an alarming rate; late diagnosis is attended by high mortality.

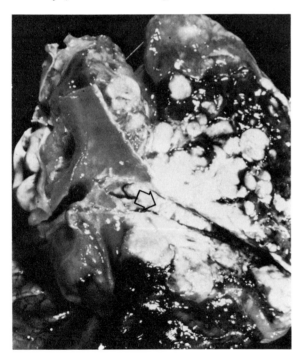

Figure 14-15 *A bronchogenic carcinoma has blocked the bronchus and is seen invading lung tissue.*

Bibliography

Ackerman, L. V., and Regato, J. A. 1970. *Cancer.* St. Louis: The C. V. Mosby Co. A standard textbook with good sections on laryngeal and lung cancers.

Armstrong, J. D., and Bragg, D. G. 1975. Radiology in lung cancer. *Ca* 25 (5). Describes typical histopathology and radiological findings of various types of lung cancer.

Cherniack, R. M. 1977. *Pulmonary Function.* Philadelphia: W. B. Saunders Co. Simple discussion of normal and diseased pulmonary function is provided with procedures and interpretation.

Cocke, E. W., and Wang, C. C. 1976. Cancer of the larynx: selecting optimal treatment. *Ca* 26 (4). A special issue on cancer of the larynx.

Eichenwald, H. F. 1976. Respiratory infections in children. *Hosp. Pract.* April, 81–90. Reviews infectious diseases of the respiratory tract of children.

Feinstein, A. R. 1964. Symptomatic patterns, biologic behavior and prognoses of cancer of the lung. *Ann. Intern. Med.* 61:27. Describes the typical clinical pattern of lung cancer.

Heard, B. E. 1969. *Pathology of chronic bronchitis and emphysema*. London: Churchill, Ltd. A monograph on pathology of chronic obstructive lung disease.

Kendig, E. L., and Chernik, V., Eds. 1977. *Disorders of the Respiratory Tract in Children*. Philadelphia: W. B. Saunders Co. A library of pediatric pulmonary disorders.

Lyon, J. L.; Klaurer, M. R.; Gardner, J. W.; and Smart, C. R. 1976. Cancer incidence in Mormons and non-Mormons in Utah. 1966–1970. *N. Engl. J. Med.* 294:129. Illustrates the value of not smoking cigarettes.

Markham, J. 1976. Occupational chest problems. *Can. Family Physician* 22:58–61. Review article on occupationally related pulmonary diseases.

McCombs, R. P. 1972. Diseases due to immunologic actions in the lung. *N. Engl. J. Med.* 286:1186. Review article on hypersensitivity reactions in the lungs.

Newhouse, M., et al. 1976. Lung defense mechanisms. *N. Engl. J. Med.* 295:990–998, 1045–1052. A scholarly discussion of mechanisms that protect our lungs.

Pepys, J. 1969. *Hypersensitivity diseases of the lungs due to fungi and organic dust*. New York: S. Carger. A monograph on organic dust-induced pulmonary disease.

Purtilo, D. T.; Brem, J.; Yang, J. P. S.; and Cassel, C. 1975. A family study of pigeon breeders disease. *J. Pediatr.* 86:569. Describes the boy who developed an allergic lung disease to his pet dove.

Seaton, A., et al. 1975. *Occupational lung diseases*. Philadelphia: W. B. Saunders Company. Focuses on industrial diseases of the lung.

Spencer, H. 1972. *Pathology of the lung*. Third Edition London: Pergamon. A standard textbook.

Tomashefski, J. F., and Mahagan, V. Managing respiratory distress syndrome in adults. *Postgrad. Med.* 59:77–82. Describes the etiology, pathophysiology, and management of this syndrome.

Wynder, E. L. 1972. Etiology of lung cancer. *Cancer* 30:1332. Discusses various causes of lung cancer.

Zapol, W. M., and Snider, M. T. 1977. Pulmonary hypertension in severe acute respiratory failure. *N. Engl. J. Med.* 296:476–480. The article describes how and why pulmonary arterial hypertension in acute respiratory failure can lead to right-sided heart failure.

Gastrointestinal Disorders

Chapter Outline

Objectives

After reading this chapter you should be able to

Define the terms dental caries, gingivitis, and peridontitis.

Know what is responsible for loss of teeth at various ages.

Name the etiologic agent of cold sore.

Define the term thrush.

Compare leukoplakia and cancer of the mouth.

Define the terms sialoadenitis and sialolithiasis.

Describe the etiology of megaesophagus and megacolon.

List several congenital obstructive lesions of the G-I tract.

Define the terms diverticuli and hernia.

List the bacteria usually causing bacterial-induced diarrhea.

List several intestinal parasites.

Describe the clinical and pathological findings of acute appendicitis.

Define the term peptic ulcer.

List common sites of peptic ulcer.

Discuss the pathophysiology of peptic ulcer.

List complications of peptic ulcers.

List causes of gastrointestinal hemorrhage.

Describe how peptic ulcers are treated.

Define the term gastritis.

Compare Crohn's disease and ulcerative colitis.

List complications of both the above diseases.

List causes of malabsorption.

Describe how biliary tract obstruction can cause rickets.

List the clinical findings for gastric cancer.

Compare the changes in the incidence in recent years of gastric, pancreatic, and colon cancers.

Know the frequency of colorectal cancer.

Describe how colorectal cancer is diagnosed.

Know the prognosis for colon cancer.

Describe how carcinoembryonic antigen is used in patients with colon cancer.

Introduction

The gastrointestinal (G-I) tract is a long hollow tube and associated glands (salivary, liver, and pancreas) which digest and absorb food as well as eliminate wastes. The G-I tract is lined with moist epithelium. The common diseases of the G-I tract result from ulceration or infection of the mucosal lining. Also, occlusion of blood vessels and neoplasia contribute significantly to diseases of the G-I tract. The G-I tract begins in the mouth which prepares food for swallowing and absorption (chewing of food by the teeth and mixing of it with saliva are important for proper digestion). Also, the salivary glands, liver, and pancreas secrete enzymes and bile, vital to digestion and absorption of food.

Oral Cavity

Virtually all of us have been plagued by the common diseases, *dental caries* or *inflamed gums (gingivitis)*. Approximately 95% of Americans have been affected by dental caries (the cost of treating caries is estimated at $2 billion per year). This chronic destructive disease of calcified tissue (enamel and dentin) of the teeth develops shortly after bicuspid eruption (at about age 10) and is a major cause of loss of teeth up to age 35. Thereafter, gingivitis is largely responsible for loss of teeth.

Dental Caries

Caries begin as *dental plaques*—deposits of debris accumulated on tooth surfaces. A swarm of bacteria grow into the plaque burrowing into the enamel of the tooth and creating caries. The bacteria release lactic acid which dissolves enamel. Plaques can develop within six hours after cleaning teeth. Individuals who habitually eat carbohydrates are apt to develop caries. Fluoridation of drinking water has decreased the incidence of caries in children because the fluoride salts deposited in enamel are resistant to bacteria.

Periodontal tissues consist of the gums (gingivae) and connective tissues that support the teeth. When the periodontal tissues become inflamed, gingivitis occurs. Loosening of the teeth and destruction of the supporting bone ensues. *Periodontitis* (also called pyorrhea or gingivitis) is responsible for nearly 80% of the loss of teeth after age 35.

Cold Sore

A common infectious disease of the mouth is caused by the *herpes simplex virus*. Infection by this virus inflames the oral mucosa, lips, and gums and a "cold sore" develops. It often recurs when an individual is stressed (when immunity becomes depressed), as occurs with a common cold (hence the term "cold sore"). A red to yellow blister appears which persists for one to two weeks. The virus is usually brought under control by the immune system. Rarely, herpes simplex disseminates throughout the body. When this happens, immuno-suppression is present, as in victims of cutaneous burns, malnutrition, or cancer.

An infection of the mouth (*moniliasis or thrush*) is caused by a fungus called *Candida albicans*. New-born infants and individuals treated with high doses of antibiotics or toxic drugs often develop oral moniliasis. White patches of fungi are seen in the back of the throat. Rarely, this fungus invades the blood stream of immunosuppressed patients and infects other organs.

Cancer

Leukoplakia (white plaque) is a common premalignant lesion occurring most often in the tongue or oral mucosa of elderly persons. Leukoplakia causes the smooth, moist squamous mucosa to become dry and roughened, and chronic inflammation is seen beneath the plaque. Leukoplakia and smoker's palate (stomatitis nicotina) can be caused by smoking cigarettes or pipes. These two disorders can, if the irritant persists, transform into carcinoma.

The lower lip is the most common site of squamous cell carcinoma involving the oral cavity. Cigarette smoking is the major cause of this carcinoma. In addition, the floor of the mouth and the base of the tongue can be involved. These cancers ulcerate and invade locally; however, the cancer can metastasize to regional lymph nodes.

Salivary Glands

The most common lesion involving the salivary glands (parotid, submandibular, and submaxillary glands) is characterized by inflammation. Mumps virus is the most common cause of infection of salivary glands (*sialadenitis*). Obstruction of the salivary ducts by stones (*sialolithiasis*) is another common cause of sialadenitis. The affected individual experiences sharp pain in the inflamed salivary gland. The stone can, if large, be palpated and is visible in an X-ray.

Neoplasms of the salivary gland are rare. The most common salivary tumor is an *adenoma* (80%), whereas *adenocarcinomas* constitute approximately 20% of salivary neoplasms. Malignant salivary tumors are troublesome because total surgical removal is difficult; the tumor tends to invade the nearby facial nerve and paralysis ensues. Repeated attempts at removal are often required to completely eradicate the tumor.

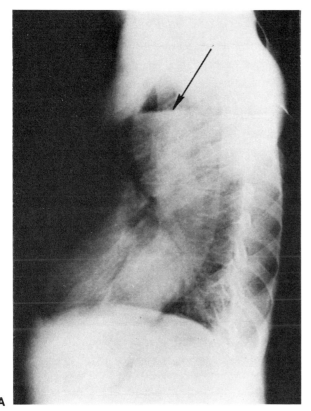 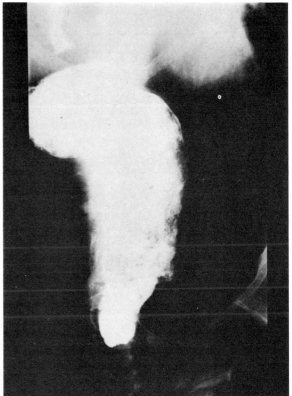

Figure 15-1   A, *Aganglionosis of esophagus causing megaesophagus. A lateral X-ray reveals a markedly enlarged esophagus with fluid* (left). **B,** *On the right, aganglionosis of the colon has resulted in dilation of the colon.*

Gastrointestinal Tract

Peristalsis, or successive autonomic waves of muscular contraction, is required for the G-I tract to propel food and process it for digestion, absorption, and elimination of feces. Disorders from *congenital defects* or *mechanical degenerative phenomena* can result in diseases in the gastrointestinal tract.

The gastrointestinal tract (alimentary canal) is a hollow tube lined by mucosa and surrounded by smooth muscle. Within this long tube, digestive juices are secreted into the lumen (passageway of the tube) and peristalsis propels the digesting food onward. The mucosa absorbs the liquids and digested food (carbohydrates, fats, protein) which is then transported through the portal vein into the liver for further processing.

The motility of the gastrointestinal tract is controlled by the autonomic nervous system. When the autonomic nerves are absent (aganglionosis), *megaesophagus* or *megacolon* occurs (Fig. 15-1). Food does not pass through the esophagus nor feces through the aganglionic colon. The latter condition is called *Hirschsprung's disease.*

Congenital Obstructive Lesions

The passageway of the gastrointestinal tract must remain open for proper digestion of food. Several conditons, however, can obstruct the lumen. For instance, obstruction occurs from narrowing in the gut of newborn infants (see Chapter 3, Development and Birth Defects) and from hernias or tumors in adults. A severe congenital abnormality in infants results from an *imperforate anus.* A child suffering from failure of the anus to open is unable to survive without surgical reconstruction of the anus. Another congenital abnormality, *atresia* (failure of the tract to form a lumen), blocks the tube. Atresia occurs at any level of the gastrointestinal tract, but is most frequently found in the esophagus and small intestines of infants.

Blockage of the G-I tract need not be entirely complete. For instance, *pyloric stenosis* (narrowing) occurs in some boys at about two months of age. These boys vomit after feeding and a firm, olive-like knot can be felt at the pyloric end of the stomach which empties food into the duodenum. The stenosis obstructs the outflow of stomach contents into the duodenum. Surgical opening of the stenotic area relieves the pressure.

Hernia

A *hernia* is the protrusion of one of the abdominal visceral organs through a wall of the cavity in which it is normally enclosed. Examples would be when a portion of the G-I tract becomes displaced through a defect in the diaphragm or through the wall of the abdominal cavity. The umbilicus, inguinal, and femoral regions are the most common sites for hernias. The stomach can herniate through the leaves of the diaphragm (hiatal hernia). Hernias can usually be reduced by application of pressure. Danger arises when a hernia becomes *incarcerated* (entrapped) in the hernia sac. When incarceration occurs, the blood supply to the trapped intestine can become *strangulated* (obstructed) and necrosis results. *Septicemia* (blood poisoning) ensues if the necrotic bowel is not resected.

Two conditions related to hernias can obstruct the G-I tract: *Volvulus* is a twisting of the bowel on itself (occurs in elderly persons), and *intussusception* is an obstructive disorder that occurs in children wherein the bowel telescopes or invaginates within itself.

Arterial Occlusion

Another cause of necrosis of the bowel is when arteries supplying the intestine become occluded (blocked). Abdominal discomfort (abdominal angina) can occur following a meal in a person with partially obstructed mesenteric

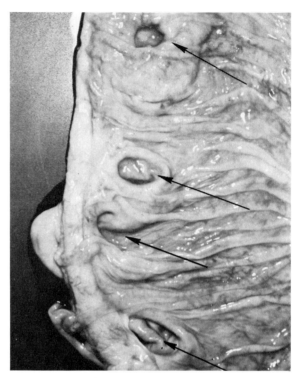

Figure 15-2   *Diverticulosis of colon. Openings into diverticuli are seen in the mucosa* (arrows).

arteries. The condition is analogous in its pathophysiology to angina pectoris. This can occur from an embolus or from thrombosis of an artery. The feces, rich in bacteria, flood into the abdominal cavity and cause *peritonitis* (acute inflammation) when the blood supply is blocked and the bowel undergoes necrosis.

Diverticulosis

Diverticuli are saclike outpouchings (usually of the colon) that arise from degeneration of the wall. They protrude from the lumen of the gut (Fig. 15-2). Diverticuli of the sigmoid occurs commonly in elderly Americans (Fig. 15-2); approximately one-third of persons beyond forty years of age experience diverticulosis. The diverticuli become packed with feces and can become infected (*diverticulitis*). The affected person develops fever, diarrhea, and abdominal discomfort. Usually diverticulitis responds to antibiotics and occasionally surgical resection is required. Diverticulosis is preventable and treatable with a diet rich in fiber.

Gastroenteritis

Gastroenteritis occurs as a result of infectious diseases and inflammatory conditions arising from toxins or unknown causes. When the inflammatory process involves the stomach, *gastritis* is present. It is signaled by epigastric pain and vomiting. By contrast, inflammation of the intestines (from any etiology) generally causes *diarrhea*, an excessive expulsion of liquid stools.

Bacterial Gastroenteritis

All experienced travelers to Latin American countries have become familiar with gastroenteritis ("Montezuma's revenge"). A variety of viruses, bacteria, and parasites can infect the intestinal tract and cause acute or chronic ulceration of the mucosa. Most frequently it is caused by *Salmonella*, *Shigella*, cholera, or *E. coli*.

Signs and symptoms of acute gastroenteritis are: (a) nausea, (b) vomiting, and (c) watery diarrhea. All the bacterial gastroenteritis diseases are responsive to antibiotics and can be prevented by good sanitation and hygiene. Antispasmodic drugs such as Lomotil and fluids restore electrolytes and stop the diarrhea.

Parasites

Amebic colitis is caused by a protozoan which is acquired by ingesting contaminated food or liquids. This parasite ulcerates the mucosa of the colon and causes acute inflammation. Diarrhea characterized by extensive mucus production and hemorrhage results. The diagnosis is achieved by identifying amebae in the stool.

Various *helminth worms* (hookworm, roundworm, tapeworm) can cause severe chronic gastroenteritis. Parasitized individuals often suffer from malnutrition and become weakened by anemia. Blood is lost from the parasitized mucosa and absorption of food is often impaired.

Acute Appendicitis

Acute appendicitis is an inflammation of the vermiform appendix. This common disease occurs most frequently in adolescent children. Typically, nausea, loss of appetite (anorexia), fever, leukocytosis, and right lower abdominal pain is experienced. Tenderness is noted when the appendix is palpated at *McBurney's point*, lateral to and below the umbilicus overlying the inflamed appendix. Many inflammatory and infectious disorders involving the intestines, urinary tract, Fallopian tubes, and ovaries can mimic acute appendicitis. Hence, the differential diagnosis of acute appendicitis can be very difficult. About 20% of the time a surgeon removes an appendix (for a diagnosis of acute appendicitis) which turns out to be normal.

The surgeon exploring the abdomen for acute appendicitis sees and removes a swollen red appendix. Microscopic examination reveals acute inflammation in the appendix (Fig. 15-3). Failure to remove the appendix can lead to rupture. The abdominal cavity is invaded by bacteria from the feces and *acute peritonitis*, which is life-threatening, ensues.★

Peptic Ulcer

Experts estimate that one American in ten will develop an ulcer at some time. Thirty years ago men were 20 times more likely than women to develop ulcers. Today the ratio is only two to one and the incidence is declining in both sexes.

Etiology

Peptic ulcer is characterized by the loss of the mucosal lining in the stomach or the first part of the duodenum. Such ulcers result from the digestive action of gastric juice on the mucous membrane when the latter is rendered susceptible to such action by local or psychosomatic factors. The extreme thinness and fragility of the G-I mucosa facilitates ulceration. Ulcers arise from many causes:

★An estimated 150 patients die yearly from ruptured appendicitis in the United States.

physical and psychological stress, trauma, stress resulting from cutaneous burns, major surgery, infections, uremia, and drugs such as aspirin, cortisone, or alcohol.

Location

Peptic ulcers occur at any level in the gastrointestinal tract where acid and enzymes damage the intestinal mucosa. Most frequently ulcers occur in the lesser curvature of the distal part of the stomach. Ulcers are localized chiefly in five areas: (a) duodenum, (b) stomach, (c) esophagus, (d) Meckel's diverticulum in the ileum, and (e) jejunum. Approximately 99% of all peptic ulcers occur in the duodenum and stomach.

Duodenal ulcers occur most frequently in middle-aged men, whereas *gastric ulcers* occur more frequently in elderly individuals. All peptic ulcers occur from peptic acid digestion of the mucosa. Usually, individuals with duodenal ulcers have excessive hydrochloric acid secretion.

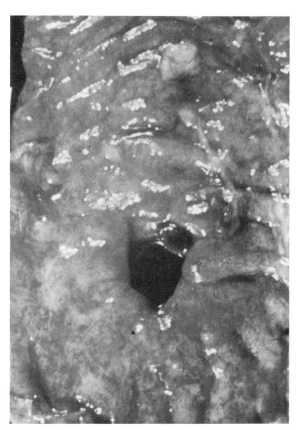

Figure 15-4 *Peptic ulcer. A punched-out sharply defined ulcer is seen in the mucosa of the duodenum. The patient died of hemorrhage.*

Acid Secretion

The production of acid is controlled (a) by stimuli from the brain (psychic phase) via the vagus nerve which stimulates the gastric mucosa to release HCl; and (b) by liberation of a hormone, gastrin, which also stimulates the release of HCl.

Peptic ulcers are round and sharply punched out with perpendicular walls (Fig. 15-4). The base of the ulcer is covered by a thin layer of fibrin and necrotic debris and beneath this layer neutrophils, granulation, and scar tissue are seen.

Complications

Complications of peptic ulcers include: (a) hemorrhage; (b) perforation; (c) obstruction of the

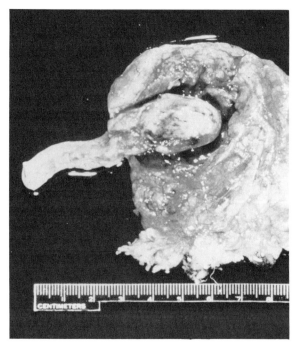

Figure 15-3 *Acute appendicitis. The tip of the appendix is necrotic and surrounded by the greater omentum, which has sealed the perforated tip.*

G-I tract from edema and scars; and (d) rarely, malignancy. Hemorrhage can be massive and is the commonest complication. It is important to determine the source of bleeding. The duodenum ranks first as the most likely source of bleeding and accounts for nearly 30% of gastrointestinal hemorrhage.

Various causes of upper gastrointestinal hemorrhage are illustrated in Figure 15-5. The mortality rate of patients with G-I hemorrhage is approximately 5%; hemorrhage causes one-fourth of deaths from peptic ulcer disease.

Perforation of ulcer is an infrequent but grave complication. The acute peritonitis which ensues

following perforation accounts for nearly two-thirds of all deaths in peptic ulcer patients. Another complication of peptic ulcer, obstruction, is often signaled by vomiting. When the outlet of the stomach and duodenum become scarred and narrowed, food is unable to pass downward and vomiting ensues.

Treatment

Following the diagnosis of a peptic ulcer a bland diet and antacids are given. More than one-half of the ulcers will respond to therapy. But when the ulcer fails to heal within a few weeks or if a complication occurs, surgical procedures are carried

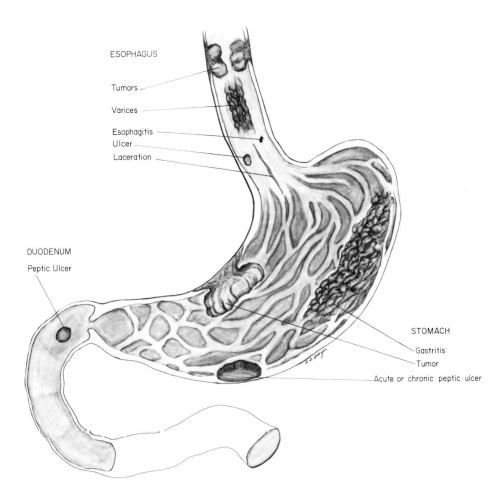

Figure 15-5   *Causes and sites of upper gastrointestinal hemorrhage.*

out to decrease secretion of HCl and exposure of the mucosa to this acid. Cutting of vagus nerves (*vagotomy*) or the removal of a portion of the stomach (*gastrectomy*) usually corrects the hyperacidity. Alternatively, widening the outlet of the stomach (*pyloroplasty*) decreases exposure of the mucosa to acid. Pyloroplasty and vagotomy are often performed together to eliminate the effects of the acid on the mucosa. Finally, for duodenal ulcers the stomach is sewed to the jejunum and an opening between them is made (gastrojejunostomy) to bypass the ulcerated duodenum.

Acute Gastritis

Inflammation of the gastric mucosa (*gastritis*, Figures 15-5, 15-6) can cause extensive hemorrhage and death. Acute hemorrhagic gastritis can sometimes be successfully treated by pouring ice water through a nasogastric tube into the stomach. Cold water constricts the blood vessels and the hemorrhage usually subsides. A major cause of acute hemorrhagic gastritis is acute alcoholism. Alcohol stimulates HCl secretion which inflames the mucosa.

Inflammatory Disorders of Unknown Etiology

In additon to the infectious diseases which cause ulceration and inflammation of the intestinal tract, two diseases of unknown etiology also commonly cause chronic ulcerative and inflammatory diseases of the intestines in Western countries. *Crohn's disease* (regional enteritis) inflames and ulcerates the small intestine, and *ulcerative colitis* inflames and ulcerates the colon and rectum. As mentioned earlier, abdominal pain with cramping, diarrhea, malabsorption, and weight loss occur when the intestines are inflamed.

Crohn's Disease

Crohn's disease is a chronic, relapsing, inflammatory disorder which usually affects the terminal end

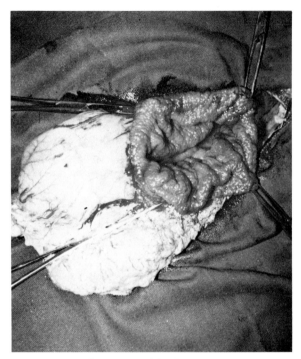

Figure 15-6   *Acute gastritis. The opened stomach mucosa is reddened and inflamed.*

of the ileum and, on occasion, the adjacent colon. This disease is thought to be caused by an infectious agent and it afflicts individuals in the third and fourth decades of life. Physical examination reveals tenderness of the abdomen and a thickened ileal bowel wall may be felt. X-rays show that the lumen of the ileum is narrowed ("string sign").

With this disease the wall of the intestine is thickened by an acute and chronic inflammatory infiltrate that extends through all layers of the bowel wall from the mucosa to the serosa (Fig. 15-7). Neutrophils, lymphocytes, histiocytes, and plasma cells invade the wall of the ileum. Their presence suggests an immune reaction to an infectious agent.

The weakened, inflamed intestinal wall can perforate and form a *fissure* (crack) around the anus or a *fistulous tract* (abnormal passageway) extending from a hole in the inflamed intestine out to the anus or nearby skin. Since this disease tends to recur, surgery is not usually performed unless fistulas are present. Sulfa drugs, rest, and fluids are given to maintain the patient until the inflammation subsides.

Ulcerative Colitis

Ulcerative colitis is an inflammatory disease of unknown etiology that commonly involves the recto-sigmoid, but it can affect the entire colon. Persons suffering from ulcerative colitis have remitting and relapsing attacks of bloody mucoid diarrhea which persist for days to months. The attacks subside but then recur when the individual is under emotional stress.

The disease is characterized by ulceration of the mucosa with an acute inflammatory infiltrate of neutrophils (Fig. 15-8). Unlike Crohn's disease, the inflammation in ulcerative colitis is limited to the mucosal surface.

Complications of ulcerative colitis can arise in patients with aggressive disease. These include: (a) *anemia* from bloody diarrhea and weight loss, (b) *arthritis,* and (c) *carcinoma,* which can arise in ulcers which have persisted for several decades.

The diagnosis of ulcerative colitis can be made clinically, but the diagnosis must be confirmed by a proctoscope (Fig. 15-8). Biopsy of lesions reveals ulceration of the mucosa and acute inflammation.

Treatment often includes the use of antibiotics and cortisone. In severe cases, the surgeon removes portions of the colon or performs a diverting colostomy. This procedure involves moving a loop of the colon or ileum up to and through the abdominal wall. An opening is made in the intestine to permit feces to be collected in a *colostomy bag*. A colostomy enables the inflamed colon to rest while the feces bypass the inflamed site. Later, the colostomy can be reduced and the flow of feces through the colon and anus can be reestablished.

Malabsorption

Malabsorption, faulty absorption of nutrient materials from the alimentary canal, can be caused by intestinal inflammation or infection, pancreatic disorders, biliary tract obstruction, or primary disease in the intestines. The small intestine, except for the duodenum, is relatively free of disease, but malabsorption of food in the ileum and jejunum is a common problem.

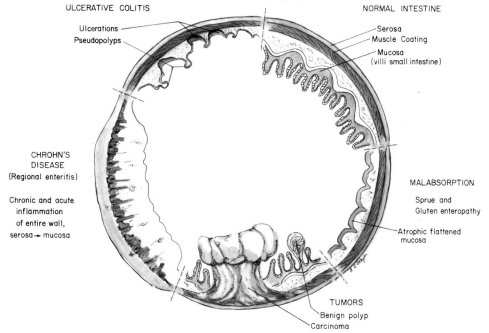

Figure 15-7   *Cross-sectional composite of diseases of the small and large intestines.*

Failure of the pancreas (see Chapter 16, Liver and Pancreatic Disorders) causes malabsorption from incomplete absorption of nutrients. For example, when the pancreas fails to produce *lipase*, fat cannot be absorbed in the ileum and the stool becomes fatty due to the presence of undigested fats. Malnutrition can develop.

When the flow of bile is obstructed, the lack of bile in the intestinal tract impairs emulsification and absorption of both fat and fat soluble vitamins A, D, E, K. *Rickets*, from deficient absorption of vitamin D, (see Chapter 10, Nutritional Diseases) occurs. Malabsorption can also be caused by allergic responses to foods or deficiencies of enzymes in intestinal mucosa cells. Two-thirds of black persons have a lactase deficiency (lactose intolerance). When drinking milk, the person fails to digest lactose, with diarrhea, bloating, and malabsorption resulting.

Celiac disease, another disorder related to malabsorption, is caused by a toxic reaction to *gluten*, a substance found in wheat. The intestinal villi become atrophic and edematous. Another disorder, *sprue*, also causes malabsorption. It is probably caused by an infectious agent. In celiac disease and sprue the intestinal villi become atrophic. Following treatment, the villi regain a normal appearance and can absorb food. The composite diagram displayed in Figure 15-7 demonstrates several common intestinal disorders.

Cancer of Gastrointestinal Tract

The causes of gastrointestinal cancer are unknown. Suspected causative agents in our diets include nitrosamines (food preservatives). Certain bacteria which can convert bile acids into carcinogens have been found in persons with diets low in fiber and high in fats. Such diets and bacteria are associated with colon cancer. Several autosomal-dominant inherited colonic polyposis cancer syndromes occur; however, inherited colon cancer constitutes only a small fraction of all colon cancers. The recent progressive decline in gastric cancer implies a change in diet has protected us against this cancer, but the increased frequency of colon and pancreatic cancers is not reassuring (see Chapter 8).

Gastric Cancer

Despite the decline in gastric cancer in the United States, it still ranks fourth as the cause of death due to cancer. When a diagnosis is made, the patient has often lost weight, experienced upper abdominal pain, and has anemia.

Physical examination often reveals a palpable tumor mass in the abdomen and anemia. The diagnosis is achieved by X-ray examination and by taking a biopsy specimen through a gastroscopy tube. If the lesion is identified early, gastrectomy (80% of the stomach is removed) can be done. But chances of surviving five years are only 10%. Death often

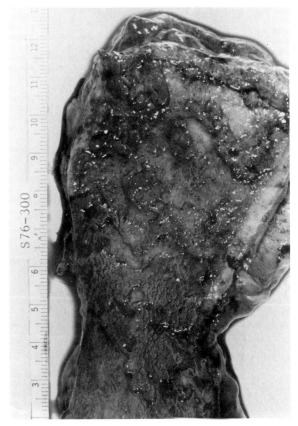

Figure 15-8 *Ulcerative colitis of the rectum and sigmoid colon. The entire mucosa is inflamed and numerous small ulcers are present.*

results from extensive metastases to the liver (Fig. 15-9) and from complicating hemorrhage or infection.

Colon and Rectal Cancer

The small intestine is not frequently involved by cancer. By contrast, the large intestine (colon) and rectum develop cancers in approximately 70,000 persons in the United States each year and 45,000 deaths occur. Cancers of the colon and rectum are the second leading cause of death from cancer in the United States (lung cancer ranks first).

A frequent symptom of G-I tract cancer is melena (blood in the stool). But both benign adenomatous or villous polyps and cancer can hemorrhage into the stool. Polyps can be identified with

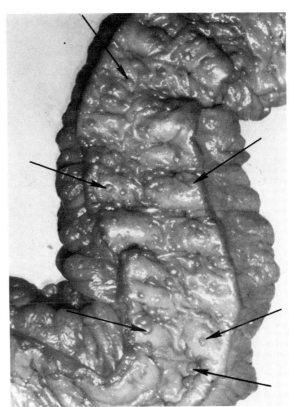

Figure 15-10   *Colonic polyps. Multiple benign adenomatous polyps are seen* (arrows).

an X-ray (lower G-I barium enema examination) or they can be seen and removed in a proctoscope (Fig. 15-10). Polyps on long stalks can sometimes become malignant. About 5% of adenomatous polyps contain carcinoma in situ in their tips. These carcinomas show no invasion of underlying tissue.

Diagnosis

Rectal bleeding with either diarrhea or constipation, abdominal pain and weight loss are commonly experienced by elderly persons with colorectal cancer. A tumor mass is often palpable in the abdomen or the tumor can be detected by simply examining the rectum with an index finger (Fig. 15-11). In fact, about 50% of the cancers can be palpated with the gloved finger. A biopsy is taken through a proctoscope for diagnosis and if malignancy is found the rectum is removed.

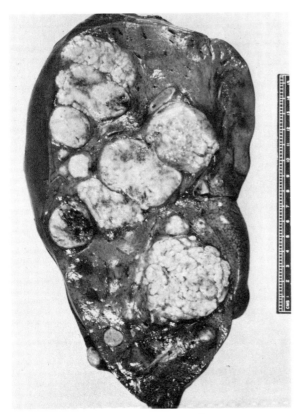

Figure 15-9   *Metastatic gastric cancer to the liver. Large white "cannon ball" tumors fill the liver. (Armed Forces Institute of Pathology, negative No. 4234.)*

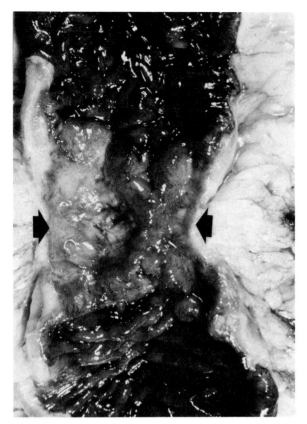

Figure 15-11   *Colonic carcinoma. This carcinoma constricted the channel and caused constipation. It was detected by barium enema X-ray examination (between arrows).*

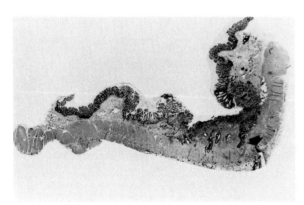

Figure 15-12   *Minute ulcerating colon cancer. The patient had been anticoagulated for pulmonary embolism and developed hemorrhage from the small artery eroded by the cancerous ulcer (arrow).*

Colonoscopy and colonoscopic polypectomy are techniques which enable clinicians to diagnose colon cancer. Colonoscopy permits direct visualization of the colonic mucosa from the rectum to the cecum; biopsies may be taken of any lesion and cytology may be collected by aspirating or brushing a lesion.

Adenomatous polyps can be completely resected (polypectomy) through a colonoscopic resectoscope. Larger (more than 2 cm diameter) lesions usually require segmental resection of the malignant segment of the colon. If the tumor is large and located in the rectum an abdominal-perineal resection is required in which the anus and rectum containing the carcinoma are removed. A colostomy or opening of the colon to permit the passage of stool into colostomy bag is made in patients with rectal or obstructing colon cancers.

Typically, tumors in the right side of the colon are annular (surround the colon in a ring-like fashion) and thereby cause constipation. By contrast, tumors occurring in the sigmoid colon often protrude as large malignant polyps into the lumen of the colon. The polypoid tumors are usually less invasive than the annular tumors. Surgical resection is the only curative method of treatment for colon and rectal cancer.

A diagnosis of colon or rectal cancer can often be further substantiated by detection of a fetal antigen, *carcinoembryonic antigen (CEA)* in the patient's serum. Carcinoembryonic antigen is produced by the colon cancer and should disappear from the patient's serum when the cancer has been totally removed. Conversely, CEA persists when tumor persists (see Chapter 8).

Prognosis

When colorectal carcinomas invade only superficially (Fig. 15-12), the five year survival rate after surgical resection is approximately 95%. By contrast, the prognosis is poor for patients who have metastases to the liver. Early diagnosis of colorectal cancer is possible by yearly proctoscopic examination. All persons over the age of 40 should have yearly proctoscopic examinations.

Summary

The gastrointestinal tract, like the respiratory tract, is exposed and vulnerable to environmental agents. Infectious diseases can ensue from contaminated food. The delicate mucosal lining can become ulcerated when HCl and enzymes digest it. Cancers probably result from chemicals ingested with food. Carcinomas of digestive organs is the leading cause of death from cancer in the United States. Within the digestive tract, carcinoma of the large intestine is the most common form.

Signs and symptoms of G-I disorders include toxic reactions, obstruction, irritation of nerves, masses, disturbed motility, hemorrhage, or malabsorption. Chemical carcinogens which are ingested are thought to be responsible for carcinomas of the G-I tract which affect the colon, rectum, and the stomach. Other sites seldom are affected by cancer.

Typical clinical patterns of weight loss and anemia signal G-I tract cancer. Diagnosis rests on X-ray demonstration of a lesion, endoscopy, and microscopic examination of a biopsy confirms the diagnosis. As for other malignancies, prognosis is predicated on the location, histologic type, and stage of the tumor at time of surgical intervention.

Bibliography

Cope, Z. 1973. *The early diagnosis of the acute abdomen*, ed. 4. New York: Oxford University Press, Inc. A book of the differential diagnosis of abdominal pain. Surgeons rely on the "pearls" contained in this book. Deciding when it is appropriate to operate is the most difficult task a surgeon faces.

Gold, P., and Friedman, S. 1973. Immunology and colon cancer: further evaluation of the radioimmunoassay for carcinoembryonic antigen of the human digestive system as an adjunct in cancer diagnosis. *Dis. Colon Rectum* 16:358. Discusses the use of carcinoembryonic antigens in colorectal cancer.

Gordon, H. E., et al. 1969. Diagnosis and management of gastrointestinal bleeding. *Ann. Inst. Med.* 71:966. Lists and discusses the differential diagnosis of gastrointestinal hemorrhage.

Hillebrand, S. S. 1975. *Dental caries*. Bethesda, Maryland. A monograph on tooth decay.

Kretchmer, N. 1972. Lactose and lactase. *Sci. Am.* 227: 1–10. The global problem of enzyme deficiency and resulting failure to absorb lactose in milk is presented.

Peterson, W. L. 1977. Healing of duodenal ulcer with an antacid regimen. *N. Engl. J. Med.* 297:341–345. This double blind study demonstrated the importance of antacids in healing ulcers.

Robbins, S. L. 1974. *Pathologic basis of disease*, 901–984. Philadelphia: W. B. Saunders Company. Summarizes the pathology of the G-I tract.

Rowe, N. H., et al. 1976. The effect of age, sex, race, and economic status on dental caries experience of the permanent dentition. *Pediatrics* 57:457–461. Discusses the prevalence of dental caries at various ages.

Schuster, M. 1976. Disorders of the aging GI system. *Hosp. Pract.* 11:95. Thorough discussion of functional or psychological G-I complaints.

Spiro, H. M. 1970. *Clinical gastroenterology*. New York: Macmillan, Inc. A standard comprehensive textbook.

Valdes-Dapena, A. M., and Stein, G. M. 1970. *Morphologic pathology of the alimentary canal*. Philadelphia: W. B. Saunders Company. Emphasis on the X-ray findings of G-I disease.

Wayne, J. D. 1973. The development of carcinoma of the colon. *Gastroenterology* 46:427–429. Reviews the pathogenesis of colon polyps as related to colon cancer.

Welch, C. E. 1975. Abdominal surgery. *N. Engl. J. Med.* 293:957–964. A review article on surgery of the abdominal viscera.

Winawer, S. J., and Sherlock, P. 1977. Detecting early colon cancer. *Hosp. Pract.* 12:49–56. Techniques for detecting colon cancer early are presented.

CHAPTER 16

Hepatic and Pancreatic Disorders

Chapter Outline

Objectives

After reading this chapter you should be able to

List the four major functions of the liver.

Describe a normal liver lobule.

Describe normal circulation of blood through the liver.

List the three major life-threatening groups of hepatic disease.

Describe the common signs and symptoms of hepatic disease.

Compare the physical examination findings which indicate acute and chronic liver
disease.

Describe the pathophysiology of portal hypertension.

Compare the clinical aspects of hepatitis B and hepatitis A types of viral hepatitis.

List the pathophysiologic events responsible for death from hepatic failure.

Describe three lesions that alcohol can cause in the liver.

Know the frequency of occurrence of cirrhosis in chronic alcoholics.

List two histopathologic features of cirrhosis.

Classify seven types of cirrhosis.

Compare micronodular and macronodular cirrhosis.

List the complications possible in a cirrhotic patient.

Describe two pathophysiologic processes responsible for ascites with cirrhosis.

Compare the frequency of metastatic versus primary cancer of the liver.

List two etiologic agents of hepatocarcinoma in Africans and compare the etiology with that of the disease in the United States.

Know what alpha-fetoprotein is and how it is used in diagnosis of liver disease.

Compare the cellular origin of hepatocarcinoma and cholangiocarcinoma.

List the uses for tests of liver function.

List the groups of functions and diseases on which liver function tests have a bearing.

List the fat soluble vitamins requiring bile for their absorption.

Define the terms cholecystitis and cholelithiasis.

Discuss why one must distinguish between diagnoses of intrahepatic and extrahepatic jaundice.

Describe the clinical findings regarding acute cholecystitis.

Know how a cholecystogram is performed and interpreted.

List three possible complications of gallstones.

List the three major diseases of the exocrine pancreas.

Describe the clinical findings regarding pancreatic deficiency.

Know what pancreatic enzymes do to tissues when they are liberated from an injured pancreas.

Describe the typical symptoms of a person with acute pancreatitis.

List two complications of acute pancreatitis.

Discuss the etiology of chronic pancreatitis and how the disease is diagnosed.

Define the term insulinoma.

Compare the clinical findings regarding a pancreatic cancer arising in the head and one arising in the tail of the pancreas.

Know the prognoses for hepatic and pancreatic cancers.

Introduction

The liver in an adult weighs between 1400 and 1600 gm. This highly vascular organ performs several vital processes: (a) synthesis of proteins (by hepatocytes); (b) detoxification of drugs and bilirubin (by hepatocytes); (c) phagocytosis of particulate material (by Kupfer cells); and (d) production and excretion of bile (hepatocytes produce bile and bile ductules excrete it). Diseases of the liver cause dysfunction of the hepatocytes and Kupfer cells.

Liver Lobule

The normal physiology of the liver depends upon a prescribed flow of blood and bile through a vascular and bile canalicular system. A *liver lobule* (Fig. 16-1) has as its center a hepatic venule, from which cords of hepatocytes radiate out to the periphery. The outer boundaries of the lobule are demarcated by the *portal triads* (hepatic artery, portal venule, and bile ductule). Hepatocytes are surrounded by hepatic *sinusoids* which are lined by specialized reticuloendothelial cells (Kupfer cells).

Blood enters the liver from the gastrointestinal tract via the portal vein at a volume of 800 ml per minute. Immediately within the substance of the liver the large portal vein divides into tiny portal venules which are connected directly to the sinusoids. Blood flows through the sinusoids in intimate contact with Kupfer cells and hepatocytes and exits from the liver via hepatic veins into the inferior vena cava. Arterial blood supply (at 600 ml per minute) comes from the hepatic artery which subdivides into hepatic arterioles that course along the portal triads and empty into the sinuses. Minute bile canaliculi are formed by adjacent hepatocytes and they unite with bile ductules which carry bile to the bile ducts.

Diseases of the Liver

Diseases of the liver that are life-threatening include three groups: (a) disorders caused by chemical toxins (like ethyl alcohol); (b) infectious diseases (like viral hepatitis); and (c) cancer (hepatocarcinoma). Other liver diseases arise from inborn errors of metabolism (see Chapter 9, Inherited Disorders), congenital defects, or injuries.

Virtually all diseases of the liver cause *necrosis* of the hepatocytes. But the liver's immense capacity for regeneration (up to 90% of the liver in humans has been removed and the remaining 10% has regenerated) makes it resistant to permanent damage. The necrosis and inflammation that occur in *acute liver disease* is termed *acute hepatitis*. When the severely injured liver heals, scar tissue and regenerative nodules produce *cirrhosis*, or *chronic liver disease*. Examples of toxins, infections, and neoplasms follow. Later they will be discussed in greater detail.

Toxic chemicals can seriously alter the function and structure of the liver. Alcohol is enjoyed socially by millions of people, but when taken in excess it can cause hepatic necrosis. Acute inflam-

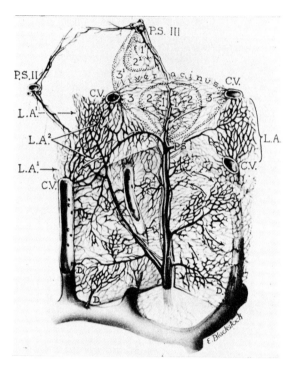

Figure 16-1   *Liver lobule (Rappaport). Vascular biliary architecture of an acinar agglomerate, see P.S.I. and P.S.III, three adjacent portal fields; L.A. and L.A.¹, simple liver acinus; L.A.², simple acinus penetrating a hexagonal field situated well above the level of origin of the acinus. C.V. (central vein), terminal hepatic venule. 1, 2, 3, circulatory zones of the simple liver acinus; D, collecting venules. (From Schiff, L. 1975. Diseases of liver, ed. 3. Philadelphia: J. B. Lippincott Company.)*

mation develops as a response to the necrosis and chronic alcoholism can cause fibrosis (cirrhosis) of the liver. Nearly 9 million chronic alcoholic persons reside in the United States, but only one in ten develops cirrhosis. Cirrhosis is the fifth ranking cause of death in middle-aged men. In addition to alcohol, other agents such as chloroform, vinyl chloride, and certain toxins in both mushrooms and fungi can destroy the liver.

Infectious diseases of the liver are caused by various parasites, bacteria, and viruses. Infectious hepatitis, for example, results from eating or drinking food contaminated with hepatitis A virus. In contrast, hepatitis B virus is generally obtained in blood transfusions and hence is termed serum hepatitis. Both diseases inflame the liver (hepatitis) and, on rare occasions, cause progressive chronic hepatic failure or cirrhosis.

The liver is vulnerable to primary and secondary *neoplasms*. Metastatic (secondary) carcinomas implant in the liver from the stomach and colon after passing through the portal vein. Less commonly, primary malignancies arise from hepatocytes (hepatocarcinoma), bile ducts (cholangiocarcinoma), or blood vessels (angiosarcoma) in the liver. Regardless of what causes liver disease, only a few stereotyped clinical signs and symptoms indicate liver disease.

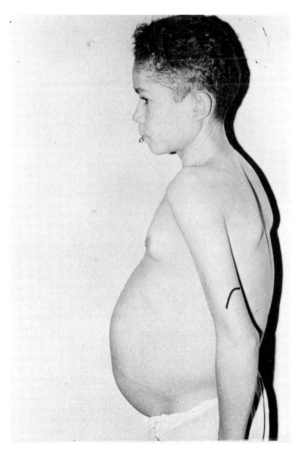

Figure 16-2 *This young man has stigmata of chronic liver disease: gynecomastia (breast enlargement), wasting, and ascites fluid distending his abdomen.*

Symptoms and Signs

A *sense of fullness* of the abdomen and a loss of appetite (*anorexia*) are initial symptoms of liver disease. *Diarrhea, constipation,* and *pale colored feces* also signal liver disease. Concurrently, the *urine* becomes *brown-green. Nausea and vomiting* as well as *weight loss* may occur. A person who smokes may lose the desire for cigarettes.

Jaundice, a yellow discoloration of the skin and sclerae, results from an accumulation of bilirubin in the blood and tissues. Bilirubin is catabolized from digested hemoglobin (see Chapter 11, Hematology) in the liver. When the liver fails to detoxify bilirubin, it accumulates and discolors the body.

Red palms and numerous small dilated blood vessels (*spider nevi*) are seen in the skin of persons with liver disease. The *testes* can become *atrophic* and the breasts of males enlarge (*gynecomastia*). The person becomes thin and the abdomen swells with ascitic fluid (Fig. 16-2).

The *physical examination* findings help determine whether the hepatic disease is acute or chronic. When the disease is *chronic* (cirrhosis), the liver is *firm* and *shrunken*. With *acute liver disease* (hepatitis), the liver is enlarged and tender upon deep palpation. Signs of *increased portal hypertension* are found in chronic liver disease: The spleen can be enlarged (*splenomegaly*) and palpable, and *engorged collateral veins* cover the abdomen. Portal hypertension also causes hemorrhoids to develop in some persons.

Clinical History   The clinical histories taken from patients thought to have hepatic disease focus on possible exposure to infectious agents (those received via contaminated blood or water) or toxins (such as alcohol). Patients are asked whether their skin has ever been yellow (jaundice), and about their diet, alcohol intake, or exposure to hepatotoxins. Typically, a person experiencing serum hepatitis becomes tired (malaise) and jaundiced six weeks after receiving a blood transfusion. In contrast, cirrhosis generally occurs in chronic alcoholics giving a long history of alcohol abuse. Jaundice, ascites (accumulation of serous fluid in the abdomen) and hematemesis (vomiting of blood) may result in their hospitalization.

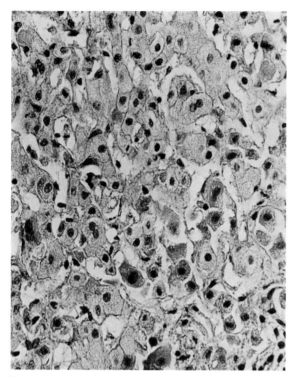

Figure 16-3 *Photomicrograph of acute hepatitis. The infected hepatocytes have become balloon-shaped and necrosis is occurring in cells with dark nuclei. × 400.*

Acute Hepatitis

Infectious agents (such as viruses) and chemical toxins (such as alcohol) cause necrosis and acute inflammation of the liver (hepatitis). Hepatitis, whatever the cause, usually implies a viral etiology. But acute hepatitis in a broad sense can also be caused by alcohol excess, drugs, and other hepatotoxic agents. What follows are descriptions of hepatitis caused by viral infections and alcohol—the most common causes of hepatitis.

Infectious Hepatitis (Hepatitis A Virus)   Acute infectious hepatitis can occur in isolated cases or in epidemics. Infectious hepatitis is caused by hepatitis A virus which is acquired by eating contaminated food or liquids. This virus enters the body by the fecal-oral route; unsanitary conditions accelerate its spread (see Chapter 7, Infectious Diseases).

The author recalls two beaches in Brazil. One beach was completely safe whereas the other was called "Hepatitis Beach." The town's sewage, laden with human excrement, flowed directly into the water of "Hepatitis Beach." Several nurses, technicians, and a medical student from the SS HOPE developed acute hepatitis from swimming there.

The incubation period (time from exposure to onset of symptoms) for infectious hepatitis is about one month. Only 1 in 20 individuals develop outward or clinical signs of hepatitis. Anorexia, malaise, nausea, vomiting, and diarrhea together with fever and chills are some of the signs. The individual becomes jaundiced, the urine is dark, and the stools are light. A feeling of fullness and tenderness to touch in the area of the liver are noted. Usually recovery provides lasting immunity. Prophylactic injections of gamma globulin containing antibodies against the virus minimize the infection.

Pathology   The hepatocytes swell and neutrophils invade the liver to remove necrotic hepatocytes (Fig. 16-3). Rarely, the infection persists and severe necrosis and cirrhosis develop. Infectious hepatitis is generally a less severe disease than serum hepatitis.

Serum Hepatitis (Hepatitis B Virus)   Hepatitis caused by the type B virus is acquired by needle pricks, transfusion of infected blood, or, rarely, by mouth. Serum hepatitis is an occupational hazard of hospital personnel who work with transplant recipients or patients who might have acquired hepatitis from blood transfusions. Likewise, individuals working in clinical laboratories can easily become infected by hepatitis B virus. When body fluids, tissues, or exudates are handled, the risk of acquiring viral hepatitis increases tenfold. For instance, during a two year period while the author was at the University of Minnesota Hospitals, 75 new cases of hepatitis occurred among personnel (laboratory staff, nurses, physicians) associated with hemodialysis transplant patients.

In view of this serious occupational hazard, health professionals such as nurses, aids, medical technologists, and especially blood bank personnel and persons working in immunology and clinical chemistry laboratories, should take precautions to avoid infection and their serum should be periodically screened for hepatitis B virus.

Dectection   Various immunological techniques can be used to detect hepatitis B virus—agar gel diffusion, counter immunoelectrophoresis, and radioimmunoassay. Blood donors, patients, and hospital workers can be screened for this virus. A vaccine should soon become available to protect us from this deadly virus.

Serum hepatitis is characterized by a more gradual onset than infectious hepatitis. Patients may not feel ill but suddenly realize they have turned yellow. Shortly thereafter a loss of appetite and weakness may be noted. Individuals who use drugs, especially heroin addicts, are often infected by hepatitis B virus. Serum hepatitis has a higher mortality than infectious hepatitis because chronic persistent hepatitis and cirrhosis ensue more often. Acute serum hepatitis can produce fulminating liver failure and death within weeks. Death results from one of three pathophysiologic events: (a) hemorrhage (the liver fails to produce clotting factors); (b) hepatic coma (nitrogenous toxic compounds depress cerebral function); or (c) renal failure (toxic agents such as bilirubin injure the kidney).

Alcoholic Hepatitis   Alcohol is a hepatotoxic agent which can cause either a *fatty liver* (Fig. 16-4) or hepatic necrosis with inflammation (alcoholic hepatitis). Severe damage to hepatocytes by alcohol causes an acute inflammatory reaction. This lesion is occasionally fatal (one in ten times); more often (one in two times) it heals with scarring and formation of regenerative nodules (cirrhosis). Several factors (alcohol, genetic susceptibility, and possibly malnutrition) combine to produce alcoholic hepatitis.

Individuals who develop alcoholic hepatitis generally subsist on distilled alcoholic beverages and eat poorly for weeks or months. (See Chapter 9, Nutritional Deficiency Diseases.) A fever, an enlarged and tender liver, and jaundice are experienced. Such individuals have marked abnormalities of liver function and coagulation defects commonly lead to hemorrhage. The microscopic examination

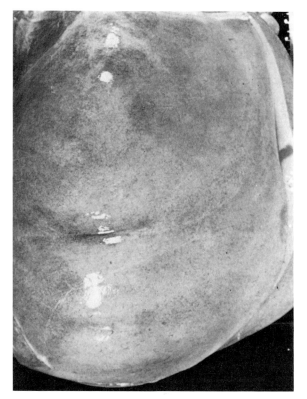

Figure 16-4   *Fatty liver from alcoholic person. It is enlarged, swollen, and greasy yellow.*

of a liver biopsy specimen reveals necrosis of the hepatocytes and an amorphous pink material in cytoplasm termed alcoholic hyalin (Fig. 16-5).

Cirrhosis (Chronic Liver Disease)

The term *cirrhosis* is derived from the Greek word, kirrhos (meaning tawny color), and it commonly refers to scarring or hardening of the liver. With this disease the liver is observed to be *fibrotic* and *nodular* (Fig. 16-6). Subsequently, surviving hepatocytes regenerate and, together with the fibrous scar tissue and regenerative nodules, interfere with the circulation of blood through the liver. Cirrhosis results from injury to hepatocytes followed by scars during the healing process.

Classification   No single histopathological classification of cirrhosis is available which is accu-

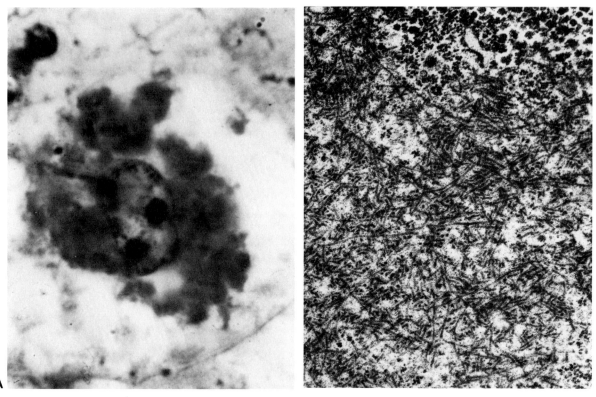

A   B

Figure 16-5   A, *Photomicrograph of liver with alcoholic hepatitis. The hepatocyte cytoplasm contains alcoholic hyalin.* × *1200.* **B,** *Electronmicrograph of alcoholic hyalin. Note the protein fibrils.* × *50,000. (Courtesy Dr. L. Gottlieb.)*

rately based on etiology. Causes of cirrhosis include alcoholism, drugs, toxins, infectious agents, bile duct obstruction, metabolic and inherited abnormalities. The simplest classification of cirrhosis is morphological and is based upon the size (micronodular or macronodular) of the regenerative nodules (Table 16-1). The key pathologic features of cirrhosis are fibrous bands connecting portal areas, and pseudolobules which obstruct blood flow through the liver (Fig. 16-7).

Complications   The complications arising from liver disease result from necrosis of hepatocytes and a loss of function. A failing liver does not produce albumin and blood clotting factors. Hypoalbuminemia and edema result and hemorrhage is apt to occur because blood clotting factor deficiencies develop.

Secondly, blockage of blood circulation through the liver by scars and regenerative nodules prevents detoxification of blood, and toxins (bilirubin and ammonia) accumulate, with jaundice and hepatic coma resulting.

Most complications of liver disease occur because of cirrhosis (Table 16-2). Portal hypertension aggravates the tendency to hemorrhage from esophageal varices. Ascites, hepatic coma, gastric hemorrhage, and renal failure may also be burdensome problems to cirrhotic patients.

Portal hypertension (increased pressure in portal vein) arises from the fibrosis within a cirrhotic liver which obstructs the portal blood flow through the liver causing the venous portal vein pressure to increase. The spleen enlarges and collateral veins form in the esophagus and abdominal wall to provide an alternate route past the fibrotic liver. Mas-

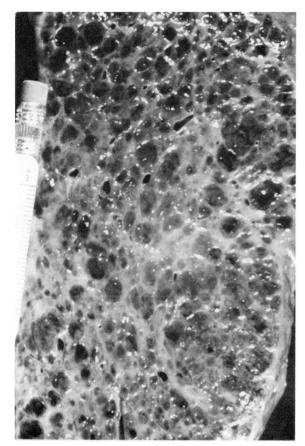

Figure 16-6   *Cirrhosis of liver. Large regenerative nodules separated by gray scar tissue are seen.*

Table 16-1
Classification of Cirrhosis*

Cirrhosis associated with alcoholism

Cirrhosis associated with hemochromatosis (iron overload)

Postnecrotic cirrhosis secondary to hepatitis

Secondary biliary cirrhosis (from bile duct obstruction)

Cirrhosis with autoimmune disorders (primary biliary cirrhosis)

α_1-antitrypsin deficiency

Miscellaneous types

*Micronodular (2 to 3 mm in diameter regenerative nodules) cirrhosis occurs as a mild type. The macronodular (3 to 10 mm nodules) type is a more severe form of cirrhosis. Either type can occur in any of the above seven subtypes.

sive hemorrhage from an *esophageal varix* (dilated collateral vein) commonly causes sudden death in cirrhotic individuals. Also, hemorrhage from the stomach and duodenum is a common complication of liver disease. The hemorrhage occurs because of two underlying pathophysiologic processes: the diseased liver fails to produce blood clotting factors and the increased portal hypertension predisposes the patient to peptic ulceration and hemorrhage. Moreover, alcohol is toxic to gastric mucosa and can induce *hemorrhagic gastritis.*

Ascites, an accumulation of fluid in the abdominal cavity (Fig. 16-2) develops when portal veins and lymphatics become compressed in the cirrhotic liver. The venous pressure increases and decreased synthesis of serum albumin by the cirrhotic liver causes water to pass from the blood and lymphatic vessels into the abdominal cavity to form ascitic fluid.

Neuropsychiatric disorders such as confusion, lethargy, inappropriate behavior, disorientation, tremor, and abnormal reflexes ensue in severe he-

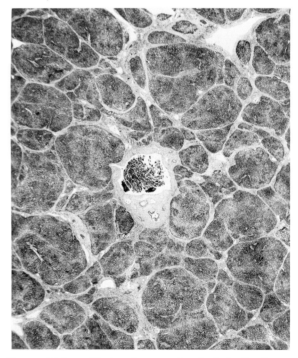

Figure 16-7   *Photomicrograph of cirrhotic liver. Regenerative nodules separated by bands of scar tissue (collagen) are seen. × 6.5.*

Table 16-2
Complications of Cirrhosis

Complications	Causes
Hemorrhage (gastrointestinal)	Decreased clotting factor synthesis and increased portal venous pressure.
Ascites	Decreased albumin synthesis and increased portal venous pressure.
Neuropsychiatric (coma or psychosis)	Accumulation of toxic nitrogenous substances or alcohol withdrawal.
Hepatorenal failure	Accumulation of toxic nitrogenous substances in the kidney.
Hepatocarcinoma	Hepatocytic necrosis with probable mutation in one hepatocyte giving rise to a malignant clone of cells.

patic disorders. Eventually *coma* can result if the liver becomes unable to detoxify ammonia and other substances noxious to the brain. The toxic blood can be removed by giving the patient blood transfusions (called exchange blood transfusion). But many patients die despite transfusions.

For unknown reasons the kidneys stop functioning in some individuals with hepatic failure. This condition is known as the *hepato-renal syndrome.* The kidneys become swollen and cease to function.

Another complication of cirrhosis is the development of *hepatocarcinoma* (hepatoma). Approximately 5% of persons with long-standing alcoholic cirrhosis develop hepatocarcinoma.

Liver Cancer

Benign and malignant hepatic neoplasms of the liver can also occur. Benign proliferation of blood vessels (hemangioma) is the most common benign tumor. Hemangiomas usually do not cause problems, but in infants they can hemorrhage and exsanguinate the child. Other benign hepatic tumors (adenoma) develop from bile ducts or hepatocytes. Adenomas seem to occur in rare instances from oral contraceptives. Such benign tumors are usually not troublesome.

By contrast, malignancies of the liver are almost always lethal. Metastatic (secondary) tumors of the liver far outnumber (20 to 1) primary hepatocarcinomas (see Chapter 15, Gastrointestinal Disorders). A metastatic tumor becomes situated in

the liver after it travels, via the portal or systemic bloodstream or lymphatics, from the stomach or colon (see Chapter 15, Gastrointestinal Disorders). Interference with liver function does not occur until approximately 80% to 90% of the liver is replaced by metastatic carcinoma.

Hepatocarcinoma accounts for the majority of primary malignancies of the liver (Fig. 16-8). The etiology of hepatocarcinoma is unknown but the 60 times greater frequency of occurrence in Mozambique than in the United States has been linked with fungal toxins that are eaten in moldy food in Africa. The toxin in the moldy food is termed aflatoxin. In addition, hepatitis B virus could be a cocarcinogen for hepatocarcinoma. In the United States, by contrast, approximately 70% of hepatocarcinomas are associated with cirrhosis. When cirrhosis persists for one or more decades, liver cancer often arises.

Hepatocarcinoma can be detected by examining the patient's serum for a fetal antigen, *alpha-fetoprotein,* which is produced by the malignant cells (Fig. 16-9). But the tumor is usually far advanced (has metastasized) before it is detected. Despite chemotherapy, the patient most often dies within months of diagnosis.

Cholangiocarcinoma is a primary cancer which develops in bile ducts within the liver. Under a microscope, cholangiocarcinomas look like malignant bile ducts. Cholangiocarcinoma is not associated with cirrhosis and occurs less commonly than does hepatocarcinoma. Both primary hepatic can-

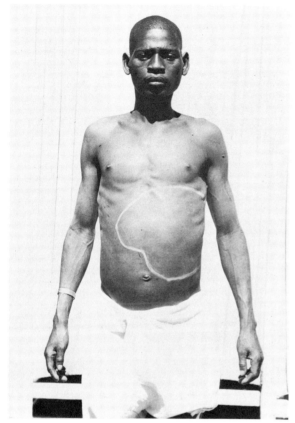

Figure 16-8   *This young African had hepatocellular carcinoma.*

cers are extremely lethal—death occurs within a few months of diagnosis.

Liver Function Tests

Since the clinical signs and symptoms of hepatic disease are nonspecific, laboratory tests of liver function are required for specific diagnosis. Liver function tests are used to: (a) detect, (b) specifically diagnose, (c) determine prognosis, and (d) evaluate the effects of various modes of therapy in liver disease. The tests answer one or more of the following questions: Is there anything wrong? What is wrong? How wrong? Rarely do single tests answer any of these questions, but in combination they may answer some. When these tests fail to provide a diagnosis, a liver biopsy specimen is taken for a de-

finitive answer. Biopsies are valuable for detecting hepatitis, cirrhosis, cancer, and rare metabolic or some inherited disorders (Fig. 16-10).

Tests of liver function are broadly divisible into tests which detect: hepatocytic necrosis (involving enzymes), obstructed bile flow (involving bilirubin), decreased synthesis of proteins (such as albumin), autoimmune diseases (involving autoantibodies), viral infections (hepatitis B virus), and hepatocarcinoma (involving alpha-fetoprotein). Tests of liver function are summarized in Table 16-3.

Hepatocytes contain numerous enzymes. When liver cells undergo necrosis, enzymes (such as transaminase) spill into the blood and become more concentrated there. When the bile ducts become obstructed another enzyme, alkaline phosphatase, elevates in the blood. Autoimmune disease of the liver (primary biliary cirrhosis) can be detected by finding autoantibodies against smooth muscle cells and mitochondria. Immunochemical tests detect hepatitis B virus and alpha-fetoprotein in serum.

To reiterate, acute inflammatory responses occur in response to hepatic necrosis. Subsequently, jaundice can occur and bilirubin and serum transaminase levels elevate in the blood. Detection of decreased synthesis of blood clotting factors and the existence of serum albumin and other proteins also signal liver disease. The decreased ability of diseased liver to form clotting factors along with increased portal hypertension often causes fatal hemorrhage into the gastrointestinal tract. Individuals who survive cirrhosis for years can develop other fatal complications—hepatic coma, failing kidneys, or hepatocarcinoma.

Gallbladder and Bile Ducts

The gallbladder is a reservoir for bile. It stores bile and contracts (following the ingestion of fats) and empties its contents into the common bile duct which leads into the duodenum. Together, bile and pancreatic enzymes digest foods. Bile is required for emulsifying fat and absorbing fat soluble vitamins A, D, E, and K. Thus, any obstruction in the flow of bile into the duodenum results in malab-

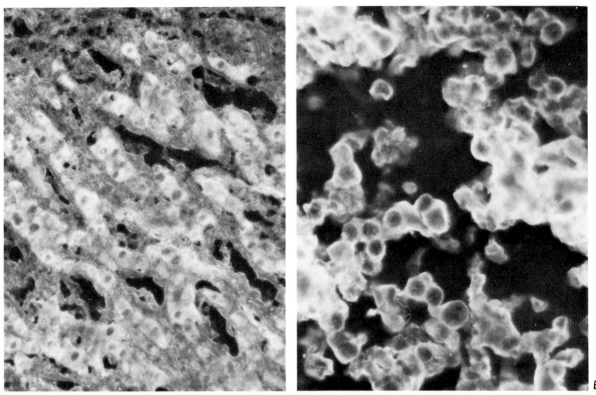

A

B

Figure 16-9   **A,** *Alpha-fetoprotein (AFP) is displayed in a hepatocarcinoma using an antibody against AFP which is fluorescent.* × 350. **B,** *Also AFP is displayed by fluorescence in a liver from a 16-week-old fetus.* × 350.

sorption in these vitamins and fat. Malnutrition can arise from the malabsorption.

Gallstones and Cholecystitis

Inflammation of the gallbladder is called cholecystitis, which can be acute or chronic. This condition often arises in association with gallstones (Fig. 16-11). Cholesterol, bilirubin, or minerals can form stones in the gallbladder. Pure bilirubin stones occur in persons with hemolytic anemias such as sickle cell or hereditary spherocytic hemolytic anemias (see Chapter 11, Hematology).

Persons with gallstones become jaundiced when stones pass out of the gallbladder and obstruct the bile ducts. The differential diagnosis of jaundice is extemely important: surgical intervention is mandatory when the obstruction is *extrahepatic*, whereas if jaundice is caused by intrahepatic diseases, as in viral hepatitis, an operation would endanger the surgical team and harm the patient. The liver function tests aid in differential diagnosis of jaundice (Table 16-3).

In patients with acute cholecystitis, chills, fever, jaundice, nausea, tenderness over the gallbladder, and pain radiating to the right shoulder may occur.

Diagnosis of cholecystitis is aided by obtaining a clinical history of intolerance to fat. A *cholecystogram* is used to confirm the diagnosis of cholecystitis. A dye is swallowed (in pill form), is absorbed by the intestine, and is normally excreted in bile into the gallbladder. If the bile duct is obstructed by a stone, the dye, which is seen with an X-ray, will not concentrate in the gallbladder. Surgical intervention (removal of stones and gallbladder) prevents complications.

Three major complications of cholecystitis and cholithiasis (gallstones) occur: (a) *biliary cirrhosis*

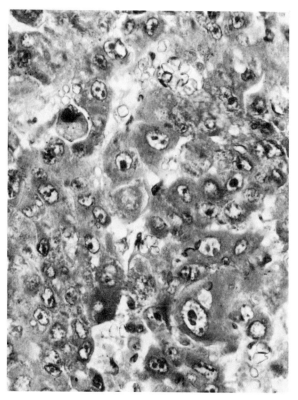

Figure 16-10   *Photomicrograph of needle biopsy of bone marrow showing metastatic hepatocarcinoma.* × *400.*

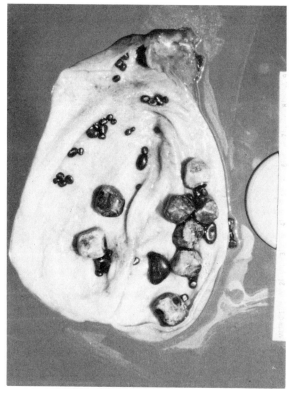

Figure 16-11   *Gallstones have provoked inflammation in this gallbladder (cholecystitis).*

Table 16-3
Tests of Liver Function

Abnormal Function	Tests
Hepatocyte necrosis	Enzyme elevation in serum: SGOT (serum glutamic oxaloacetic transaminase) and other hepatic enzymes.
Cholestasis (bile duct obstruction)	Elevations of serum alkaline phosphatase and bilirubin.
Cell synthesizing capacity	Serum albumin and blood clotting factors decrease (coagulation times are prolonged).
Immunologic disorders	Serum antibodies to smooth muscle, mitochondria or antinuclear antibody.
Virus detection	Hepatitis B virus by immunodiffusion or radioimmunoassay.
Tumor antigens	Alpha-fotoprotein with hepatocarcinoma. Carcinoembryonic antigen with colon carcinoma metastases to liver.
Liver biopsy	Detection of hepatitis, cirrhosis, tumors, or genetic disorders.

can develop when bile accumulates in the liver and this causes necrosis and fibrosis around bile ductules; (b) life-threatening, ascending infection by *Gram-negative bacteria* can induce shock; (c) a third complication, *acute pancreatitis*, is provoked when stones obstruct the pancreatic duct. Necrosis of the pancreas causes inflammation and destruction when pancreatic enzymes spill from damaged cells.

Rarely, carcinomas can occur in the gallbladder or in the common bile duct or tributaries. When carcinomas occur in the gallbladder, gallstones are present in 95% of the cases.

Pancreatic Disorders

The three major diseases of the pancreas are: (a) inherited pancreatic enzyme deficiencies, (b) pancreatitis, and (c) neoplasms. These disorders tend to occur at three periods of life: infancy (deficiency), adulthood (pancreatitis), and old age (neoplasms, especially pancreatic cancer).

Inherited Pancreatic Deficiency

The pancreas can be affected by inherited deficiencies of enzymes (proteases, amylase, or lipase) which leads to maldigestion, malabsorption, and retarded growth. Pancreatic enzyme deficiency causes failure of an infant to thrive. Diarrhea with foul smelling, frothy stools occurs because of failure to digest and absorb fat. The administration of pancreatic extracts with food corrects the deficiency. Cystic fibrosis, another inherited disorder (of secretory glands), leads to fibrosis of the pancreas and liver, with malabsorption of food subsequently occurring.

Pancreatitis

The pancreas is a fragile organ with great potential danger to the body because it is filled with potent digestive enzymes. Injury of any sort to pancreatic exocrine cells causes enzymes to spill out, digest tissue, and provoke inflammation. Inflammation of the pancreas may be either acute or chronic. Acute pancreatitis is generally caused by one of two agents: obstruction of pancreatic ducts by gallstones or alcohol abuse.

The outstanding symptom of *acute pancreatitis* is severe, knife-like, upper abdominal pain; its location corresponds to the area of the pancreas that is inflamed. Patients occasionally seek relief by sitting with the trunk flexed and the knees drawn up in the fetal position.

On physical examination the patient is obviously distressed, anxious, febrile (38C to 38.5C), hypotensive, and has tachycardia and a tender abdomen. When hemorrhagic necrosis occurs in the pancreas and surrounding tissues the condition worsens. Diagnosis of acute pancreatitis is made by noting the type of pain and by detecting elevated lipase and amylase enzymes in the patient's serum and urine.

The patient can develop two severe complications. *Tetany* develops from lowered serum calcium when calcium binds with fat being digested by lipase. Treatment involves administration of calcium gluconate and transfusion of blood. Secondly, the acute pancreatitis can become *hemorrhagic;* the patient goes into cardiogenic shock and intravenous plasma and blood are required to sustain life.

Chronic pancreatitis usually occurs either from chronic alcoholism or hemochromatosis (excessive deposition of iron in liver, pancreas, and endocrine organs). Two signs of chronic pancreatitis arising from the damage to the pancreas are malabsorption and diabetes mellitus. An X-ray of the abdomen of a person with chronic pancreatitis usually reveals calcified areas in the pancreas. Both exocrine (enzymes) and endocrine (insulin) secretion of the pancreas are impaired and hence treatment requires giving extracts of pancreas (with meals), and insulin to the patient.

Tumors

Cysts, adenomas, and carcinomas are common lesions of the pancreas. *Adenomas* of the islet cells (insulinoma) can produce excessive amounts of insulin (hyperinsulinism), which elicits hypoglycemia (low blood sugar), nervousness, sweating, and even a loss of consciousness. Surgical removal of pancreatic adenomas correct the hypoglycemia.

Carcinoma of the pancreas is now the fourth most common death-causing cancer in the United States, with only cancer of the lung, colon and rectum, and breast more frequently fatal. The threefold increase in incidence of pancreatic cancer since 1920 is alarming.

The etiology of pancreatic cancer is unknown. Epidemiological studies, however, demonstrate that incidence of the disease in cigarette smokers is twice that in nonsmokers. In countries with a high per capita consumption of fat, the national incidence is high. The incidence is increased twofold in patients with diabetes mellitus. Methylnitrosourea causes pancreatic cancer in animals fed this compound. Similar compounds are used in preserving cold cuts of meat and sausage; some believe these additives are carcinogenic.

The diagnosis is based on the existence of symptoms such as abdominal pain (25% to 60%), jaundice (20% to 60%), and loss of weight (70% to 90%). On physical examination a tender mass is found in 60% of patients. No specific laboratory studies are available for diagnosis, so an exploratory laparotomy and biopsy are required for diagnosis.

Prognosis for pancreatic cancer is grim; the average survival after diagnosis is less than six months because the tumor metastasizes early. Rarely, small lesions detected early which are in the head of the pancreas can be resected, allowing the patient to survive.

Summary

The liver's major functions are: synthesis of blood proteins and fats; storage of carbohydrate as glycogen; secretion of bile; phagocytosis of particulate matter; and detoxification of ethyl alcohol and other drugs. Hepatic disorders induced by toxins, infectious hepatitis, or neoplasms cause dysfunction.

Persons with hepatic disease often exhibit jaundice and have tenderness of the liver with acute hepatitis. Chronic liver disease such as cirrhosis is associated with jaundice, plus problems associated with increased portal venous pressure including ascites, edema, and increased collateral venous channels. Profound acute or chronic hepatic failure is associated with hemorrhage, and hepatorenal syndrome with renal failure or coma.

Diagnosis of liver disease is based on clinical history of exposure to toxins or infectious agents, and tests of liver function document the extent of hepatic dysfunction and the source of the injury. Occasionally a needle biopsy of the liver is required for microscopic evaluation and definitive diagnosis.

Jaundice poses a vexing problem in differential diagnosis. It can be caused by hemolytic anemia, hepatocytic necrosis, or obstruction of the bile ducts; all cause elevated bilirubin in the blood. Only obstruction by a gallstone or tumor requires surgical intervention. Special X-ray studies (cholecystogram) indicate gallstones or defective function of the gallbladder, and the alkaline phosphatase level becomes elevated in the blood due to obstruction of the bile ducts. Surgery is indicated to correct such obstruction. By contrast, if jaundice is caused by viral hepatitis, surgery would be contraindicated.

Pancreatic cancer is increasing in frequency at an alarming rate. This tumor metastasizes early and few patients survive beyond one year following diagnosis.

Bibliography

Burke, M. D. 1975. Liver function. *Hum. Pathol.* 6:273–286. Discusses the use of tests of liver function in the differential diagnosis of liver disease.

Davidson, M. 1976. GI problems in children. *Hosp. Prac.* 11:47–55. Describes GI problems commonly occurring in children.

Di Magno, E. P. 1977. A prospective comparison of current diagnostic tests for pancreatic cancer. *N. Engl. J. Med.* 297:737–742. No single laboratory test is diagnostic of pancreatic cancer; a battery of tests is required.

Gall, E. A., and Mostofi, F. K., eds. 1973. *The liver.* Baltimore: The Williams & Wilkins Company. A comprehensive discussion of the liver and its diseases.

Jukes, T. H. 1977. Food additives. *New Eng. J. Med.* 297: 427–430. Food additives are on the enemy list along with kepone, strip mining, offshore oil wells, and supersonic transports. This article demythologizes some of our notions about dangers of food additives.

Leiber, C. S. 1976. The metabolism of alcohol. *Sci. Am.* 234:25–33. Emphasizes that alcohol can be toxic.

Morgan, R. G., and Wormsley, K. G. 1977. Progress report on cancer of the pancreas. *Gut* 18:580–596. Comprehensive discussion of epidemiology, etiology, diagnosis, treatment, and prognosis of this important problem.

Popper, H. 1972. Diseases of the liver. *Hum. Pathol.* 3:3. Entire issue devoted to liver diseases and describes the pathology of liver diseases.

Purtilo, D. T., et al. 1973. Alpha-fetoprotein: diagnostic and prognostic use in patients with hepatoma. *Am. J. Clin. Pathol.* 59:295–299. Describes the use of AFP in patients with hepatocarcinoma.

Purtilo, D. T., and Gottlieb, L. S. 1973. Cirrhosis and hepatoma occurring at Boston City Hospital (1917–1968). *Cancer* 32:458–463. Alcoholism was responsible for cirrhosis and hepatocarcinoma in two-thirds of patients with these diseases.

Purtilo, D. T. 1976. Clonorchiasis and hepatic neoplasms. *Trop. Geogr. Med.* 28:21–27. A liver fluke (*Clonorchis sinensis*) is linked with cancer of bile ducts in patients from Hong Kong.

Sherlock, S. 1975. *Diseases of liver and biliary system*, ed. 5. F. A. Davis Company. The standard clinical textbook on liver diseases.

CHAPTER 17

Urology and Renal Medicine

Chapter Outline

Objectives

After reading this chapter you should be able to

Define the term nephron.

List the five major signs and symptoms of urinary tract diseases.

Define the terms renal failure, azotemia, uremia, and acute tubular necrosis.

Describe the processes of renal regeneration.

Describe the two types of chronic renal failure.

List the major birth defects of the urinary tract.

Describe the pathogenesis of acute glomerulonephritis.

List several inherited defects of renal structure or function.

Describe three consequences of obstructed urine flow.

Define the terms cystitis and dysuria.

Compare acute and chronic pyelonephritis.

Describe the symptoms of urolithiasis.

Compare Wilms' tumor with renal carcinoma.

Discuss the etiology of bladder cancer.

Name the most common cause of acute prostatitis in young men.

Describe the common symptom of benign prostatic hyperplasia.

Discuss the diagnosis and treatment of prostatic cancer.

Define the term hydrocele.

Introduction

The *genitourinary tract* consists of the kidneys, ureters, urinary bladder, urethra, and gonads (Fig. 17-1). Each kidney weighs about 250 gm and is composed of approximately one and one-half million nephrons. The basic unit of the kidney is the *nephron*, composed of a glomerulus (blood filter) and a long tubule (concentrator and collector of urine).

Blood filters through glomeruli and is concentrated in tubules which empty into the ureters (Fig. 17-2). The glomerulus is supplied by an arteriole which divides into numerous small capillaries. These capillaries are covered by epithelial cells which permit the passage of fluid from the blood into the urinary space. The endothelium lining the capillaries of the glomerulus is perforated by minute (700 Å) holes. These small openings permit water to pass, but large (greater than 70,000 molecular weight) proteins are retained. Albumin and other large proteins in blood plasma are retained. The total area of the glomerular capillary filter is one square meter. Absorption and secretion of compounds occurs at various levels of the tubule.

Approximately 85% of the fluid filtered through glomeruli is reabsorbed in the proximal tubule and the remaining amount is concentrated distally. The concentration and volume of the urine is controlled by an antidiuretic hormone (ADH) which causes the distal tubule to reabsorb water.

The composition of our bodies is determined not so much by what we eat, but by what the kidneys excrete. The kidneys establish the electrolyte (Ca, Na, K, PO_4, Cl, HCO_3, NH_4) balance in our bodies and excrete toxic substances.

Symptoms of Urogenital Disorders*

There are five major signs and symptoms that signal urinary tract disease:

1. Blood in the urine (*hematuria*) may be detected with the naked eye or by seeing erythrocytes in urinary sediment under a microscope (*microscopic hematuria*).

Individuals experiencing *hematuria* often have lesions in their urinary tracts that must be diagnosed

---

*Three medical specialists cope with diseases of the urogenital tract. *Urologists* diagnose and surgically treat disorders of the urinary tract and also male genitalia. *Gynecologists* specialize in problems of the female genital tract. *Nephrologists* are concerned with renal medicine or problems related to renal failure.

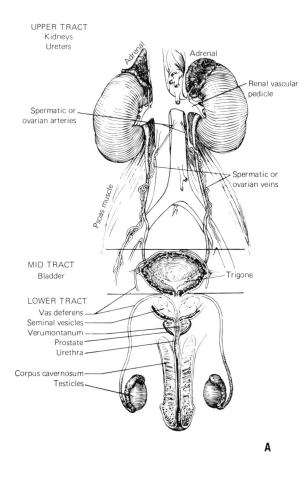

UPPER TRACT
Kidneys
Ureters

Adrenal

Adrenal

Renal vascular
pedicle

Spermatic or
ovarian arteries

Spermatic or
ovarian veins

Psoas muscle

MID TRACT
Bladder

Trigone

LOWER TRACT
Vas deferens
Seminal vesicles
Verumontanum
Prostate
Urethra

Corpus cavernosum
Testicles

A

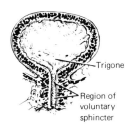

Trigone

Region of
voluntary
sphincter

B

Figure 17-1   A, *Anatomy of the male genitourinary tract.* **B,** *Female tract. (Reproduced, with permission, from Smith, D.R.:* General Urology, *ed. 8. Lange, 1975.)*

and treated. Hemorrhage can occur at any level in the urinary tract, from the kidney to the urethra. Blood from the upper urinary tract might be caused by an immunologic reaction (glomerulonephritis), a malignancy, infection, trauma, or a stone. Lower urinary tract hemorrhage (in the bladder or urethra) can be likewise associated with infection, malignancy, stone, or with infection of the urethra (urethritis).

2. *Edema* (accumulation of fluid in tissues) is another common sign of renal disease (Fig. 17-3). The edema of renal failure results because albumin is passed from the blood into the urine. The pressure that the albumin exerts to retain fluid in the bloodstream is lost and consequently fluid flows from the capillaries into tissue spaces producing edema. Edema of renal failure affects the face and all parts of the body (is generalized), whereas *congestive heart failure* causes edema only in dependent areas, like the lower extremities. Similarly, edema occurring because of *failure of the liver* to produce albumin results in a generalized edema; however, signs diagnostic of liver failure are often seen in patients with hepatic disease (see Chapter 13, Cardiology, and Chapter 16, Hepatic and Pancreatic Disorders).

3. *Pain* is another manifestation of urinary tract disease. The pain arises either from an infection that inflames the kidneys, ureters, or urinary bladder, or from a tumor which produces pain when nerves are invaded. Excruciating pain occurs when a stone obstructs a ureter (urolithiasis).

4. *Enlargement of the kidneys* occurs with inflammation (nephritis) and thus the swollen kidneys may be felt in the abdomen. Moreover, pain can also be elicited when the back is tapped over the location of the inflamed kidneys.

5. Finally, *anemia* arises from severe urinary tract disease when blood passes into the urine (hematuria) or when blood formation in the bone marrow is suppressed by chronic renal failure.

Renal Failure

The term *renal failure* implies a loss of renal function. *Azotemia* results when kidneys fail to excrete

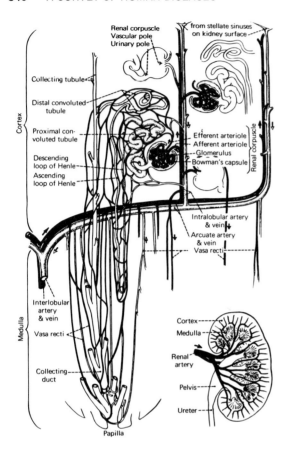

Renal corpuscle
Vascular pole
Urinary pole

from stellate sinuses
on kidney surface

Collecting tubule

Distal convoluted
tubule

Proximal con-
voluted tubule

Efferent arteriole
Afferent arteriole
Glomerulus
Bowman's capsule

Descending
loop of Henle

Ascending
loop of Henle

Cortex

Renal corpuscle

Intralobular artery
& vein

Arcuate artery
& vein

Vasa recti

Interlobular
artery
& vein

Vasa recti

Cortex

Medulla

Renal
artery

Collecting
duct

Pelvis

Ureter

Medulla

Papilla

Figure 17-2 *Structure of normal nephron. (From Geschickter, C.F., and Antonovych, T.T. 1971. The kidney in health and disease. Philadelphia; J.B. Lippincott Company.)*

nitrogen substances, with *blood urea nitrogen* (BUN) and creatinine accumulating in the blood. These nitrogenous substances are metabolic breakdown products of proteins (from diet and muscles in our body). The concentration of BUN and creatinine rises in the blood when the kidneys fail. Detection of azotemia provides laboratory confirmation that renal failure has occurred.

The clinical counterpart of azotemia is *uremia*, a condition characterized by reduced renal function and disturbances in the gastrointestinal, neuro-muscular, and cardiovascular systems. The abnormal functioning of these systems results from the toxicity of excessive nitrogenous substances and the imbalance of electrolytes in the blood.

Acute Renal Failure

The sudden loss of renal function (*acute renal failure*) is caused by shock (prolonged hypotension, associated with surgery or hemorrhage in two-thirds of cases). Thrombosis, trauma, or acute nephritis (acute glomerulonephritis or acute pyelonephritis) are other causes of *acute renal tubular necrosis* (ATN). Each of them causes nephrons to die (Fig. 17-4).

Within a few days following injury to the kidneys the individual develops *oliguria* (urinary output of only 400 ml daily). Oliguria occasionally progresses to *anuria* (less than 200 ml of urine daily). Ordinarily, an adult excretes approximately 1300 ml of urine daily.

The kidneys may sustain a loss of up to 90% of their nephrons without obvious loss of function. When the vast majority of nephrons are injured, uremia ensues. But the nephrons have an excellent capacity to regenerate. Usually by the tenth day following injury, regeneration of tubular cells occurs and *diuresis* (an increased excretion of urine) occurs. During this phase up to 4 liters of urine are urinated daily. Diuresis is a favorable sign of kidney regeneration. Persons who live through the diuretic phase return to near normal renal function.

Chronic Renal Failure

Many diseases lead to chronic renal failure, chiefly infectious, traumatic, vascular, or immunologic diseases. The kidneys and nephrons become injured and die. The organ becomes shrunken and loses electrolytes and albumin; toxic nitrogenous substances are not excreted. To reiterate, persons with chronic renal failure exhibit various degrees of uremia, with gastrointestinal, neuromuscular, and cardiovascular disturbances ensuing.

Treatment

Failing kidneys are unable to maintain electrolyte balance and eliminate nitrogenous wastes. Chronic renal failure is treated by *hemodialysis* or *renal transplantation*. In renal hemodialysis, the blood of the patient is cleansed in a machine with physiologic solutions. The toxic substances and excessive elec-

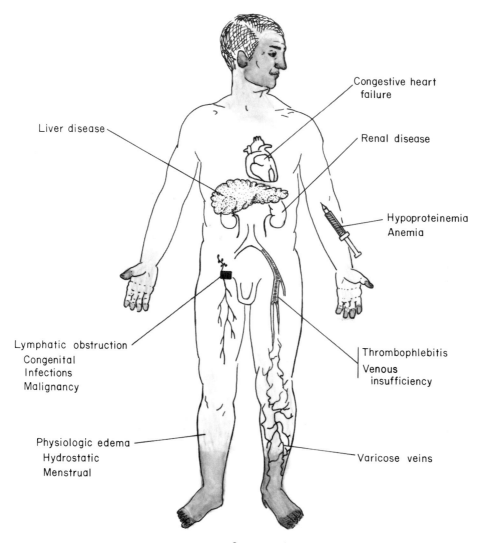

Figure 17-3   *Causes of edema.*

trolytes pass from the patient's blood into the solution through a selectively permeable dialysis membrane. This process is costly in time (up to ten hours a week), emotions, and money.

Renal transplantation is possible because tissues can be typed and matched for donor and recipient. In addition the immune responses which cause rejection of foreign tissues can be suppressed (see Chapter 6, Immunology). The procedure is costly and donors matching the tissue type of the patient are difficult to find. Many complications occur with transplantation—rejection of the transplant, infections, psychiatric illness, or malignancy can result. Transplantation will undoubtedly be further perfected and provide an answer for victims of chronic renal failure.

Congenital Anomalies

The urinary tract is afflicted more commonly by defects in development (congenital anomalies) than are other organs (see Chapter 3, Development and Birth Defects). Kidneys can be absent (*agenesis*) or undersized (*hypoplastic*). They can be displaced (*ectopic*) from their normal position and extra ureters or renal arteries may be found. These displaced organs or extra parts can cross the ureters and obstruct the urine flow and predispose the individual to infections. The kidneys can fuse during organogenesis across the midline of the abdomen giving a horseshoe shape, or be filled with cysts (*polycystic renal disease*). This latter condition is usually associated with hypertension and progressive renal failure.

Immunologic Injury of Kidneys

Nearly one-half of renal diseases are caused by immunologic hypersensitivity reactions in glomeruli. There are two main types of glomerular disease that are caused by immunologic hypersensitivity reactions: (a) antibodies can form against the patient's own basement membranes in the kidneys and lungs (*Goodpasture's syndrome*) and (b) immune complexes, consisting of antigen-antibody, can circulate in the blood and become trapped in the glomerulus with inflammation of the glomerulus (*glomerulonephritis*) resulting (see Chapter 6, Immunology).

Acute Glomerulonephritis

The most common hypersensitivity glomerular disease is *acute glomerulonephritis* (AGN). Typically, a group A β hemolytic streptococcal infection occurs in the pharynx ("strep throat") approximately one to four weeks before edema, hypertension, and hematuria occur. The kidneys trap streptococcal antigen-antibody immune complexes in the glomeruli and thereby provoke AGN.

The prognosis with AGN is excellent; the vast majority (99%) of individuals afflicted with AGN experience a return to normal renal function within a few months. If a renal biopsy specimen is taken early in the disease, the glomeruli are large and contain numerous neutrophils. The neutrophils invade glomeruli in response to the immune complex deposits. Staining for the immune complexes by

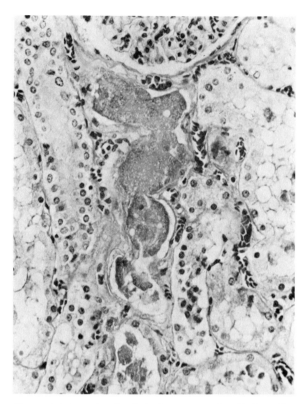

Figure 17-4   *Acute tubular necrosis. Below the glomerulus the proximal tubule contains cast material of dead tubular cells. (From Kashgarian, M.; Hayslett, J.P.; and Spargo, B.H. 1974. Renal Disease. Bethesda, Maryland: Universities Associated for Research and Education in Pathology, Inc.)*

immunofluorescence reveals antibodies (immunoglobulins) deposited in glomeruli and electron microscopy studies reveal deposits of immune complexes (Fig. 17-5).

Chronic Glomerulonephritis

The causes of chronic glomerulonephritis (CGN) are multiple; about 10% of the cases arise following AGN. The onset of CGN is slow and subtle. Hypertension and proteinuria persist. From the time the disease begins to the time a diagnosis is made, a long period (1 to 3 decades) usually transpires during which the patient enjoys good health.

Later, CGN is characterized by progressive renal insufficiency. The kidneys become small, scarred, and atrophic. The glomeruli become thickened and bloodless and the tubules become atrophic.

The glomerulus can also be injured by immune complexes in diseases such as systemic lupus erythematosus (SLE) (see Chapter 6, Immunology). In SLE, antibodies form against the body's own DNA (autoantibody). Immune complexes consisting of antibodies to DNA and DNA antigen circulate in the blood and become trapped in the glomeruli, with glomerulonephritis ensuing. If this process continues the kidneys become small, scarred, and renal failure can develop.

Genetic And Metabolic Diseases of the Kidney

Patients with inherited forms of renal disease are quite numerous, and occasionally some of these inherited forms can cause chronic renal failure and require hemodialysis or renal transplantation to cope with irreversible lesions. The great majority of these patients suffer from diabetes mellitus, hypertension, or gout—disorders which affect many tissues including those of the kidney. These conditions are inherited in a variety of ways and are present throughout life but are not usually evident until adulthood. More than 30 specific inherited renal diseases are recognized. A few of these are listed in Table 17-1.

One example of an inherited renal disease, *cystinuria*, is shown in Figure 17-6. Cystinuria is an inborn defect in the tubular reabsorption of four amino acids—cystine, lysine, ornithine, and arginine. Individuals with this disease form stones from the excessively excreted cystine, and renal failure can ensue.

The kidneys are targets for destruction in a variety of systemic diseases. Diabetes mellitus causes arteriosclerosis which affects the kidneys and other organs (see Chapters 12, Endocrine and Metabolic Disorders, and Chapter 13, Cardiology). Other acquired metabolic disorders such as liver failure also impair renal function.

Hypertension causes arteriosclerosis in the kidney and elsewhere. Approximately 8% of persons with hypertension develop marked hypertension

(malignant hypertension) which can lead to death because the renal arterioles undergo necrosis, become blocked, and the kidneys fail to filter blood.

Obstruction of the Genitourinary Tract

Obstruction of the flow of urine leads to severe renal disease. A variety of congenital and acquired lesions obstruct the flow of urine. When obstruction occurs, muscles in the bladder wall or ureter proximal to the obstruction undergo hypertrophy. The muscle in the bladder wall undergoes hyper-

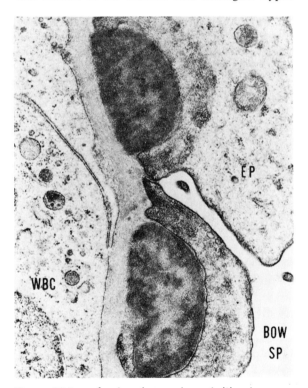

Figure 17-5   *Acute glomerulonephritis. Immune complexes trapped in a glomerulus have characteristic dome-shaped (hump) appearance between the basement membrane and the epithelial cells (EP). Related to these humps, leukocytes adhere (WBC), degranulate and erode the endothelium. Bowman's Space (BOW SP) is shown. × 23,000. (From Kashgarian, M.: Hayslett, J.P.; and Spargo, B.H. 1974. Renal Disease. Bethesda, Maryland: Universities Associated for Research and Education in Pathology, Inc.)*

Table 17-1
Inherited Renal Diseases

Structural Defects	Inheritance
1. Nephritis with deafness or ocular disorders (Alport's syndrome)	Autosomal dominant
2. Fabry's disease	X-linked recessive
3. Infantile and adult polycystic diseases	Autosomal recessive
4. Renal agenesis	Autosomal recessive

Functional Defects	Inheritance
1. Cystinuria	Autosomal recessive
2. Renal glycosuria	Autosomal recessive
3. Fanconi syndrome	Autosomal recessive
4. Renal rickets (hypophosphatemic rickets)	X-linked dominant

trophy and the pressure of urine causes the ureters to dilate (*hydroureter*) or kidney to dilate (*hydronephrosis*). Figure 17-7 illustrates hydronephrosis which resulted when a blood vessel compressed the ureter. Often the obstruction gives rise to urinary tract infections.

Urinary Tract Infections

The major complication of obstruction of the urinary tract is *acute urinary tract infection*. The urinary bladder can become infected and inflamed (*cystitis*), as can the ureter (*ureteritis*), or the kidney (*pyelonephritis*).

Cystitis

Cystitis occurs most often in women. It commonly occurs following initial intercourse ("honeymoon cystitis") or during pregnancy. In both men and children the presence of cystitis more often signals an obstruction in the urinary tract than it does in women. Usually the bacteria infecting the kidney are Gram-negative bacteria including *E coli, Proteus,* or *Klebsiella,* but staphylococcus and other microorganisms also infect the urinary tract (see Chapter 7, Infectious Diseases).

The symptoms of acute cystitis are annoying—burning upon urination (*dysuria*), increased frequency of urination, and even hematuria can result.

The major danger of cystitis is that the infection can ascend to the kidneys and cause pyelonephritis. The diagnosis of cystitis is made, as in other urinary tract infections, by finding pus and bacteria in the urine on microscopic examination. The urine is cultured for bacteria and tested for sensitivity to antibiotics so appropriate antibiotics can be given.

Acute Pyelonephritis

Individuals with acute pyelonephritis experience pain in the flanks, chills, fever, and weakness. The finding of leukocyte casts which have formed in infected renal tubules in the urine indicates the existence of pyelonephritis. Depending on the extent of involvement of the kidney, renal function can be reduced. Acute pyelonephritis frequently remits spontaneously, but it can persist for years. The infected kidney usually becomes swollen and contains multiple small abscesses on the external surfaces. An intensive infiltrate consisting of neutrophils, bacteria, and damaged tubules and glomeruli is seen within the kidney.

Chronic Pyelonephritis

Repeated episodes of acute pyelonephritis may directly lead to chronic pyelonephritis. Otherwise, the onset of chronic pyelonephritis is gradual—asymptomatic azotemia and hypertension are usually detected during a routine examination.

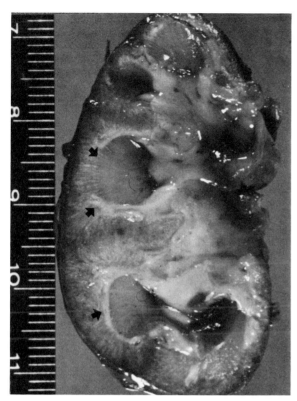

Figure 17-6   *Cystinuric kidney showing a marked decrease in size due to injury by cystine crystals (arrows)* in the substance of the kidney.

With chronic pyelonephritis the kidney becomes shrunken because tubules are destroyed. Fibrous tissue accumulates between tubules and chokes glomeruli, which become fibrotic (Fig. 17-8). The lesions are seldom reversible and when the damage is severe, uremia can ensue.

Urinary tract infections should be suspected in patients with symptoms and conditions prediposing to infection. Pregnancy, sickle cell trait, diabetes, hypertension, prostatic enlargement, renal or bladder stones, or indwelling urinary catheters often lead to urinary tract infection.

Urinary Tract Stones

One in one thousand persons residing in the United States has been hospitalized for *urinary tract stones*

(calculi). Urinary tract stones occur most frequently in individuals between the ages of 20 and 55.

Symptoms can be entirely absent (the individual is asymptomatic) or vague abdominal and flank pain may persist. The stone can be discovered during a routine X-ray examination of the abdomen. When a ureter becomes suddenly obstructed, severe knife-like pain *(colic)* occurs. This intense pain is felt in the renal (flank) and ureteral areas and often radiates into the groin.

Stones formed in the kidney often pass into the bladder. But the bladder can also be obstructed by prostatic hypertrophy or strictures of the urethra, leading to the development of infections and the formation of bladder stones. The symptoms usually associated with bladder stones are cystitis and hematuria.

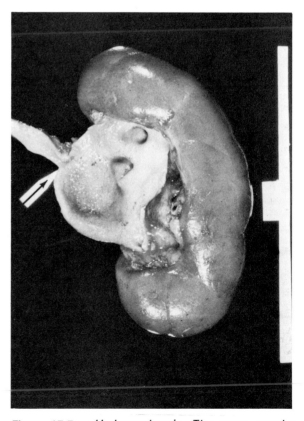

Figure 17-7   *Hydronephrosis. The arrow marks where a vessel compressed the ureter. The renal pelvis is dilated and kidney compressed.*

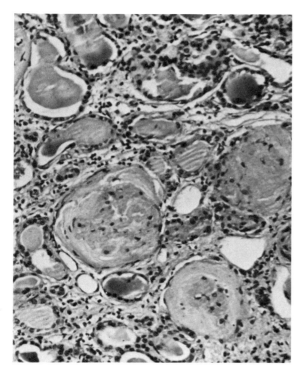

Figure 17-8   *Chronic pyelonephritis. The glomeruli are hyalinized, tubules atrophic, and lymphocytes (black dots) inflame the kidney.*

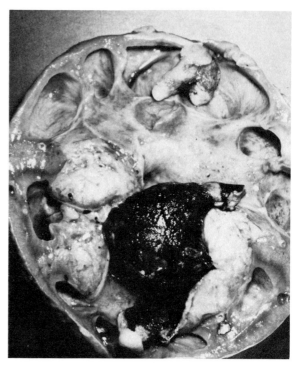

Figure 17-9   *A large black stone (staghorn calculus) fills and obstructs a renal pelvis. The kidney has been cut open to demonstrate the stone.*

Etiology

Most stones form in the kidneys (Fig. 17-9). They are a chemical mixture of proteins, calcium, oxalate, phosphate, magnesium, ammonium, and other salts. Certain metabolic diseases (such as cystinuria) are associated with the formation of stones. Persons unable to absorb certain amino acids or who have excessive excretion of calcium or oxalate are most likely to form stones. In addition, 10% of urinary stones are caused by hyperparathyroidism. Individuals afflicted with this endocrine disease have excess calcium in their urine and form calcified stones (see Chapter 12, Endocrine and Metabolic Diseases).

Treatment

Surgical excision of stones is frequently required. But occasionally a bladder stone can be removed through a cystoscope or is spontaneously passed upon urination. In addition, affected individuals are put on diets deficient in minerals and informed of the necessity of drinking large amounts of demineralized water (at least 2 liters daily).

Neoplasms of Genitourinary Tract

Neoplasms of the urogenital tract can be either benign (*adenoma*) or malignant (*carcinoma*). Benign renal tumors and cysts can mimic malignant tumors, so it is important that they be distinguished from cancer of the kidney. Most cysts and adenomas are of no consequence. Renal adenomas are small nodules that occur in the cortex of the kidney. Cysts also occur in the cortex. Malignancies, as always, are of greater concern than adenomas and cysts.

Nephroblastoma (Wilms' Tumor)

Wilms' tumor is a renal malignancy found in young children (Fig. 17-10). Typically, affected infants have an abdominal mass which is detected by the mother. This malignancy may metastasize to the lungs, liver, lymph nodes, and, less frequently, to the bones. It is treated by surgical resection, however, actinomycin D chemotherapy is given to destroy tumor not removed surgically. In general, prognoses of patients with nephroblastoma are not good.

Renal Carcinoma

Cancer of the kidney can arise in the kidney or renal pelvis. Three-fourths of all cancers in the kidney are adenocarcinomas (hypernephroma, or clear cell carcinoma). The cause is unknown, but cigarette smoking has been linked with a higher frequency of renal cancers that occur in males over 50 years old.

Few symptoms are noted, except that a mass can occasionally be palpated in the flank. The tumor can also be initially discovered by observing red blood cells in a routine urine examination. The person might experience fever, weight loss, and anemia. The diagnosis is achieved by injecting dye into the renal artery (arteriogram), and abnormal blood vessels supplying the tumor can be seen in the X-ray.

Renal carcinomas are solid and lobulated. The cells comprising the tumor are clear and not bizarre. Treatment is by surgical excision. Prognosis depends upon the stage of the carcinoma at the time of diagnosis. When the tumor metastasizes through the blood stream into the lungs, the prognosis is usually unfavorable.

Approximately 8% of all renal tumors arise in the renal pelvis or ureters. These tumors have finger-like (papillary) projections which may obstruct the flow of urine. Hematuria or infection in the urinary tract often result from the obstructing tumor. The diagnosis is established by cytological examination of the urine and an intravenous pyelogram X-ray which shows the tumor in the renal pelvis or ureter. Treatment is by excision.

Bladder Carcinoma

Carcinomas of the urinary bladder cause 5% of all deaths by malignancies. Most bladder tumors arise

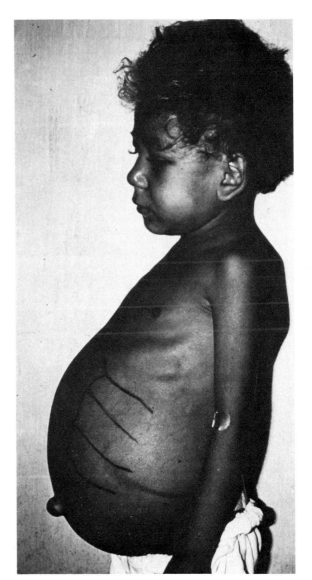

Figure 17-10   *Child with Wilms' renal tumor. Note the protruding abdomen.*

from the transitional epithelium that lines the collecting system of the urinary tract (Fig. 17-11, *A*). As with cancer of the kidney, bladder cancer principally occurs in elderly men who smoke cigarettes.

Etiology   Certain chemicals (benzidine and aniline dyes) are known to cause bladder cancer. This fact was discovered by noting the high occurrence of bladder cancer in workers in dye and rubber tire industries.

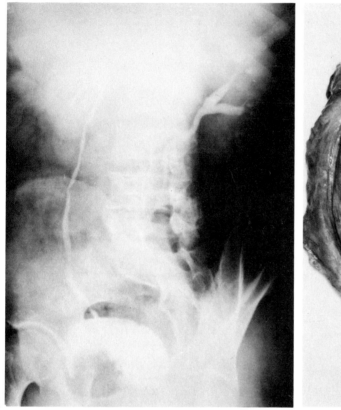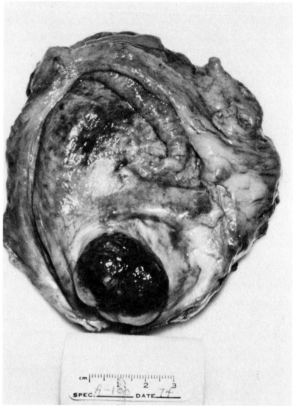

A B

Figure 17-11 *Bladder cancer. The tumor protrudes from the bladder mucosa.* **A,** *X-ray;* **B,** *gross specimen.*

The majority of bladder tumors are papillomas (Fig. 17-11, *B* and *C*) that protrude into the lumen of the bladder. The papillomas are composed of atypical urothelial cells. In more advanced bladder cancers, sheets of tumor cells can be seen invading the bladder wall (see Chapter 8).

Bladder cancers usually bleed with hematuria resulting. The tumors can be visualized through a urologist's cystoscope and small cancers can be easily resected through a resectoscope. The tumors often recur and are notoriously unpredictable in behavior. Carcinomas can act in a benign fashion for years and then suddenly invade the bladder wall or metastasize.* These latter cancers are associated with poor prognoses.

*Senator Hubert Humphrey in 1976 was found to have metastasis of a bladder cancer after eight years of apparent cure. Senator Humphrey subsequently died from this condition.

Treatment Treatment of bladder cancer depends upon the extent of the disease. Noninfiltrating tumors can be coagulated with heat (fulgerized) by an electric probe passed through a cystoscope. Patients are thereafter monitored every three months for tumor recurrence. In contrast, cancers that deeply infiltrate the bladder wall necessitate removal of a part or all of the bladder by cystectomy. Radiotherapy or chemotherapy is used when surgical therapy fails.

Prostate Gland

The prostate gland surrounds the urethra at the base of the urinary bladder (Fig. 17-1). Three disorders commonly affect the gland: (a) acute prostatitis, (b) benign prostatic hyperplasia, and (c) carcinoma of the prostate.

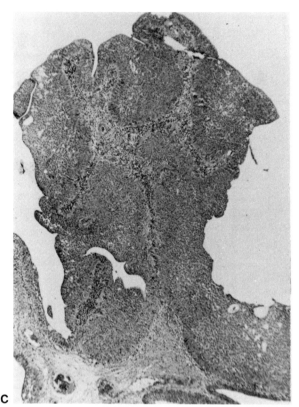

Figure 17-11 **C,** Photomicrograph of papillary carcinoma.

Acute Prostatitis

Sexually active young men often develop acute urethritis and prostatitis from infection by the gonococcus bacterium (see Chapters 7 and 18). Pain and burning upon urination are experienced and tenderness of the prostate may be noted. Pus can often be seen dripping from the penis and a culture and Gram's stain reveal gonococcus. Treatment is with penicillin.

Prostatic Hyperplasia

Middle-aged and elderly men frequently experience prostatic hyperplasia when their testosterone levels decline. The estrogen produced in the adrenals then stimulates the prostatic epithelium to grow and hyperplasia occurs. Subsequently, the prostate gland enlarges and obstructs the outflow of urine through the urethra (Fig. 17-12).

Commonly, aging men with prostatic hyperplasia must urinate in the middle of the night (*nocturia*). They may experience difficulty in initiating a stream of urine and complete obstruction can ensue. A urinary tract infection is a frequent complication of this disease.

Treatment of prostatic hyperplasia by urologists consists of curetting (removing by cutting small fragments) the hyperplastic prostate tissue through the urethra (transurethral resection). The pathologist examining the specimen observes a marked increase in the size and number of epithelial cells lining the glands of the prostate.

Prostatic Carcinoma

Prostatic cancer causes obstruction of the urinary tract. Prostatic carcinoma occurs most commonly in men beyond the age of 50. This cancer is one of the most common malignancies, but most are small and asymptomatic. In contrast, large invasive carcinomas can cause pain when they invade nerves surrounding the prostate. In addition, metastases to the spine or brain can arise and kill the patient.

Typically, men with prostatic carcinoma have signs nearly identical to those with prostatic hypertrophy—nocturia and urinary tract infections. But they can also have urinary incontinence and pain. Prostatic gland examination by rectal palpation with a gloved finger reveals a hard cancer mass in contrast with the enlarged, soft prostate which signals the existence of prostatic hypertrophy.

Treatment of carcinoma of the prostate is by prostatectomy. In addition to an orchiectomy (resection of the testes), estrogen is commonly given to suppress the growth of the cancer. As with other malignancies, the prognosis depends upon two features, the histologic appearance of the tumor and extent (stage) of the tumor.

Penis and Testes

Except for venereal infections in young males (see Chapter 7, Infectious Diseases, and Chapter 18, Gynecology and Breast Diseases) and squamous

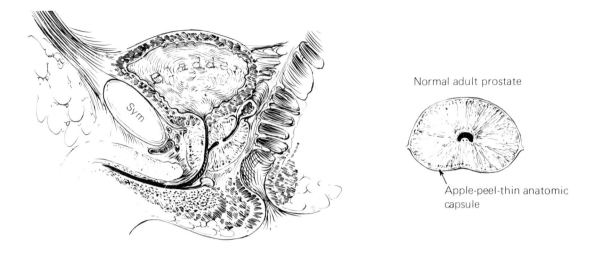

Normal adult prostate

Apple-peel-thin anatomic capsule

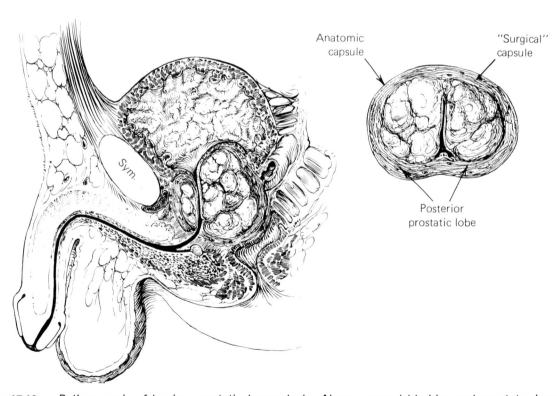

Anatomic capsule

"Surgical" capsule

Posterior prostatic lobe

Figure 17-12 *Pathogenesis of benign prostatic hyperplasia. Above, normal bladder and prostate. Inset shows normal prostate (containing prostatic urethra) and thin capsule. Below, enlarged prostate enclosed by thick capsule composed of the posterior prostatic lobe. (Reproduced, with permission, from Smith, D.R.: General urology, 8th ed. Lange, 1975.)*

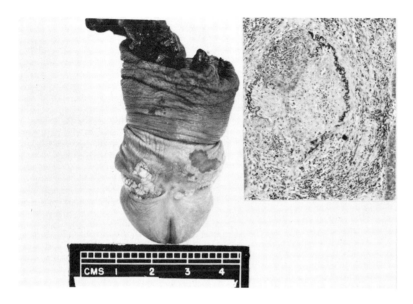

Figure 17-13 *Squamous cell carcinoma of shaft of penis. The inset shows the cancer has invaded a blood vessel. × 150*

cell carcinoma in elderly males (Fig. 17-13), the penis is not often involved by disease.

Testicular masses are rather common. For instance, fluid can collect in the sac surrounding the testis (hydrocele) producing a mass that can be easily removed. By contrast, carcinomas are rare but when they strike it is often during the second decade of life. Enlargement of a testis with metastases to the lungs or bone can mark the appearance of a malignant testicular tumor. Many testicular carcinomas are responsive to chemotherapy or radiotherapy.

Summary

Five major signs and symptoms that signal urinary tract disease are hematuria, edema, pain, enlarged kidneys, and anemia. Acute or chronic renal failure is recognized by analyzing the blood and urine. Characteristically, nitrogenous substances accumulate in blood and azotemia is thus recognized by the elevated blood urea nitrogen and creatinine. Uremia is the clinical expression of renal failure. It is characterized by reduced renal function and pathophysiologic changes in neuromuscular, gastrointestinal, and cardiovascular systems.

Acute renal failure can result from a variety of insults. Acute tubular necrosis is a common cause of acute failure, but fortunately if the patient is maintained on renal dialysis, the renal tubules can often regenerate. Chronic renal failure can result from the same events that cause acute failure, but the kidneys are usually unable to regenerate because they are damaged by scars.

Glomerulonephritis is often caused by deposits of immune complexes of antigen-antibody in the glomeruli, which provoke acute inflammation and damage. Generally, acute glomerulonephritis completely heals leaving no impairment.

Obstruction of the flow of urine, whatever the cause, induces stasis of urine and predisposes to urinary tract infection. Cystitis is very common in girls and women because the urethra is short and bacteria gain ready access to the bladder. Unfortunately, the infection can ascend to the kidneys and pyelonephritis can develop. The most common cause of stasis in males is from obstruction of the urethra by a hyperplastic prostate gland. Urinary tract infections are diagnosed by urine analysis and culture. Antibiotics and correction of the obstruction can prevent chronic infection and permanent renal damage.

Cancers of the urinary tract are found at all sites and they are in increasing order of frequency: renal cell carcinomas, bladder cancer, and prostatic cancer. They are diagnosed by history, physical exam, X-ray, cytology, and biopsy and treated surgically. Chemotherapy and radiotherapy serve as other measures for treating patients with urogenital cancers.

Bibliography

Bennett, W. M., and Singer, I. 1977. Guidelines for drug therapy in acute renal failure. *Ann. Intern. Med.* 86: 754–783. Comprehensive approach to treatment of renal failure with drugs.

Bergsma, D. ed. 1970. Genetic and cellular bases of congenital renal dysfunction. In *Birth defects,* vol. VI. A thorough discussion of inherited renal diseases.

Campbell, M. F., and Harrison, J. H. 1974. *Urology.* Philadelphia: W. B. Saunders Company. A seven-volume set used by urologists and others as a definitive reference source.

Chapman, W. H., and Bulger, R. E., et al. 1973. *The urinary system.* Philadelphia: W. B. Saunders Company. Pathophysiologic emphasis, 250 pages.

Cooper, E. H., and Williams, R. E., eds. 1975. *The biology and clinical management of bladder cancer.* Oxford: Blackwell Scientific Publishers. Describes virtually all aspects of bladder cancer.

Gersmith, F. G., and Rodriguez, E. *Immunopathology of the renal glomerulus.* Boston: Little, Brown and Company. A synopsis of diseases caused by immune mechanisms.

Harwood, T. H., Hiesterman, D. R. 1976. Prognosis for recovery of function in acute renal failure. *Archives Internal Medicine* 136:916–919. Describes the chances for survival and recovery of patients with acute renal failure.

Heptinstall, R. H. 1974. *Pathology of the kidney,* ed. 2. Boston: Little, Brown and Company. The standard textbook for pathologists and nephrologists.

Kashgarian, M., et at. 1974. *Renal disease.* Kalamazoo: The Upjohn Co. A monograph describing the pathology of renal disease, 52 pages.

Levinsky, N. G. 1977. Pathophysiology of acute renal failure. *New England Journal of Medicine* 296:1453–1458. Describes renal tubular necrosis and vasoconstriction as the major causes of acute renal failure.

Mostofi, F. K., and Price, E. G. 1973. *Tumors of the male genital system.* Fascicle 8. Armed Forces Institute of Pathology, Washington, D.C. Standard reference for pathologists. Excellent photographs.

Netter, F. H. 1973. *Kidneys, ureters, urinary bladder.* The Ciba Collection of Medical Illustrations, Vol. 6. Summit, New Jersey: Ciba Pharmaceutical Company. Conceptually clear presentation with magnificent colored illustrations.

Newsam, J. E., and Petrie, J. J. B. 1971. *Urology and renal medicine.* London: E. E. Livingston. A simplified 250-page summary of this subject with a clinical emphasis.

Pengelley, E. T. 1974. *Sex and human life.* Reading, Massachusetts: Addison-Wesley Publishing Company. Up-to-date practical summary of information we should all know about.

Smith, D. R. 1972. *General urology,* ed. 7. Los Altos, California: Lange Medical Publishers. A thorough presentation covering virtually all aspects of urology.

CHAPTER 18

Gynecology and Breast Diseases

Chapter Outline

Objectives

After reading this chapter you should be able to
Describe the medical specialty which encompasses gynecology and obstetrics.
Identify the organs comprising the female reproductive tract.
Identify the six microbes chiefly responsible for vulvovaginitis.

Recognize the signs and symptoms of vulvovaginitis.

Discuss the basis for diagnosis of vulvovaginitis.

Know the antibiotics most commonly used for treating vulvovaginitis.

Identify the common pyogenic bacterium responsible for endometritis.

Describe the frequency of occurrence of gonorrhea in the United States.

Identify the signs and symptoms of gonorrhea.

Understand the basis for diagnosis of gonorrhea.

Know the treatment for gonorrhea.

Describe the complications accompanying gonorrhea.

Define what an ectopic pregnancy is.

Recognize why surgical intervention is the only treatment for an ectopic pregnancy.

Distinguish hydatidiform mole from choriocarcinoma.

Define endometriosis.

Recognize the symptoms and potential consequences of endometriosis.

Identify the most common uterine tumor.

List the benign and malignant causes of vaginal hemorrhage.

Recognize the relationship between frequent intercourse and a virus to cervical cancer.

Compare the prognosis for various stages of uterine cancer.

Understand that vaginal hemorrhage in a postmenopausal woman could signal endometrial cancer.

List the major complication accompanying uterine cancer.

Know the age distribution of women who develop ovarian cancer.

Understand the frequency and significance of bilateral ovarian cancer.

Define the components of a teratoma.

List features which help determine the prognosis with ovarian cancers.

Recognize how benign and malignant tumors can cause ill-defined lumps in the breast.

Know how to do a monthly breast examination.

List the breast tumors most common during each decade of life.

Understand how cystic disease and hereditary factors increase chances for breast cancer.

Define the term dysplasia including fibrosis, cystic disease, and adenosis in your definition.

List the five common signs and symptoms of breast cancer.

Know the frequency of occurrence of breast cancer in women and men.

Recognize the importance of biopsy and frozen section diagnosis in cases of breast cancer.

Recognize the characteristic appearance of breast cancer observed in a gross specimen and with a microscope.

Define lumpectomy (excisional biopsy), simple mastectomy, and radical mastectomy.

List the six factors determining the prognosis for women with breast cancer.

Define lymphedema.

List other complications of breast cancer and treatment.

Introduction

Many medical problems unique to women arise from disorders of the reproductive tract and breasts. During each phase of life women are faced with special potential gynecologic problems. The *menarche* or onset of menstruation occurs when the endometrial lining is shed in a young woman, usually between the ages of 11 and 14. This event signals the onset of the reproductive years and *menopause* ends them. The medical specialties of obstetrics and gynecology have been developed to help women cope with disorders of the reproductive tract. The objective of the *obstetrician* is to help with each pregnancy, labor, and delivery to provide a normal mother with a normal baby. The aim of the *gynecologist* is to treat and prevent gyencologic diseases. In recent years the obstetrician-gynecologist has become the primary care physician for many women.

The female genital tract consists of the labia majora and minora, vagina, uterine cervix, uterus, oviducts, and ovaries. The genital tract permits sperm to travel to where it can unite with the ovum that has traveled downward from the ovaries. Fertilization usually occurs within an oviduct approximately 24 hours following intercourse. Implantation of the fertilized ovum in the endometrium of the uterus occurs four days later. Hormonal changes governed by the endocrine system determine when ovulation occurs and prepare the endometrium for receiving the fertilized egg. Normally the menstrual cycle occurs every 28 days. Ovulation usually occurs roughly midway through the cycle.

Diseases involving the female genital tract can occur at many levels in this passageway. In young women, infectious agents, hormonal imbalances, or abnormalities in reproduction are responsible for most diseases. In contrast, malignancies occur chiefly in women beyond the reproductive age.

Infectious Diseases

Whether an infectious disease occurs (anywhere) depends upon several factors: (a) number of microorganisms and their virulence (ability to estab-lish themselves as infectious agents); (b) portal of entry, such as an abrasion; (c) prior exposure to the microbe and immune defenses against the invading microbes (see Chapter 7, Infectious Diseases).

Infectious agents can cause minor irritation or morbidity in nonpregnant women, but can kill a fetus when they pass from a woman to her fetus through the placenta. The various infectious agents which can threaten the fetus are discussed in detail in Chapter 7. These important microbes include toxoplasma, syphilis, rubella, cytomegalovirus, and herpes simplex virus. The agents infecting the genital tracts of women include viruses, bacteria, protozoa, and fungi (yeast).

Infectious vulvovaginitis

Vaginitis or vulvovaginitis is a vexing gynecological problem. The major symptoms of vaginitis are *leukorrhea* (an abnormal discharge of white pus) and *pruritus* (itching). Local swelling or pain upon intercourse *dyspareunia* occur less frequently. The causes of vaginitis are multiple (Table 18-1).

Vulvovaginitis is frequently caused by a protozoan, *Trichomonas vaginalis* or a yeast, *Candida albicans*, a yeast (fungus). When trichomonas infects the vagina and urethra it causes a burning sensation upon urination (dysuria). A watery vaginal discharge is usually experienced. A diagnosis is achieved by examining a wet smear of the fluid from the vagina. The protozoan microorganisms can be seen swimming in the fluid. Treatment is with metronidazole (Flagyl).

Monilia (candida) vaginitis is characterized by a white, cheesy discharge. Severe itching may occur because of the acute inflammatory response that arises from the fungus. Monilial vaginitis is common in pregnant women and has been associated with the use of oral contraceptives. The diagnosis can be achieved by observing the fungus in a vaginal smear. Treatment is by inserting Mycostatin suppositories into the infected vagina. This antifungal agent is usually effective.

The uterine cervix, urethra, and surrounding structures can be infected by syphilis, which is caused by *Treponema pallidum* (See Chapter 7, Infectious Diseases). Also gonococcus, staphylococ-

Table 18-1
Common Causes of Vulvovaginitis

Microbe	Character of discharge	Symptoms	Treatment
Trichomonas vaginalis	Green-white foamy	Profuse discharge and irritation	Metronidazole (Flagyl)
Candida albicans	Thick yellow curd	Moderate discharge with severe irritation	Nystatin (Mycostatin)
Hemophilus vaginalis	Purulent (pus)	Profuse discharge with minimal irritation	Local sulfa
Treponema pallidum	Ulcer (chancre) with red base or rash	Ulcer (chancre) in primary stage; rash in secondary stage	Penicillin
Neisseria gonorrhoeae	Purulent	Burning on urination	Penicillin
Herpes simplex	None	Red-white, raised, painful vesicles	None

cus, or streptococcus may infect the genital tract. All of these infectious agents, except for syphilis, are pyogenic infectious agents—they elicit a pyogenic (acute inflammatory) response and leukorrhea. The best treatment for all of these venereal infections is penicillin.

Chronic cervicitis is found to some degree in all women. Type II herpes simplex virus is usually responsible for cervicitis. An intensive lymphocytic and plasma cell infiltration is seen under the squamous epithelium that lines the cervix. Currently, no definitive treatment is available for treating this or any viral infection. In addition, herpes simplex infection has been linked with uterine cervical cancer.

Pelvic Inflammatory Disease

The term pelvic inflammatory disease (PID) refers to infection of the pelvic organs of the female genital tract. The importance of pelvic infection in general is measurable not only by its high frequency, but also by the amount of damage it causes to the reproductive potential of infected women.

Endometritis is an uncommon inflammatory condition of the endometrium that lines the uterus. This disease is caused by pyogenic bacteria, intrauterine contraceptive devices, or may occur following pregnancy. Typically, an individual with endometritis has vaginal spotting with blood or fluid, pelvic discomfort, or infertility. Treatment involves the use of appropriate antibiotics, and dila-

tation and curettage (D and C) may be attempted by some gynecologists. The pathologist examining the biopsy specimen of the endometrium observes irregularly shaped endometrial glands and chronic inflammatory cells including plasma cells and lymphocytes.

Gonorrhea

By far the most common cause of PID is *N gonorrhoeae*: Approximately 60% of acute PID is caused by gonococci. In the United States approximately 1.5 million cases are thought to occur annually. This organism invades the mucosal lining of the oviducts after passing up the uterine cavity from the vagina, and it induces an acute inflammatory response. The disease is transmitted by sexual intercourse. The diagnosis can be made by observing a Gram stained smear from pus of the male or female urethra. The bacterium is a Gram-negative oval or spherical coccus measuring 0.8 by 0.6μ, frequently found in pairs within neutrophils. Culture of the pus confirms the diagnosis. The incubation period or time from contact to onset of disease varies from two to ten days.

Most women with gonorrhea are asymptomatic. Some may have dysuria (lower urinary tract pain upon urination) and vaginal discharge. It is only when the disease spreads upward from the cervix to the Fallopian tubes that the classical features of acute PID arise: chills, fever (38 to 39C), weakness, loss of appetite, nausea, and vomiting can ensue. The cervix becomes painful to touch. This symptom is sometimes called the "chandelier sign"—the infected woman almost jumps off the table for the chandelier when the inflamed cervix is gently touched.

If the acute PID is not treated, chronic PID can develop. Abscesses in the Fallopian tubes and adjacent ovaries can produce pain, fever, and sterility. Later, healing induces scars which may block the lumen of the tube. The obstruction may cause an *ectopic pregnancy*—the implantation of a fertilized ovum at a site other than the uterus. Ideally, gonorrhea should be treated with penicillin and the sexual contacts of the patient should also be treated. The person should be cultured ten days later to be sure the gonococci have been eradicated.

Syphilis caused by *Treponema pallidum* often occurs together with gonorrhea and thus ulcers and rash should be searched for. Special laboratory tests discussed in Chapter 7, Infectious Diseases, are used for diagnosing syphilis. The treatment, penicillin, is the same as for gonorrhea.

Ectopic Pregancy

The ovum is usually fertilized in the oviduct and a stricture in the oviduct caused by an infection thus traps the embryo (Fig. 18-1). In such in-

stances an ectopic pregnancy occurs. Symptoms of ectopic pregnancies occur in the oviducts three to six weeks after fertilization. The developing embryo enlarges and explodes the oviduct. Intense pain may be experienced and shock can ensue as blood rushes into the abdominal cavity. The diagnosis must be made quickly and the oviduct and fetus removed. If the ectopic pregnancy occurs on the right side, a mistaken diagnosis of acute appendicitis is often made. The gynecologist or surgeon should check to see whether the woman has missed a menstrual period, has a positive pregnancy test, and has endometrial changes compatible with pregnancy. Following removal of the ectopic pregnancy with the Fallopian tube, placental tissues can be seen within the oviduct and very infrequently, a fetus may be visible (Fig. 18-2).

Tumors of Placenta

Benign or malignant tumors can arise in placental tissue. A benign tumor, *hydatidiform mole*, and its malignant counterpart, *choriocarcinoma*, may arise from the chorionic villi. Both of these placental tumors are common in Southeast Asia, but uncommon in the United States. They often develop associated with or shortly following a pregnancy.

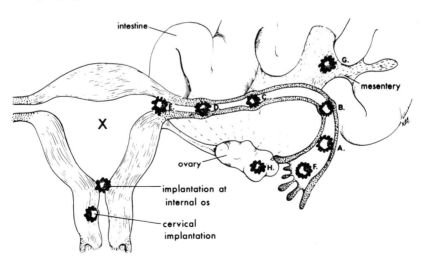

Figure 18-1 *Sites of ectopic pregnancy. The usual site of implantation is indicated by an X. The appropriate order of frequency of ectopic (extrauterine) implantation is indicated alphabetically. (From Moore: THE DEVELOPING HUMAN, © 1973 by the W. B. Saunders Company, Philadelphia.)*

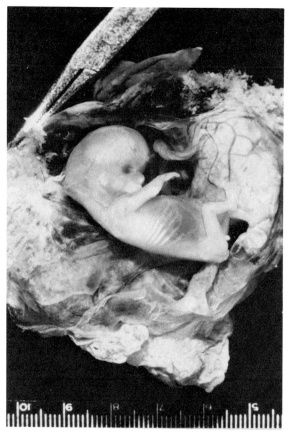

Figure 18-2 *An ectopic pregnancy (fetus) in fallopian tube.*

Bleeding, enlargement of the uterus beyond the expected size for a normal pregnancy, and softening of the uterus are observed. The individual may have a watery discharge, and bits of tissue resembling grapes (moles) may be seen. The hormone that is responsible for a positive pregnancy test, chorionic gonadotropin hormone (CGT) which is produced by the placental tumor, is markedly elevated in these individuals. Treatment is by a D and C.

Approximately 2% of moles transform into choriocarcinomas. Hence, persons with hydatidiform mole must be monitored for complete removal of the mole. This is done by noting disappearance of the positive pregnancy test when the tumor is completely removed. Choriocarcinoma usually arises following a mole or pregnancy. Choriocarcinoma,

in contrast with hydatidiform mole, is a small but malignant tumor. The tumor consists of sheets of malignant cells resembling placental tissue. These tumors often metastasize to the lungs, vagina, brain, liver, and kidneys. Elevated CGT is also found in the serum and urine of patients with choriocarcinoma. Fortunately, this tumor is very responsive to a drug called Methotrexate. The response of the tumor to the therapy can be monitored by testing the level of the CGT. When the tumor is completely removed, CGT disappears from the blood of the patient.

Endometriosis

Endometriosis is a disease characterized by the presence of endometrial tissue at a site other than the uterine endometrial cavity (ectopic endometrium). Dysmenorrhea occurs when the endometrial tissue hemorrhages during menstruation.

The ovary and the lower abdominal peritoneum are the sites most frequently affected. The endometrial tissue probably becomes implanted in ectopic sites after being flushed backwards from the uterus during menstruation. Endometrial tissue passes out through oviducts and implants on the ovary and on the peritoneum.

Successful treatment of endometriosis is usually achieved by suppressing the endometrial tissues with oral contraceptive pills containing estrogen and progesterone (creating pseudopregnancy which suppresses the endometriosis). Occasionally, however, an exploratory operation must be done when the endometriosis hemorrhages in the ovary. Blood which spills into the abdominal cavity causes acute abdominal pain. The surgeon removes blood-filled cysts ("chocolate" cysts). Following menopause the disease subsides when the estrogen supporting the growth of the ectopic endometrial tissue becomes deficient.

Vaginal Neoplasms

Vaginal tumors occur in old or young women. Elderly women develop squamous cell carcinoma of

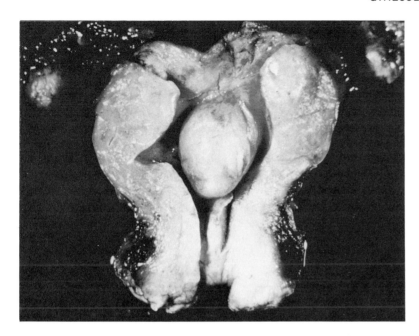

Figure 18-3   *A leiomyoma is seen filling the uterine cavity.*

the vulva or vagina on rare occasions. Generally radical surgical removal is required for cure.

Young women whose mothers had been given stilbestrol during pregnancy to prevent threatened abortion can show a rare clear-cell cervico-vaginal adenocarcinoma. More commonly the women will experience benign vaginal adenosis. Thus, women born of mothers given stilbestrol ought to be evaluated for these tumors by a gynecologist who can provide surgical extirpation (removal) of the neoplasms.

Uterine Neoplasms

Benign uterine tumors occur much more commonly than do malignant tumors. Cysts, polyps, and smooth muscle tumors, or *leiomyomas,* are commonly causes of uterine masses and hemorrhage in women (Fig. 18-3).

Fibroid (Leiomyoma)

A fibroid (leiomyoma) is a benign tumor of smooth muscle. It arises frequently from the smooth muscle in the uterus. Fibroids are the most common

uterine tumor, being present in 20% or more of women over the age of 30.

Fibroids may provoke hemorrhage, cause infertility, or when they are massive (Fig. 18-4) can produce pressure on pelvic organs. The diagnosis is made by acquiring a thorough history and by palpating the tumor, which feels like a round mass. If the fibroid is symptomatic, a partial or complete hysterectomy (removal of the uterus) is performed. Fibroids, like endometriotic tissue, require estrogen for their growth, so during menopause the tumors atrophy as the estrogen diminishes.

Polyps   Benign polyps occur within the endocervical canal and within the endometrium. Polyps may cause hemorrhage ("spotting"). These benign tumors are covered by hyperplastic glands. Treatment is by surgical excision. Hemorrhage is the major sign of malignancy in postmenopausal women; however, polyps and other benign conditions may also induce vaginal bleeding (Fig. 18-4).

Two major forms of cancer commonly occur in the uterus. These are squamous cell carcinoma of the uterine cervix and endometrial adenocarcinoma. These cancers usually occur in middle-aged and elderly women respectively.

Malignant   Nonmalignant

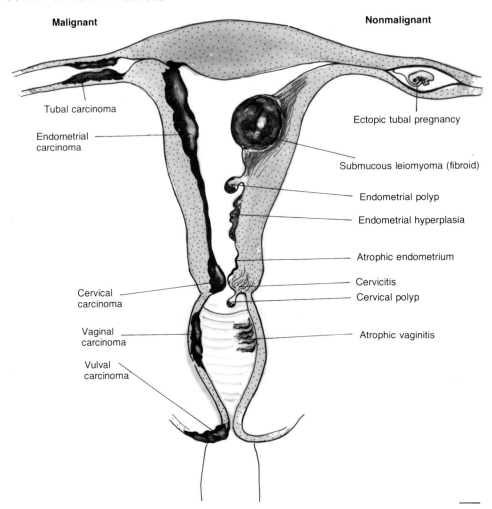

Tubal carcinoma

Endometrial carcinoma

Ectopic tubal pregnancy

Submucous leiomyoma (fibroid)

Endometrial polyp

Endometrial hyperplasia

Atrophic endometrium

Cervicitis

Cervical polyp

Cervical carcinoma

Vaginal carcinoma

Atrophic vaginitis

Vulval carcinoma

Figure 18-4   *Causes of uterine hemorrhage.*

Carcinoma of Cervix

The cause of cervical carcinoma is unknown; however, it occurs commonly in women who have frequent intercourse with multiple partners during their youth and onward. The disease has been linked with type II herpes simplex virus. It takes approximately 10 to 20 years from detection of the earliest evidence of atypical (dysplastic) cells in a Pap smear of the cervix to the appearance of invasive cancer. *Carcinoma-in-situ* is a lesion that involves only the cervical mucosa and occurs generally around age 35, whereas invasive carcinoma occurs approximately 10 years later at age 45. A

yearly Pap smear often enables detection of cancer at an early, treatable stage. A premalignant lesion can be treated by excisional biopsy (see Chapter 8).

Spotting of blood is the usual sign of cervical cancer (Fig. 18-4). The diagnosis of cervical cancer is made with a Pap smear followed by biopsy. The prognosis depends upon the stage the tumor is in when diagnosed. Stage 0 is carcinoma-in-situ and when treated in this early stage the survival rate is 100%. Stage I is when the tumor is confined to the cervix. The five-year survival drops to 85%. With stage II, infiltration into surrounding tissues has occurred. Then only 50% of persons are cured. Stage III is when the invading tumor reaches the pelvic wall or surrounding tissues. The cure rate drops to 25%. Stage IV, the most advanced uterine cervical cancer, occurs when the rectum and urinary bladder become involved by tumor.

Treatment of uterine cancer consists of hysterectomy for stage 0 and 1 disease. For the more advanced stages pelvic radiation is given by implanting radioactive needles in the uterus and by external deep irradiation.

Endometrial Cancer

Prior to the onset of adenocarcinoma, hyperplasia of the endometrial glands is often seen. The cause of endometrial adenocarcinoma is unknown, but excessive sensitivity to estrogen or exposure to excessive exogenous (given to perpetuate youthfulness) or endogenous estrogen may in some unknown way induce endometrial cancer.

Cancer of the endometrium affects postmenopausal women with low or no fertility and often occurs in elderly individuals. For instance, endometrial cancer is inordinately frequent in elderly nuns who experience uterine hemorrhage many years following menopause. A Pap smear reveals tumor cells and a D and C reveals adenocarcinoma. Treatment involves implantation of radiation seeds into the uterine cavity and later a hysterectomy. In contrast with cervical cancer this tumor is less aggressive, hence the survival rate is better.

Major complications of uterine cancer (cervical and endometrial) arise from invasion of surrounding structures and metastases. Especially vulnerable are the ureters, which can be obstructed by infiltrating tumors and fibrosis induced by radiotherapy. Thus the patient can die of renal failure from infected kidneys due to obstruction of the ureters, even when there is no residual cancer.

Ovarian Neoplasms

Tumors of the ovaries arise from the surface epithelium, germ cells, and stroma of the ovaries. Most tumors of the ovary are simply cysts lined by cuboidal epithelium and filled with clear fluid. These tumors can often be palpated on pelvic ex-

amination. If these tumors exceed 4 cm in diameter they require surgical removal because they can twist and cause infarction to occur, blocking the flow of blood. Furthermore, it is impossible to distinguish by physical examination alone (palpation) whether the mass is malignant or benign.

Malignant tumors of the ovary occur chiefly in elderly women between the ages of 60 and 80. Ovarian tumors may reach massive size. In very rare cases 300 lb ovarian tumors have been reported. The most common malignant ovarian tumor is *papillary cystadenocarcinoma* (usually weighing 50 to 5000 gm). *Solid adenocarcinoma* also is common, but has a poorer prognosis. In approximately 10% to 25% of instances, malignant tumors are bilateral (Fig. 18-5). The prognosis worsens when the tumors are bilateral.

Some of the tumors may arise from germ cells and form a mass composed of body parts including teeth, hair, thyroid, bone, and brain tissues. These tumors, which contain the primary germ elements (ectoderm, mesoderm, and endoderm), are called benign *teratomas*. Rarely are teratomas malignant.

Some tumors may produce estrogen and thus may feminize an elderly woman. She may recommence having menstrual periods signaling the existence of an ovarian tumor. Rarely, ovarian tumors may secrete male hormones and masculinize a woman. Ovarian tumors are treated by surgical removal.

The prognosis for various ovarian tumors depends upon: (a) the histologic type of the tumor, and (b) the stage of the tumor. The major question to answer is whether metastasis or seeding of the peritoneal cavity has occurred. When metastasis occurs or when seeds of tumors are implanted in the peritoneum, fluid fills the abdominal cavity. When this occurs, chemotherapy is the last resort.

Diseases of the Breast

Diseases involving the breast produce masses. These masses are always sources of alarm because they may be malignant. Therefore, virtually all breast masses need to be biopsied and examined microscopically to determine whether cancer is present.

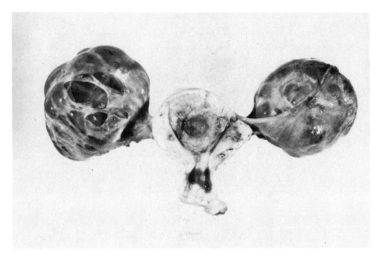

Figure 18-5 *Bilateral ovarian adenocarcinoma. (Armed Forces Institute of Pathology negative No. 57-7233-2.)*

However, when multiple nodules or cysts occur that vary considerably in size during the menstrual cycle or when they decrease in size, they probably need not be biopsied.

Every woman should examine herself each month on the first day of her menstrual cycle and, during the postmenopausal period, examination should be done on the first day of each month.

The American Cancer Society suggests that women establish the following routine. Once a month, check your breasts in front of a mirror. "Look at your breasts. Arms at your sides. Arms up. Do you look the same as always? Lie down. Put a pillow under your left shoulder and your left hand under your head. Use the other hand, fingers flattened to check your left breast. Think of your breasts as a spiral. Begin feeling gently for a lump or thickening. It's important to be thorough. Now repeat the same procedure sitting up. Repeat the check on the other breast."

Depicted in Figure 18-6 are the most common diseases occurring in the female breast. The normal female breast is composed of glandular tissue derived from modified sweat glands, fat, supporting ligaments, and ducts that drain into the nipple. The relative frequency and age of occurrence of common breast diseases are listed in Table 18-2.

Fibroadenoma

Fibroadenoma is a common, benign tumor that occurs in women under the age of 35. As the name suggests, it consists of both fibrous and adenomatous ductal tissue. Fibroadenomas measure from several millimeters to 4 or 5 cm in diameter and have a rubbery consistency. Microscopically, the tumor is clearly demarcated from the normal glands by a capsule. This tumor has no association with cancer but should be biopsied to completely rule cancer out.

Dysplasia of Breast Tissue

Dysplasia, or abnormal growth of breast tissue, is the most common benign tumor that produces a

Table 18-2
Age of Occurrence and Relative Frequency of Common Breast Diseases

Disease	Age period (median age)	Relative frequency (percent)
Fibrocystic disease	20–50 years (30)	40
Fibroadenoma	15–40 (20)	20
Intraductal papilloma	35–55 (40)	5
Cancer	40–70 (55)	25
Other	15–80	10

mass in the female breast. Approximately one-half of adult women have mild mammary dysplasia. The three different types of abnormal (dysplastic) breast tissue are encompassed by the diagnostic categories of fibrosis, adenosis, and cystic disease (Fig. 18-6).

Fibrosis

Fibrosis of the breast results from a proliferation of the fibroblasts that produce collagen between the ducts and lobules. Ordinarily, fibrosis is limited to the upper outer quadrant of one breast, but on occasion may be bilateral. It has a rubbery consistency and is gray-white. This lesion has no malignant predisposition.

Cystic Disease

Cystic disease (fibrocystic disease) is another common dysplastic lesion that develops about the time of menopause (fifth decade). Unlike fibrosis, it is associated with an increased (four-fold) occurrence of cancer. Pathologically, this condition consists of cysts that are formed from dilated ducts surrounded by fibrous tissue. On cut section the cysts vary in size (up to 4 cm in diameter) and may be filled with blood (Fig. 18-5). The mucosal lining of the cysts is often hyperplastic.

Adenosis

Adenosis, the third variety of dysplasia of the breast, frequently occurs in women during their fourth and fifth decades of life. The lesion is rubbery or hard and can mimic cancer, both in consistency and gross appearance. Adenosis consists of tightly compressed glands which are two cell layers in thickness and surrounded by dense fibrous tissue. When the lesion occurs in only one breast, a biopsy is required to rule out carcinoma. This form of dysplasia involves no increased risk of cancer (Fig. 18-6).

Women between the ages of 35 and 50 are commonly affected by mammary dysplasia, but carcinoma of the breast is by no means uncommon. Carcinoma is the major cause of a mass in the breast

in women over 50. Rarely, fat can become necrotic due to injury or infection of the breast and mimic a carcinoma. Infection of the breast (mastitis) is caused by *Staphylococcus aureus* and most often occurs during lactation. Acute inflammation with redness, swelling, and pain are noted at the site involved by mastitis and in the axillary lymph nodes. Treatment is with penicillin.

Breast Cancer

Breast cancer is the most common malignancy in women. One out of every 13 women, or about seven percent, will develop breast cancer during her lifetime. In 1975, there were nearly 90,000 new cases in the United States. Breast cancer is the leading cause of cancer death in women and is the leading cause of death from all causes in women 40 to 44 years of age.

The cause of carcinoma of the breast is unknown, however, studies in mice have demonstrated transmission of breast cancer by a virus in milk (Bittner factor) from mother to female offspring. Although a virus has not been found in women, there is a tendency for breast cancer to run in families. Approximately a two-fold increase above the normal frequency of breast cancer occurs in close relatives of patients with breast cancer. An inherited predisposition to breast, endometrial, ovarian, and colon carcinoma can also occur in various members of some families. Carcinoma of the breast occurs more often in women who have not been pregnant. Factors associated with increased risk of breast cancer are summarized in Table 18-3.

Clinical Findings

Characteristically, a woman with breast cancer accidently discovers a mass in her breast while bathing, or the mass may be found by her husband or physician. It is unfortunate that many women, out of fear or denial, fail to report the discovery to a physician.

The examining physician looks for signs of breast cancer: (a) retraction of the nipple, (b) dimpling of

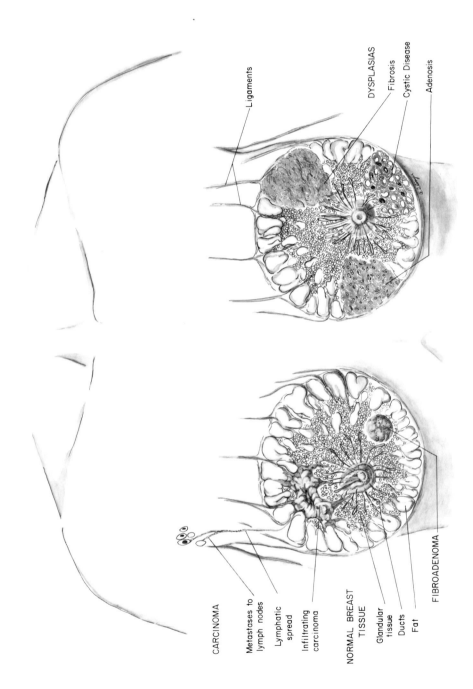

Ligaments

DYSPLASIAS
Fibrosis
Cystic Disease
Adenosis

CARCINOMA

Metastases to
lymph nodes

Lymphatic
spread

Infiltrating
carcinoma

NORMAL BREAST
TISSUE

Glandular
tissue

Ducts

Fat

FIBROADENOMA

Figure 18-6   *Common diseases of the breast in women.*

the skin, (c) fixation of the mass to skin or chest wall, (d) enlargement of axillary lymph nodes draining the mass, and (e) discharge from the nipple. Surprisingly, approximately five years transpire from the occurrence of mutant cancer cells to the accumulation of cells sufficient to attain 1-cm diameter in size, a size that can be felt with the fingers. So a tumor can exist for five years before it is detected!

Cancer of the female breast affects 5 in 100 women and rarely occurs under the age of 25 years. The disease is primarily one of middle and late years of life. The cancers can arise in either lobules or ducts. Over 90% of breast cancers arise in the ducts. Approximately 50% begin in the upper outer quadrant and the remaining are distributed evenly in the other quadrants. Only 10% of breast carcinomas form in the lobules. This tumor, however, is apt to be bilateral (20% bilaterality). Infiltrating carcinomas carry the worst prognosis and, unfortunately, most tumors have infiltrated by the time a diagnosis is achieved. Other tumors such as medullary and colloid carcinomas are rare and have more favorable prognoses.

Usually when lesions are discovered they measure an average of 4 cm in diameter. Approximately two-thirds have already spread to axillary or other lymph nodes. The intraductal cancers, in contrast, do not usually produce masses but come to the attention of the patient because of discharge from the nipple (Fig. 18-6).

Table 18-3
Risk Factors of Breast Cancer

Women
Over 40 years
Family history of breast cancer
Nonpregnant women or pregnancy after 34
Cancer in the other breast
Cancer of endometrium
Fibrocystic disease
Excessive exposure to radiation
Psychosocial features of stress and upper
   socioeconomic group

Diagnosis

The diagnosis is based upon clinical history, physical examination, mammography, and examination of the tissue histopathologically. A *mammograph* consists of an X-ray examination of the breast (see Chapter 8). It is useful in detecting approximately 80% of breast cancers. Characteristically, a fine stripping of calcium is seen within the tumor mass in the mammograph. And calcification may also occur in dysplasia of the breast, leading to a false positive diagnosis. However, this technique is not sufficiently sensitive to detect all breast cancers. Moreover, in 1976 an epidemiologist from the National Cancer Institute presented convincing evidence that mammographs and their associated radiation could cause as many breast cancers as they detect. Screening for breast cancer using self-examination, physician evaluation on a semiannual basis, and mammography in selected instances has resulted in reduction of advanced breast cancer and has improved the survival rates in thousands of women.

Frozen Section Examination   Following evaluation of the mass by the above procedures, a *frozen section* is performed and the specimen is examined microscopically. In this procedure, a woman is prepared for a biopsy of the breast. The surgeon removes the lump, which is examined by a pathologist. Characteristically, carcinomas have a fibrous, white-yellow appearance (Fig. 18-7). When the specimen is cut the cancer feels gritty due to calcification and dense fibrosis of the tumor. The calcification can be seen on the mammograph. The pathologist freezes a small portion of the tumor in a refrigerated compartment (cryostat). He or she makes a thin section of the tissue, stains it, and examines it with a microscope.

Characteristically, a malignant tumor consists of anaplastic tumor cells that have increased nuclear size. Tumor cells can be seen invading the connective tissue of the breast (Fig. 18-7). Based upon the pathologist's diagnosis the surgeon may or may not proceed with an operation. Approximately one in five biopsy specimens examined by frozen section are found to be malignant. The remaining benign

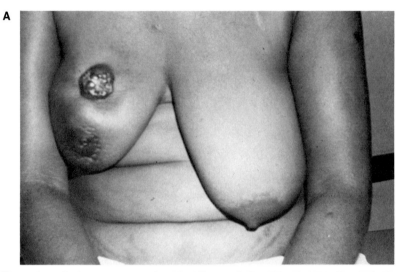

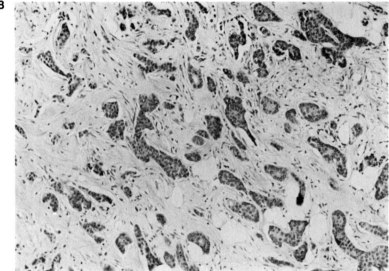

Figure 18-7 **A,** *Carcinoma of breast.* **B,** *Tumor cells are seen invading the connective tissue.* × 400.

lesions are thoroughly examined and the biopsy site closed by suture.

Treatment

If the breast biopsy shows a malignant tumor a mastectomy procedure should follow. A *radical mastectomy* consists of removing the breast, including the overlying skin and the pectoralis major and minor muscles. In addition, an axillary "tail" of tissue which contains axillary lymph nodes is removed for pathological examination. Occasionally

only the tumor, overlying skin, and breast tissue must be removed. This is a *simple mastectomy* (Fig. 18-8). Recent preferences for a simple mastectomy together with irradiation and possibly chemotherapy has been voiced by some physicians. Efforts are finally being made on a wide scale to reconstruct the breast after surgery.

Prognosis

The prognosis for patients with breast cancer is based upon the following factors: (a) large tumors

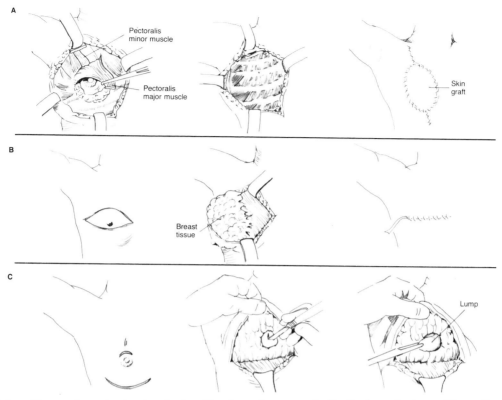

Figure 18-8 *Types of mastectomies for treating breast cancer.* **A,** Radical mastectomy. *The entire breast, portion of skin, the nipple, pectoralis major and minor muscles, axillary fat pad, and lymph nodes are removed. A skin graft is usually not needed.* **B,** Total or simple mastectomy. *Like radical, but muscles are not removed.* **C,** Lumpectomy or segmentectomy. *Removal of lump and 3 to 5 cm margin of normal breast.*

measuring over 2.5 cm in diameter are associated with poorer prognosis than smaller tumors; (b) infiltration of the skin, breast tissue, underlying pectoralis muscle, or bone is associated with a poorer prognosis than are noninfiltrating tumors; (c) restriction of tumor to the breast is associated with a more favorable prognosis; (d) when four or more lymph nodes contain metastatic tumor the prognosis worsens; (e) When the tumors are bilateral the prognosis worsens. There is approximately a 7% to 10% risk of developing a second primary cancer in the opposite breast; and (f) carcinomas arising during pregnancy are associated with poorer survival.

In summary, small lesions which have not infiltrated or metastasized are associated with an 85% five-year survival. Unfortunately, the five-year survival for patients with large tumors that infiltrate and metastasize is only approximately 15%. Overall, most patients with treated breast cancer have an approximately 50% to 60% five-year survival. Treatment by radical mastectomy or simple mastectomy with irradiation in patients with more advanced disease does not appear to significantly change the prognosis. Relentless persistence of the tumor despite therapeutic efforts suggests that the individual tumors have a predetermined and unmeasurable malignant potential.

Complications

Lymphedema (swollen arm) following a radical mastectomy is a serious complication that occurs in approximately 20% of women. Elephantiasis of the extremity with progressive increase in dermal connective tissue may severely incapacitate the person. The lymphedema often requires physical therapy such as massage to reduce the edema. In addition, irradiation can cause poor wound healing and predispose to infection. Obesity may add to the edema.

The use of super voltage radiotherapy can inflict damage to the lungs (radiation pneumonitis) and the heart (carditis), causing congestion and cough. On rare occasion *sarcomas* (cancer of connective tissue in the scar) have appeared following radiation.

A common complication following mastectomy is recurrence of tumor. This may occur in the scar or in the axilla. Also, the tumor could have already metastasized to the lungs or other organs. The tumor may also metastasize to the brain and cause abnormalities of cerebral function. Metastatic breast cancer to the brain is the most common cause of brain tumors in women.

The radiotherapy and chemotherapy depress the patient's immunity and render her susceptible to infections. Furthermore, she may suffer from hemorrhage when the platelet count becomes low (thrombocytopenia) due to suppression of bone marrow arising from chemotherapy. Paradoxically, some individuals with cancer tend to clot (thrombose) blood vessels.

Male Breast

The male breast is affected by cancer only approximately 1% as often as the female breast. When breast cancer occurs in males, however, the prognosis is worse than in females. Curiously, a 20-fold increase in occurrence appears in dysgenetic men with an extra X chromosome (XXY). This is termed Klinefelter's syndrome (see Chapter 9, Inherited Disorders).

A benign disorder of the male breast common in adolescent boys or in individuals with cirrhosis of the liver is *gynecomastia*. It occurs when the breast tissue responds to estrogen and becomes hyperplastic and edematous. Examination of these boys or men reveals a button-like nubbin of breast tissue beneath the nipple. Spontaneous subsidence of gynecomastia normally occurs in adolescent boys, but the condition tends to persist in individuals with

cirrhosis. The excessive breast tissue is removed surgically if it is disfiguring.

Summary

Women, because they possess reproductive tracts and childbearing capabilities, are subject to a group of diseases to which men are not vulnerable. Most of these disorders involve hormonal imbalance which lead to uterine hemorrhage, infertility, or neoplasms. The reproductive tract is vulnerable to various infectious diseases that do not occur in males. For example, vulvovaginitis is an extremely common group of infectious diseases in women caused by viruses, bacteria, protozoa and fungi.

Disorders of reproduction most commonly seen are ectopic pregnancy, infertility, spontaneous abortion, and benign placental tumors. In nonfertile women, endometrial tissue in sites outside the uterus (endometriosis) can cause pain and obstruction of fallopian tubes. Fibroids (leiomyomas) are common benign tumors arising in the muscular wall of the uterus. Cervical or endometrial adenomatous polyps are common and cause vaginal spotting.

Vaginal hemorrhage deserves medical evaluation especially in women near or beyond menopause. Women beyond the fourth decade with postmenopausal hemorrhage are likely to have a carcinoma of the uterus (cervix or endometrial).

Carcinoma of the cervix usually undergoes a gradual (usually 10 to 20 years) transformation from mild dysplasia, to carcinoma-in-situ, to invasive carcinoma. Hence, detection of early lesions by a Pap smear can lead to effective cure and obviate prospects for cancer. Cervical cancer occurs more often in women who are quite active sexually, and is associated with herpes simplex type II virus. By contrast, endometrial cancer is a disease of elderly women who usually have never been pregnant. Ovarian malignancies are also apt to occur in women beyond 50 years.

Most diseases of the breast produce lumps that require biopsy and microscopic examination to rule out carcinoma. For each age group a certain breast disorder is common: fibroadenoma (younger than

35 years); dysplasias including fibrosis, fibrocystic disease, and adenosis (35 to 50 years); and carcinoma (30 to 70 years).

The prognosis associated with breast cancer is based on the size, histologic type, and presence or absence of metastases. Traditional radical mastectomy is now being challenged as the optimal mode of therapy. The five-year survival rate of women treated for breast cancer has remained at 50% to 60% during this century. Thus efforts are being made to achieve earlier diagnosis (self examination and mammograph) and treatment with simple mastectomy plus radiotherapy, with or without chemotherapy.

Bibliography

Dilts, P. V., et al. 1971. *Core studies in obstetrics and gynecology.* Baltimore: The Williams & Wilkins Company. A 234 page introductory textbook.

Green, T. H. 1971. *Gynecology.* Boston: Little, Brown and Company. Comprehensive discussion.

Haagensen, C. D. 1971. *Diseases of the breast.* Philadelphia: W. B. Saunders Company. Standard clinical textbook.

Herbst, A. L., et al. 1975. Prenatal exposure to stilbestrol. *N. Engl. J. Med.* 292: 334–339. Describes the development of vaginal cancer in young women born of mothers who had received stilbestrol while pregnant.

Leis, H. P. 1977. The diagnosis of breast cancer. CA 27: 209–232. The scope of this problem is discussed and illustrated with photographs of patients with breast cancer.

McDivitt, R. W.; Stewart, F. W.; and Berg, J. W. 1969. *Atlas of tumor pathology: tumors of the breast.* Fascicle 2. Washington, D. C.: Armed Forces Institute of Pathology. Excellent photographs and the definitive reference for pathologists.

Norris, H. J.; Hertig, A. T.; and Abell, M. R., eds. 1973. *The uterus.* Baltimore: The Williams & Wilkins Company. Thorough presentation on endometrial cancer.

Novak, E. R., and Woodruff, J. D. 1974. *Novak's gynecologic and obstetric pathology*, ed. 7. Philadelphia: W. B. Saunders Company. Standard textbook.

Our bodies ourselves. 1973. New York: Simon & Schuster, Inc. A book by and for women. Basic handbook written in lay language.

Purtilo, D. T. 1975. Fatal mycotic infections in pregnant women. *Am. J. Obstet. Gynecol.* 122: 607–610. Describes fatal fungal infections in a group of pregnant women.

Treating the woman with breast cancer. 1975. *Nursing Update* 8, November. Lucid description of various surgical procedures.

Wolfe, J. N. 1967. A study of breast parenchyma mammography in the normal woman and those with benign and malignant disease. *Radiology* 89:201–205. Describes use of mammography in diagnosing breast cancer.

CHAPTER 19

Dermatology and Dermatopathology

Chapter Outline

Objectives

After reading this chapter you should be able to

Describe senses perceived by the skin and the emotions expressed in the skin.

List the three layers of skin as seen with a microscope.

Compare keratinocytes with melanocytes.

List the three disorders involving abnormal pigmentation.

List the cell types within the dermis.

Describe the appendages of skin.

List the questions asked of a patient with a dermatologic problem.

List the four major features of a skin lesion noted during the physical examination.

Compare and list primary and secondary skin lesions.

List laboratory tests commonly employed in the diagnosis of skin diseases.

Know the two large groups of skin disorders.

List several disorders of the keratinocyte.

Describe changes in the color of the skin that mirror systemic diseases.

List signs of internal malignancy detectable in the skin.

Describe and compare cutaneous manifestations of endocrine disorders.

Define the terms eczema and atopy.

Discuss the frequency and cause of drug allergies.

List common allergic reactions to penicillin.

Know the pathophysiologic bases of drug allergies.

Describe the immunologic basis for vasculitis.

Explain how pemphigus vulgaris can kill a patient.

Define dermatitis herpetiformis.

List examples of cutaneous infections.

Compare herpes simplex and herpes zoster infections.

List the two infectious agents responsible for impetigo.

Compare the three stages of syphilis with respect to types of skin lesions and their communicability.

Name the microbe responsible for leprosy.

Compare the two major forms of leprosy.

Describe how a claw hand can develop from leprosy.

List types of superficial fungal infections.

Describe techniques used for diagnosing fungal infections.

Recognize scabes dermatitis.

Discuss the appearance of psoriatic lesions.

Distinguish seborrheic keratosis from melanoma.

Compare epidermal cyst and pilonidal sinus.

Describe the etiology of warts.

Compare condyloma acuminatum with molluscum contagiosum.

List benign tumors of the skin.

Describe a premalignant skin lesion.

Compare the cells of origin for squamous carcinoma, basal cell carcinoma and melanoma.

Know how squamous cell carcinomas are treated.

State the prognosis for malignant melanoma.

Introduction

Without the protection of the skin, we would be traumatized by heat, chemicals, and radiant energy. Our abilities to regulate heat, water, and mineral balance would be upset by excessive evaporation. The nerve endings in the skin allow us to perceive sensations of touch, pain, pressure, heat, and cold. In addition, some skin reactions allow us to show emotions—we blush with shame, turn red with anger, blanche with fear, and perspire with anxiety. These expressions are only possible because the skin is a highly organized structure responsive to internal and external stimuli.

The normal histology of the skin will be described as a basis for you to comprehend the diseases of the skin. General pathologic processes, manifestations of systemic diseases in skin, and terms used to describe lesions will then be considered. Important infectious, immunologic hypersensitivity, and neoplastic skin diseases will then be discussed.

Histology of Skin

The skin is divided into three layers (see Chapter 2, Normal Cells, Tissues, and Organs) which extend from the outside inward (Fig. 19-1).

The *epidermis* is paper thin and composed of a special protein, keratin. The *dermis* is formed by dense collagen tissue and other connective tissues that lie beneath the epidermis. The *subcutaneous tissue* comprises the thickest layer of the skin and is composed of blood vessels, fat, and nerves.

Up until the fifth week of fetal life, the ectodermally derived epidermis is only a single layer of cells; thereafter many layers form and this layer thickens. At approximately six months of gestation epidermal appendages form (sweat glands, hair follicles, nails, and sebaceous glands).

Epidermal Layer

The epidermis is a thin, cellular membrane devoid of blood vessels and connective tissue. It grows from basal cells that rest upon the underlying dermis and it derives its nutrition by diffusion from blood vessels within the dermis (Fig. 19-2). As basal cells grow and mature, they migrate outward to form squamous cells or *keratinocytes* that make *keratin*, a tough fibrous protein that prevents drying of the body and invasion by bacteria. Hair and nails are specialized keratin that becomes dry and firm.

Melanocytes are the other major cell of the epidermis (Fig. 19-2). Melanocytes are derived from

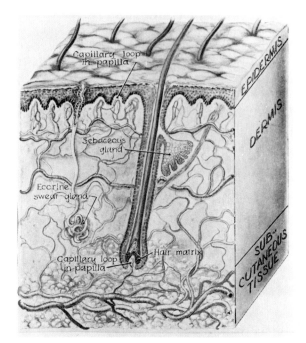

Figure 19-1 *Diagram of skin. (Courtesy Ciba Foundation.)*

neuroectodermal crest cells in the embryo. They produce melanin pigment which is distributed throughout the epidermis. Melanin prevents cancer from developing in the skin by shielding it from excessive exposure to sunlight. The process of tanning results from increased synthesis of melanin upon exposure to ultraviolent light. Surprisingly, black persons do not contain more melanocytes than light persons; their melanin pigment granules are simply larger. By contrast, when no pigmentation is present, *albinism*, an autosomal recessive disorder, occurs (see Chapter 9, Inherited Disorders). Figure 19-3 shows an inherited disorder (LEOPARD syndrome) involving abnormal migration and concentration of melanocytes along nerves (dermatotomes).

Dermal Layer

The dermis consists of collagen fibers traversed by nerves, blood vessels, and lymphatics. Also embedded in the dermis are hairs, sebaceous, and sweat glands. *Sebaceous (oil) glands* located in the dermis

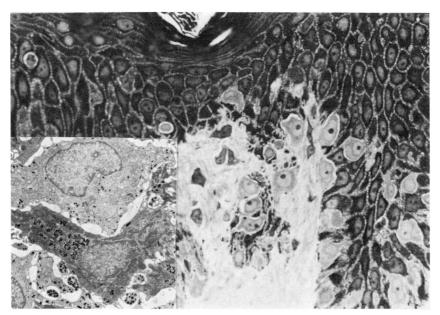

Figure 19-2 *Photomicrograph of skin demonstrating keratinocytes and melanocytes (light cells) in epidermis. × 600. Inset at higher magnification shows a melanocyte and keratinocyte. Note the black melanin granules in both cell types. × 5000. (Courtesy of Dr. Jag Bhawan.)*

are attached to hair shafts; they secrete oil which moistens skin. Intimately connected with sebaceous glands is the condition of *acne*, which occurs when the hair follicle is plugged by keratin and/or concentrated oil (sebum) to form *comedomes*, or blackheads. Often, acute inflammation and infection ensue in acne (see Chapter 7, Infectious Diseases).

The *sweat glands* help to control body temperature and are distributed throughout the dermis. There are two types. *Eccrine sweat glands* are located all over the cutaneous surface, especially on the forehead, palm, and soles. The eccrine glands are stimulated by heat and emotional stress. *Apocrine sweat glands* are found in the axillae, anogenital areas, and nipples. They do not develop fully until puberty.

Subcutaneous Layer

The subcutaneous tissue constitutes most of the substance that we consider the skin; by contrast, the epidermis is paper thin. Within the subcutaneous layer lie the skin appendage glands described above, nerves, blood vessels, collagen, lymphatics, elastin, fat, mast cells, lymphocytes, and histiocytes of the immune system.

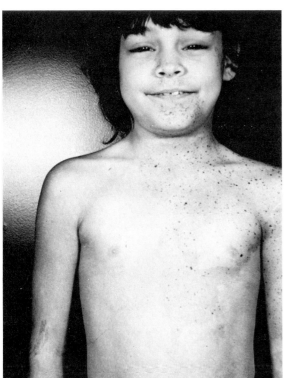

Figure 19-3 *Leopard syndrome. This child has melanotic spots confined in a dermatomal distribution.*

Diagnosis of Skin Disorders

Dermatologists are physicians who specialize in the diagnosis and treatment of skin disorders. They use the three approaches outlined in Chapter 1 to diagnose skin disorders: (a) clinical history, (b) physical examination, and (c) laboratory determinations.

Clinical History

The chief complaint of a patient (for example, "I have a lump on my arm") is investigated by asking questions: When did it appear? Where did it appear? Did it spread? Does it come and go? Is it wet or dry? Does it itch?

A personal history with questions concerning sleep, anxiety, allergies, drugs, occupation, use of cosmetics, inherited disorders, travel, and skin contact with others is obtained.

Physical Examination

The examiner's eye is the single most important instrument for diagnosis. Four important observations to be made are: (a) the *type* of lesion; (b) *distribution;* (c) *shape;* and (d) the *arrangement* of lesions.

Types of lesions are classified by considering whether the lesion protrudes or is superimposed above or below the level of normal skin (Fig. 19-4). *Primary lesions* of the skin (defined in Table 19-1) include macules, papules, wheals, nodules, tumors, vesicles, bullae, and pustules. *Secondary lesions* (defined in Table 19-1) include scales, crusts, ulcers, and scars.

Laboratory Determinations

The skin can be examined in detail using a magnifying glass. Ultraviolet light is used to detect fungal infections because they fluoresce. Scrapings of skin can also reveal fungi and other microbes. Culture of the lesions can reveal pathologic bacteria or fungi. Finally, cutaneous lesions can be biopsied with a "punch biopsy," which removes a 4-mm diameter disk of skin for microscopic study. Punch biopsies are usually done for small lesions; larger lesions are either biopsied with a scalpel or the lesion is entirely removed. The microscopic findings for most skin lesions are limited to a few pathologic responses.

Basic Pathologic Responses

Hundreds of diseases of the skin arise from just a few basic pathologic responses. The two largest groups of skin disorders include *inflammatory-infectious* dermatitis and *proliferative-neoplastic* skin lesions. Most of the pathologic responses involve one of the two major cell types—the keratinocytes and the melanocytes.

Disorders Involving Keratinocytes   The keratinocyte (Fig. 19-2) produces keratin which forms the corneum. Rare, inherited defects in the keratinocytes can occur. The inherited disease, *congenital ichthyosis* is characterized by an excessive growth of keratinocytes and keratin giving the skin a fish-scale appearance (Fig. 19-5). Corns and calluses result from adaptive hyperplasia. Stimulation of the epidermis by intermittent pressure elicits hyperkeratosis (callus). By contrast, atrophy of epidermis can arise from a decreased blood supply.

Benign or malignant neoplasms commonly arise from keratinocytes. Warts (verrucae), for instance, are caused by a virus which provokes a benign proliferation of keratinocytes. Squamous cell carcinomas (arising from keratinocytes) often occur in areas of skin excessively exposed to sunlight.

Disorders Involving Melanocytes   Melanocytes produce melanin pigment. In normal persons melanin synthesis is stimulated by exposure to sunlight. A total absence of melanin arises as an inborn error in metabolism in persons with albinism. Vitiligo (leucoderma) is a condition in which pigment disappears from a patch of skin (Fig. 19-6). The onset is sudden and is frequently associated with autoimmune diseases (such as pernicious anemia, hyperthyroidism, or diabetes mellitus).

Melanocytes can undergo benign or malignant proliferation. The common *mole* (nevus) arises from

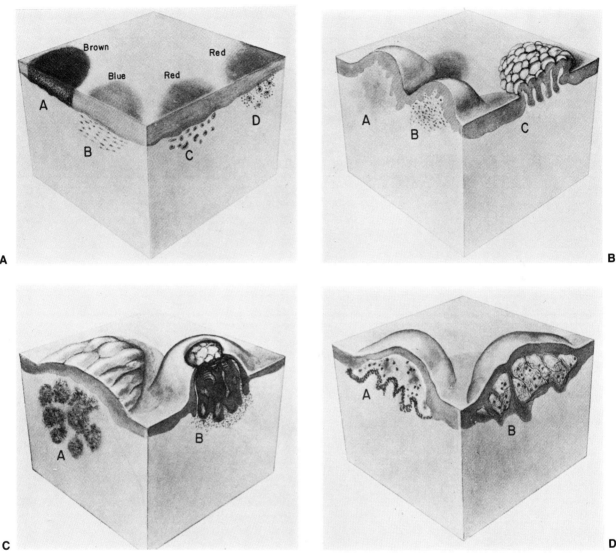

Figure 19-4   *Types of skin lesions based on their relationship to the surface of normal skin.* **A,** Macule *(flat lesion): variations include hyperpigmentation from excessive melanin,* A, *and iron deposits,* D. *Vascular abnormalities give blue,* B, *or red,* C, *appearance.* **B,** Papule *(raised lesion): papules result from deposits of metabolic substances, eg, cholesterol,* A; *excessive growth of dermal cells,* B; *or excessive growth of epidermal cells.* **C,** Nodule *(solid lesion projecting above and below the surface): nodules result from infiltrates,* A *or neoplasms,* B. **D,** Vesicle *(fluid-filled blister in epidermis): it results from a loss of intercellular bridges, or desmosomes,* A; *or from degeneration caused by viral or other injurious agents. (From* Harrison's Principles of Internal Medicine, *ed. 7, by M. M. Wintrobe, et al. Copyright © 1974 McGraw-Hill Book Company. Used with permission of McGraw-Hill Book Company.)*

Table 19-1
Primary and Secondary Skin Lesions

Primary Lesions	
Macule	A circumscribed, nonelevated discoloration, up to 1 cm in diameter
Papule	A circumscribed, superficial, solid elevation, up to 1 cm in diameter
Nodule	A solid, circumscribed dermal or hypodermal lesion, often projecting above the surface of the skin, up to 1 cm in diameter
Vesicle	A papule containing fluid, from 0.1 to 1 cm
Bulla	A vesicle over 1 cm in diameter
Pustule	A pus-filled vesicle
Secondary Lesions	
Excoriation	A traumatized, superficial ulceration from scratching
Fissure	A linear break in the skin surface bounded by abrupt sides
Scales or squames	A collection of horny material ranging from small, thin flakes to large sheets
Crust	A mass of dried exudate
Ulcer	An irregularly shaped excavation of the skin
Scar (cicatrice)	The connective tissue replacement following the loss of dermal tissue

a benign proliferation of melanocytes. Rarely, moles undergo a malignant change to become malignant melanomas.

Other components of the skin—fibroblasts, histiocytes, fat cells, hair follicles, sebaceous glands, blood vessels, and nerves—can also become neoplastic. Invariably, neoplasms produce a lump in the skin. Lumps which increase rapidly in size, change color, ulcerate, or bleed should be biopsied and examined microscopically to rule out malignancy.

The Skin in Systemic Disease

The skin reflects the status of many organ systems —endocrine, cardiopulmonary, renal, and hepatic dysfunctions are manifested in the skin. Metabolic disorders (diabetes mellitus) and internal malignancies also cause cutaneous alterations. These alter-

ations are in color, texture, and composition of the skin.

Color

Color changes in the skin can signal the existence of systemic disease.* To illustrate this point, let us go through the rainbow of possible color changes in the skin and give examples of systemic diseases responsible for these changes. The spectrum of colors is red, orange, yellow, green, blue, indigo, and violet. (Remember "ROY G BIV.")

Redness can be generalized as with carbon monoxide poisoning, or be generalized or localized in rashes or on the palms. *Orange* discoloration can occur from the deposition of carotene. A friend who was an excellent athelete came to the author

*Color changes are more difficult to see in darkly pigmented persons so one must rely on subjective signs such as itching, pain, or warmth. Mucous membranes of the mouth and eyes, however, may show some color changes.

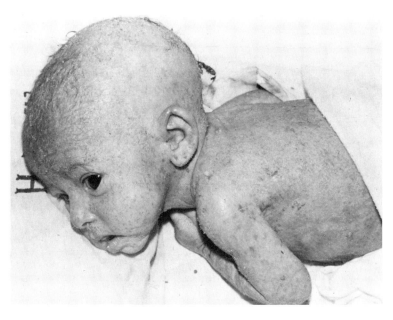

Figure 19-5   *Congenital ichthyosis. The infant is covered with flakes of keratin, which resemble fish scales.*

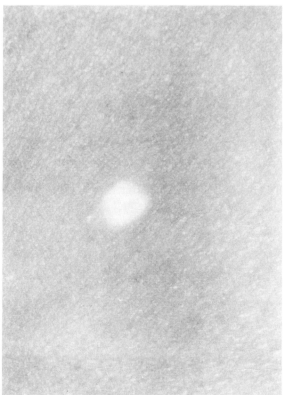

Figure 19-6   *Vitiligo. A depigmented patch has occurred on the forearm.*

complaining of darkening of his skin. I thought he had liver disease. Fortunately, it turned out that he was consuming large quantities of carrots and carotene had deposited in his skin. Also, protein-calorie malnutrition can cause hypopigmentation in black children and cause the hair and skin to appear orange.

Yellow discoloration can occur locally when lipids deposit in skin (xanthomatosis), secondary to a metabolic defect in blood lipids (such as hypercholesterolemia). More commonly, a generalized yellow or jaundiced appearance arises because of liver disease. Bilirubin accumulates in blood and saturates the tissues (see Chapter 16, Hepatic and Pancreatic Disorders). When jaundice is severe, biliverdin also accumulates. A person with obstructed bile ducts can become green-yellow due to biliverdin.

Blueness of the skin (cyanosis) often occurs on the *acral* (tips of fingers, feet, nose, and lips) parts in persons having cardiac or pulmonary disorders that prevent oxygenation of blood. Localized blueness with pain of the fingers upon exposure to cold is termed *Raynaud's phenomenon*. It frequently arises from cryoglobulins which solidify in the cold and is associated with disorders of the immune system (autoimmunity or lymphoma).

Indigo discoloration occurs locally as in gangrene of the toes from severe generalized arteriosclerosis. The skin can darken from increased melanin synthesis as in chronic adrenal insufficiency (Addison's disease). Also, silver poisoning, *argyria*, can make the skin dusky.

White (the absence of all color) skin occurs locally from vitiligo arising from autoimmunity, or the condition can be generalized in albinism. Anemia causes pallor (whitening) of the skin (see Chapter 11, Hematology). Occasionally, profound renal failure causes white uric acid crystals (uremic frost) on the skin (Fig. 19-7). Deposits of white urate crystals (tophi) likewise can accumulate in the skin of persons suffering from gout.

Violet colored palms (palmar erythema) can be seen in some persons with liver diseases and occasionally in pregnant women as a response to hyperestrogenism. Shades of violet occur in the legs from vascular insufficiency or when cardiopulmonary function is compromised.

Internal Malignancy

The manifestations of internal malignancies in the skin can be obvious. The late appearing features of cachexia (wasting), pallor, and cutaneous metastases are obvious signs of malignancy. Other diverse manifestations are also seen.

These manifestations of internal malignancies will be discussed alphabetically. *Acanthosis nigricans* is a pigmentation and thickening of skin in the axillae and groin. In patients beyond age 40, gastrointestinal malignancies may be found. *Bullous eruptions* also appear more commonly in persons with visceral (internal) malignancies.

Cushing's syndrome arising from excessive cortisol production can be caused by adrenal, lung, and pituitary tumors. *Dermatomyositis* is an autoimmune process often provoked by an internal malignancy. *Erythroderma* and itching (pruritus) can be manifestations of Hodgkin's disease.

Jaundice can signal hepatic cancer. *Keratosis* of the hands and feet is associated with lung and esophageal cancer. *Melanosis* (darkening of skin) appears with adrenal insufficiency that can arise

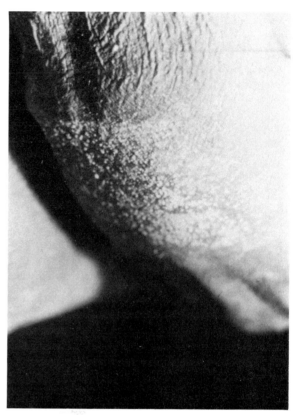

Figure 19-7   *Uremic frost has crystalized on the arm of this patient with renal failure.*

from destruction of the adrenals by metastases. *Orange peel skin* of the breast is caused by invasion of dermal lymphatics by tumor.

Sex changes manifested in the skin, such as the development of breasts in men or hairiness (hirsutism) in women, can be caused by neoplasms. *Zoster* (shingles) vesicles in a dermatomal distribution sometimes signal the presence of lymphoma or leukemia.

Endocrine Disease

Abnormalities of endocrine function (see Chapter 12, Endocrine and Metabolic Disorders) produce a myriad of cutaneous changes. The epidermal color, texture, and distribution of subcutaneous tissues are altered in endocrinopathies. These are briefly discussed (again alphabetically).

Acromegaly (arising from pituitary adenoma) is characterized by skin which is coarse, thick, oily, and hairy. Lantern jaw and thick hands are more specific clues for diagnosis of acromegaly.

Addison's disease arises from destruction of adrenals. Widespread melanosis occurs most prominantly on sun exposed areas, but the mucosa of the mouth and scars also darken.

Cushing's syndrome (excessive cortisol production) causes a maldistribution of fat—the face is round (moon face), the trunk is obese (but extremities are normal), and a hump of fat overlies the upper spine ("buffalo hump"). The complexion is ruddy and purple stretch marks (striae) are seen in the skin (see Chapter 12, Endocrine and Metabolic Disorders).

Diabetes mellitus is characterized by complications arising from arteriosclerosis (such as gangrene and ulcers) and infections occur with relative ease.

Thyroid disorders cause variable cutaneous changes. *Hyperthyroidism* causes perspiration, flushing, fine skin texture, fine hair, itching, and deposits of tissue over the tibia (pretibial myxedema) and in the orbit (exophthalmos, causing the eyes to bulge outward). *Hypothyroidism* causes general pallor with redness of cheeks. The hair and skin become coarse. When the condition is severe, *myxedema* occurs and subcutaneous tissues are deposited in the face and shins.

Common Skin Diseases

Armed with the foregoing information, we are ready for a discussion of common skin diseases (Fig. 19-8). The diseases are divided into two large categories: (a) *inflammatory* (dermatitis) diseases caused by immunologic hypersensitivity or infectious agents; and (b) *neoplastic* diseases. Emphasis here will be on malignant neoplasms because they can be life-threatening. These two groups of skin disorders will not begin to encompass all of the 1200 different skin diseases, but discussion of them will provide the reader with a conceptual basis for understanding many important diseases. Nor does space permit a discussion of the response of the

skin to injury by various environmental agents (see Chapters 4 and 5).

Immunologic and Infectious Inflammatory Skin Diseases

The common feature of various forms of *dermatitis* (inflammation of the skin) is an infiltration by blood leukocytes. The etiologic basis can be specifically identified in infectious diseases of the skin, but the etiology of immunologic hypersensitivity reactions in the skin is often obscure.

Immunologic Hypersensitivity Diseases of Skin Certain individuals easily become sensitized to foreign proteins (antigens). These *atopic* individuals have an inherited predisposition to develop immunologic hypersensitivity reactions such as asthma, hay fever, drug and food allergies, hives, and eczema. These diseases result from exposure and hypersensitivity responses to various environmental agents and are expressed as cutaneous anaphylaxis (hives), immune complex deposition, or cell-mediated immunity responses (see Chapter 6, Immunology).

Eczema Eczema is an acute or chronic, noncontagious, inflammatory condition of the skin that is characterized by redness, itching, and oozing vesicular lesions which become scaly, crusted, and dry. Eczema is often associated with exposure to chemical or other irritants. Eczema, or contact dermatitis, can be caused by contact sensitivity to a variety of chemicals, metals, fat solvents, alkaloids, hot water, turpentine, detergents containing enzymes, and certain plants.

An atopic person, upon contact with certain chemicals (such as *poison ivy*), becomes sensitized and forms long-lived memory lymphocytes that, upon reexposure to the antigen, react and inflame the skin producing eczema (Fig. 19-9 and 19-10). Contact dermatitis is usually caused by a cell-mediated immune reaction.

Redness results from dilated venules and itching and vesicles are caused by edema fluid liberated from the venules (see Chapter 5, Acute Inflam-

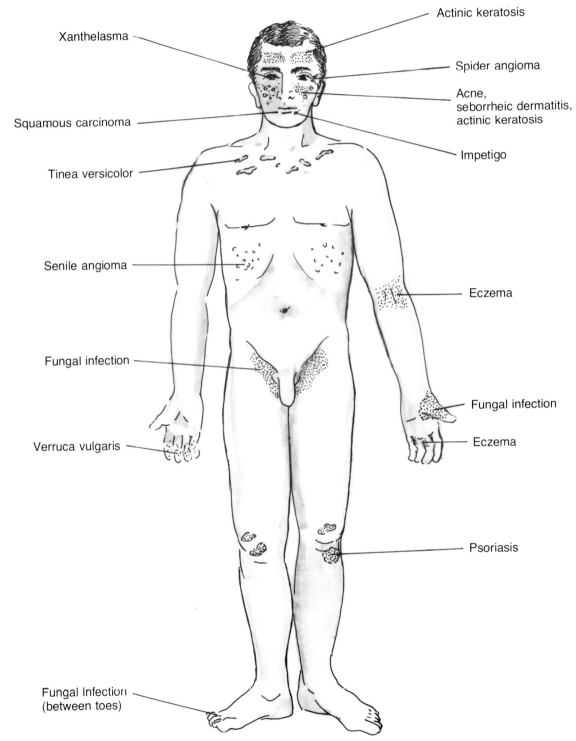

Figure 19-8   *Common skin lesions are shown in their usual sites of occurrence.*

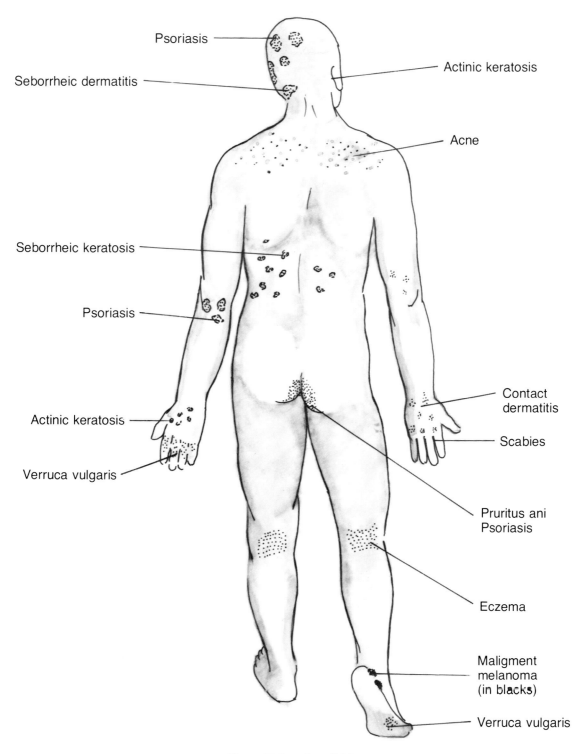

Figure 19-8   *(cont'd.)*

mation and Repair). The inflammation is usually relieved by topical steroid; however, the patient shown in Figure 19-9 required cortisone by mouth because the poison ivy was spreading all over her skin.

Drug Allergies   A *drug reaction* is an adverse effect (a nonbeneficial, unintended effect). About 15% of hospitalized patients develop adverse effects to drugs and of these about 7% are life-threatening or fatal effects (Fig. 19-11). Many adverse drug reactions occur from immunologic hypersensitivity reactions. Penicillin allergy is responsible for about 20% of adverse drug reactions (Fig. 19-12). The commonly occurring allergic reactions to penicillin are listed in Table 19-2.

Table 19-2
Common Allergic Reactions to Penicillin

Urticarial (hives)

Serum sickness-like (fever, proteinuria arthritis)

Eczema (contact)

Anaphylactic (life-threatening)

Exanthematic (rash)

Erythematous nodules and plaques

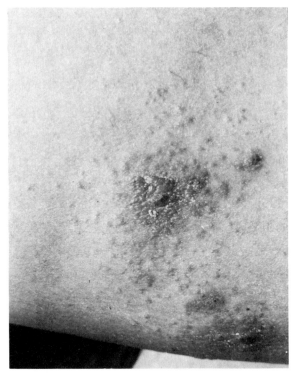

Figure 19-9   *Contact dermatitis from poison ivy. Initially numerous vesicles were present. This lesion was subsiding in response to prednisone.*

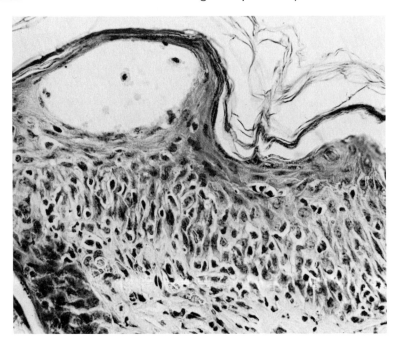

Figure 19-10   *Photomicrograph. A small vesicle filled with edema fluid is seen in the epidermis. The dermis is slightly inflamed by leukocytes.*

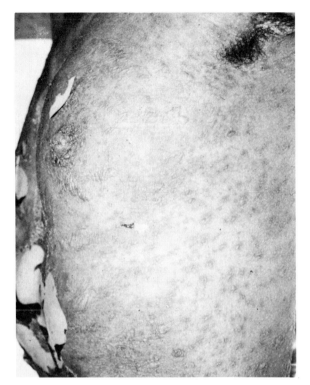

Figure 19-11 *Toxic epidermal necrolysis and death resulted from an allergy to a sulfa drug.*

Penicillin and other drug hypersensitivity reactions occur in atopic patients. These individuals form antibodies against penicillin which binds as a *hapten* (incomplete antigen) with serum proteins making it an antigen. The sensitized person has memory lymphocytes and circulating antibodies of the immunoglobulin classes—IgE (which triggers anaphylaxis and urticaria upon contact with a subsequent exposure to penicillin) and IgG and IgM which can cause a serum sickness-like illness. Nurses and persons handling penicillin can develop a cell-mediated contact dermatitis.

Thus far, no effective laboratory tests are available for simply detecting allergy to penicillin. Persons allergic to this drug should never receive it as anaphylaxis and death can ensue.

Vasculitis When antigen and antibody react in blood vessels in the skin, severe necrotizing inflammation (vasculitis) can appear (Fig. 19-13). This can occur from drug allergies, autoimmune disor-

ders (systemic lupus erythematosus, rheumatoid arthritis, and glomerulonephritis), and certain infectious diseases (such as *hepatitis B virus infection*). *Polyarteritis nodosum* is a form of systemic vasculitis which can inflame arteries in visceral organs, brain, and skin.

Immunofluorescent studies will reveal antibodies and serum immunoglobulins trapped in the wall of the blood vessel which is inflamed by neutrophils. Acute vasculitis can cause damage not only to skin but also to the brain and visceral organs. When vasculitis is severe, systemic cortisone is administered in high doses.

Pemphigus Group A group of related disorders (*pemphigus group* of vulgaris, vegetans, foliaceus, and erythematous types) is characterized by *bullous eruptions* (blisters) (Fig. 19-14). These disorders are

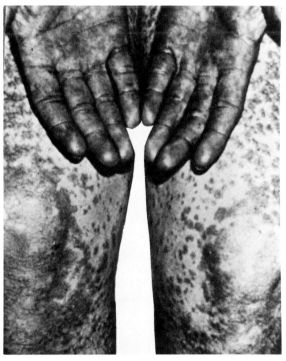

Figure 19-12 *Allergy to penicillin has caused a generalized rash on this patient's extremities and hands. (From Okun, M.R., and Edelstein, L.M. 1973. Differential Diagnosis Series. Set 2. Gross and Microscopic Differential Diagnosis of Cutaneous Lymphomas and Inflamatory Dermatoses. Dermatopathology Foundation.)*

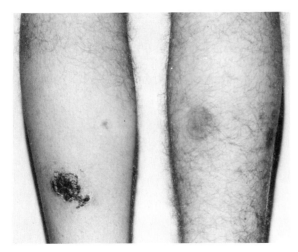

Figure 19-13 *Vasculitis of legs of a 19-year-old man. The lesion on the left is recent, and remote scars are seen in the right calf. Immune complexes deposited in walls of blood vessels and also in his glomeruli causing vasculitis and glomerulonephritis.*

thought to be caused by autoimmune reactions. The patients show antibodies against keratinocytes and basement membranes. The autoantibodies perhaps cause the keratinocytes to separate from one another to form blisters. Of the group of related diseases, *pemphigus vulgaris* has the worst prognosis. Bullae can erupt on the skin and mucous membranes (for example, esophagus) and toxemia and infection can cause death if proper treatment (cortisone) is not administered.

Dermatitis herpetiformis is another autoimmune disorder that causes bullae in the skin. Intense itching is common. Eosinophils and antibodies of the IgA class are seen in biopsy specimens of skin. The drug of choice is a sulphone (dapsone).

Infectious Diseases of Skin   It is not surprising that the skin frequently becomes infected. What is surprising is that this thin envelope does not become infected more frequently (see Chapter 7, Infectious Diseases). In this section, groups of infectious agents and examples of cutaneous infections that are discussed include *viruses* such as herpes simplex (cold sore) and childhood viral infections (measles and chicken pox); *bacteria* such as staphylococcus (impetigo); venereal diseases (syphilis);

leprosy; fungi (dermatophyte ringworm, candida, and coccidioidomycosis); and insects (scabes).

Viral Infection   *Herpes simplex* commonly causes cold sore (Fig. 19-15), an acute erythematous and vesicular eruption with lesions on any part of the body. The lips and genital regions most often become infected. The virus can remain dormant in the ganglia of the fifth cranial nerve or sacral sympathetic ganglia until the person's immunity becomes depressed. The diagnosis is made by observing characteristic intranuclear herpes viral

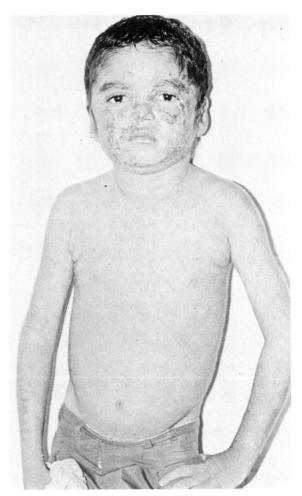

Figure 19-14 *Pemphigus vulgaris in a boy. Note the bullae on his face. A cushingoid appearance (moon face) has resulted from treatment with cortisone.*

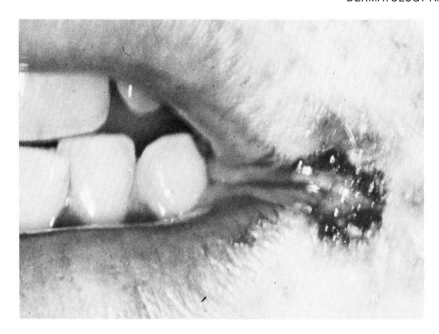

Figure 19-15 *Cold sore. The ulcer on the lip resulted from herpes simplex infection.*

inclusions in cells scraped from the lesions. The disease can spread and kill an immunosuppressed person. No treatment is available.

Herpes zoster (varicella) is characterized by activation of the zoster-varicella virus in adults. "Shingles" is a patch of inflamed vesicles along a dermatomal distribution. This condition can be painful, especially when the cornea is involved. No treatment is available.

Childhood viral infections are characterized by a rash (exanthem). The rash for each virus has a special distribution and appearance. For example, measles (rubeola) involves the entire cutaneous surface (Fig. 19-16) and appears faint. The feverish child also suffers from photophobia (eye discomfort is experienced in bright light).

Bacterial Infection   Impetigo is an acute, contagious skin disease characterized by the formation of vesicles, pustules, and yellowish crusts. It is the most common cause of infection of the skin and is caused by staphylococci or streptococci bacteria (see Chapter 7, Infectious Diseases). Approximately 5% of persons sustain staphylococcus infections each year of a severity sufficient to require medical attention. Approximately 20% of adults are chronic carriers of the bacterium, *Staphylococcus*

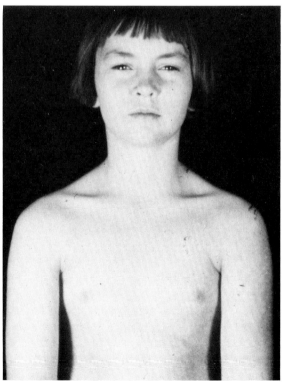

Figure 19-16   *Measles rash, which is generalized and faint, is shown. Note the boy is squinting because he has photophobia.*

aureus and another 60% are intermittent carriers. The bacterium is carried in the nasal area and may pass onto the skin producing a disease. Infections by staphylococci are a special problem for hospitalized patients who become infected from the infected staff of the hospital.

Venereal diseases are acquired during sexual intercourse. A variety of infectious diseases can infect the genitalia, the most serious is syphilis* (see Chapter 7, Infectious Diseases). Syphilis is caused by *Treponema pallidum* and, if untreated, three stages can occur. In primary syphilis a chancre (ulcer) generally occurs as a single lesion on the genitalia; the spirochettal microorganism which causes syphilis can be seen in a scraping of the chancre. Secondary syphilis is characterized by a disseminated rash which cannot be clearly distinguished from other rashes. Both the primary and secondary stages of syphilis are contagious. Studies to detect serum antibodies against syphilis (such as VDRL) and examination of the pustules for the spirochete are required to achieve a diagnosis. Penicillin is very effective in eradicating syphilis in the primary and secondary stages, but unfortunately, the damage caused by tertiary syphilis occurring in the cardiovascular and central nervous systems is permanent.

Leprosy is a chronic infectious disease of the skin caused by the intracellular bacillus, *Mycobacterium leprae*. Approximately 11 million persons in the world have leprosy.

The cell-mediated immunity (CMI) of the patient determines which form of leprosy will occur. When CMI is vigorous, *tuberculoid leprosy* (Fig. 19-17) occurs. By contrast, when CMI is deficient, *lepromatous leprosy* occurs. *M leprae* tends to infect cool areas of the body. Involvement of nerves (such as the ulnar nerve) causes a "claw hand." The anesthesia resulting from infection of the nerves makes patients especially susceptible to injury because they feel no pain. Diagnosis is by skin biopsy.

*Syphilis has been considered the great masquerader of skin diseases and hence until recent years the major medical journal of dermatology was called *The Journal of Syphilology and Dermatology*.

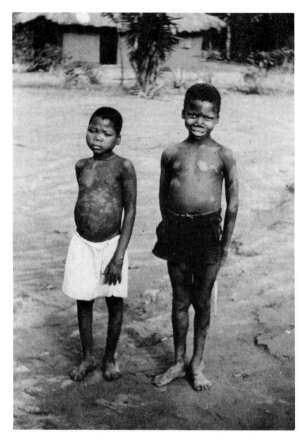

Figure 19-17 *Tuberculoid leprosy. The lesions are hypopigmented and anesthetic. (Courtesy Dr. Clitus Olson.)*

Leprosy has a low rate of infectivity and is usually responsive to sulfone drugs like dapsone. For chronic deformities, corrective orthopedic surgery is required.

Fungal Infection Fungal infections tend to be either *superficial* or spread to become *deep*. The superficial fungal diseases are caused by *dermatophytes* and result in ringworm, athlete's foot (tinea pedis), "jock" itch (tinea cruris), and a fungus causing a brawny discoloration of the skin, termed *tinea versicolor*. The diagnosis of dermatophyte fungal infections can be made by using a Wood's ultraviolet lamp. The fungi fluoresce. Microscopic study of scrapings or culture of the skin will often reveal the fungus.

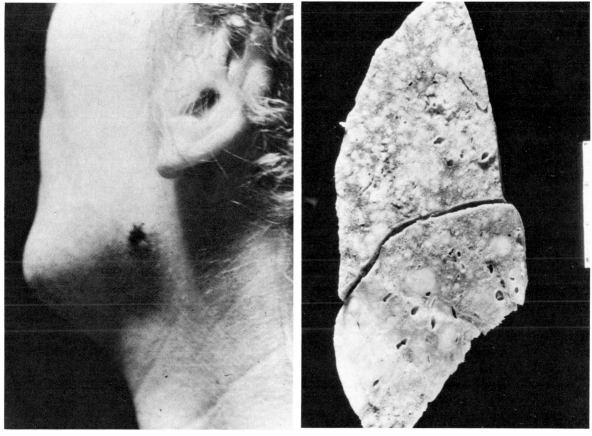

Figure 19-18   **A,** *Skin ulcer from coccidioidomycosis.* **B,** *The patient died of severe pulmonary infection during the eighth month of pregnancy. The lungs were severely infected. Note the white granulomas.*

The deep fungal infections blastomycosis, cryptococcosis, coccidioidomycosis, and histoplasmosis either begin in the skin or are inhaled. They can cause profound disseminated illness in immunosuppressed persons. The person depicted in Figure 19-18 had moved to Arizona and was exposed to fungal spores and developed "valley fever." She was pregnant and apparently the accompanying immunosuppression permitted fatal coccidioidomycosis.

Insects   Insects and parasites can bite or invade the skin producing itching lesions. *Scabies*, a chronic contagious dermatoses, is caused by the itch mite, *Acarus scabiei* (Fig. 19-19). The female mite burrows between the fingers into folds of skin. Chronic

inflammation results. We all fear stings by bees, hornets, and other stinging insects, but a few hypersensitized people can die from anaphylaxis following a sting (see Chapter 6, Immunology).

Proliferative Diseases

Both benign and malignant proliferative (neoplastic) diseases are very common in the skin. For example, all of us have at least eight pigmented moles (nevi) composed of a benign neoplastic growth of melanocytes in our skin. Also cysts and benign viral infections producing tumors are seen in many persons. Other important common proliferative disorders, such as psoriasis, are not neoplastic.

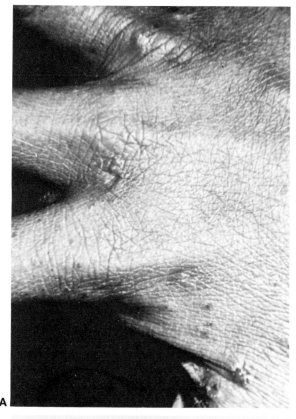

A

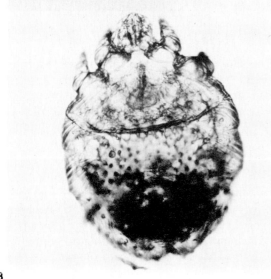

B

Figure 19-19 **A,** *Scabies of hand. Mites have burrowed into the epidermis between the fingers and caused inflammation.* **B,** *A mite is shown at 80× .*

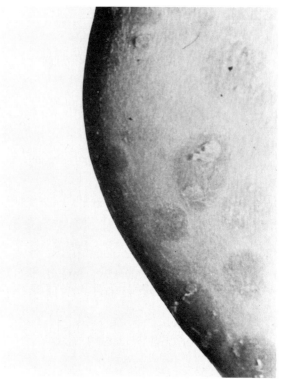

Figure 19-20 *Psoriasis. White thin flakes of keratin over red blotches. (From Okun, M.R., and Edelstein, L.M. 1973. Differential Diagnosis Series. Set 2. Gross and Microscopic Differential Diagnosis of Cutaneous Lymphomas and Inflamatory Dermatoses. Dermatopathology Foundation.)*

Psoriasis Psoriasis is a chronic skin disease characterized by circumscribed red patches covered with white scales (Fig. 19-20). It usually occurs in adults over the extensor surfaces and in the scalp and nails. Psoriasis can be hereditary, and it plagues approximately nine million persons in the United States. The disease may produce a great deal of morbidity, and psoriatic arthritis can occur.

Microscopically, psoriasis shows hyperkeratosis and thinning of the epidermis. Small microabscesses can be seen in the epidermis. There is an acceleration of the epidermal metabolism; the skin becomes unable to stop producing keratinocytes.

Seborrheic Keratosis Seborrheic keratosis is characterized by a benign proliferation of keratinocytes and occurs in middle-aged or older patients.

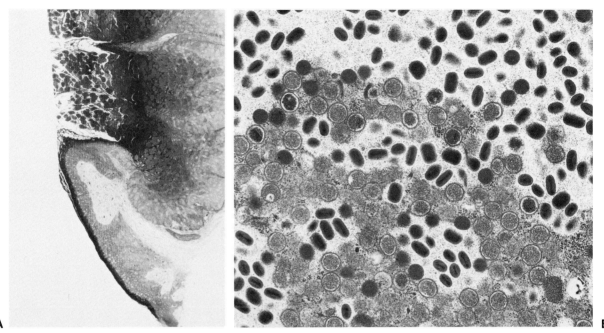

Figure 19-21 **A,** *Photomicrograph of skin lesion of molluscum contagiosum.* × *300.* **B,** *Electron micrograph showing hundreds of pox viruses. The virus causes molluscum contagiosum.* × *37,000 (Courtesy Dr. Jag Bhawan.)*

The number of keratinocytes varies from a few to hundreds. The lesions are raised above the level of the skin and appear to be pasted on the skin surface. They vary from light yellow, to tan, to brown, to black depending on the amount of melanin pigment they contain. Microscopically they consist of a benign growth of basal cells. Ordinarily, no treatment is required, except for cosmetic purposes.

Cysts   Two cysts (hollow, epithelium-lined sacs) that commonly bother patients are *epidermal inclusion cysts* (which cause disfiguration) and *pilonidal cysts* (which become inflamed).

Epidermal inclusion cysts (wens, sebaceous cysts) are lined by squamous epithelium. They fill up with plugs of keratin producing subcutaneous masses that are raised above the skin surface. Most often they are located in the scalp, face, or back. The cysts can rupture or become infected. They are usually surgically excised.

Pilonidal cysts are epidermal inclusion cysts located in the natal crease between the buttocks. They may arise from pinched off epidermis or in-

grown hairs. When they become infected they drain pus and are painful. Treatment is by surgical excision.

Viral-Induced Proliferation   Viruses can infect the keratinocytes and cause three kinds of benign neoplasms: (a) warts, (b) condyloma acuminatum, and (c) molluscum contagiosum (Fig. 19-21).

Verruca vulgaris, the common wart and *verruca plantaris,* the wart of the plantar surface of the sole of the foot are caused by virally infected keratinocytes. These lesions are papules measuring 1 to 10 mm in diameter and have a rough, keratinized surface. Warts are usually easy to excise, but plantar warts are imbedded deep in the sole and thus are difficult to resect. Microscopically, hyperkeratosis and vacuolated keratinocytes with intranuclear viral inclusions can be seen.

Condyloma acuminatum (venereal warts, synon.) occur chiefly in the warm, moist, anogenital region. Sexual partners often both show genital warts. Treatment is by excision or by painting the warts with podophyllin.

Molluscum contagiosum is a benign virus-induced papular tumor of keratinocytes. Several 3 to 8 mm papules with depression centrally are seen. Microscopically large dark inclusion bodies are seen with light microscopy and electron microscopy reveals the pox virus (Fig. 19-21). Treatment is by applying phenol or nitric acid, or they are excised.

Benign Skin Tumors   Each cell type of the skin can give rise to either benign or malignant tumors. Benign tumors including squamous papillomas arise from keratinocytes; nevi arise from melanocytes; lipomas (Fig. 19-22) from adipose cells; vascular tumors (hemangiomas) from blood vessels; dermatofibromas from fibroblasts; and neuromas from nerves.

Skin Cancers

Cancer of the skin is common—300,000 new cases of skin cancer occur each year in the United States. Most skin cancers are trivial, but certain types can be lethal. Excessive exposure to sunlight in a person with fair skin often leads to skin cancer. Besides sunlight, exposure to irritating chemicals, recurrent trauma, and irradiation are associated with a high risk of skin cancer.

Precancerous changes in the skin can usually be identified and hence cancer is avoidable. For example, a shiny, scaly, sunken lesion, *actinic keratosis*, results from excessive exposure to actinic ultraviolet rays of sunlight and may progress to squamous cell carcinoma. Areas damaged by radiation and chronically inflamed ulcers and scars should be watched for.

The three main histologic types of skin cancer in order of increasing severity are: (a) basal cell carcinoma, (b) squamous cell carcinoma, and (c) malignant melanoma. Each type of skin cancer has a different prognosis, and premalignant lesions are detectable (Table 19-3).

Basal Cell Carcinoma

By far the most common malignant tumor of the skin is basal cell carcinoma which arises from basal

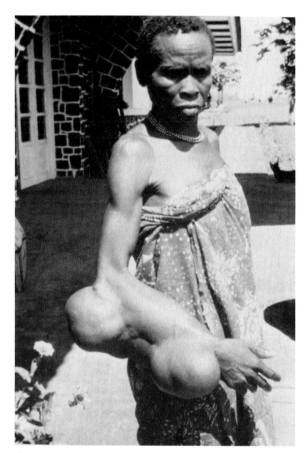

Figure 19-22   *Lipomas are prominently seen in the subcutaneous tissue. (Courtesy Dr. Clitus Olson.)*

cells in the epidermis. It appears mostly on the face and trunk of elderly adults. It begins as a painless, slow-growing scale which may later become depressed or ulcerated (Fig. 19-23). This tumor is sensitive to radiotherapy or can be easily excised. It seldom metastasizes.

Squamous Cell Carcinoma

Squamous cell carcinoma (SCC) arises from keratinocytes in the epidermis of elderly individuals who have been excessively exposed to the sun. SCC often gradually develops from premalignant actinic keratosis lesions. A nodule forms and later an ulcer develops, surrounded by rolled-up edges. SCC is commonly found in other organs lined by squamous epithelium such as the mouth, esophagus, larynx, lung, uterine cervix, and anus. SCC can in-

Table 19-3
*Premalignant Conditions and Malignant Neoplasms of Skin**

Disorder	Frequent location	Estimated Malignant potential
I. Premalignant		
Dermatitis (radiation-induced)	Face and breast exposed to radiation	10% or more
Dermatitis (sun-induced)	Sun exposed skin	High with severe repeated exposure
Keratosis (senile)	Face, arms	20% to 25%
Albinism	Sun exposed skin	About 10%
Chronic ulcer	Leg, face	Low
Leukoplakia	Mouth, vagina	2% to 12%
Erythroplasia	Penis or vulva	14%
Benign pigmented nevus	Sun exposed skin	<0.0001%
Bathing trunk nevus	Trunk	10% to 60%
Basal cell nevus syndrome	Skin (autosomal dominant)	Up to 100%
Xeroderma pigmentosum	Skin exposed to sun (autosomal recessive)	Up to 100%, develop all types of skin cancer
II. Malignant		
Bowen's disease	Skin, glans penis, vulva, mouth	Carcinoma in situ
Paget's disease	Nipple, vulva	Associated with carcinoma of breast or vulval glands
Basal cell carcinoma	Sun exposed skin	Almost never metastasizes
Squamous cell carcinoma	Sun exposed skin	About 0.5% metastasize
Malignant melanoma	Sun exposed skin, eye	About 50% metastasize

*Summarized from Dunham, L. J. 1972. Cancer in man at site of prior benign lesion of skin or mucous membrane: a review. *Cancer Res.* 32:1359–1374.

filtrate underlying tissues or metastasize in lymphatic channels; prognoses are, therefore, worse than for basal cell carcinomas.

Treatment consists of complete removal. Small tumors can be locally excised with a scalpel or by electrocoagulation surgery. A new experimental technique consists of painting a chemical on small tumors; a vigorous immune response develops and destroys the tumor. Radiotherapy is sometimes used for large squamous cancers.

Malignant Melanoma

Malignant melanomas arise from melanocytes in the epidermis. They are highly malignant skin tumors (Fig. 19-24 to 19-26). Approximately 4400 persons in the United States died of malignant melanoma during 1976. Many cases occur in places like Texas and Australia, where the climate is hot and sunny. Roughly one-half of the individuals affected will die of the melanoma within five years. The majority (estimated at 85%) of melanomas arise from pre-existing benign moles (nevi). Each person has an average of eight moles on his or her body. In blacks, melanomas tend to occur on the border between dark skin and the light skin on the palms and soles. The prognosis for melanoma depends on the depth of invasion, completeness of surgical resection, and whether metastasis has occurred.

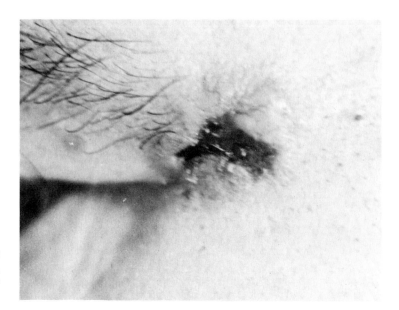

Figure 19-23 *Ulcerating basal cell carcinoma near left eye of a 52-year-old man who worked on highway construction.*

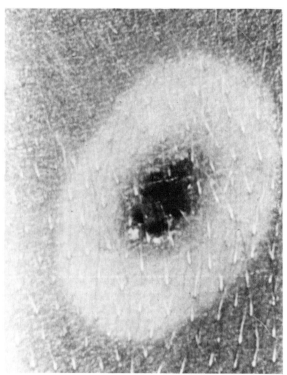

Figure 19-24 *Halo nevus. The light zone (halo) surrounding this nevus (mole) was caused by an immune response to the premalignant lesion. Malignant melanoma was probably prevented by this response.*

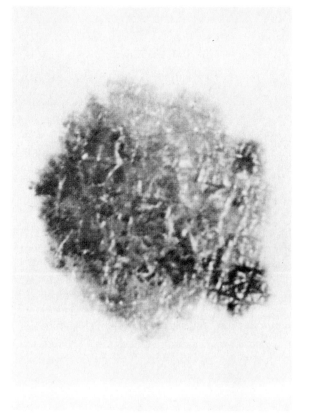

Figure 19-25 *Malignant melonoma. Note the variation in the intensity of the pigment.*

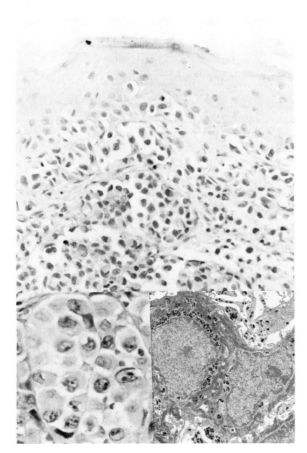

Figure 19-26 *Photomicrograph of malignant melanoma. The tumor has invaded the epidermis. The insets show the malignant melanocytes (left) (× 600) and black melanin granules (right) (× 10,000). (Courtesy Dr. Jag Bhawan.)*

Summary

The skin is a large organ containing highly developed appendages and receptors that are specialized for receiving stimuli and displaying emotions. Skin is composed of epidermis, dermis, and subcutaneous layers. Keratinocytes and melanocytes are the two types of cells in the epidermis. In systemic diseases the color, texture, and composition of the skin mirror and participate in widespread pathophysiologic events. Because the skin is a mirror it is important in the physical diagnosis of diseases.

Diseases of the skin are divisible into two broad categories: inflammatory-infectious and neoplastic diseases. Inflammatory disorders of the skin (dermatitis) often occur in individuals who have hypersensitivity reactions to substances in the environment; eczema is a commonly occurring example. Other examples include drug allergy and vasculitis of unknown etiology. Pemphigus, psoriasis, and dermatitis herpetiformis are autoimmune hypersensitivity diseases.

Infectious agents ranging in size from viruses to insects often infect skin. Herpes simplex and zoster viruses cause problems in adults whereas a variety of other viruses cause rashes associated with childhood disorders. Bacterial infections of skin commonly are caused by Staphylococcus, Streptococcus, Treponema, and in the Third World, *Mycobacterium leprae*.

Benign keratinocytic proliferative disorders include psoriasis, seborrheic keratosis, cysts, warts, and papillomas. Other benign tumors arise from other cells in skin: nevi, lipomas, dermatofibromas, neuromas, and hemangiomas.

Skin cancer is the most common malignancy in the United States, but except for malignant melanoma and a few squamous carcinomas skin cancers are not life-threatening. Ultraviolet light damages sun-exposed skin and is a major factor in causing skin cancer. Basal cell carcinomas are the commonest skin tumors and the most benign. Squamous cell carcinomas are the next most common malignancy. They can occasionally metastasize. By contrast, malignant melanoma is rare but can be highly malignant. Melanoma is notoriously unpredictable; however, prognosis is based on the size, depth of invasion of the tumor, and presence of metastasis. Complete surgical excision is the treatment of choice for all skin cancers.

Bibliography

Bluefarb, S. M. 1974. *Dermatology*. Kalamazoo, Michigan. Upjohn Company. Excellent photographs of common diseases are displayed.

Giannelli, F. 1977. DNA repair and tumors of the skin: xeroderma pigmentosum as a model. Proceedings of the Royal Society of Medicine 70: 388–395. Describes how ultraviolet light damages chromosomes and how defective DNA repair mechanisms in this disease predispose to cancer.

Helwig, E. B., and Mostofi, F. K., eds. 1971. *The skin.* Baltimore: The Williams & Wilkins Company. A thorough treatise on the embryology, anatomy, physiology and diseases of skin.

Lever, W. F. 1975. *Histopathology of the skin*, ed. 5. Philadelphia: J.B. Lippincott Company. A standard reference for pathologists and dermatologists.

Maddin, S., ed. 1975. *Current dermatologic management*, ed. 2. St. Louis: The C.V. Mosby Co. Describes treatment of skin disorders.

Okun, M. R., and Edelstein, L. M. 1976. *Gross and microscopic pathology of the skin*. Boston: Dermatopathology Foundation Press. Illustrates more than 1000 diseases in 1333 illustrations.

Pillsbury, D. M.; Shelley, W.D.; and Kligman, A. M. 1964. *Cutaneous medicine*. Philadelphia: W.B. Saunders Company. A brief standard textbook.

Smith, P. H., et. al. 1973. *Dermatology*. London: Crosby Lockwood Staples. Beautiful photographs and easy to read.

Solomons, B. 1973. *Lecture notes on dermatology*, ed. 3. Philadelphia: F.A. Davis Company. An excellent introductory textbook.

Vasconez, L. O.; Schneider, W. J.; Jurkiewicz, W. J. 1977. Pressure sores. *Curr. Probl. Surg.* 14(4): 1–62. Summarizes pathogenesis, prevention, and treatment of this common disorder.

Westbury, G. 1977. Strategy in the management of melanoma. Proceedings of the Royal Society of Medicine 70: 395–397. Describes surgical treatment for various types of malignant melanoma.

CHAPTER 20

Diseases of Muscles, Bones, and Joints

Chapter Outline

Objectives

After reading this chapter you should be able to
Know the frequency of occurrence of arthritis.
Define rheumatic disease.
List the fibers in connective tissues.

Describe the basic cell of connective tissues.

List rheumatic diseases.

Define rheumatoid arthritis.

Describe the typical apprearance of a person with rheumatoid arthritis.

Describe the pathologic lesion in the joints in rheumatoid arthritis.

Know the role of lysosomes in injury to joints.

Define Felty's syndrome.

Explain why ankylosing spondylitis occurs in families.

Predict the prognosis for a patient with rheumatoid arthritis.

List modes of treatment for rheumatoid arthritis.

Define osteoarthritis.

Compare rheumatoid arthritis with osteoarthritis both clinically and pathologically.

Know the frequency of occurrence of osteoarthritis of the hip.

Define the terms chondrocyte, osteophyte, and ankylose.

Describe the physical deformities accompanying osteoarthritis.

Understand the intervertebral disc syndrome.

List methods of treating osteoarthritis.

Define Charcot joint.

Compare simple, compound, and comminuted bone fractures.

Describe the process of healing of bone.

List reasons why bones fail to heal.

Recognize gonococcal arthritis.

Define osteomyelitis.

Know causes of rickets and scurvy.

List the endocrine glands and the diseases linking endocrine and bone dysfunction.

Define osteoporosis.

List factors causing osteoporosis.

Describe Paget's disease.

List two complications of Paget's disease.

Define fibrous dysplasia.

Know the substance found in the joints of patients with gout.

Define pseudogout.

List benign and malignant bone tumors.

List signs and symptoms of bone tumors.

Describe osteoma.

Know the prognosis for osteogenic sarcoma.

Compare various cartilagenous tumors.

List the basic pathological changes of skeletal muscle.

Describe clinical features of muscle disease.

Classify muscle diseases.

Know how patients with muscle diseases are diagnosed.

Define muscular dystrophy.

Compare the two leading theories of muscular dystrophy.

List the types of muscular dystrophy and compare their inheritance, age of onset,
    muscles involved, and prognoses.
Define the term atrophy.
Describe the disease polydermatomyositis.
List common metabolic muscle diseases.
Compare rhabdomyoma and rhabdomyosarcoma.

Introduction

A recent national health survey revealed that 1 in 13 persons in the United States believes he or she has arthritis. In fact, signs of rheumatoid arthritis were demonstrated by X-rays in 3% of individuals screened randomly for arthritis. Also, millions of adults have degenerative joint disease (osteoarthritis). Thus health professionals will assist many patients with these chronic disorders.

Rheumatic diseases involve the diarthrodial (movable) joints and surrounding structures. Although the causes of most rheumatic diseases are unknown, several result from abnormal immune responses to self; persons affected possess autoantibodies in their sera (see Chapter 6, Immunology). Rheumatoid arthritis, systemic lupus erythematosus, and rheumatic fever are important examples of autoimmune connective tissue disease.

Normal Connective Tissues

The connective tissues of the body include bone, cartilage, tendon sheaths, aponeuroses, ligaments, joint structures, bursae, and skeletal muscle. Connective tissues come from primitive mesoderm in the embryo. Connective tissue cells (*fibroblasts*) produce three characteristic fibrillar proteins: (a) collagen, (b) elastin, and (c) reticulin. These three fibers are embedded in the ground substance. Each type of connective tissue has distinctive properties suited best for specific functions (see Chapter 2, Normal Cells, Tissues, and Organs).

Tendons, aponeuroses, and ligaments contain strong collagen fibers that are arranged in parallel bundles. By contrast, fascial membranes, the dermis, and periosteum are woven from collagen fibers. These tissue fabrics are capable of withstanding stress from any direction.

The fibroblast is the basic cell of connective tissue. It has a large nucleus, scanty cytoplasm, and is responsible for forming ground substance and various fibrillar proteins. When mature, these primitive mesenchymal cells can become *chondroblasts* that form cartilage or *synoviocytes* that form the lining (synovium) of joints.

Collagen, the most abundant component of connective tissue, is woven into thick sheaths that have a high tensile strength. Collagen is composed of two strands of protein spun in a double helix. Based on the chemical composition there are four types of collagen in the body (Table 20-1). It accounts for approximately 25% of the protein in our

Table 20-1
Types and Distribution of Collagen

Type	Composition	Normal distribution	Abnormal distribution
I	α Chains	Bone, tendon, skin, etc.	Scars of cirrhosis; osteoarthritis
II	α Chains and other compounds	Cartilage	Ectopic cartilage
III	α Chains and reticulin	Internal organs, skin, blood vessels	Wounds in early phases
Basement membrane	Protocollagenlike	Subepithelial basement membrane	Proliferative glomerulonephritis

body. Other types of connective tissue have different chemicals in their ground substance. For example, chondroitin is abundant in cartilage, whereas osteoid traps calcium salts in order to cement bones.

Rheumatic Disease

Diseases of connective tissue are collectively termed *collagen* or *rheumatic diseases*, some of which are listed in Table 20-2. The feature which collagen diseases have in common is their predilection for destroying connective tissue by inflammation. The joints, small calibre blood vessels, and organs such

Table 20-2
Classification of Rheumatic (Collagen) Diseases

Arthritis
Rheumatoid arthritis
Felty's syndrome
Ankylosing spondylitis
Osteoarthritis
Infectious arthritis
Gouty arthritis

Autoimmune Connective Tissue Disorders
Systemic lupus erythematosus
Scleroderma
Necrotizing arteritis
Amyloidosis
Rheumatic fever
Rheumatoid arthritis

Nonarticular Rheumatism
Fibrositis
Intervertebral disc syndrome
Myositis
Tendonitis
Bursitis

Inherited Connective Tissue Disorders
Ehlers-Danlos syndrome
Osteogenesis imperfecta
Various types of clubfoot
Gout
Ankylosing spondylitis
Cutis laxis

as the skin, lungs, and kidneys, which are rich in connective tissue, are commonly involved. Also, serosal membranes (pleura, pericardium, and peritoneum) can be affected. Organs affected by collagen diseases show *fibrinoid** necrosis.

Rheumatoid Arthritis

Rheumatoid arthritis (RA) is a chronic inflammatory disease that is unpredictable in its course, being characterized by recurring exacerbations and remissions. With each successive attack, additional joints may become involved. The cause of RA is as yet unknown. However, viruses and other infectious agents are most likely involved. The disease has both juvenile and adult forms.

Clinical Picture In many patients, RA begins slowly and is characterized by exacerbations and remissions over the years. A small fraction of patients begin with an acute polyarthritis which is unremitting and difficult to control with medical treatment. The most distinctive diagnostic features of RA include *symmetrical (bilateral) polyarthritis* involving more than four or five joints and associated with *morning stiffness* of at least one or two hours duration, and *systemic symptoms* such as fatigue, weakness, and weight loss (Fig. 20-1).

Pathologic Findings The synovium of the small joints of the hand is most often affected initially. During the acute phase the synovium becomes edematous, the small blood vessels engorge with blood, fibrin is found on the synovial surface, and neutrophils infiltrate the underlying connective tissue. Later, the synovium thickens as a result of proliferation of synovial cells and fibroblasts. Lymphocytes, histiocytes, and plasma cells invade the synovium (Fig. 20-2). At the junction of the synovium and articular cartilage, granulation tissue proliferates, forming a thick pad termed the *pannus*. This pad extends over the surface of the cartilage, burrowing into and destroying the underlying bone (see Chapter 6, Immunology).

*The adjective, fibrinoid (Greek *oid*, like), is so named because it stains bright pink, like fibrin, with the eosin stain.

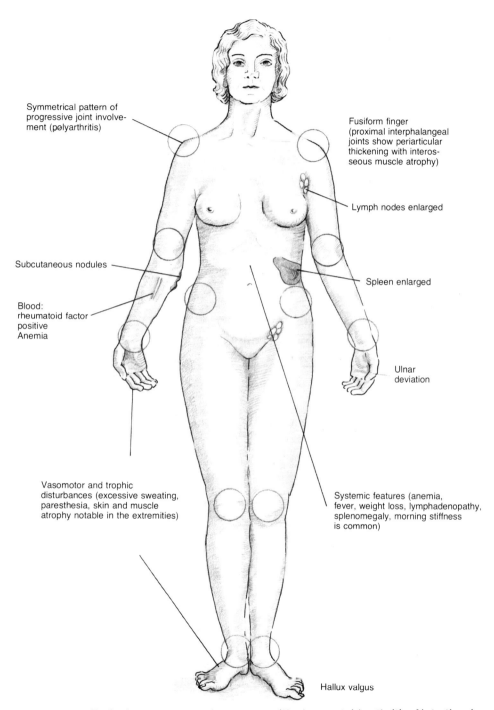

Symmetrical pattern of progressive joint involvement (polyarthritis)

Fusiform finger (proximal interphalangeal joints show periarticular thickening with interosseous muscle atrophy)

Lymph nodes enlarged

Subcutaneous nodules

Spleen enlarged

Blood: rheumatoid factor positive Anemia

Ulnar deviation

Vasomotor and trophic disturbances (excessive sweating, paresthesia, skin and muscle atrophy notable in the extremities)

Systemic features (anemia, fever, weight loss, lymphadenopathy, splenomegaly, morning stiffness is common)

Hallux valgus

Figure 20-1 *Typical appearance of a person with rheumatoid arthritis. Note the deformities and swelling at proximal interphalangeal joints, boney deformities, and enlarged lymphoid organs.*

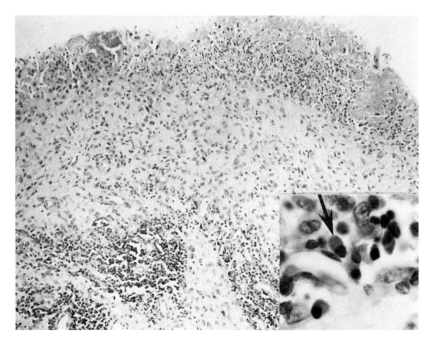

Figure 20-2 *Photomicrograph of synovitis of rheumatoid arthritis. The surface is covered with fibrin.* × 200. *Lymphocytes, histiocytes, and plasma cells* (arrow) *are seen at high magnification.* × 450.

Enzymes released from lysosomes carried into the synovium within neutrophils initiate the injury in RA. They digest the articular cartilage. The underlying bone is also absorbed, thereby weakening tendons, ligaments, and supporting structures; the joint becomes unstable and dislocation or subluxation may occur. Furthermore, subcutaneous nodules develop in approximately 25% of patients with RA (Fig. 20-1). Often, these nodules appear over the ulna or form on the sclera (white portion) of the eye. The center of the nodules contain rheumatoid factor, an autoantibody against one's own immunoglobulin.

Felty's Syndrome Felty's syndrome is a variant of rheumatoid arthritis. In order to diagnose Felty's syndrome, the patient must have RA, a low WBC (leukopenia), and an enlarged spleen (splenomegaly). Other features of this syndrome include subcutaneous nodules and a high serum concentration of rheumatiod factor; occasionally, a low platelet count (thrombocytopenia) is observed. Both white blood cells and platelets are reduced because blood is trapped in the enlarged spleen. However, the greatest danger lies in the leukopenia which may lead to serious or recurrent infections.

Ankylosing Spondylitis (Marie-Strümpell Disease) Ankylosing spondylitis is primarily a disease of young men that may result in progressive inflammation, fibrosis, and fusion (ankylosis) of the spine, especially in the lumbar area and in the sacroiliac joints. It can cause a peripheral arthritis. This disorder is frequently inherited by a specific gene (see Chapter 9, Inherited Disorders).

Prognosis and Treatment of Rheumatoid Arthritis Approximately 60% of RA patients show no clinical or radiographic progression during the first ten years of their disease and approximately two-thirds of these are capable of employment 15 years following initial diagnosis. Unfortunately, 10% of RA patients become incapacitated because of progressive polyarthritis.

The aim of treatment is to maintain good joint function. Maintenance of joint motion by exercise, heat, and anti-inflammatory medications may prevent destruction of joints. Aspirin remains the most effective, safest, and cheapest anti-inflammatory drug for the treatment of RA. It is given in high doses to reduce inflammation and pain. Up to 4 gm of aspirin per day, or a dose sufficient to produce ringing (tinnitus) in the ears, is given. Cortisone is reserved for RA patients who have been resistant to treatment with nonsteroidal anti-inflammatory medications. The beneficial anti-inflammatory effects of cortisone are outweighed by the serious complications that may arise from their use, including hemorrhage into the gastrointestinal tract, demineralization of bone (osteoporosis), psychiatric disturbances, and untoward cosmetic effects. Orthopedic surgery may be required to prevent or correct deformities and to relieve pain.

Degenerative Joint Disease (Osteoarthritis)

Degenerative joint disease is a relatively common, noninflammatory disorder of movable joints. Weight-bearing joints and the distal joints of the fingers are especially vulnerable. Osteoarthritis is pathologically characterized by deterioration of articular cartilage and the formation of new bone in and about the joints. Nearly 200,000 persons in the United States aged 65 or older are incapacitated by degenerative arthritis of the hip.

Destruction occurs in the articular surface of the cartilage which lines diarthrodial joints. The cartilage fragments, reducing the number of cartilage cells (chondrocytes) and thereby altering the ground substance. The underlying subchondral bone becomes hardened and the articular surface becomes smooth and shiny. Boney spurs (osteophytes) form at the outer margin of the joints and may fuse (ankylose) across a joint (Fig. 20-3). The lumbar vertebra bodies are also vulnerable to boney spurs and ankylosis.

Etiology   The etiology of osteoarthritis is unknown, but enzymes such as hyaluronidase may digest the articular cartilage when it is released into traumatized joints. Also, during aging, arteriosclerosis fails to supply blood to the chondrocytes,

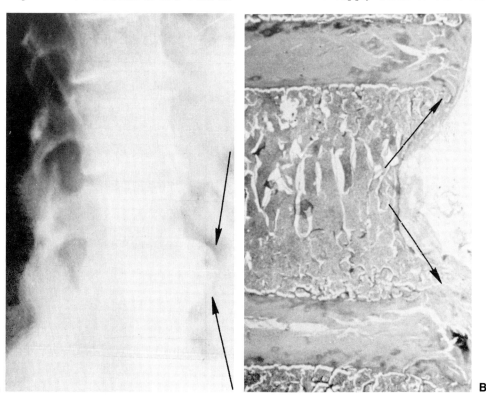

Figure 20-3   *Osteoarthritis. Bone spurs have fused across the intervetebral discs (arrows).* **A,** *X-ray;* **B,** *cross-section. (Courtesy the Arthritis Foundation, 1972.)*

causing these cells to fail. There is also a form of osteoarthritis which is caused by trauma or overuse of the involved joint.

Clinical Signs   Symptoms of degenerative joint disease include joint pain, particularly upon motion of weight-bearing joints such as the hip, and stiffness or "gelling" after a period of rest or on a cold, damp day.

Physical Findings   Physical examination demonstrates crepitation (feeling of crushed bone fragments), decreased range of motion, and pain upon movement of the involved joint. Spasm and atrophy of surrounding muscles, malalignment of the extremity, and changes in the shape of joints may also be detected. *Heberden's nodes* are osteoarthritic deformities that occur in the distal interphalangeal joints of the fingers.

The femur is often involved by osteoarthritis. Destruction of the head of the femur and fracture of the neck of the femur may occur. The latter is often termed a hip fracture.

The lumbar vertebral column is vulnerable to degeneration of the articular surfaces between the bodies and processes. The resulting narrowing of the spinal cord impinges upon the spinal cord and causes neurological dysfunction. When the nerve roots are pinched, pain radiates down the extremity, a condition termed *radiculitis*, or *sciatica*.

Intervertebral Disc Syndrome   Osteoarthritis in the lumbar spine is often associated with herniation of one or more intervertebral discs. During the aging process the central portion of the disc, the nucleus pulposus, becomes dehydrated and brittle. Thereafter, when force is exerted on the dry disc, it herniates. The herniation most often occurs laterally or can compress the spinal cord or nerve roots (Fig. 20-4). Degenerative changes of the vertebral bodies (spondylosis) also contribute to this pathological process.

Pain with the intervertebral disc syndrome radiates down the sciatic nerve from the lower back into the posterior thigh when the hip is flexed. The patient has limited lumbar motion, localized tenderness, spasm of lower back muscles, and a reversal of the normal lumbar curvature. The common sites of the intervertebral disc syndrome are L4-5, L5-S1. Cervical disc syndromes involving C6-7 are also common.

Treatment of Osteoarthritis   The main objective of therapy for osteoarthritis is to relieve pain since most forms of this disease do not lead to joint destruction. Restoration of joint function and prevention of progression of the disease is also important. Patients should be reassured that osteoarthritis is likely to remain confined to a few joints. In contrast, rheumatoid arthritis may progress and cause crippling joint destruction.

Approaches to the treatment of cervical and lumbar intervetebral disc syndromes depends upon the extent of involvement and the age and occupation of the patient. Physical therapy including traction, massage, heat, and the use of a cervical collar to stabilize the neck joints may relieve pain. Lumbar involvement can demand bed rest, support by corset, massage, and exercises to strengthen the back. If these conservative measures fail, *laminectomy*, a surgical procedure that fuses (arthrodesis) the joint may be required.

Orthopedic surgical procedures are of great value when osteoarthritis involves the hip. Total replacement of the involved hip with a prosthesis provides relief of pain and increased joint stability. Most importantly, the patient is once again able to ambulate.

Neuropathic Joint Disease

Charcot joints are a variety of osteoarthritis that results when the nerve supply to a joint is lost. Awareness of position (proprioception) of a joint is lost in some persons with advanced syphilis who have a damaged spinal cord. Marked destruction of the distal femur and proximal tibia occurs. New bone forms and osteoarthritis develops as the person slaps and bangs his insensitive legs and feet while walking. Syphilis can also infect the bone, or cause injury to fetuses in pregnant women. The periosteum becomes infected and new bone forms in the skull, tibia, and clavicles. Other diseases

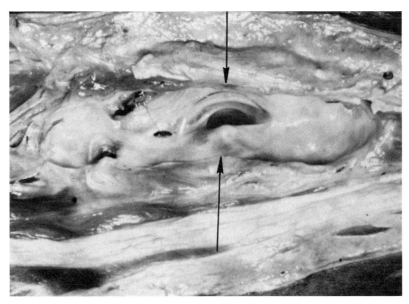

Figure 20-4   *"Slipped disc." Herniation of the intervetebral disc has oc-curred in spinal canal* (arrows).

which may result in Charcot or neuropathic joint disease include septic arthritis (particularly tuberculosis) and syringomyelia (see Chapter 21, Neurology and Neuropathology).

Response to Injury

Bone is injured by trauma or fractures as described above. In addition, infections of the bone and synovium may cause dysfunction, deformity, and pain.

Following an injury, bone generally has a good capacity for repair. Osteoblast cells capable of proliferation (to fill the defect), are located both in the periosteum that surrounds the outside of the bone and also in the endosteum in the shaft of a bone. The osteoblasts create new bone to fill the defect.

Bone Fractures

Fractures result when excessive stress is placed on bones. Fractures are classified as either *simple* or *compound*. The former describes fracture of a bone without the bone protruding through the skin, in the latter situation the broken bone does extend

through the skin. A *comminuted* fracture refers to fragmentation of bone into many pieces.

Healing of a fracture requires the formation of granulation tissue. This is composed of blood vessels and proliferating fibroblasts that organize the blood clot which forms at the fracture site (Fig. 20-5). A *callus* begins to form from osteoblasts after about 48 hours and blood vessels invade the callus after three to four days. The bone at the edges of the fracture dies and is resorbed. New bone is also formed by osteoblasts in the endosteum. The time required for the union of a fracture varies with the age of the individual. Union is complete within one month in infants, two months in adolescents, and four months in adults. Ideal union of bone occurs when the bone is immobilized with the fractured ends closely approximated.

Nonunion of Fractures

Fractures fail to heal (nonunion) for four reasons: (a) *ischemia:* the navicular bone of the wrist, the femoral neck and the lower third of the tibia are all poorly vascularized and therefore are subject to ischemic necrosis after a fracture; (b) *excessive mo-*

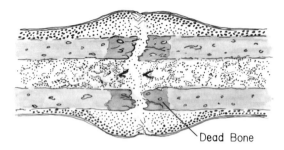

Formation of Primary Cellular Callus

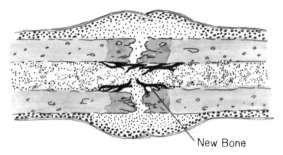

Ossification of Cellular Callus

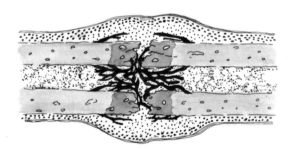

Remodelling of Primary Bone

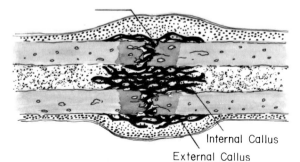

Figure 20-5 *Stages in healing of a bone fracture.*

bility: healing is prevented and pseudoarthrosis or a pseudojoint may result; (c) *interposition of soft tissues between the fractured ends;* and (d) *infection:* compound fractures have a tendency to become infected.

Pathological fractures can occur at the site of a metastatic cancer to bone or in the substance of a bone cancer. Osteoporosis is another source of pathological fractures which may occur with only minimal or normal activity.

Infectious Arthritis

Pyogenic microorganisms (staphylococcus, gonococcus, pneumococcus, streptococcus, and others) may spread to the synovium from infectious foci in the respiratory or genitourinary tracts. In contrast to RA or osteoarthritis, infectious arthritis usually involves only one joint. Gonococcal arthritis occurs primarily in young adults following intercourse with an infected partner. Several days later, sudden onset of swelling and pain in a joint occurs. Painful urination (dysuria), fever, chills, and skin rash usually provide a clue that one is dealing with a gonococcal infection arising in the genitourinary tract. Aspiration of fluid from the affected joint reveals numerous neutrophils and a Gram stain shows the gonococci. The arthritis usually subsides following the administration of penicillin or other suitable antibiotics to which the gonococcus is sensitive.

Infection of Bone (Osteomyelitis)

Osteomyelitis arises at the end of a shaft (metaphysis) of a long bone. *Staphylococcus aureus,* which has been carried to the bone by the blood stream from infected skin, lungs, or other foci is often responsible. Trauma (fracture) predisposes to osteomyelitis. The process begins in the bone marrow cavity where an abscess forms, expanding and compressing the nearby bone. The adjacent blood vessels thrombose and bone dies. The dead bone (sequestrum) is resorbed, replaced, and surrounded by new bone (involucrum).

Treatment is two-fold: (a) Surgical curettage is used to ream out the dead and infected bone, and (b) antibiotics such as penicillin are given to destroy the staphylococcus.

Metabolic Disorders of Bone

For bone to form, several nutrients are required: calcium, vitamins D and C, and protein. *Rickets* (in children) and *osteomalacia* (in adults) both arise from a deficiency of vitamin D. When this vitamin is lacking, calcium is not absorbed in the gut causing inadequate calcification of bone. *Scurvy* results from the inadequate intake of vitamin C and causes a failure to form collagen. The bone becomes thin and fractures easily (see Chapter 10, Nutritional Diseases). In contrast to rickets, calcium deposition is adequate.

Endocrine Diseases

Endocrine diseases and associated hormonal alterations are described in detail in Chapter 12, Endocrine and Metabolic Disorders. Since the impact of hormones on the growth of bone is great, a few endocrine disorders causing boney abnormalities deserve description. A tumor of the acidophil cells of the pituitary gland results in the excessive secretion of growth hormone. This leads to *gigantism* in young persons (before fusion of their epiphyseal growth plates occur) and *acromegaly* in adults. The mandible, vertebra, and the bones of the hands and feet become enlarged in acromegaly (G. acros = ends, megaly = large). In contrast, hypofunction of the pituitary gland can lead to dwarfism.

Nonendocrine failure of growth may result from inherited diseases such as *osteogenesis imperfecta*. With this disorder fractures are common even at birth. The disease is characterized by an increased production of type III collagen. *Achondroplastic dwarfism*, an autosomal dominant condition, leads to the failure of long bones to grow properly. The membranous bones of the skull, however, form normally and hence the skull is normal. *Ehlers-Danlos* syndrome is characterized by hyperextensibility of joints and skin. It arises from an inherited hydroxylase enzyme deficiency which interferes with the normal cross linking of collagen.

Hyperfunction of the adrenal gland (Cushing's syndrome) leads to excessive production of cortisol which demineralizes bone and leads to osteoporosis, or demineralization of bone. This frequently results in compression fractures of the vertebrae. Also, poor healing of fractures and wounds occurs because collagen is not produced. Likewise, hyperfunction of the thyroid gland can lead to osteoporosis. In contrast, *hypothyroidism* or *cretinism* (extreme hypothyroidism of infancy) can lead to early closure of epiphyseal growth plates causing stunted growth.

The hypersecretion of parathormone in *hyperparathyroidism* stimulates osteoblasts to resorb bone. Calcium is excreted in the urine as calcium and phosphorus stones. Generalized osteoporosis and compression fractures occur (see Chapter 12, Endocrine and Metabolic Disorders).

Osteoporosis

An elderly, postmenopausal woman seeking medical attention for pain in her back often has a compression fracture of one or more of the lumbar vertebrae (Fig. 20-6). Osteoporosis, a disorder characterized by marked demineralization of bone, is common in postmenopausal patients.

The causes of osteoporosis include aging, prolonged immunobilization (disuse atrophy), malnutrition, and excessive secretion of hormones (as described earlier). Another factor responsible for osteoporosis is inadequate calcium intake (insufficient to replace bone undergoing resorption and remodeling). Underlying causative factors should be corrected and immobilized individuals should be encouraged to exercise if possible. Vitamin D, in addition to calcium and fluoride salts, may have beneficial effects in persons with osteoporosis.

Osteitis Deformans (Paget's Disease)

Repeated episodes of bone resorption closely followed by extraordinary attempts at repair produce weakened, deformed bones that fracture easily despite their bulkiness.

Paget's disease is most commonly seen in elderly individuals, most of whom are asymptomatic. However, Paget's disease of the skull may compress cranial nerves exiting from holes (foramina) in the skull resulting in palsies and deafness. Generalized involvement of the skull and the axial and peripheral skeleton causes a triangular-shaped head, scoliosis or kyphosis of the spine, and bowed legs.

Pathologic fractures are frequent. The most serious complication is the finding of *osteogenic sarcoma* of affected bones (Fig. 20-7). Osteogenic sarcoma occurs in approximately 2% to 3% of persons with Paget's disease.

Fibrous Dysplasia

This metabolic disorder, which is more commonly seen in young persons, results in circumscribed fibrous islands of tissue that replace bone. Long bones, especially the femur, tibia, ribs, and facial bones, are most frequently involved. Severe distortion of facial bones may result. Treatment involves surgical removal of the abnormal tissue.

Gout

Gout is an autosomal dominant inherited metabolic disease (see Chapter 12, Endocrine and Metabolic Disorders). Pain in the joint of the big toe (podagra) may signal an acute gouty episode. Trauma or overindulgence in rich foods are often precipitating factors. The diagnosis is made by detecting monosodium urate crystals in synovial fluid from the involved joint (with or without an increased serum uric acid). Pain occurs as a result of deposition of uric acid crystals in the synovium and soft tissues. The uric acid crystals provoke an acute inflammatory response in the joints. Relief of pain occurs when colchicine, indomethocin, or phenylbutazone are given.

Pseudogout

The presence of calcium pyrophosphate crystals in the joint space also causes acute pain and swelling. The diagnosis of pseudogout is made by observation of such crystals in synovial fluid along with the

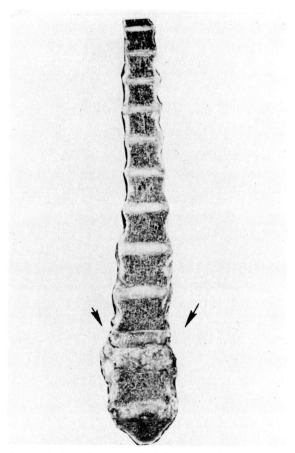

Figure 20-6 *Compression fracture of lumbar vertebra* (arrows) *in elderly woman with osteoporosis.*

finding of subchondral calcifications in a joint X-ray. Pseudogout may accompany hyperparathyroidism, hemochromatosis, diabetes, or gout. Types of arthritis are summarized in Table 20-1.

Neoplasms of Bone

Bone, cartilage, bone marrow, connective tissues, blood vessels, lymphatic vessels, and nerves may undergo neoplastic transformation. Malignant bone tumors outnumber benign tumors three to one.

A clinical feature common to almost all bone tumors is pain. Although pain may sometimes not be present in a benign bone tumor, the pain usually associated with malignant bone tumors is deep, aching, and persistent. A mass can be seen in some tumors. A mass without pain usually signals a benign tumor. Pathological fractures and impairment of function are additional clinical features of bone tumors.

An *osteoma* is the most frequent benign tumor of bone. It often involves the skull and produces thickening of the forehead which is of no consequence. In contrast, *osteoid osteoma* produces pain which is usually relieved by aspirin. It often affects the long bones, ribs, femur, and humerus of children or young adults. On X-ray film, a target-like pattern with a central radiodensity is seen. The treatment of choice to relieve pain is orthopedic surgery. The central area of the tumor, or the dense "bull's eye" area, consists of thickened bone spicules.

Osteogenic Sarcoma

One of the most virulent bone malignancies is osteogenic sarcoma. Early metastasis through blood vessels to the lung is common. The five-year survival rate is only 30%. This malignancy occurs in the long bones of young individuals or in elderly persons as a complication of Paget's disease. Typically, the symptoms at onset consist of pain in the involved extremity and weight loss.

The X-ray often shows a sunburst pattern surrounding the tumor (Fig. 20-7). Surgical biopsy reveals bizzare, malignant osteoblasts that form bone spicules. Amputation of the involved extremity is required. Recently, favorable results for treating early pulmonary metastases with chemotherapy have been achieved.

Cartilagenous Tumors

Chondrocytes present in the ends of bones may form malignant or benign tumors including *osteochondroma* (exotosis). This benign tumor occurs at the metaphysis of bones and results from the proliferation of an ectopic (displaced) epiphyseal plate. An exostosis is also called a boney spur and is covered by a cartilagenous cap. This growth may produce discomfort by impinging upon a tendon or a nerve, making surgical removal mandatory.

Enchondromas are like exostoses except that they occur in the central cavity of bones. Rarely, they become malignant. *Chondrosarcomas* comprise less than 10% of malignant bone tumors and have a more favorable prognosis than osteogenic sarcomas.

Diseases of Muscle

Basic pathological changes of skeletal muscles are atrophy, hypertrophy, degeneration, and regeneration. *Atrophy* refers to abnormally small myofibrils or muscle mass and may result from disuse, dystrophy, or denervation. *Hypertrophy* is enlargement of muscle mass caused by an increase in both size and number of individual fibers. It is an adaptive reaction to work rather than a pathological reaction. *Degeneration* refers to progressive destruction of a muscle fiber and occurs in a variety of conditions. *Regeneration* restores the continuity of my-

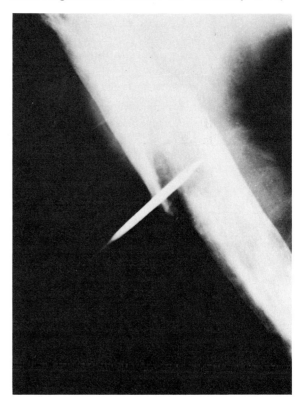

Figure 20-7   *Osteogenic sarcoma with fracture in Paget's disease. A pin secures the fracture.*

ofibrils. It occurs to a variable extent following degeneration.

The clinical features of muscle disease are usually weakness, wasting, and pain. The extent of these symptoms and others depends on the type of muscle disease.

A classification of primary diseases of muscles according to etiology includes six broad categories: (a) dystrophy, (b) atrophy, (c) inflammatory-autoimmune, (d) congenital myopathy, (e) metabolic myopathy, and (f) neoplasms. Except for disuse atrophy, diseases of muscles are uncommon.

Skeletal muscle dysfunction and disease is assessed by: (a) clinical examination of the patient; (b) the use of an electromyography (EMG) to measure conduction rates of nerve impulses and electrical activity in muscles; (c) serum enzyme assays that reflect destruction of muscle (creatinine phosphokinase and aldolase); and (d) muscle biopsy examination under the microscope.

Often all of the above techniques are needed for diagnosis of muscle disease. Muscle biopsy can be the most definitive source of diagnostic information and is especially valuable in diagnosing: (a) progressive dystrophy and atrophy; (b) localized or diffuse inflammatory autoimmune diseases, such as polymyositis; and (c) metabolic diseases. Changes are seen in muscle biopsy specimens in the connective tissues, blood vessels, nerves, and muscle.

Muscular Dystrophies

Unknown factors cause progressive destruction of muscle fibers unassociated with inflammatory reactions in a group of muscle diseases called dystrophies (Table 20-3). Muscular dystrophies often have a hereditary basis and begin during childhood. These diseases are characterized by variable age of onset and selective weakness of certain muscle groups.

The histological appearances of the various muscular dystrophies are similar and involve: (a) a loss of the normal polygonal contour of the muscle fibers due to ballooning of the cell; (b) necrosis and loss of cross-striations; (c) regeneration of muscle fibers with prominent nucleoli and nuclei, and migration of the nucleus into the center of the fiber; and (d) a proliferation of connective tissue, espe-

Table 20-3
The Muscular Dystrophies

Type	Inheritance
Duchenne muscular dystrophy	X-linked recessive
Facioscapulohumeral dystrophy	Autosomal dominant
Limb-girdle muscular dystrophy	Autosomal recessive
Congenital myotonic dystrophy	Autosomal dominant

cially the ingrowth of fat between the damaged muscle cells (Fig. 20-8).

Theories of Muscular Dystrophy

The *dystrophic theory* proposes that when dystrophies occur there is something intrinsically abnormal in the metabolism of the muscle fibers, leading to degeneration. However, no abnormality of the plasma membrane of the skeletal muscle has been identified. The other theory, the *neurogenic theory,* is based upon the demonstration of a loss of functional motor nerve units in EMG studies. In addition, abnormalities in the anterior motor nerve roots of animals with muscular dystrophy have been identified.

Duchenne's Muscular Dystrophy A sex-linked recessive form, *Duchenne's muscular dystrophy,* begins before age 5, progresses relentlessly from the pelvic girdle to the shoulder girdle, and typically leads to death in the third decade of life. Affected individuals have pseudohypertrophy of the calf muscle due to infiltration of fat between the damaged cells and hypertrophy of surviving muscle fibers. In addition, the heart is often involved—cardiac muscle fibers are destroyed and connective tissue infiltrates the heart. Intellectual impairment can occur in late stages of this disease and mental retardation has also been found.

Facioscapulohumeral Dystrophy Facioscapulohumeral dystrophy has an autosomal dominant inheritance, hence both sexes are affected. The disease may begin either in childhood or adulthood. The muscles of the face and shoulder girdles are affected initially, hence the name. Later, the disease may spread to the pelvic girdle after remaining quiet for long periods of time. Muscle hypertrophy

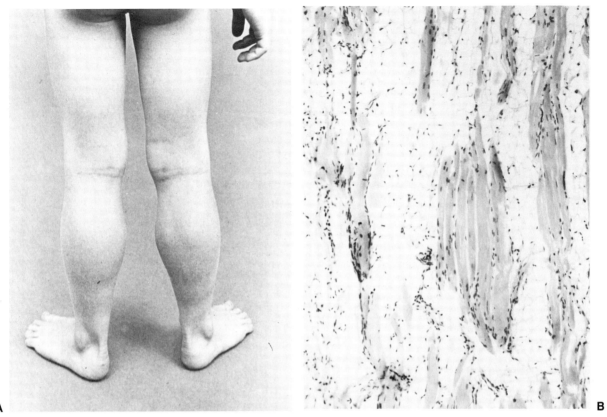

A

B

Figure 20-8   *Muscular dystrophy.* **A,** *Pseudohypertrophy of calf muscles.* **B,** *Muscle fibers are degenerating (dystrophic) and fat has grown between muscle fibers in this muscle biopsy specimen.* × 150.

and cardiac involvement are rare and therefore the outlook is favorable.

Limb-Girdle Dystrophy   This rare autosomal recessive or sporadically recurring disease arises from a mutation. It shows marked variability in its onset and prognosis. However, it generally begins in the third decade of life and involves either the shoulder or pelvic girdle and may later spread. Disability is usually not marked until 20 years after the onset. Cardiac involvement can occur.

Myotonic Dystrophy   Myotonic dystrophy is separable from the other muscular dystrophies because it is transmitted as an autosomal dominant disease that occurs in individuals between the ages of 20 and 40. Ninety percent of the individuals afflicted by myotonic dystrophy have cataracts and abnormalities of the endocrine system, including atrophy of the gonads and frontal balding. Abnormalities of the heart have also been noted.

Since myotonic dystrophy immobilizes facial muscles, the capacity for facial expression is lost. Moreover, the distal muscles of the upper and lower extremities may become involved. Myotonia refers to sustained involuntary contraction of a group of muscles. This can easily be demonstrated by tapping the tongue or hand of the patient. Vigorous contractions also result from exposure to the cold. A unique pathological muscle fiber, the ring fiber, is found upon microscopic study of a muscle biopsy specimen and helps in diagnosis of this disorder.

Atrophy of Muscle

When the nerves that supply muscles are blocked or interrupted, *neuropathic (neurogenic) muscular disease* occurs. The muscle fibers reduce in size (atrophy) and eventually die. Abnormalities of the neuromuscular plate or the myelin sheaths of nerves, or damage to the anterior horn cell within the spinal cord, all result in small, weak muscles. For unknown reasons, atrophy usually begins within a week or two following nerve disruption. Distal muscles become atrophic prior to proximal involvement. In anterior horn neuron disease (polio) and disorders of the neuromuscular junction (myesthenia gravis), sensation remains. But when nerves carrying sensory and motor fibers are injured, both motor and sensory functions are lost.

Nerve conduction and EMG studies help to evaluate the lesions. They determine whether the lesion is localized (a) in the muscle, (b) along the peripheral nerve, or (c) in the spinal cord.

The histopathologic changes occurring in neurogenic atrophy are uniform. The polygonal contours of muscle fibers on cross section change to angular forms. In addition, the diameters of the fibers decrease (Fig. 20-9). Inflammation, necrosis, phagocytosis, and regeneration are not observed.

Autoimmune-Inflammatory Myopathy

Polymyositis and *dermatomyositis* are diseases that affect skeletal muscles, the skin, and other connective tissues of the body. The etiologies of the disorders are unknown; however, they are autoimmune-collagen vascular diseases. An autoimmune response is thought to be responsible for the diseases because marked inflammation is observed in the muscle and skin and autoantibodies are often found in the serum. Viruses can trigger autoimmunity, however, viruses have not been identified in this disease.

Polymyositis and Dermatomyositis   *Polymyositis* most often involves women between the ages of 20 and 40. *Dermatomyositis* also occurs most frequently in women. But, when it is associated with malignancy, it frequently occurs in elderly men. Dermatomyositis occurring in childhood is associated with inflammation of blood vessels (angitis) that involves the skin and gastrointestinal tract.

Pain and tenderness are noted in the affected muscles, and weakness and difficulty in swallowing

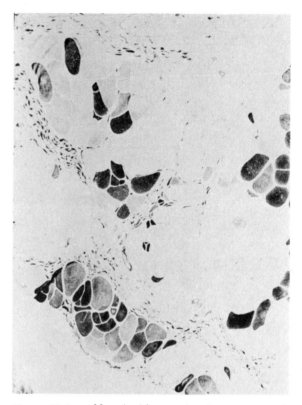

Figure 20-9   *Muscle biopsy showing neurogenic atrophy. Centrally minute atrophic fibers are seen on cross-section. Dark and light staining of fibers is due to reaction for acid phosphatase in the muscle fibers. × 150. (Courtesy Dr. Umberto DeGirolami.)*

(dysphagia) are also often noted. Proximal muscles of the arms and thighs are involved in the vast majority of instances. Next, flexors are involved. Usually facial muscles and muscles of the eyes are spared. The skin lesions are typically dark red, shiny, and sometimes scaly and atrophic over the face, neck, chest, extensor surfaces of joints, hands, and forearms. The clinical course of dermatomyositis is variable; spontaneous remissions and exacerbations have been noted. Approximately two-thirds of the individuals show improvement when given cortisone.

A muscle biopsy is usually obtained to rule out other causes of myositis. *Cortisone-induced myopathy*, for instance, can cause myopathy characterized by myofibril necrosis with inflammatory cells. With electron microscopy, characteristic abnormalities in mitochondria and muscle bands are seen. Ectopic bone formation in muscles gives rise to a condition termed *myositis ossificans* which is diagnosable by biopsy. Finally, *trichinosis*, a parasitic infection acquired by eating undercooked pork, causes myositis. *Trichinella spiralis* larvae can be seen in the muscle.

Microscopically, a biopsy specimen of muscle in dermatomyositis reveals pools of leukocytes — especially macrophages, lymphocytes, and plasma cells—scattered among dying muscle fibers and small blood vessels. The muscle fibers undergoing necrosis have a glassy and pink appearance.

Myasthenia Gravis   Myasthenia gravis is a disease characterized by defective transmission of impulses from nerves to muscles at the neuromuscular plate. Typically, myasthenia gravis affects women between the ages of 20 and 40. Its presence is signaled by progressive weakness during exercise.

Autoantibodies that react against the neuromuscular plate are found in the patient's serum. They interfere with the function of acetylcholamine, the chemical that transmits the nerve impulses to muscle. Hence, nerve impulses fail to pass across the neuromuscular junction and stimulate contraction of the muscle.

Neostigmine and related drugs are given to affected individuals to temporarily restore neuromuscular function. Myasthenia gravis may progress and lead to respiratory paralysis and death.

Autoimmunity is believed to be the cause of myasthenia gravis because the thymus gland of persons with the disease is usually abnormal and autoantibodies to motor endplates and muscle are found in the patient's serum. A neoplasm of the thymus (thymoma), or enlargement is often seen. Moreover, muscles contain numerous lymphocytes that invade the neuromuscular plate. Removal of the thymus glands or thymoma often results in the remission of the disease. Bleeding the patient to remove antibodies against motor endplates also relieves the disease. All of these features point to an autoimmune basis for myasthenia gravis.

Metabolic Myopathy

A group of diseases characterized by muscle weakness involving the proximal regions of extremities is associated with changes in potassium or glycogen metabolism.

Glycogen Storage Diseases   Glycogen storage diseases (glycogenoses) encompass at least six different inherited inborn errors of metabolism (see Chapter 9, Inherited Disorders). Glycogenoses result from the absence of enzymes that metabolize glycogen. Excessive accumulation of glycogen occurs within skeletal muscle and causes dysfunction.

Hypokalemic Periodic Paralysis   This disease is an autosomal dominant hereditary condition of persons between the ages of 20 and 25. Affected individuals experience sudden generalized attacks of weakness and paralysis of proximal muscle groups. The attacks usually occur during the night or are precipitated by strenuous exercise, a meal rich in carbohydrates, or exposure to cold. The attacks last approximately 6 to 24 hours. During the attack the serum potassium concentration becomes very low. Muscle biopsies taken during the attack reveal extensive vacuolization of fibers. The cause of this abnormality is not understood, but the permeability of the skeletal muscles to potassium is abnormal.

Neoplasms of Muscle

All neoplasms of muscle are rare, but when encountered they are usually malignant. The benign variety, *rhabdomyoma*, can arise in any striated muscle of the body. This benign tumor produces a mass (swelling) in the muscle. It must be biopsied and examined with the microscope to rule out a malignant muscle tumor. Rhabdomyomas are composed of numerous enlarged skeletal muscle fibers. No mitotic figures are seen. *Rhabdomyosarcoma* is a malignant tumor of the skeletal muscle that can arise in any skeletal muscle in the body. Most often young children and elderly individuals are afflicted by rhabdomyosarcoma. In children and adolescents the rhabdomyosarcoma occurs chiefly in the head, neck, or genitourinary tract. In adults (usually aged 30 to 60) the tumor arises in places where striated muscle are present, for instance within large skeletal muscles or in unusual places such as the middle ear muscles that move the auditory ossicles (bones), or the heart.

Rhabdomyosarcoma is of unknown etiology and is usually far advanced by the time a diagnosis is achieved. It metastasizes early and the prognosis for survival in most cases is very poor, irrespective of the treatment employed.

Summary

Collagen is the major protein in the body and consists of two chains of protein spun in a double helix. It is especially prominent in connective tissues and bone. Diseases arising in connective tissues have, therefore, been termed collagen diseases, but since they often have an autoimmune basis they are classified with autoimmune disorders. They are also called rheumatic diseases because the disorders involve joints.

Rheumatic diseases are classified in several overlapping groups based on the location of the disease, and common pathophysiology or inheritance: arthritis, nonarticular rheumatism, and autoimmune or inherited connective tissues disorders.

The etiology of rheumatoid arthritis is unknown. Patients have autoantibodies against their own immunoglobulins and lysozymes released from neutrophils are thought to participate in destroying joints. Related to rheumatoid arthritis are Felty's syndrome, juvenile rheumatoid arthritis, and ankylosing spondylitis.

Osteoarthritis is the most common of the rheumatic disorders. It induces much morbidity and profound disorders such as fractures of the hip and spine. Neoplasms of bone are rare; malignant tumors outnumber the benign three to one.

Diseases of muscle can arise from primary defects in muscle as with the inherited muscular dystrophies. Rarely, autoimmune disorders damage blood vessels and affect muscles, or autoantibodies against the motor endplate of muscle can prevent transmission of nerve impulses from nerve to muscle resulting in myasthenia gravis. Most often muscle disorders result in atrophy of muscle fibers either from disuse or from injury to motor nerve fibers. Metabolic and neoplastic disorders of muscle are rare.

Bibliography

Bethlem, J. 1970. *Muscle pathology introduction and atlas.* New York: North Holland Publishing Co. Color photographs of histopathology of muscle diseases are displayed.

Compere, E. L. 1974. *Orthopedic surgery.* Chicago: Year Book Medical Publishers, Inc. Concise description of orthopedics.

Dahlin, D. 1973. *Bone tumors,* ed. 2. Springfield, Illinois: C. C Thomas, Publisher. Contains X-rays, gross, and microscopic photographs of tumors from 4000 cases at the Mayo clinic.

Dubowitz, V. 1975. Neuromuscular disorders of childhood. *Arch. Dis. Child.* 50:335–346. Review article by an expert.

Farfan, H. F. 1973. *Mechanical disorders of the low back.* Philadelphia: Lea & Febiger. Describes mechanisms responsible for low-back pain.

Fessel, W. J. 1975. *Rheumatology for clinicians.* New York: Stratton Intercontinental Medical Book Corporation. Briefly discusses diseases affecting joints and connective tissues.

Fox, A. T. 1966. *Manual of orthopaedic surgery.* Am. Orthop. Assoc. Standard handbook, excellent for terminology.

Jaffe, H. L. 1972. *Metabolic, degenerative and inflammatory diseases of bones and joints.* Philadelphia: Lea & Febiger. Standard reference.

Primer on the rheumatic diseases, ed. 7. 1973. Arthritis Foundation. Can be obtained gratis from the Arthritis Foundation. Excellent reference for classification.

Rodman, G. P. 1975. Gout and other crystalline forms of arthritis. Postgrad. Med. 58:4–12. Describes metabolic basis and treatment of gout.

Schneider, F. R. 1972. *Handbook for the orthopaedic assistant.* St. Louis: The C. V. Mosby Co. Practical clinical information for allied health professionals.

Waldvogel, F. A.; Medoff, G.; and Swartz; M. N. 1971. *Osteomyelitis.* Springfield, Illinois: C. C Thomas, Publisher. Monograph on bone infections.

Walton, J. N., ed. 1974. *Disorders of voluntary muscle.* London: Churchill-Livingstone. Standard textbook.

Wilson, F. C. 1975. *The musculoskeletal system.* Philadelphia: J. B. Lippincott Company. The best overall introduction to normal and abnormal structure and function of bones, joints, and muscles.

CHAPTER 21

Neurology and Neuropathology

Chapter Outline

Objectives

After reading this chapter you should be able to

Describe the morphologic unit of the central nervous system (CNS).

Discuss the concept of localization of neurological function.

List features unique to the CNS.

Describe the supporting cells of the CNS.

Define the terms atrophy, ischemia, chromatolysis, and necrosis.

List the sequential changes occurring during axonal reaction.

Define the term gliosis.

List synonyms for cerebrovascular accidents.

Describe the major life-threatening complication of cerebral edema.

Know the pathogenesis of hydrocephalus.

Describe the potential impact on the brain of malnutrition.

List the TORCH infectious agents that can damage the brain of the fetus.

Define the terms agenesis, anencephaly, and spina bifida.

Define the terms paraplegia and syringomyelia.

List lesions that can result from trauma to the head.

Compare subdural hematoma and subarachnoid hemorrhage.

Define the terms concussion and contusion.

Describe the location of a lesion that results in quadriplegia.

List three types of infectious processes occurring in the CNS.

List the bacteria that cause meningitis.

Know how meningitis is diagnosed.

Compare the mortality rates associated with meningitis and cerebral abscesses.

Describe the origin of tuberculous meningitis.

List fungi that can infect the brain.

Describe how aseptic meningitis is diagnosed.

Know the pathogenesis of poliomyelitis.

Define the term shingles.

Describe the part of the brain infected by herpes simplex.

List examples of slow viral infections.

Describe the etiology of postinfectious encephalomyelitis.

Describe the clinical pattern of multiple sclerosis.

Define the term senility.

Compare Alzheimer's and Pick's diseases.

Describe the clinical findings of Huntington's chorea.

Discuss the etiology of Parkinson's disease.

Describe the pathologic basis of Parkinson's disease.

Define Friedreich's ataxia.

Describe the pathologic lesions of amyotrophic lateral sclerosis.

Know how Werdnig-Hoffmann disease is inherited.

Discuss the role copper plays in Wilson's disease.

List the clinical findings associated with pellagra.

Describe the degenerative changes that pernicious anemia causes in the spinal cord.

Know how frequently cerebrovascular disease causes death in the United States.

List the arteries supplying the brain.

Describe the cause of and clinical findings regarding transient ischemic attacks.

List the two major factors that determine necrosis in the CNS.

Describe the pathogenesis of necrosis in the brain.

List three causes of CVA.

Compare the clinical aspects of CVA according to etiology.

Describe where arteriosclerosis tends to occur.

Know the prognosis following cerebral infarction.

Compare the clinical syndromes arising from lesions in the internal carotid, middle cerebral, anterior cerebral, posterior or cerebellar arteries.

List the three regions in the cerebrum that serve language.

Define the terms motor aphasia and central aphasia.

Describe the terms dysarthria and dysphagia.

Know what condition predisposes an individual to intracerebral hemorrhage.

Describe the term aneurysm.

List the factors that determine prognoses for brain tumors.

Describe the three syndromes resulting from brain tumors.

Know how brain tumors are diagnosed.

Describe the cerebrospinal fluid taken from a person with brain tumor.

Describe how X-rays assist in the diagnosis of brain tumors.

List the major histologic types of brain tumors.

Describe the location and prognosis for meningiomas.

Compare the frequency of and prognosis for brain tumors.

Know the prognosis for glioma.

Describe how brain tumors are treated.

Describe two tumors of nerves.

Introduction

The *neuron is the morphological and functional unit of the nervous system and is the only cell in the central nervous system* (CNS) capable of conducting nervous impulses. Neurons of adults are incapable of mitosis, hence death of a neuron results in a permanent loss of function.

A typical neuron of the cerebral cortex is shaped like a pyramid. The nucleus is centered within the cytoplasm, is round, and has dispersed DNA and a prominent nuclear membrane and nucleolus. The cytoplasm contains Nissl substance. Many dendrites (branches) go outward from the cell body, and the axon (nerve fiber) extends from one end of the neuron (Fig. 21-1). The gray matter of the

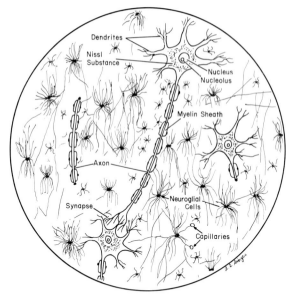

Figure 21-1   *Cells of the central nervous system.*

brain contains neurons and the white matter contains axons covered by myelin sheaths composed of white "fat." The junction where axons and dendrites meet in the CNS is call a *synapse*. Glial cells surround the neurons and support or bind the CNS together.

Localization of Function

Specific functions of the body are localized anatomically within specific groups of neurons. Our knowledge about the localization of function within the CNS has resulted from the careful observing, recording, and correlating of clinical neurological deficits with the pathological findings seen within the brain at autopsy (Fig. 21-2). For example, when a person loses the ability to speak (becomes aphasic), a lesion in the temporal lobe speech area can be responsible for the deficit. Furthermore, depending upon the cause of the disease, a predictable pattern of onset, progression, and termination of deficits occurs (Fig. 21-3).

The patterns of response of the nervous system to injury are predictable because of features unique to the CNS: (a) the brain is enclosed in a fixed space (skull); (b) the brain has limited mobility within the skull; (c) the dural covering of the brain is immobile; (d) most lesions progress in a predictable manner; and (e) neurons cannot regenerate. Furthermore, special functional, metabolic, and structural features of certain groups of neurons enable specific diseases to strike neurons having common features.

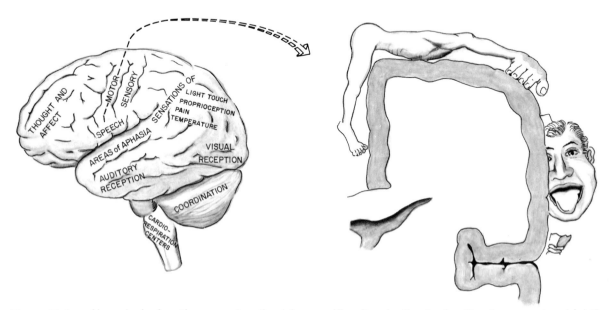

Figure 21-2   *Neurologic functions are localized in specific sites in the brain. The homunculus* (right) *illustrates the precise sites in the motor or sensory cortex responsible for certain functions.*

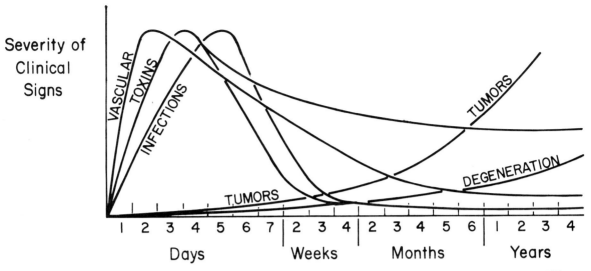

Figure 21-3   *The relative rate of onset and progression of neurologic diseases is predictable for different disorders.*

Supporting Cells

The neuron maintains itself by relying on the supporting, insulating, stimulating, and nutritional contributions of neighboring cells. The cellular components of the brain include not only neurons, but also the *connective tissue cells*—astrocytes, microglia, and oligodendrocytes. The latter cells manufacture the insulating sheaths that surround nerve fibers within the CNS. Neurons are highly specialized and the types of reactions to injury are limited; thus diverse diseases may show an indentical lesion. Neuronal cell necrosis constitutes the end stage of all pathological processes involving nerve cells.

Neuronal Cell Lesions

Atrophy is a common pathologic change occurring in neurons and accompanies numerous progressive degenerative processes. The most common cause of neuronal atrophy is deficiency in blood supply *(ischemia)*. Nerve cells undergoing atrophy decrease in cell size and their cytoplasm shrinks. Both the cytoplasm and nuclei become dark, and clumping of the neurofibrils occurs. Often persons suffering with senility (loss of recent memory with inappropriate behavior) have experienced a generalized atrophy of the cerebral cortex. Another disorder characterized by atrophy is *Alzheimer's disease,* where the frontal lobes of the cerebral cortex become atrophic in a person of 40 to 55 years.

Necrosis results when a sudden interference with oxygenation or metabolism of the neurons occurs, causing acute cell injury and death of cells. These acute cellular changes are similar to the process of atrophy described above, except the cytoplasm becomes red and the nucleus becomes displaced to the side. The latter process is called *chromatolysis* and is often found in lower motor neuron lesions involving the anterior horn cells of the spinal cord. Chromatolysis also occurs in upper motor neuron lesions involving cranial nerve nuclei and the motor portion of the cerebral cortex.

Neurons may also become damaged when lipids or other substances accumulate in the neurons of persons having inborn errors of metabolism (see Chapter 9, Inherited Disorders, and Chapter 12, Endocrine and Metabolic Disorders). Another group, *degenerative neurological diseases*, results in a loss of neurons and produces functional changes resulting in senility. Finally, the nervous system is subject to *infectious diseases* and to *neoplasia* (tumors).

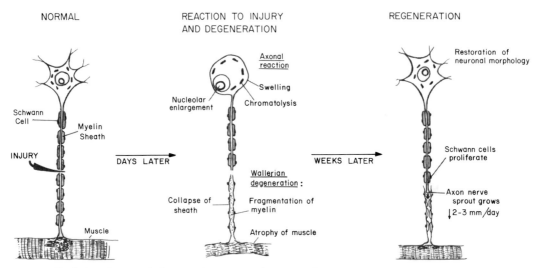

Figure 21-4   *Peripheral nerve injury and regeneration. The time required for the nerve to regenerate may be estimated. The nerve sprout grows 2 to 3 mm/day.*

Axonal Reaction

The changes that occur in the nerve cell body following cutting of an axon are called axonal reaction. This process, called wallerian degeneration, occurs in the axon stump and the neuron cell body. Axonal reaction occurs sequentially within nerve bodies within days after an axon is severed. The reaction involves (a) rounding of the neuron; (b) migration of the nucleus from its central position to the periphery of the cell; (c) enlargement of the nucleolus; and (d) dispersion of the Nissl substance from the center of the cell to the edge or chromatolysis (Fig. 21-4).

In wallerian degeneration, the myelin fragments and Schwann's cells which surround axons proliferate. The axon remaining attached to the neuron body undergoes atrophy and chromatolysis ensues. When the axon begins to regenerate, an axon nerve sprout grows within the nerve tube at the rate of several millimeters per day and may rejoin the cut nerve. One can estimate how long it will take for the nerve to regenerate. However, if a scar results a painful *traumatic neuroma* may develop. In addition, following an amputation of a limb, "phantom" limb (the feeling that the extremity remains attached) can develop.

Neuroglia (*"nerve glue"*) is comprised of three types of cells that support and bind neurons together. *Astrocytes* are the largest neuroglia cells of the CNS, and *oligodendrocytes* and *microglia* are small neuroglial cells. Astrocytes may contain numerous short processes (protoplasmic astrocytes) and others (such as fibrous astrocytes) have long dendritic, tree-like, processes. The processes surround small blood vessels and transmit nutrients to the neurons. Following injury, astrocytes proliferate to form glial scars which are vital in healing wounds in the brain. *Gliosis* (scar formation in the CNS) is a fundamental reaction of nervous tissue to injury.

Glial Cell Reaction

Gliosis produces a disorderly array of glial cells within the injured site, and may accompany degenerative processes afflicting nerve tracts. Subsequently, numerous stout fibers from cell processes and glial cell bodies become reduced in size. Gliosis is seen in disorders affecting the white matter: multiple sclerosis, leukodystrophies, and subacute sclerosing panencephalitis are examples. Gliosis can occur following injury to the brain and may disrupt transmission of nerve impulses. Posttraumatic epilepsy (seizures) arises when nerve impulses are discharged chaotically while passing through the glial scar.

Oligodendrocytes are special glial cells that reside in white matter. They line up adjacent to myelinated nerve fibers and form the myelin sheaths that wrap around nerves and insulate and protect them. In the peripheral nerve, Schwann's cells serve the same myelinating function. The oligodendrocytes are vulnerable to anoxia and hence demyelination occurs when they die. When the myelin sheath is destroyed as in postinfectious encephalomyelitis, the oligodendrocytes disappear.

Central Nervous System Lesions

The neuronal lesions described above (atrophy, necrosis, gliosis, and demyelination) affect the CNS. Lesions are often of sufficient size to be observed with the naked eye. For example, cerebral atrophy is characterized by narrowing of the gyri (convexities) and widening of the sulci (valleys) over the cerebral convexity (Fig. 21-5). A loss of neurons associated with gliosis is seen in an atrophic brain and the underlying ventricular chambers become dilated.

Cerebrovascular disorders are the most frequent cause of death from CNS lesions. Stroke results from hemorrhage directly into the substance of the brain or because of thrombosis (formation of a clot) in a cerebral artery. Following necrosis of brain tissue, scars do not form to bridge the area of necrosis, rather liquefaction necrosis ensues (Fig. 21-6). Scar tissue (gliosis) only forms adjacent to the cavities filled with liquid, which continue to exist.

Edema of the Brain

Cerebral edema swells the cerebral hemispheres and the result is flattening of the gyri and compression of the ventricular spaces. When extensive, edema produces devastating consequences, including shifting of brain tissue within the skull and disruption of vital respiratory control centers. Edema arises from trauma and other conditions that increase the permeability of the blood vessels to fluid. The brain, rigidly encased within the skull and

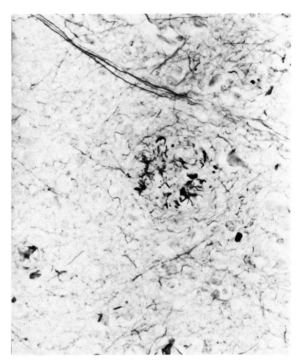

Figure 21-5 *Cerebral atrophy from severe Alzheimer's disease. The gyri (convexities) are narrowed and sulci (valleys) deepened (See Figure 4-3). The photomicrograph shows degenerative neurofibrillary tangles. ×400. (Courtesy Dr. Umberto DeGirolami.)*

dura mater is vulnerable to increased pressure from edema when it expands within this enclosed area. Thus, when expansion occurs the blood supply becomes compressed and the brain shifts (herniates) from its normal position. Multiple small hemorrhages into the white matter resulting from trauma are seen both in the cerebral and cerebellar hemispheres. The hemorrhages further aggravate the problem brought about by cerebral edema.

Ordinarily a blood brain barrier (BBB) restricts the passage of substances from the blood vessels into the nervous tissue. The blood vessel walls form the BBB. When a blood vessel wall is injured, the spaces between the cells separate and fluid readily passes from the vessel into the brain substance (see Chapter 5, Acute Inflammation and Repair). In the skull, the fluid volume in the brain, cerebrospinal fluid (CSF), and blood must be kept constant. But when the brain swells, it is pushed toward several possible exits (Fig. 21-7). *Herniation* through the

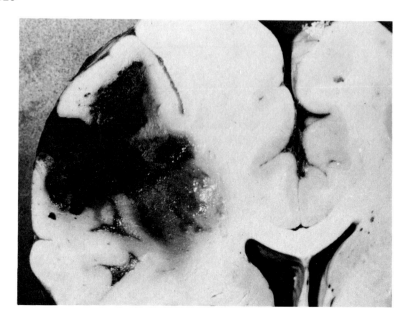

Figure 21-6 *Hemorrhagic cerebral infarction. Liquefaction necrosis is beginning.*

foramen magnum proves fatal. Cerebral edema is treated with corticosteroids, which decrease the permeability of the BBB to fluid. Secondly, diuretic drugs are given to eliminate excessive fluid from the circulation and brain via the kidneys.

Hydrocephalus

Cerebrospinal fluid (CSF) is secreted in the vascular choroid plexus which lines the ventricles of the brain. Ordinarily, 0.4 ml/min. of CSF is produced, circulates, and is reabsorbed into veins within the meninges. CSF cushions and prevents the brain from being damaged by trauma.

In hydrocephalus the ventricular chambers enlarge from blocked circulation or impaired absorption of CSF by the meninges. Obstruction of CSF circulation is the major problem. Hydrocephalus is either communicating or noncommunicating. In the latter instance, the elevated CSF pressure within the ventricular system dilates the ventricular chambers, but the pressure is not transmitted to the subarachnoid space and thus increased CSF pressure is not evident when a lumbar puncture is performed. Communicating hydrocephalus results most often from congenital or acquired lesions (as with meningitis) that block the drainage of CSF. Tumors also produce similar effects. A tube (shunt) can be inserted between the blocked ventricle or subarachnoid space and the heart, thereby returning CSF into circulation.

Disorders of Development

In the middle of an embryo's back, a neural groove forms which migrates to the midline and eventually fuses into a neural tube (see Chapter 3, Development and Birth Defects). Clusters of neural crest cells group on both sides of the neural tube to form the dorsal root ganglion. Simultaneously, peripheral nerves develop. Overlying vertebral bone and skin fuse to protect the spinal cord. The brain develops much more rapidly in the embryo than the trunk and limbs; it comprises nearly one-half of the embryo for several months following conception.

Normally, the brain reaches a maximal rate of growth at about 38 weeks of gestation. This growth spurt occurs simultaneously with the physical and nutritional stresses of birth rendering the brain vulnerable to damage during birth.

Myelination of nerves begins in the head and in the upper thoracic region, and then spreads distally. Within weeks following birth, the nerves supplying the eyes and ear become myelinated. The

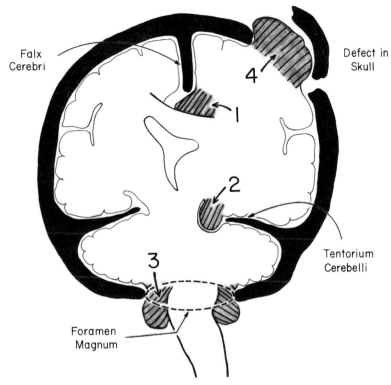

Figure 21-7   *Increased pressure of edematous brain herniates brain substance. 1, under falx cerebri; 2, tentorium cerebelli; 3, through foramen magnum; or, 4, defect in skull.*

newborn is thus soon able to coordinate eye movements and to hear; senses essential for feeding are available. Various normal developmental milestones like sitting, standing, and walking are dependent upon the extent of myelination.

Malnutrition occurring in utero can severely retard the growth of the brain. The brain grows to approximately 80% of its adult weight by 2 years of age, and by 5 it approaches its final weight. Thus, malnutrition in young children can also retard the growth of the brain and impair mental capacity (see Chapter 10, Nutritional Diseases).

Infectious Diseases of the Fetus and Neonate

Approximately one-half of all congenital defects occur in the central nervous system. Genetic dis-

orders, fetal infections, irradiation, lack of blood supply to the fetus, drugs (like alcohol or thalidomide), or trauma can induce congenital defects of the CNS. During gestation, the fetal brain may be the site of infections without any evidence of an inflammatory response. Later, lymphocytes may infiltrate the infected brain.

The TORCH complex of infections (see Chapter 7, Infectious Diseases) are *toxoplasmosis, other* (syphilis), and *rubella*, which can cause deafness, cataracts, and other defects including mental retardation; *cytomegalovirus*, which can result in necrosis and calcification of the brain producing mental retardation; and finally, *herpes simplex*, which can infect the baby as it passes through an infected cervix. Neonatal meningitis is usually caused by the colon bacillus *Escherichia coli*, and results from a lack of acquired immunity to this common bacterium. The TORCH agents are most likely to cause malformation in the brain when infection occurs prior to 12 weeks of gestation because this is the period of formation of brain structures.

CNS Malformations

Agenesis (absence of a structure) ranges from *anencephaly* (lack of brain) to a failure in development of a single structure, as in agenesis of the cerebellum. Furthermore, there may be a failure of the skull or vertebral arches to fuse (see Chapter 3, Development and Birth Defects). When the calvaria (skull vault) remains intact and the brain fails to fully develop, CSF fills the empty space (hydrocephaly). This condition can be detected by holding a flashlight against the side of the skull in a dark room. If brain tissue is lacking, light passes through the CSF. A pink glow is observed.

Abnormal closure of the neural tube in the lumbosacral region is rather common; incomplete closure of the bony vertebral arches results in *spina bifida*. Herniation of the meninges and nervous tissue through a bony defect is called *meningomyelocele*. This can occur also in the occipital bone of the skull resulting in herniation of meninges and brain tissue, or *meningoencephalocele*.

The *Arnold-Chiari malformation* is a partial agenesis (hypoplasia) of the base of the brainstem. The malformed medulla oblongata and a portion of the cerebellum slip downward into the opening (foramen magnum) at the base of the skull. Pressure on the base of the brain then produces hydrocephalus and causes death when pressure is exerted on vital respiratory centers.

Failure of the neural tube to fully close renders individuals vulnerable to infections and *meningitis* often results. In addition, deficits of peripheral nerve function result and even complete paralysis below the waist (*paraplegia*) can occur.

Inadequate formation of the neural tube in children or spinal cord tumors (gliomas) in adults can produce *syringomyelia* which is characterized by a dilatation of the central canal of the spinal cord. Syringomyelia may also be associated with inflammation or infarction. This lesion frequently causes impingement on surrounding spinal cord tracts and results in permanent neurological deficits. Combined sensory and motor function impairment often ensue.

Trauma

Traumatic injury to the head produces lesions of: (a) the skull, (b) epidural space, (c) meninges, (d) subdural space (between the dura and leptomeninges), (e) the subarachnoid space, and (f) the brain.

Patients with head injuries usually show a variety of neurological symptoms such as unequal pupils; dilated, fixed pupils; or paralysis on one side (hemiplegia). Increased respiration, blood pressure, and perspiration may occur. If blood collects in large quantities in the subdural space, confusion progressive to *coma* (loss of consciousness with failure to awaken to painful stimuli) can ensue. Skull fractures are often not serious, but a fractured temporal bone can lacerate the middle meningeal artery and cause extensive hemorrhage. Blood accumulates in the epidural space (epidural hematoma) and compresses the brain. Eventual herniation of the brain tissue and death may ensue. Therefore, large blood clots must be surgically removed before compression occurs.

Subdural hematomas arise from ruptured veins that bridge between the arachnoid and dura mater (Fig. 21-8). When the resulting hematoma reaches about 100 ml or greater, the underlying cerebral cortex is displaced and herniation of brain tissue can arise. The clot becomes organized by granulation tissue as times passes, but immediate surgical removal is required to prevent herniation.

Subarachnoid hemorrhage often results from a defect in the wall of meningeal blood vessels, especially in vessels at the base of the brain comprising the circle of Willis. Here a ruptured *aneurysm* (dilated or ballooned-out artery) is often found to be the cause of sudden death (Figs. 21-9 and 21-10). The thin arterial wall suddenly ruptures; a severe headache and loss of consciousness follow. A lumbar tap reveals blood within the CSF. The hemorrhaging vessels can be clipped surgically; however, aneurysms subsequently rebleed in one-half of patients, and neurological impairment almost always results.

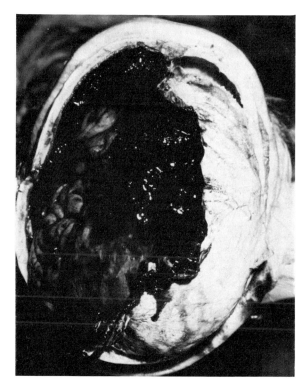

Figure 21-8 *Subdural hematoma over left cerebral hemisphere. The alcoholic person struck his head on pavement.*

Concussion and Contusion

Concussion is a transient neurological disorder caused by injury to the head. It is characterized by an instantaneous, widespread paralysis, and amnesia about the events of the accident. No obvious lesion of the brain is demonstrable following a concussion. This syndrome is probably brought about by rapid to-and-fro movements of the brain within the CSF.

Contusion is a bruise on the surface of the brain where the dura remains intact. Typically, a wedge-shaped area of necrosis of neurons with the apex extending several millimeters into the white matter is seen. Later, a glial scar can form at the site which may be the local point of posttraumatic epilepsy.

The main types of contusion are coup and contre-coup lesions. The *coup* contusion underlies the blow (directly impacted area) and the *contre-coup* lies opposite the line of the force. The contre-coup

lesions occur when the brain strikes bone and hard meningeal surfaces at the opposite side.

Trauma to the CNS may elicit herniation of brain tissue as described above, and acute hydrocephalus arises from blockage of CSF. Furthermore, bacteria can invade the brain through a skull fracture site.

Whatever the cause, the typical clinical course of a lesion of the CNS resolves as follows (Fig. 21-3). Damage ensues from direct destruction or from indirect effects of vascular thrombosis, hemorrhage, infection, or edema caused by tumor or injury. Then, a phase of clearing of tissue debris by neutrophils and macrophages occurs. Finally, a repair phase ensues and glial cells proliferate, sometimes leaving a mutilating glial scar. Many lesions never resolve but rather progress, and death can occur if medical or surgical intervention is not provided.

Spinal Cord Injuries

The spinal cord and nerve roots are frequently injured when sudden movements fracture or *sublux (dislocate)* the vertebral column. The common sites of vertebral injury are in vertebrae C4-6 and L1-2. Following a fracture, hemorrhage and necrosis of the spinal cord often ensue. Compression of the cord and disruption of the cord blood vessels may follow (Fig. 21-11). Extreme hyperextension or hyperflexion of the neck can result in a fracture and dislocation; *quadriplegia* (loss of motor and sensory function of the trunk and upper and lower extremities) is often the result of a high (C4-6) cervical lesion.

The cord develops an hourglass narrowing at the site of the injury and a bulging and softening above and below the level of injury. The same pathological features observed in a brain damaged by trauma are seen in the cord. In contrast to severe cerebral injuries, spinal cord injuries are seldom fatal, but they leave a permanent paraplegia or quadriplegia with a loss of motor and sensory function below the spinal cord segment that is functionally or anatomically severed.

The spinal cord of an infant can, while passing through the birth canal, be injured. Breech deliveries cause hyperextension of the head, and injury to the spinal cord and brain can result. The overstretched cord develops an hourglass narrowing at the cervical-thoracic juncture. In adults, especially in middle-aged to elderly individuals, the spinal cord can also be compressed by herniated intervertebral discs (slipped discs) or by spurs of bone that protrude between vertebral bodies degenerated by osteoarthritis (see Chapter 20, Diseases of Muscles, Bones, and Joints).

Infections of the CNS

Infections of the CNS are caused by a wide variety of microorganisms (see Chapter 7, Infectious Dis-

eases). Typically fever, weakness, headache, and stiff neck signal infection in the CNS. The immune and inflammatory reactions to the microorganisms elicit: (a) meningitis, (b) abscess or granulomatous response, or (c) encephalitis. The latter is provoked by viral infections and the former two are caused chiefly by pyogenic bacteria.

Meningeal infections occur in several spaces surrounding the brain: (a) the epidural space (epidural abscess); (b) subdural space (subdural empyema or abscess); and (c) subarachnoid space (meningitis). Involvement of the first two spaces of membranes is considered pachymeningitis (external-epidural, internal-subdural).

The subarachnoid space is infected most commonly. Meningitis is an inflammation of the pi-

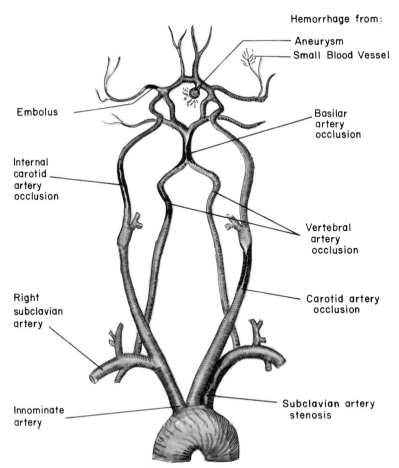

Figure   21-9   *Vascular lesions producing strokes.*

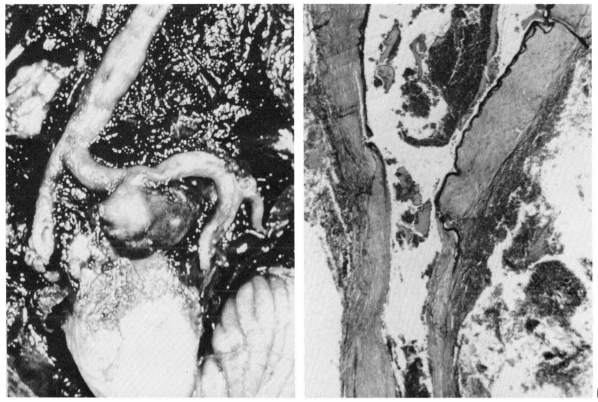

Figure 21-10   A, *Berry aneurysm of base of brain which has hemorrhaged.* **B,** *Photomicrograph of wall of aneurysm in cerebral artery. Note the absence of an elastic membrane* (arrow). *Rupture occurs through this weak site. (Courtesy Dr. Umberto DeGirolami.)*

arachnoid meninges and the CSF bathing the brain and spinal cord. Bacteria reach the CNS via the bloodstream or by direct extension from surrounding bones of the middle ear (otitis media), osteomyelitis of the skull, penetrating wounds, or sinusitis. Recurrent meningitis is usually the result of direct reinfection from an open wound.

Pyogenic Meningitis

Purulent bacterial meningitis (see Chapter 7, Infectious Diseases) is most often caused by *E coli* in the newborn, *H influenzae* in infants and young children, *N meningitidis* in young adults, and *S pneumoniae* in adults and aged persons. Cardinal manifestations of meningitis are chills, fever, headache in the back of the neck, vomiting, and deterioration of mental function progressing to stupor

and coma. Individuals at the extreme ages of life, however, may lack obvious signs of meningitis.

Laboratory evaluation of the CSF fluid of the patient reveals elevated pressure, increased protein, and a decrease in sugar content. A Gram stain of the CSF sediment is a useful diagnostic test to detect the presence of bacteria. Numerous neutrophils can also be present in the fluid as a result of acute inflammation. The patient is treated vigorously with specific antibiotics and is also given intravenous fluids.

If the individual dies of meningitis, examination of the brain reveals pus over the surface of the brain within the subarachnoid space. The distribution of pus depends upon the duration of the infection, effectiveness of antibiotic treatment, virulence of the organisms, and the inflammatory response of the person (see Chapter 7, Infectious Diseases).

The acute neutrophil inflammatory reaction begins immediately when bacteria invade. Microorganisms can be seen both inside and outside the neutrophils. At about one week, the subacute phase, characterized by degenerating leukocytes and layers of fibrin, begins. The innermost layer becomes composed mainly of plasma cells, lymphocytes, histiocytes, and macrophages; the latter remove cellular debris. When exudate at the base of the brain blocks CSF flow, hydrocephalus appears.

In the chronic stage the ventricles become enlarged, the convolutions flattened, and subdural membranes form as a marked fibroblastic proliferation ensues. Necrosis of gray and white matter may proceed, but permanent damage rarely occurs.

Other permanent sequela may include dementia (loss of intellectual functions), blindness, deafness, and focal paralysis. Death can result from the meningitis itself or from subdural empyema or hydrocephalus.

Brain Abscess

Abscesses of the brain account for approximately 10% of CNS infections. Delay in diagnosis or complications resulting from attempts to drain abscesses result in a mortality rate approaching 50%. Patients frequently experience fever, headache, and often have infections in the bones (osteomyelitis) of the skull or ear, or may have underlying pneumonia or endocarditis. Bacteria travel to the brain from infected lungs or heart valves and brain abscess ensues.

The CSF in persons with cerebral abscesses is characterized by elevated pressure, numerous neutrophils and lymphocytes, and abundant protein. The common bacteria responsible for abscesses are hemolytic streptococcus, staphylococcus, *E coli*, and various fungi.

Abscesses form most often in the subcortical white matter and progressively invade deep white matter. The first insult is neuronal necrosis secondary to thrombosis of infected vessels, and within four to five days liquefaction necrosis of the brain occurs and the bacteria multiply within the pus. Later, mononuclear cells and granulation tissue form the abscess wall. The entire lesion then becomes surrounded by reactive astrocytes.

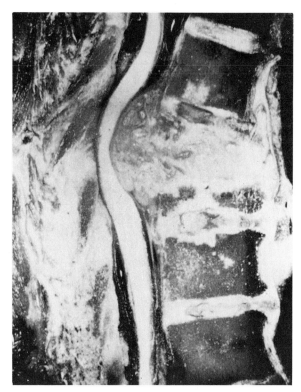

Figure 21-11 *Compression fracture, dislocation and compression of lumbar spinal cord.*

Epidural empyema often occurs due to penetrating osteomyelitis of the skull or from infection of the middle ear or sinuses. Pus collects in the epidural space as the infection penetrates the bone. In the spinal cord this may also result from osteomyelitis of the spine. Subdural empyema or subdural abscess arises also from otitis media, sinusitis, or infected wounds. Treatment of brain abscesses and empyema involves surgical drainage and antibiotics.

Tuberculous Meningitis

Tuberculosis of the brain results from spreading in the blood of tubercle bacilli from infected lungs. The base of the brain often contains a gelatinous, gray-white exudate mixed with tiny tubercles. The tubercles are composed of granulomas that contain Langhans giant cells and macrophages (see Chapter 7, Infectious Diseases) and tubercle bacilli are observed in the granulomas. Examination of the CSF fluid reveals lymphocytes, histiocytes, occasional plasma cells, and neutrophils.

Individuals afflicted by tuberculous meningitis frequently develop paralysis of cranial nerves because these nerves become compressed by the scars formed at the base of the infected brain. In addition, the ventricles become dilated (hydrocephalus) because the drainage of CSF fluid becomes obstructed. Treatment involves administration of isoniazid, streptomycin, or other drugs. Tuberculous meningitis is uncommon in the United States, however, in India, Central Africa, and South America tuberculosis of the CNS accounts for approximately one-half of the cases of meningitis. Also, children, immunosuppressed individuals, alcoholics, and the aged can suffer from tuberculous meningitis.

Fungal Infections of the Brain

Fungi invade the nervous system of debilitated, immunosuppressed individuals. Two pathological inflammatory responses occur: (a) granulomatous necrotizing inflammation of the brain and meninges, or (b) abscesses. Fungal organisms in the yeast phase tend to produce granulomatous inflammation, whereas those having mycelia (filaments) produce abscesses. The granulomatous forms are caused by *Cryptococcus, Coccidioides, Histoplasma,* and *Blastomyces.* In contrast, abscesses arise from Aspergillus, Mucor, or Candida.

Affected individuals suffer from headache and stiff neck as in other conditions that inflame the meninges. The CSF is under increasing pressure

and the protein content also increases. On occasion, the fungi can be seen in the CSF sediment. Following diagnosis, treatment of fungal infections is with amphotercin B.

Neurosyphilis, a tertiary stage of syphilis that occurs 10 to 20 years following the onset of infection by *Treponema pallidum* is described in detail in Chapter 7, Infectious Diseases.

Viral Infections of the Brain

Viral infections of the CNS can cause meningitis (aseptic meningitis) or may involve the brain and spinal cord (meningoencephalomyelitis).

Aseptic meningitis occurs when the virus infects the meninges. This disorder is characterized by signs of fever, irritability, and stiffness of the neck. A slight elevation in CSF protein with a normal sugar content and mononuclear cells is seen. The most frequent causes are enteroviruses (Coxsackie and poliomyelitis), mumps, and lymphocytic choriomeningitis. Brains infected by viruses show lymphocytes and plasma cells surrounding blood vessels (perivascular cuffing).

Viral encephalitis, or encephalomyelitis, usually begins suddenly with fever, meningeal irritation, generalized seizures, disorders of involuntary movement, and confusion progressive to coma. The individual may even develop decerebration (Fig. 21-12). Nearly 20% of viral encephalidities are fatal. Antibiotics are of no use against any viral infection. They are, however, effective in cases of bacterial infection.

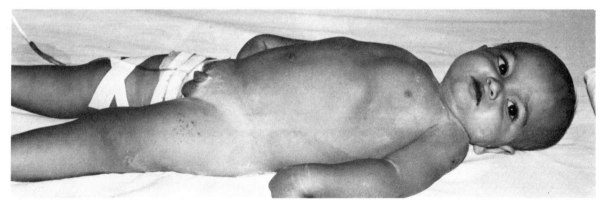

Figure 21-12   *Boy with decerebration from encephalitis. He was unable to move. Note clenched fists.*

Small necrotic lesions of the white and gray matter are seen with encephalomyelitis. Groups of dead nerve cells are often seen surrounded by reacting glial cells, and cuffing of lymphocytes and plasma cells around blood vessels is characteristic. The most deadly (nearly 100%) form of acute viral encephalitis is rabies. Negri bodies can be seen in neurons of persons or animals who die of rabies. Vaccination can protect against rabies and polio.

Poliomyelitis is neurotropic. The virus enters the body by way of the intestinal tract and via the bloodstream into the nervous system. The individual infected with polio has fever, a stiff neck, may experience fasciculations (twitching) of small groups of muscles, and eventually may develop paralysis of muscles supplied by cranial or peripheral nerves.

The anterior horn motor cells of the spinal cord are destroyed by the poliomyelitis virus. Lesions may also be present in motor neurons of the brain stem nuclei (bulbar polio). In addition to loss of motor neurons, perivascular cuffing by lymphocytes and plasma cells is seen, as well as gliosis and cavitation of the tissue.

Herpes zoster (shingles) is caused by varicella-zoster, the virus that also causes chickenpox. This virus infects the sensory dorsal root ganglion cells and produces lesions in the skin (dermatome) supplied by the affected sensory nerve.

Shingles usually occur in older persons or in immunosuppressed patients. They experience a sudden onset of sharp pain and increased sensitivity (hyperesthesia) in the involved dermatome and small blisters erupt in the skin. The virus remains dormant in the dorsal root ganglion for many years following an episode of chickenpox and becomes activated when the individual's immune system becomes compromised.

Herpes simplex

Herpes simplex virus can infect individuals of all ages, however, neonates and immunosuppressed patients are extremely vulnerable. This disease develops several days to weeks following exposure to the virus. The infected person often develops amnesia, especially when the temporal lobes and orbital areas of the frontal lobes are involved. Intra-nuclear inclusions can be seen in the brain, but not in the CSF. Approximately one-third of affected individuals die, or psychosis may ensue. Treatment with adenine arabinoside became available experimentally in 1977 and shows promise as a cure for herpes simplex encephalitis.

Subacute sclerosing panencephalitis (SSPE) is a chronic, slow, viral infection that produces progressive neurological deterioration. The white matter rather than the gray matter degenerates. Individuals affected by this illness have elevated antibodies to measles virus, and electron microscopy reveals measles-like viral inclusions in the CNS. Probably an inappropriate immune response to measles virus occurs. The chronic viral infection★ demyelinates the brain, and gliosis and infiltration by lymphocytes and plasma cells ensues.

Demyelinating Diseases

Demyelination refers to a loss of myelin surrounding nerve fibers that results from SSPE, postinfectious encephalomyelitis, multiple sclerosis, and progressive multifocal leukoencephalopathy.

Postinfectious encephalomyelitis occurs rarely (less than 1 in 2000 cases) following acute viral illnesses like measles or chickenpox. It may also occur following vaccination against smallpox or rabies. An autoimmune response against the protein in myelin is probably responsible for the demyelination of nerve fibers in the CNS. Lesions occur in the white matter of the brain and spinal cord consisting of a perivascular infiltration of lymphocytes, plasma cells and histiocytes, and demyelinated axons.

Affected patients have profound neurological symptoms which may persist for days to weeks, and the demyelinative process may even be fatal. In severe cases, coma ensues followed by decortication, decerebration, or paraplegia.

Acute idiopathic polyneuritis (Guillain-Barré Syndrome) is a demyelinative disease characterized by an abrupt onset of paralysis that most often remits

★The Nobel Prize was awarded in 1976 to Dr. D. C. Gajdusek for discovering that viruses slowly cause certain demyelinating diseases. Someday we may be able to prevent such diseases with vaccines.

spontaneously leaving no significant impairment. This syndrome is thought to be caused by a variety of viruses. Segments of the peripheral nerves become demyelinated. Lymphocytes can be seen infiltrating the peripheral nerve sheaths, suggesting an immune response to a virus or altered myelin protein.

Multiple Sclerosis (Disseminated Sclerosis)

Multiple sclerosis (MS) is a demyelinative disease characterized by either acute or chronic remitting and relapsing involvement of the white matter of the CNS. The etiology is unknown; however, slow viruses such as unusual types of measles have been suggested as the cause. Furthermore, a genetic predisposition can occasionally render families vulnerable to MS, especially to the rapidly progressive form.

The clinical course of MS is variable; some individuals may die within weeks to months of onset. Paresthesias, double vision (diplopia), and cerebellar motor involvement may produce uncoordination. Furthermore, involvement of the lumbosacral spinal cord supplying the urinary bladder leads to urinary dysfunction or incontinence.

Clinically and pathologically, acute and chronic forms of MS occur. Acute MS lesions are characterized by a perivascular lymphocytic and plasma cellular infiltration surrounding small patches of demyelination. In contrast, the chronic variety of MS is characterized by larger lesions, occasionally located surrounding blood vessels. The lesions are multiple and the axons are frequently spared. When the optic nerves are affected, blindness can occur. The inflammatory reaction in the chronic form of MS is much less prominent than in the acute form, but is also lymphocytic. The myelin breaks down and gliosis occurs. The resulting demyelination can easily be seen (Fig. 21-13). No effective treatment of MS is available. Rehabilitation and medical and psychological support are very important.

Progressive Multifocal Leukoencephalopathy (PML)

This syndrome occurs in patients suffering from malignancies, especially lymphomas. The patients develop signs of cerebral white matter disease, including hemiplegia and the unilateral loss of vision, and they often die within weeks to months. The demyelinative lesions of PML are often multifocal and usually merge. Oligodendrocytes disappear

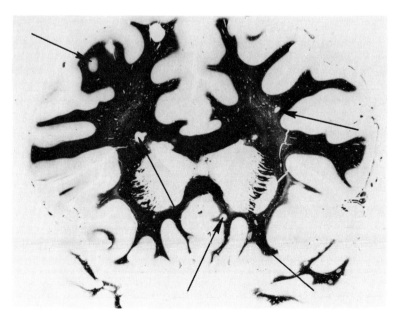

Figure 21-13 *White demyelinated patches* (arrows) *are seen in a cerebrum from a person with multiple sclerosis. (Courtesy Dr. Umberto DeGirolami.)*

within these lesions while the demyelination occurs. The astrocytes become multinucleated and inclusion bodies characteristic of papova viruses are seen.

Degenerative Diseases of the CNS

Degenerative illnesses are characterized by progressive, symmetrical deterioration of certain functional units of the CNS. The etiology of these degenerative processes is unknown, but may have genetic bases. These diseases begin gradually, and in early stages only one side of the body is involved, but symmetrical involvement ensues.

Degenerative Diseases Causing Dementia

Senility in adults is characterized by confusion and loss of memory, especially recent memory. The normal adult cerebral cortex is comprised of 14 billion neurons. Numerous neurons die daily, never to be replaced. Senility is often correlated with a loss of neurons.

The normal brain of a man weighs approximately 1400 gm; a woman's brain weighs approximately 125 gm less. In contrast, brains of aged individuals are frequently decreased in weight and atrophy is manifested in widened sulci ("valleys") and narrowed gyri ("hills") over the convexities of the cerebrum (Fig. 21-4). The ventricles become dilated when neurons are lost. The number of neurons is reduced and aged neurons characteristically contain abundant lipomelanin pigment. Additionally, neurofibrillary tangles or senile glial plaques may be seen in the cerebrum.

Alzheimer's disease is characterized by premature mental deterioration. The frontal lobes of the brain become atrophic and senile plaques and tangles of neurofibrils abound. The frontal lobes contain areas for memory and other intellectual functions.

Pick's disease is clinically indistinguishable from Alzheimer's disease; severe disproportionate atrophy of the temporal and frontal lobes occurs. The posterior two-thirds of the superior temporal gyrus, however, are spared of atrophy. Senile plaques,

neurofibril tangles, and intracytoplasmic inclusions are seen.

Huntington's Chorea

Huntington's chorea is a rare autosomal dominant inherited disease that usually begins in middle adult life. Gradually progressive dementia (mental deterioration) and chorea (slow, writhing movements of the hands) develop and the person dies within 10 to 15 years following onset. Marked atrophy due to a loss of neurons in the basal ganglia and cortex of the brain are seen. This disease is thought to result from imbalanced transmission of nerve impulses due to abnormalities in neurochemicals (dopamine and acetylcholine) important for the transmission of nerve impulses. A recently described hormone, endomorphin, may be associated with schizophrenia.

Parkinson's Disease

Victims of *Parkinson's disease (paralysis agitans)* experience stiffness of muscles; slowness of movement; a stiff, rigid mask-like facial expression; and a "pill rolling" tremor (4 to 6 cycles per second) of the fingers that subsides upon voluntary movement (Fig. 21-14). This disease gradually strikes persons in middle to late life and intellectual deterioration may become evident as the disease advances. It has occurred decades after the epidemic of influenza-induced encephalitis in 1917, and hence one form is called *postencephalitic Parkinsonism*. This form is distinguishable from *paralysis agitans* by a clinical history including prior encephalitis and because the affected person shows spasms of the eyes and extremities.

The brains of individuals afflicted with Parkinson's disease show depigmentation of the lipomelanin-bearing neurons, especially in the substantia nigra. Within the depigmented areas, neurons die and gliosis appears.

Progress in the understanding of Parkinson's disease has focused on the transmission of nerve impulses and imbalances of the neurotransmitter, dopamine. The results from treatment with L-dopa have been gratifying. This drug reduces the person's rigidity and pill-rolling tremor, and has virtually replaced neurosurgical treatment of the disease.

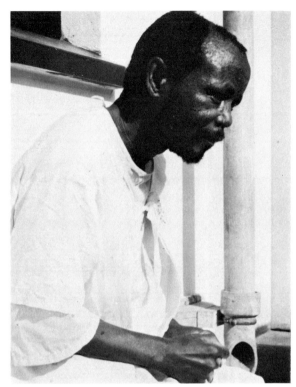

Figure 21-14 *Parkinson's disease. Note the stooped posture, immobile face, and position of hands.*

Spinocerebellar Degeneration

Friedreich's ataxia is a slowly progressive autosomal recessive inherited illness that begins in the first or second decade of life. Weakness, uncoordination of speech and walking (ataxia), high arching of each foot (pes cavus), and absence of deep tendon reflexes occur. In addition, the heart becomes progressively impaired.

The spinal cord degenerates as do the dorsal root ganglion and peripheral nerve fibers. Specifically, the corticospinal tracts, posterior column, and spinocerebellar tracts of the spinal cord degenerate. Eventually, neurons of the cerebellum degenerate and ataxia occurs.

Diseases of Motor Neurons

Several diseases selectively involve motor neurons causing progressive weakness, atrophy of muscles,

fasciculation (twitching), and hyperactive reflexes to develop.

Amyotrophic lateral sclerosis (ALS or Lou Gehrig's disease) involves motor neurons of the cerebral cortex, brain stem, and spinal cord (anterior horn cells). Fibrous astrocytes replace the motor neurons and then the corticospinal tracts and anterior roots degenerate. Concurrently, muscles show atrophy of denervation. Involvement of motor neurons of both the brain and spinal cord results in the characteristic upper and lower motor neuron impairment.

Werdnig-Hoffmann Disease

Werdnig-Hoffmann disease is an autosomally recessive inherited motor neuron disorder that can be manifested at birth. These "floppy" infants are extremely weak and have poor reflexes. They are unable to maintain an upright posture and the legs become abducted and flexed at the hips (frog posture). The muscular impairment results from degeneration and loss of the anterior horn cells in the spinal cord and other motor nuclei in the brain stem. No definitive treatment is available.

Wilson's Disease

Wilson's disease (hepatolenticular degeneration) is also an autosomal recessively transmitted disease, characterized by abnormal metabolism of copper. The individuals affected by this disease experience progressive spasticity and mental deterioration. Copper accumulates in the iris of the eye producing a pale ring, which is a sign of the disease. Also copper deposits in the lenticular nucleus of the brain and elicits degeneration of neurons. The liver becomes fibrotic, or cirrhosis develops from the accumulation of copper. The disease is caused by a failure to produce ceruloplasm, a protein that ordinarily carries copper in the blood and thus prevents copper from invading the brain and liver. If the diagnosis is made at an early age, a drug, penicillamine, which firmly binds copper can be given to prevent progressive, permanent neurological impairment.

Nutritional Disorders of the CNS

A dietary deficiency of niacin produces *pellagra*. Typically, affected patients have dementia, diarrhea, and dermatitis (the three Ds). The dementia or psychosis results from degeneration of neurons within the cerebral cortex. Furthermore, the posterior columns of the spinal cord undergo degeneration and the peripheral nerves become affected secondary to degeneration of dorsal root ganglia.

Subacute combined degeneration of the spinal cord occurs in persons suffering from pernicious anemia (see Chapter 11, Hematology). Vitamin B_{12} is not absorbed because these patients lack intrinsic factor. The formation of myelin surrounding the spinal nerve tracts in the posterior and lateral columns of the spinal cord becomes impaired because vitamin B_{12} is lacking and later demyelination occurs. Slipping and sliding ambulation results. The disease, including the accompanying anemia and neurological problems, is corrected by giving vitamin B_{12} by intramuscular injection. The vitamin B_{12} injection must be given throughout life.

Cerebrovascular Disease

Arteriosclerosis is the most common cause of organic disease of the brain. A cerebral vascular accident (CVA) occurs from thrombosis of an artery or hemorrhage into the CNS. Cerebral vascular accident accounts for approximately 13% of all deaths in the United States. In 1975 the death rate from stroke was 91.8 deaths per 10,000 persons at risk. In 1969 about 810,000 persons with some degree of functional impairment and 900,000 persons without impairment following stroke lived in the United States. Overall, deaths from cardiovascular disease have dramatically declined during the period 1960 to 1975. In 1976, strokes killed people 20% less frequently than in 1963 (Fig. 21-15).

Blood Supply to the Brain

The brain requires approximately 20% of the total cardiac output and receives blood from the internal carotid and vertebral arteries. The internal carotid

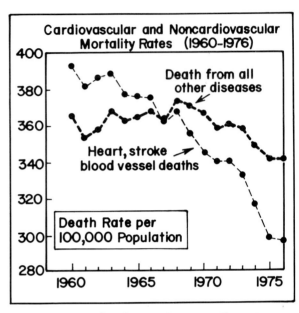

Figure 21-15 *Cardiovascular mortality rates are declining, for unknown reasons, more rapidly than noncardiovascular mortality rates. (From National Center for Health Statistics 1977.)*

artery branches from the common carotid artery and the vertebral arteries from the subclavian arteries. These arteries form the circle of Willis at the base of the brain (Fig. 21-16). The collateral blood vessels joining the carotid and vertebral basilar arteries are small and hence blockage of blood flow in a major artery usually results in an infarction (death of tissue due to lack of O_2 supply) of the CNS.

Anoxia

Occlusion of a major cerebral artery elicits anoxia (absence of O_2) of the CNS and can provoke necrosis of neurons within three to five minutes. Infrequently, low cardiac output due to heart failure or shock causes anoxia of the brain. The brain requires an enormous supply of oxygen and glucose to function and is vulnerable to deprivation of O_2 because of the poorly developed collateral vessels forming the circle of Willis. The segregation of neurological function within specific sites of the brain explains why specific functions are lost when an area of the brain is injured.

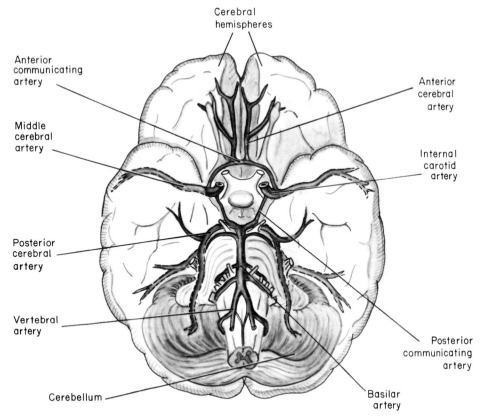

The major cerebral arterial vessels

Figure 21-16   *Arterial supply to the brain as viewed from the inferior surface.*

Preceding the occurrence of a CVA, a *transient ischemic attack* (TIA)★ occurs in about 35% of patients. These attacks occur as sudden blackouts or loss of consciousness. Dizziness, slight residual weakness of the face, leg, or arm, blurring of vision, or slurring of speech is variously noted. These symptoms are transient, remitting within 24 hours to a few days, with no obvious functional deficits remaining. However, recurrent TIA contributes progressively to the mental and motor deterioration of the individual and the chances of experiencing CVA within one year is about 25%. Reversible ischemic neurological deficit (RIND) is characterized by an episode similar to that associated with TIA but in

★Angina pectoris and intermittent claudication are pains resulting from narrowing of arteries in the heart and legs. TIA results from narrowing of arteries in the neck or brain.

which the deficit does not clear within 24 hours, but from which there is eventual recovery.

In *completed stroke* necrosis of neurons occurs in the brain following prolonged ischemia (a decreased blood supply). The pathologic findings at autopsy depend on the duration and extent of hypoxia and the length of time the individual survives following the insult. If the individual dies within minutes to a few hours, no changes are seen upon gross inspection of the brain, regardless of the severity of stroke. The initial changes are only apparent after survival of 12 to 24 hours. The swollen brain becomes softened and neutrophils can be seen surrounding degenerating neurons. At two to four days the usually distinct border between the gray and white matter becomes blurred and macrophages appear. By ten days, new blood vessels grow into the area of infarction. In addition, astrocytes can be seen forming scars surrounding the infarct. One to two months following the infarction, the central region of the lesion becomes liquefied (Fig. 21-6). Infarction of the brain is often termed *encephalomalacia* (Greek, *malakia*, softening).

Cerebrovascular Accident (CVA)

Various terms are used synonymously for CVA, including apoplexy, shock, or stroke. This condition arises from the: (a) complete occlusion of an artery by an embolus; (b) gradual occlusion of an artery by arteriosclerosis; (c) thrombosis of a cerebral artery (internal carotid artery); and (d) bleeding into the substance of the brain (Fig. 21-9). Observation of characteristic clinical aspects of stroke by etiology enable the observer to determine whether the stroke was caused by thrombosis, embolization, or hemorrhage (Table 21-1).

Three factors determine whether infarction occurs: (a) the general status of the individual's cardiovascular system; (b) the anatomic pattern of the vascular supply, including the distribution and size of the collateral circulation;* and (c) the selected vulnerability of specific regions of the brain to ischemia.

Arteriosclerosis occurs predominantly at the division (bifurcation) of arteries (see Chapter 13, Cardiology). The bifurcation of internal and external carotid arteries, for instance, are frequently severely arteriosclerotic (Fig. 21-9). Arteriosclerosis is also often severe where the internal carotid arteries divide into the anterior and middle cerebral arteries within the brain. Occlusion of the internal carotid artery accounts for approximately 20% of CVAs. An operative procedure, *endarterectomy*, can be performed to remove an arteriosclerotic plaque from a pulseless internal carotid artery. Alternatively, a bypass graft can be inserted.

Infarction is the end point of occlusion of cerebral arteries and may be either ischemic or hemorrhagic. Within 48 to 72 hours following occlusion, necrosis becomes visible and liquefaction occurs.

*Collateral circulation refers to alternate passageways (vessels) where blood can travel to circumvent a blocked vessel.

Pronounced swelling of the brain due to accumulation of edema fluid often herniates the brain through the foramen magnum and death ensues.

Approximately one-third of victims of CVA live for three or more years following initial damage. These patients, while having permanent neurological impairment, can often be rehabilitated and taught to walk, dress, and perform other important activities of daily living. Depending on the region of injury of the brain by a CVA, nonspecific and specific neurological deficits appear.

Cerebral Arterial Syndromes

Knowing that neurological functions are localized (Fig. 21-2) in specific regions of the brain supplied by specific arteries (Fig. 21-16) facilitates our understanding and diagnosis of various cerebral arterial syndromes (Table 21-2). The clinical signs that develop following a CVA depend chiefly upon the location and size of the lesion. *Hemiplegia* (loss of motor function on the opposite or contralateral side of the body) results from middle cerebral artery occlusion and loss of consciousness invariably occurs.

Internal Carotid Artery Syndrome

The internal carotid and middle cerebral arteries are the most common arteries to thrombose. The internal carotid artery divides into the anterior and middle cerebral arteries, and hence occlusion of the internal carotid artery causes neurological defects encompassing both arteries. Most of the defects occurring in the middle cerebral artery are described below.

Middle Cerebral Artery Syndrome

The middle cerebral artery supplies an enormous region of the brain—the entire cerebral convexity with the exception of small areas of the frontal and occipital poles and a thin midline rim of cerebrum supplied by the anterior cerebral arteries. Furthermore, penetrating branches from the middle cere-

Table 21-1
Clinical Aspects of Stroke by Etiology

	Thrombotic	Embolic	Hemorrhagic
History of transient ischemic attacks	Frequent	Occasional	Rare
Onset	Acute or in steps over hours to a couple of days	Acute	Acute, usually with progressive worsening or coma
Associated headache	Occasional, usually not severe	More often, moderately severe	Frequent, severe
Stiff neck	Rare	Rare	Frequent
Coma (loss of consciousness)	Occasional, usually not at onset	Occasional, usually brief at onset	Frequent

bral artery supply the basal ganglia of the brain, including the caudate, lenticular, and thalamic nuclei.

Cerebral infarction involving the total distribution of the middle cerebral artery produces *acute deficits* similar to those involved in total occlusion of internal carotid artery including unconsciousness and loss of all motor, sensory, and visual functions contralateral to the side of the lesion. Marked cerebral edema and herniation of tissue can cause death. If consciousness is regained, severe and permanent *residual deficits* are often seen including unconsciousness and loss of all or motor, sensory, and visual functions contralateral to the side of the lesion. The person can, however, sometimes be rehabilitated to perform normal activities of daily living.

Resulting Loss of Language Skills

The ability to communicate orally, visually, and in written language is a fundamental capacity of human beings. Human language depends upon maintaining the integrity of the anatomic region situated between the primary input zones of the temporal and occipital lobes and the output zones in the inferior frontal lobe of the dominant hemisphere (the left side is dominant in 90% of persons).

Three regions usually situated in the left (dominant) cerebral hemisphere serve language. Two regions (Fig. 21-2) are *receptive* and one is *expressive* (executive).

The two receptive areas are closely integrated: (a) *auditory language* is situated posteriorly in the first and second temporal convolutions (Broca's areas 41 and 42) and; (b) the *visual and comprehensive aspects of language* occupy the angular convolution (area 39 and the area immediately posterior).

Expressive, or motor, aspects of speech are situated at the posterior end of the third (inferior) frontal convolution (referred to as Broca's area 44).

Aphasia

Following an extensive lesion in the dominant temporal-parietal language centers, aphasia ensues. Aphasia refers to the loss or impairment, resulting from a brain lesion, of the power to use words as symbols or ideas. A patient can have one of several types of aphasia: *total (global) aphasia*, with loss of all or nearly all speech functions; *motor aphasia*, sometimes called verbal or expressive aphasia due to a deficit in motor speech production; *central aphasia*, with impairment of all language dependent behavior; or a *dissociative speech defect*, such as word deafness (auditory verbal aphasia), word blindness (alexia), amnesia (loss of memory), or mutism (inability to speak). Both right-sided hemiparesis (paresis means weakness) or hemiplegia (plegia means paralysis), and an impaired ability to communicate by writing (agraphia) are found to some degree in all types of aphasia.

The clinical courses of aphasic patients and their responses to speech therapy are variable. Aphasic patients with vascular disease of the internal carotid or middle cerebral arteries nearly always show some spontaneous improvement in the days, weeks, and months that follow the stroke.

Anterior Cerebral Artery Syndrome

Cerebral infarction resulting from occlusion of the anterior cerebral artery usually produces unconsciousness or mental deterioration as well as hemiplegia involving the leg. The anterior cerebral artery supplies much of the orbital surface of the tip of the frontal lobe and the entire mesial surface of the parietal-occipital juncture. Hence, following a CVA the patient can have an altered affect—inappropriate crying or laughing may result from the damage to the frontal lobes where centers of the higher intellectual functions are located.

Posterior Cerebral Artery Syndrome

The posterior cerebral artery branches from the basilar artery to supply the midbrain and portions of the cerebellum and basal ganglion. Cases of infarction can result in loss of cranial nerve function because cranial neurons located in the brain stem may be destroyed. The nucleus of the third cranial nerve is especially vulnerable to infarction. Furthermore, loss of vision and hemiplegia can also result when corticospinal tracts become damaged by thrombosis or hemorrhage of the posterior cerebral artery.

Vertebral Basilar Artery Syndrome

The arteries of the vertebral-basilar system supply the medulla, pons, midbrain, and cerebellum. Complete infarction of this region is incompatible with life; bilateral paralysis of the body ensues. Occasionally selective paralysis of a cranial nerve occurs when the infarct is small.

Posterior-Inferior Cerebellar Artery Syndrome

This artery supplies the dorsal lateral portion of the medulla oblongota which, upon infarction, produces *dysarthria* (garbled speech), *dysphagia* (difficulty in swallowing), and *cerebellar ataxia* (uncoordinated movement such as unsteadiness upon walking). These symptoms arise from involvement of the cranial nerves and also from damage to the cerebellum.

Intracerebral Hemorrhage

Hypertension is the most common predisposing factor to intracerebral hemorrhage. Hypertensive persons have two to four times more frequent occurrence of intracranial hemorrhage than do persons with normal blood pressure. Trauma, rupture of aneurysms, thrombocytopenia, or tumors can also cause intracerebral hemorrhage. A hemorrhagic infarct generally remains within the area of the tissue supplied by the involved artery; occasionally the hemorrhage extends beyond the boundaries the artery supplies.

The cerebral hemispheres are involved by intracranial hemorrhage in 80% of cases, the midbrain in 10%, and the cerebellum in the remaining 10%. *Hypertensive cerebrovascular disease* is a disorder of small arteries, especially arterioles. The *lenticulostriate* branch ("artery of stroke") is a small branch of the middle cerebral artery that supplies the basal ganglia. It very often ruptures, and hemorrhage and death often result because blood from the damaged brain flows directly into the ventricles increasing intracranial pressure, edema, and herniation of brain tissue.

Subarachnoid Hemorrhage

A ruptured aneurysm (dilated, sac-like region in the wall of a blood vessel) of the circle of Willis is the most common cause of subarachnoid hemorrhage (Fig. 21-10). Trauma can also elicit the same problem. Aneurysms most frequently occur at the juncture of the anterior communicating and anterior cerebral arteries and where the internal carotid and middle cerebral arteries branch.

Characteristically, a person with a ruptured berry aneurysm experiences a sudden, excruciating headache and stiffness of the neck. Loss of conscious-

Table 21-2
Regions Supplied by Cerebral Arteries

Artery	Branches	Territory supplied
Internal carotid	Ophthalmic	Eye, optic tract
	Tympanic	Ear
	Anterior cerebral	(see below)
	Middle cerebral	(see below)
Middle cerebral	Central lenticulostriate "artery of stroke"	Basal ganglia
	Cortical branches	Cortex under temporal-parietal lobes
	Anterior branches	Frontal lobes
	Middle and posterior branches	Cerebral convexity
Anterior cerebral	Central branches	Optic tract, inferior central portion of brain
	Cortical branches	Frontal lobes
		Olfactory bulbs
	Midline branches	Midline structures of cortex
Posterior cerebral	Cortical branches	Posterior inferior cortex, brain stem, cranial nerves
Cerebellar	Anterior and posterior-inferior cerebellar	Corresponding areas of cerebellum and medulla oblongata

ness rapidly ensues and a lumbar puncture reveals blood within the CSF. Patients can be treated neurosurgically by placing a silver clip about the ruptured aneurysm. If the hemorrhage spontaneously subsides, recurrence of hemorrhage occurs within weeks in nearly 50% of patients.

Brain Tumors

Tumors of the CNS (brain and spinal cord), because of their variable size, location, histologic type, and invasive qualities, destroy or displace tissues around them. They frequently are lethal because brain tumors cause increased intracranial pressure and herniation can result. Unlike other malignancies they seldom metastasize; they are encased in the skull. Brain tumors can occur at all ages but few persons realize that tumors of the CNS are, with the exception of leukemia, the most common neoplasms of childhood.

Clinical Features

Three syndromes are commonly encountered with brain tumors: (a) The patient experiences declining mental capacity or seizure (convulsion). (b) There is unmistakable evidence of raised intracranial pressure. Headache associated with vomiting and seizures is highly suggestive of brain tumor. Inspection of the eye with an ophthalmoscope confirms the suspicion of raised intracranial pressure; edema of the optic discs (papilledema) is seen. (c) Specific intracranial tumor syndromes causing localizing signs can occur. Localization of a tumor to the cerebellum, for instance, is possible by knowing that a loss of coordination can arise from a lesion in the cerebellum (Fig. 21-17).

Diagnosis

The clinical history, neurological deficits, and laboratory assessment together lead to diagnosis of CNS tumors. Often before launching an extensive

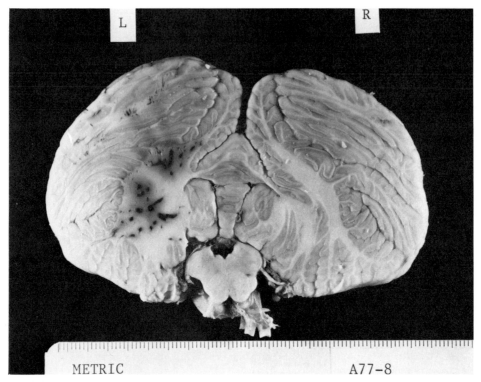

Figure 21-17   *Cerebellum showing hemangioma and hemorrhage through the thin walls of the tumor. An ataxic gait and incoordination is seen with tumors in the cerebellum.*

diagnostic study of the patient, the physician will repeatedly examine the patient over a period of several weeks. The reasons for this conservative approach are twofold. The signs and symptoms of CNS tumors are nonspecific and many other lesions such as abscesses and infarcts can mimic brain tumors. Secondly, the studies carry some risk to the patient and are expensive. Studies often employed are described below.

A needle can be introduced into the lumbar spinal canal (lumbar tap) and cerebrospinal fluid can be examined for: (a) increased pressure, (b) increased protein concentration, and (c) tumor cells. An X-ray of the skull will occasionally reveal a tumor. Adult males are evaluated for metastatic lung cancer with chest X-ray and females for metastatic breast cancer. Surprisingly, these are by far the most common tumors affecting the brain.

More specialized X-ray studies include the use of a *brain scan* (wherein radioactive dye is injected into a vein and is absorbed by the tumor and displayed in the photographed scan); *carotid angiography*, where dye injected into the carotid artery can reveal a tumor vascular "blush" in an X-ray when numerous tumoral vessels are present or normal arteries are displaced by the tumor; and finally, *computerized axial tomography* ("CAT")*, a sensitive X-ray instrument, provides views of specific slices of the brain tumor. The CAT can distinguish infarcts and abscesses from brain tumors (Fig. 21-18). An *electroencephalogram* (EEG) is used to localize regions in the brain responsible for seizures and can assist in locating a brain tumor.

Classification of Brain Tumors

Traditionally, brain tumors have been classified histologically according to their cell of origin (Table

*Instrument manufactured by a company owned primarily by the former musical group, The Beatles.

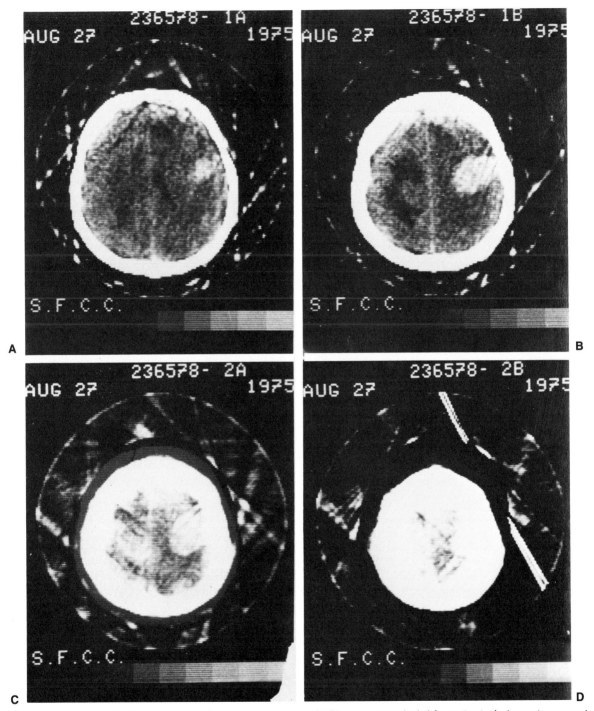

Figure 21-18   **A** to **D**, *Computerized axial tomography (CAT) scan revealed this metastatic breast cancer to the parietal lobe. The CAT scan makes images at 13 mm levels through the brain. A metastatic breast cancer shows up as a white area in the right cerebral hemisphere.*

21-3). Only two tumors—one benign (*meningioma*) and the other malignant (*glioma*)—will be discussed in some detail.

Meningioma

Approximately 20% of intracranial tumors are caused by meningiomas (benign tumors) which arise from arachnoid meningeal epithelium. Oftentimes they are located in the midline adjacent to the skull, for instance in the olfactory groove or on the sphenoidal ridge of the skull. These tumors compress brain tissues and signs of brain tumor ensue. Meningiomas are usually curable by surgical intervention.

Glioma

Astrocytomas, or gliomas, constitute approximately one-fourth of brain tumors. These tumors arise from malignant astrocytes and are the most common primary brain tumor. Metastatic brain tumors are more common. Malignant tumors of the brain are unique; they do not metastasize outside the brain whereas malignancies elsewhere in the body metastasize more widely. The prognosis for gliomas are usually grim, but if they are small and localized in accessible sites, a cure is possible. Some have a bizarre appearance (Fig. 21-19).

Treatment and Clinical Course

Neurosurgical resection is the treatment used for most brain tumors following surgical biopsy. X-ray treatment is attempted on most brain tumors, but is of questionable value for gliomas. Clearly, radiotherapy is excellent for treating children with medulloblastoma, lymphoma, and a few other histologic types. The intracranial pressure is controlled by the use of dexamethosone (a cortisol-like drug).

Nonresectable brain tumors, by virtue of their location (most important), size, and histologic type, can produce progressive neurological defects. Worsening of seizures, headache progressive to drowsiness, and stupor signal, in most cases, poor prognoses. Death usually results from herniation of brain tissue and compression of vital respiratory centers in the brain.

Tumors of Peripheral Nerves

Neoplasms can arise in peripheral and cranial nerves from Schwann cells that surround nerves. When the eighth cranial nerve is involved by a neoplastic proliferation of Schwann cells an *acoustic neuroma* occurs. This expanding tumor impairs hearing and may cause dizziness. This tumor can often be removed surgically. In addition, peripheral nerves can be affected by tumors. These tumors may be

Table 21-3
Classification of Some Brain Tumors

Type	Relative frequency	Age
Astrocytoma	25%	Adults
Meningioma	20%	All ages
Metastatic carcinomas (lung—♂, breast—♀)	35%–40%	Adults
Oligodendroglioma	5%–10%	Adults
Ependymoma	4%	All ages
Medulloblastoma	3%	Children (cerebellar)
Hemangioblastoma	1%	Children
Lymphoma	1%	All ages
Pituitary	1%	Young adults
Miscellaneous	10%	All ages

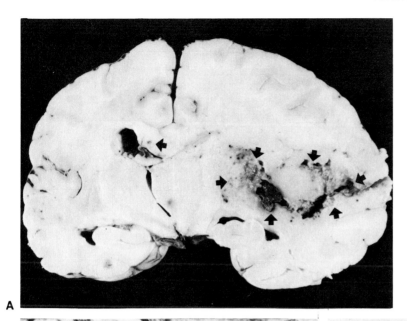

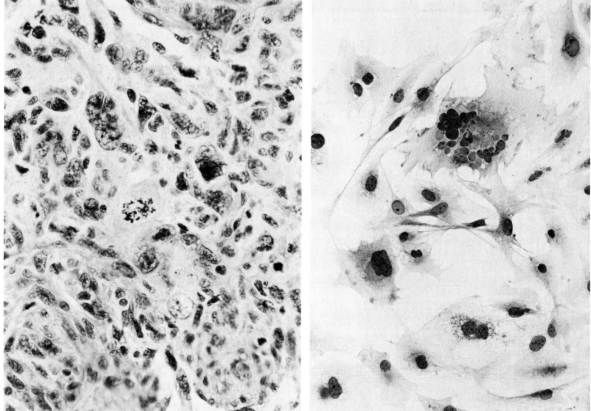

Figure 21-19   **A,** *Brain of a young boy showing necrotic and hemorrhagic astrocytoma. Edema has pushed brain substance to the left.* **B,** *Photomicrograph of this bizzare astrocytoma.* **C,** *Photomicrograph of multinucleated astrocytoma giant cells in tissue culture. (Courtesy Dr. James Yang.)*

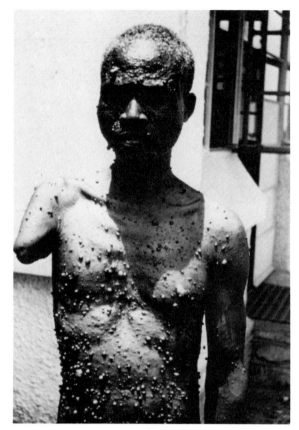

Figure 21-20 *Neurofibromatosis. Note the numerous cutaneous neurofibromas. His right arm was amputated because a neurosarcoma developed. (Courtesy Dr. Clitus Olson.)*

benign (*neurofibroma*) or malignant (*neurosarcoma*). Both tumors commonly occur in persons suffering from the autosomal dominantly inherited neurofibromatosis syndrome (von Recklinghausen's syndrome). Treatment is by surgical resection (Fig. 21-20).

Summary

Neurologic disorders are diagnosable and prognosticable because of localization of function in specific anatomic sites in the CNS, specific characteristic clinical patterns of signs and symptoms of certain disorders, and vulnerability of selected age groups to a limited number of pathologic processes and infectious agents. The brain is extraordinarily vulnerable to anoxia, and neurons do not proliferate. Edema of the brain arising from various etiologies can be fatal when the brain substance herniates and compresses vital centers. Congenital malformations in the CNS arise from toxic agents including the TORCH complex of infectious agents. Many other diseases including some progressive demyelinating are caused by slow viral infections.

Cerebrovascular disease from arteriosclerosis and associated stroke is a major cause of morbidity and mortality in the United States. Predisposing transient ischemic attacks and hypertension are treatable and stroke can be prevented. Endarterectomy, for instance, removes arteriosclerotic plaques and reestablishes blood supply through arteriosclerotic carotid arteries.

Brain tumors are most commonly due to metastatic lung and breast cancers. Unfortunately, most primary brain tumors are highly malignant, but if detected early and when localized in nonvital sites, cure is possible by surgical excision of the tumor.

Bibliography

Bergsma, D., ed. 1971. *The clinical delineation of birth defects*, part 6. Nervous system. Baltimore: The Williams & Wilkins Company. Catalogues and illustrates birth defects of the central nervous system.

Blackwood, W., and Corsellis, J. A. N. 1976. *Greenfield's neuropathology*. Chicago: Year Book Medical Publishers, Inc. Classic textbook.

Crome, L., and Stern, J. 1967. *The pathology of mental retardation*. London: J. and A. Churchill. Describes and depicts pathologic lesions responsible for mental retardation.

Escourolle, R., and Poirier, J. 1973. *Manual of basic neuropathology*. Philadelphia: W. B. Saunders Company. The best reference for beginners.

Fields, W. S., ed. 1961. *Pathogenesis and treatment of cerebrovascular disease*. Springfield, Illinois: C. C Thomas, Publisher. Overview of arteriosclerotic disorders of the brain.

Gajdusek, D. C. 1977. Unconventional viruses and the origin and disappearance of Kuru. *Science* 197: 943–960. Nobel lecture on slow viruses of the CNS.

McAlpine, D. 1972. *Multiple sclerosis: a reappraisal*. Baltimore: The Williams & Wilkins Company. Monograph on this disease.

Mumenthaler, M. 1977. *Neurology Year Book*. Chicago: Medical Publishers, Inc. Outstanding, comprehensive, intelligible compendium of clinical neurology.

Ranson, S. W., and Clark, S. L. 1972. *The anatomy of the nervous system*. Philadelphia: W. B. Saunders Company. Standard neuroanatomy textbook.

Robbins, S. 1976. Stroke in the geriatric patient. *Hosp. Prac.* 11:33–40. Describes problems in diagnosis and management of stroke.

Rubinstein, J. J. 1972. *Tumors of the central nervous system*, series 2. Armed Forces Institute of Pathology, Washington, D.C. Standard reference for pathologists. Excellent photographs.

Sahs, A. L.; Hartman, E. C.; Aronson, S. M., eds. 1976. Guidelines for stroke care. DHEW Publication no. (HRA) 76-14017. A concise, complete, and inexpensive monograph on most aspects of stroke.

Schade, J. P., and Ford, Donald H. 1973. *Basic neurology*. New York: Elsevier Scientific Publishing Co., Inc. Good clinical textbook.

Schochet, S. S., Jr., and McCormic, W. F. 1976. *Neuropathology case studies*. Flushing, New York: Medical Examination Publishing Company, Inc. Illustrates typical clinical and pathological findings of common neurologic disorders.

Stone, B. H. 1977. Computerized transaxial brain scans. *Am. J. Nurs.* 77: 1601–1605. This noninvasive X-ray procedure provides fast, accurate, and somewhat expensive diagnosis.

Thompson, R. A., and Green, J. R. 1974. *Advances in neurology*. Vol. 6. Infectious diseases of the central nervous system, New York: Raven Press. Summarizes infectious diseases of fetus, children, and adults.

Williams, P. L., and Warwick, R. 1975. *Functional neuroanatomy of man*. Philadelphia: W. B. Saunders Company. Provides anatomical and clinical pathologic correlations.

Wintrobe, M. M.; Thorn, G. W.; Adams, R. D.; Braunwald, E.; Isselbacker, K. J.; and Petersdorf, R. G., eds. 1974. *Harrison's principles of internal medicine, disorders of the nervous system*, pp. 1704–1870. New York: McGraw-Hill Book Company. Thorough clinical presentation discussing onset, diagnosis, course, and treatment of neurologic disorders.

Index